XXX. *Extract of a letter from Mr.* Lambert, *surgeon at Newcastle upon Tyne, to Dr.* Hunter; *giving an Account of a new Method of treating an* Aneurysm. *Read June* 15, 1761.

. . . I considered the coats and motions of arteries, and compared their wounds with the wounds of veins and other parts. I reflected upon the process of nature in the cure of wounds in general, and...Upon the whole, I was in hopes that a future of the wound in the artery might be successful; and if so, it would certainly be preferable to tying up the trunk of the vessel.

If it should be found by experience, that a large artery, when wounded, may be healed up by this kind of future, without becoming impervious, it would be an important discovery in surgery. It would make the operation for the A͟ successful in the arm, wh is wounded; and by this we might be able to cure the wounds of some arteries that would otherwise require amputation, or be altogether incurable.

Atlas of
VASCULAR SURGERY

Third edition

Atlas of
VASCULAR SURGERY

FALLS B. HERSHEY, M.D., F.A.C.S.

Associate Professor of Clinical Surgery, Washington University School of Medicine, St. Louis, Mo.; Chief of Vascular Surgery, St. John's Mercy Medical Center; formerly Director, St. Louis Heart Association Artery Bank; formerly Chairman, Department of Surgery, Michael Reese Hospital and Medical Center, Chicago, Ill.; Diplomate, American Board of Surgery

CARL H. CALMAN, M.D., F.A.C.S.

Formerly Assistant in Clinical Surgery, Washington University School of Medicine, St. Louis, Mo.; Diplomate, American Board of Surgery

With 681 illustrations, including original drawings by Kathryn Murphy Masterson and William R. Schwarz

Saint Louis

THE C. V. MOSBY COMPANY

1973

Third edition

Copyright © 1973 by The C. V. Mosby Company

All rights reserved. No part of this book may be reproduced
in any manner without written permission of the publisher.

Previous editions copyrighted 1963, 1967

Printed in the United States of America

Distributed in Great Britain by Henry Kimpton, London

Library of Congress Cataloging in Publication Data

Hershey, Falls B
   Atlas of vascular surgery.

   1. Blood-vessels—Surgery. I. Calman, Carl H.,
joint author. II. Title. [DNLM: 1. Vascular
surgery—Atlases. WG17 H572a 1973]
RD598.H46 1973   617'.41   73-8662
ISBN 0-8016-2153-4

To our wives, Julie and Marty, *and the patient, loyal, and loving wives of surgeons everywhere*

F. B. H. and C. H. C.

Preface to third edition

During the ten years since the first edition of *Atlas of Vascular Surgery* there has been intense activity, innovation, and recently, much critical evaluation in this field.[1-3]

In 1972 DeWeese and a committee formed from the vascular societies evaluated the scope of vascular surgery, estimated the number of operations performed, and assessed the optimal results obtainable.[4] They also defined the hospital resources necessary for optimal results and discussed the training and possible certification of vascular surgeons.

More cooperative registries similar to the renovascular hypertension and cerebrovascular insufficiency studies are needed to compare accurately the results of vascular operations. The "life table" method of reporting results is most helpful.

We are pleased to see that many suggestions made ten years ago in the first edition have become accepted procedures.

This third edition includes some helpful references as a guide to further reading and to acknowledge these notable contributions. Unfortunately, the mention of all would require another book, so rapidly has vascular surgery advanced. We do not cite the long and multitudinous reference lists supplied by computerized bibliographic services. We have reviewed each reference quoted.

In the last ten years, measurement and estimation of blood flow have improved. This has always been a difficult field in physiology. Some methods, such as the Doppler technique, have been brought into the operating room and the clinic, and we anticipate that more will follow.

Some vascular surgery is poorly done, and sometimes the indications are not clear. Improved training in vascular surgery is needed, since many vascular emergencies must necessarily be treated by general surgeons. We hope that this book will be helpful to residents and other surgeons as they confront the problems of vascular surgery. Hippocrates' first aphorism still reminds us that "life is short and the art is long; the occasion fleeting; experience fallacious, and judgment difficult. The physician must

---

[1]Cannon, J. A.: Surgical judgment in vascular surgery, Arch. Surg. **103**:521-524, 1971.
[2]Hanlon, C. R.: Presidential address. Standards in vascular surgery, Surgery **67**:1-4, 1970.
[3]Wylie, E. J.: Vascular surgery: a quest for excellence, Arch. Surg. **101**:645-648, 1970.
[4]Committee on Vascular Surgery (J. A. DeWeese, Chairman): Optimal resources for vascular surgery, Circulation **46**:A-305–A-324, 1972.

not only be prepared to do what is right himself, but also to make the patient, the attendants, and the externals cooperate."

This atlas emphasizes established operations, but some operations that are under trial and appear to be promising are also included. X-ray films have been added where they are helpful. Discussion of peripheral vascular diseases has been augmented throughout the text. Some procedures that are seldom needed but that have a proved value have been added to this edition. These include femorofemoral or axillofemoral bypass and venous bypass into the lower portion of the leg. More material has been added on microsurgery and new instruments. The natural history of diseases and the long-term results of surgery are summarized.

On some matters we have strong personal opinions and choices and are frank about these. In other instances where our experience is limited, we refer to the publications of others. Consequently, we are deeply indebted to our friends and to many other surgeons for their careful observations and reports.

It is impossible to acknowledge our indebtedness to all those who have contributed their time and talent to this book. A partial list must include the following: Mrs. Kay Masterson for her superb illustrations. Mr. Roger White, Executive Director; the Board of Directors; the X-Ray Staff and Department; and Mr. Baker of the Printing Department of Morton Plant Hospital for help with records, cases, and the reproduction of x-ray films in the files of the hospital. Mrs. Joyce Cola and Mrs. Margaret Garwood for help in preparing the manuscript. Mrs. Mildred Winn, Medical Librarian, St. John's Mercy Medical Center, for her expert library assistance. Mr. William Pilling, Mr. Leon King, and Mr. Theodore Grau of the Pilling Company for help in producing special instruments. Dr. Arthur I. Auer for his expert phlebography, for his suggestions about the Mobin-Uddin umbrella filter, and for his technique of distal tibial bypass with the saphenous vein; and Dr. Walter M. Golaski for extensive information and help with regard to technical advice and the development of a superior knitted Dacron graft.

Other credits and acknowledgements are made in the text or in legends of illustrations. Our sincere thanks to all of them.

Falls B. Hershey
Carl H. Calman

Preface to second edition

This book was written to instruct residents as well as practicing surgeons in the methods and techniques of vascular surgery. It is dedicated to them, with the hope that it will be a guide to successful and safe technique, sound judgment, and an understanding of the scope, applications, and limitations of vascular operations.

In addition to surgical procedures, short descriptions of disease patterns, both pathological and physiological, together with outlines of the various diagnostic procedures, are included. The discussions of surgical technique emphasize only those matters that are peculiar to the vascular system, avoiding the repetition of that already familiar to the general surgeon.

The chapter on arteriography outlines the major techniques that find frequent application. In addition to the methods presented herein, numerous additional basic methods and variations are available. With a little experience, innovation in this field is not difficult. Radiography frequently provides structural anatomical information for vascular reconstructive procedures. Since the vascular surgeon will usually perform and interpret his own angiograms, knowledge of these procedures is essential.

Accurate preoperative diagnosis and careful postoperative management are an integral part of the surgical procedures described and are essential to success. However, since the amount of such information that can be included in an atlas is necessarily limited, the reader must add his own knowledge of pathology, physiology, and surgery, his own evaluation of new techniques and results reported in the surgical literature, and his own personal observations and experiences.

If this atlas is successful in communicating to the experienced vascular surgeon some helpful idea or in guiding a resident more safely through his first vascular operation, it will have justified our efforts.

In the four years since the first edition was published, a great deal of practical and experimental work, as well as a great deal of clinical experience in vascular surgery, has been accumulated by many groups throughout the country. In this second edition we observe more standardization and better definition of procedures and indications. A number of ingenious innovations in technique, such as use of the Fogarty balloon catheter and the partial occluding Teflon clip for the vena cava, have been devised. As a result, vascular surgery in all of its facets has been more widely accepted and applied. Morbidity rates, as well as mortality rates, have decreased.

A number of unsolved or poorly solved problems remain. The greatest of these is possibly the problem of inadequate arterial circulation below the bifurcation of the common femoral artery. The very number of procedures proposed, such as onlay vein grafts and in situ saphenous vein transplantation, all attest to the difficulties in restoring arterial flow in this area.

We have reviewed a great deal of experimental and clinical published work, as well as our own experiences, in this edition. It has been encouraging indeed to note that a great many of the suggestions advanced four years ago are now in wide use. The continued work of many skilled surgeons in this field will assure continued progress.

We are permanently indebted to many teachers and friends. A partial list must include Dr. Robert H. Linton, whose rigorous admonition, "You've got to do it *right*," still echoes to former residents, and Dr. Michael E. DeBakey, whose bold attack and elegant and simple techniques for aneurysm and occlusive disease have been inspiring examples.

Our own early arterial replacements would not have been possible without the inspiration, encouragement, and financial support of Dr. Carl A. Moyer, formerly Bixby Professor of Surgery, Washington University School of Medicine, who helped us establish the St. Louis Heart Association Artery Bank. This organization supplied arterial homografts until satisfactory synthetic prostheses were developed. Dr. Cyril A. Costello was also most helpful.

Dr. Eric Carlsson and Dr. Hokan Arvidsson devised or introduced many arteriographic techniques during their tenures at Barnes Hospital. These contributions include the Seldinger apparatus and the "up-and-around" retrograde injection of the femoral artery.

The technique of transmetatarsal amputation is that of Dr. Leland S. McKittrick. His unparalleled success with transmetatarsal amputation is due to experience and surgical judgment not completely communicable in an atlas.

These surgeons will recognize some of their precepts and techniques but are in no way responsible for deficiencies or shortcomings.

We are grateful to Dr. Thomas Sheridan for the description of the Nakayama stapler and to Dr. Norman Brill and Dr. Gonzalo Magsaysay for assistance with the discussions on phlebography, the vein eraser, and brachiocerebral arteriography.

The usefulness of this book is due in large part to the fine drawings of Mrs. Kathryn Murphy Masterson and William R. Schwarz. Some new drawings have been made by Michael K. Meyers and Wesley Bloom.

Falls B. Hershey
Carl H. Calman

Contents

Atlas of
VASCULAR SURGERY

1

Introduction

HISTORICAL REVIEW

Medical history began with Hippocrates, but as Lancisi (1745) tells us in his work on aneurysms, Hippocrates was silent on this subject. In ancient times the term *aneurysm* was interchangeable with the phrase *wound of an artery.*

Hippocrates had some knowledge of human anatomy. For example, he cautioned against making incisions in the temple because of the "vein" there that may bleed. The manner of incision is unclear, since he also noted that this incision can cause a convulsion on the opposite side.

Therefore, all the vascular surgery of note concerned itself with wounds and with aneurysms until Lambert reported in 1762 the closure of a wound of the brachial artery without ligation carried out by his colleague Hallowell in 1759.

A great era of experimental arterial and venous surgery, grafting of blood vessels, and experimental transplantation of organs began with Eck's fistula accomplished in 1877 and drew to a close with the publication by Guthrie of his monograph *Blood Vessel Surgery and Its Applications* in 1912 and by Bernheim of *Surgery of the Vascular System* in 1913.

According to Garrison (1913), Heliodorus antedated Celsus in the treatment of aneurysms by ligation or torsion. He also cited the ancient operation of Antyllus of Alexandria. This operation consisted of both proximal and distal ligation above and below the aneurysm, after which the aneurysm was cut between the ligatures. Celsus described his operation as follows: "If pressure and astringents are ineffectual to restrain the hemorrhage, the bleeding vessel is to be taken up, and a ligature having been applied on each side of the wound in it, the vessel is then to be divided; the two parts of the vessel will become united by anastomosing branches, and the orifices will become obliterated." The distinction between a wound and what we would today call an aneurysm is unclear. Lancisi made the distinction, and rejected applying the term *aneurysm* to an arterial wound, but Hallowell clearly closed a wound in the brachial artery and called it an aneurysm.

The operation of Heliodorus, Celsus, and Antyllus remained the standard operation according to Garrison until Hunter devised proximal ligation in 1786. Hunter's reasoning was that the single proximal ligature would be placed only through sound tissue; therefore, one can presume that this usually meant a more proximal ligation than practiced before. However, proximal ligation has an older origin. Garrison himself cited the earlier employment of single ligature, presumably proximal, by Guillimeau in 1594 and Anel in 1710. Lancisi described such proceedures for true aneurysms almost casually.

In his work on aneurysms, Lancisi was well acquainted with case reports of an-

1

cient authors from Galen to Avicenna. Galen's concern with the best material to employ for the ligature of arteries evidences a familiarity with the operation. Lancisi wondered why Hippocrates and other ancients were silent on the treatment of aneurysm but never answered his question. Lancisi's pathology is largely unintelligible, but he realized that arteries do not pump and called the thesis that arteries do pump a "silly old woman's tale."

Nevertheless, there was dispute among anatomists about the nature of the arterial coats. Lancisi did not deny that the arteries are contractile and noted that they are distended by the "force and weight of blood that issues from the heart." With regard to the arteries, one receives the impression that he really did not believe in a muscular coat but that he would not contradict the authority of Galen who pointed out the similarity of this coat to the muscles of the stomach.

In his dissections Lancisi came across atherosclerosis: "Not everywhere, but in certain places, and above all in the large branches of the arteries, we find distributed fatty follicles, so to speak, which in the aorta are distinctly visible without the microscope."

He obviously knew that distal gangrene can follow the ligation of an artery, particularly the popliteal.

Some of the descriptions of his dissections are of large arch aneurysms that are unbelievable today. They fill the chest, erode the sternum and third costal cartilages, and can hemorrhage to the outside; the fatal outcome was well known. Between classical times and the seventeeth century, with the date still debatable, syphillis appeared in Europe, and it was to Lancisi, the "French disease." He recognized the relation to aneurysm, but not necessarily any relation to frightfully large arch and thoracic aneurysms that he described so well. The patient's history of primary disease and an indulgent nature established the etiological diagnosis in a limb or in the abdominal aorta.

The cause of aneurysms previously was any of the usual causes seen today, but Lancisi probably identified a common source when he discusses a soldier who developed an aneurysm after a "slight" wound of the carotid. An operation for ligature was performed. Lancisi discussed the technical difficulties. The surgery was immediately fatal. It would seem a valid assumption that warfare carried on with spears and thrusting Roman short swords would result in numerous arterial injuries, and it is not difficult to imagine that professional soldiers were well acquainted with the locations of the major arteries, if only from experience.

Paré instituted by accident, the use of ligature in major amputations on the battlefield after running out of boiling oil. This was a major advance in 1564 and established his reputation.

Harvey published his great work on the circulation in 1628. With the exception of the earliest closure in continuity of the brachial artery by Hallowell in 1759, most of the history of vascular surgery revolves about aneurysm and ligature until the late nineteenth century. Hallowell's achievement certainly deserves more praise than it has received. He was completely ignored by Garrison. Lambert's account of the operation is reproduced on the endpapers of this book. Essentially it is that, being dissatisfied with the results of ligation, Lambert considered suture. He borrowed his ideas, considering "how the union of divided parts was brought about in the operation of hare lip, and in horses' necks that are bled by farriers." He shared his ideas with his colleagues, and the next case fell, as he related, to Hallowell's lot. The operation was planned in advance, deliberately executed, and was successful; and the potentiality for avoiding gangrene was immediately recognized.

Many heroic ligations were recounted by Garrison. No artery was immune. Cooper ligated the abdominal aorta in 1817, but his patient, who had a distal iliac aneurysm, died forty hours later.

Kocher quoted Keen as having collected thirteen such heroic ligations of the aorta by 1900; in all cases the operation was fatal.

Garrison credited Dupuytren with the treatment of aneurysm by compression in 1818, but both Celsus and Lancisi mentioned this treatment, the latter for a large thoracic aneurysm and with some contempt.

Ballance and Edmunds in 1886 produced an excellent experimental study of ligation of the larger arteries in continuity. They avoided damage to the arterial wall and recognized that rupture of the coats of an artery during ligation was not only useless, but dangerous. Atheroma was an indication for a more proximal ligation. Formation of clot and secondary hemorrhage were thus avoided. A small round aseptic ligature that would not become absorbed in less than three weeks was advocated, along with complete antiseptic precautions. The preferred ligature material was chromic catgut or Kangaroo tendon. Cooper had used and advocated catgut, but to Galen and earlier surgeons it was second choice to various nonabsorbable materials.

Thus closes the era of ligation and aneurysm surgery based on ligation. The first experimental vascular anastomosis was achieved by Eck in 1877, to show that the portal vein in dogs could indeed be successfully ligated provided that the splanchnic return was diverted to the vena cava. The reference is inaccessible, and we cite a more recently published translation.

Both clinical and experimental advances in blood vessel surgery followed. Jaboulay and Briau (1896) accomplished a circular end-to-end anastomosis of the carotid artery in the donkey. They used an everting type of interrupted suture, and obviously it was a relatively large vessel. In an inaugural dissertation Jassinowski in 1899 reported numerous cases of experimentally sutured arteries in animals. We cannot find the original of this reference, but it was well known to older writers and was cited frequently. In other experiments that followed, usually the intima was avoided; this method of suture is still appropriate at times when constriction of a small arterial laceration is undesirable—for instance, in suturing the radial artery after catheterization.

Many of these early experimental attempts at suture were plagued with frequent thrombosis. The problem was solved by Dörfler, who in 1899 published his method of circular suture of the artery, including the intima. He advocated using fine needles and fine silk.

Dorrence in 1906 reviewed extensively the methods then in use for the repair of arteries. In this review, which is interesting to peruse, he described adhesive methods, which are being reintroduced; the use of rigid tubes; the use of special arterial clamps; experimental suture of the aorta; and his own method of double-suturing or back-suturing the artery, using a continuous mattress suture and interlocking stitches and recovering the area with an overhand continuous suture. Recent experimental evidence has demonstrated that this type of suture is actually weaker than a continuous running everting type of suture.

Using the advances of Dörfler, surgeons accomplished a great many experimental procedures of note in the next ten to fifteen years. In the earliest of these, Ullman in 1902 succeeded in transplanting a kidney, and Carrel in the same year mentioned the possibility of the transplantation of organs. Hopfner in 1903 not only gave an excellent bibliographic review of early work, but also reported the successful reimplantation of an amputated extremity in a dog. Those interested should refer to the historical and experimental publications of Carrel and Watts in 1907. Yamanouchi in 1911 published an excellent review detailing his work and covering most of the work to that date. Finally there is the outstanding work of Guthrie *Blood Vessel Surgery and Its Applications* published in 1912.

Under investigation, in addition to arterial suture alone, were homografts and heterografts of fresh, frozen, and otherwise preserved arteries and veins. Guthrie and Carrel working at the University of Chicago in 1905 performed renal, cardiac, and thyroid transplantations, but Guthrie credited Ullman with the first renal transplant in 1902. Borst and Enderlen in 1909 published an extensive study of the transplantation of organs, mostly the kidney, with survival of up to 100 days after ablation of the animal's own kidneys.

Guthrie left Chicago in 1905 and became Professor of Physiology at Washington University in St. Louis. It was apparently there that he transplanted on an acute basis entire canine heads and the combined heart and lungs.

Of all these pioneers, Garrison mentioned only Eck and Carrel. Much of the early work was quite ignored, and the commanding position of Guthrie seems to be completely overlooked.

The basis of arterial surgery had been firmly established by the experimental work cited, but again, except for aneurysm surgery, there was little application to clinical medicine. Some authorities say that there were no human cases before 1900, but Lambert's concept and Hallowell's execution of it are too clear to be omitted as a remarkable first.

Human cases were indeed mentioned. The first cardiac suture was reported by Farina in 1896, with the first successful case described a year later by Rehn. Arterial-venous fistulas were used by San Martin y Satrustegui in 1902. Matas, in reviewing his operation of endoaneurysmorraphy, which he called a "radical cure of aneurysm," cited one of his own case reports published in 1888. Review of this case report reveals that there was a brachial artery aneurysm that did not regress after either proximal or distal ligation. Matas was therefore forced to open it and oversew the communication between the artery and the aneurysm sac, the aneurysm still being pulsatile and fed by collateral vessels that were not included in the previous ligatures. Matas also cited a case of treatment of fully established arterial venous aneurysm by separate suture of the openings of the arteries and veins by von Manteuffel as early as 1895.

Matas' method is well known; he could cure the aneurysm if it were sacciform, by simply closing the small opening into it. He described this operation in detail and also operations on larger fusiform aneurysms. The lumen of the parent artery was not always preserved, the end result depending on the circumstances.

Embolectomy also is a relatively old operation. Key in 1923 without giving his source assigned the first case to Suabanejeu in 1895 and the first completely successful case to Labey in 1911. Bauer in 1913 reported a successful embolectomy from the abdominal aorta.

After this period there was a remarkable hiatus in the reports of arterial surgery. We find occasional reports of cases or illustrations of techniques in surgical textbooks that indicate that some operations were done. Bernheim (1920) believed that the great war might provide opportunities to apply the newly developed techniques; however, the problem of infection was apparently too great for any spectacular success. Goodman in 1914 reported some more successful cases of suture of the peripheral arteries during this period, apparently at the time of initial traumatic surgery. In some cases a muscle flap was used to check the blood loss from the sutured vessels. Goodman furthermore stated that Weitung and Vollbrecht had also sutured wounded blood vessels whenever possible in the Balkan war from 1912 to 1913.

Horsley in 1921 expressed the opinion that the field for suturing blood vessels had greatly *contracted* and summarized the experience of World War I as being more favorable to ligation than to the suture of blood vessels. He reported however, a case of suture of the brachial artery.

Holman in 1927 contributed his observations on the surgery of the large arteries and reported cases of the treatment of aneurysm by proximal ligation.

Leriche in 1923 and 1940 and Leriche and Morel in 1948 first reported and then continued to report on the surgery of the Leriche syndrome. The favored operation was sympathectomy and resection of the occluded terminal aorta and proximal iliac arteries. However, resection of arteriosclerotic and obstructed arteries was popular, particularly in France, not too many years ago. There seems to be no adequate physiological reason for this procedure. Only when there is distal embolization from an occluded or almost occluded aneurysmal artery would excision seem to be justified. Arnulf in 1950 recorded many such cases; they are of historical interest only. Leriche in 1948 wrote that the ideal treatment of this condition would be to resect the obliterated zone and bridge the vascular defect by a graft. In spite of his visualization of the definitive operation, Leriche believed that "in the present state of techniques such an achievement seems impossible."

Further development of vascular surgery awaited an x-ray technique for visualization of the blood vessels. With aneurysm, arterial injury, and even embolism, arteriograms were not entirely necessary, but they became necessary for other applications.

Reboul published a definitive work on the arteriography of the limbs and the abdominal aorta in 1935 and credited the first arteriography with Lipiodol to Sicard and Forestier. Brooks at Washington University in St. Louis used sodium iodide in the same year, 1923, but his publication did not appear until 1924. Other early media were strontium bromide and Thorotrast. The first organic compounds containing iodine and adaptable for arteriography were introduced about 1929.

Reversal of the circulation has been largely an experimental operation. The concept of revascularization of ischemic tissue has been with us from the careful experimental studies of Carrel and Guthrie (1906) in a canine limb, to Beck's operation for revascularization of the heart (1948) and the cerebral circulation (1949).

The first cases were done in human beings reported by San Martin y Satrustegui in 1902. He performed lateral arteriovenous anastomosis for gangrene in two elderly patients; one case was considered successful, and the progression of gangrene was stopped. This work was cited by Goyanes in 1906, who also credited Jaboulay with two similar cases of lateral arteriovenous anastomosis, and as he related, the results were slightly favorable. Goyanes published his own innovation, which is rather startling for the date. He simply transposed an entire section of the femoral vein in the femoral canal, substituting it for the artery. A further report on this work was promised in the original publication. We cannot find this, but the vein transplant

5

was not neglected; Lexer (1912) used a vein graft after excision of a popliteal aneurysm. In one patient, an automobile accident caused an aneurysm.

Most of the "reversal" operations fall into two categories: arteriovenous fistula or arterialization of the superficial femoral vein, which after division, is circularly sutured to the proximal artery. The vein is not similarly transposed but is ligated proximally.

In 1912 Davies and Morriston reported thirty-six cases, and Bernheim reviewed fifty-two cases in the same year. In 1931 Bernheim published an eighteen-year follow-up study of a young woman in whom the circulation had been "reversed" in all four limbs for Raynaud's disease. There was no further gangrene, but the patient then consumed 0.5 Gm. of morphine by hypodermic injection daily. Goodman reported additional cases in 1914.

Insofar as the leg was concerned, the subject was more or less finished by Horsley (1916), who presented some cases and finally concluded that the operation was no better than proximal venous ligation for arterial insufficiency, which he believed was beneficial. Horsley, like writers before him, did not clearly distinguish at all times one occlusive vascular disease from another, so that Buerger's disease, arteriosclerosis, and Raynaud's disease were all taken together. Horsley's influence must have prevailed, although there was lively discussion following his paper. Reversal was defended.

The reversal reports and experiments are impressive, and they may deserve additional experimental study and evaluation with modern methods. In a few instances we have personal knowledge of the "rediscovery" of the reversal operation in the leg by surgeons apparently ignorant of the previous history. Anastomoses were made at the groin level and consisted of complete end-to-end exchange of the vessels. The result was moist gangrene. This is similar to the early Beck II operation. Beck found that an unrestricted aortic–coronary sinus anastomosis led to about the same condition in the heart, and thereafter he limited the size of the anastomosis. Early operations of this general type in the leg were done distally, and many, but not all, were small lateral anastomoses with variations.

There were other notable individual advances. Gross and Hubbard in 1939 reported the first ligation of a patent ductus arteriosus. The first resection for coarctation of the aorta was carried out by Crafoord in 1944; Gross also reported a successful case about one year afterward.

Thereafter, to solve the problem of coarctation, human homografts were used; they were used successfully in the surgery for coarctation and later in the resection and grafting for a thoracic aortic aneurysm by Swan and associates (1950) and by Lam (1951). Lowenberg (1950) treated two cases of abdominal aortic aneurysm by "cutis grafting." Oudot in 1951 reported successful resection and grafting of the distal aorta for Leriche syndrome, using preserved homologous aorta to restore vascular continuity. The cases of Dubost were reported about a year later. Julian and associates in 1953 and DeBakey and associates in 1954 reported similar operations.

Other early operations of note include the endarterectomies of dos Santos (1947) and Bazy and associates (1949). The development of heterografts, homografts, and methods of preserving them have been in and out of the literature since the time of Guthrie and Carrel. Cloth prostheses began to be used about 1950, and there has been intense development since that time. Also since about 1950 we have witnessed the determined and enthusiastic attack on arterial disease of all types. Those items of further and special interest are developed in other sections of this book.

Cardiac surgery made similar progress. Morgagni speculated on the effects of cardiac tamponade by blood in 1761, and Larrey in 1810 drained the pericardium. An experimental heart-lung bypass was in existence in 1885, developed by von Frey and Gruber. The first human mechanical bypass was carried out by Gibbon in 1954. The earliest suture of a cardiac wound is attributed to Farina in 1896. Other cases followed rapidly. Some of the first cardiac sutures for stab wounds of the heart were performed in this country by Nietert at the City Hospital in St. Louis in 1901. These and others were reported by Kirchner in 1910. By this time over 100 cases were known, and the survival rate was about one-third, a remarkable achievement for the time. The 1911 edition of Kocher's text discusses cardiac massage and the restoration of heart contraction by electrical stimulation.

Ancillary developments such as better instrumentation and sutures, blood transfusions, better anesthesia, antibiotics, and angiography have greatly contributed to the continued development of vascular surgery in the modern era.

Other historical items of note may be found in the remainder of this text.

SURGICAL PRINCIPLES AND BASIC TECHNIQUES
General surgical principles and their applications in vascular surgery

The successful outcome of vascular operations depends on thorough understanding and conscientious application of the principles of general surgery and on careful diagnosis and preoperative and postoperative care. It must be recognized, for example, that the most meticulous repair of a gunshot wound of the femoral artery may fail because of insufficient debridement of damaged muscle, improper fixation of an associated fracture, inadequate blood replacement, and the like.

Infection is one of the most serious complications that can occur in vascular surgery. The infected arterial wall becomes soft and friable so that suture lines leak or are disrupted, and the surgeon may be compelled to ligate a blood vessel or to sacrifice a limb.

When synthetic materials are used, the problems of infection are somewhat different. These materials are, of course, unaffected by the infectious process itself and can function as conduits in the presence of infection. However, like other foreign bodies, prosthetic grafts maintain an infectious process that otherwise might be eradicated. Ultimately, if infection extends to the anastomosis, disruption can result.

Treatment of such infections is always very difficult. In most cases the prosthesis must be removed. If the prosthesis is in the aorta or another similarly critical area, it is imperative that a new and infection-free route for bypass be sought through sound tissues and uncontaminated tissue planes. Each such event poses a unique surgical problem; a recurring example, however, is the use of axillary femoral bypass when the aorta is the artery involved. Occasionally the microorganisms from an infected peripheral wound can be cultured, and the wound can be healed with appropriate antibiotics and careful local treatment.

Because of the catastrophic consequences of infection in vascular surgery, prevention is of the utmost importance. All the details of aseptic technique should receive meticulous attention. Hematomas or fluid collections invite abscess formation; drains should be employed when necessary, always if the surgery is superficial and if anticoagulants are to be used. Careful closure eliminates dead space in the wound and about prosthetic materials.

The surgeon has usually mastered these problems and is able to secure adequate exposure and hemostasis. Experience demonstrates that skill and practice in general, traumatic, and even thoracic surgery and open-heart surgery do not, in themselves, confer the knowledge needed to master the problems of vascular reconstructive procedures. Vascular surgery is, however, not obscure or unusually difficult—it is merely different.

The axioms in vascular surgery are adequate exposure, proximal and distal control of blood vessels prior to arteriotomy, and prevention of thrombosis. With good technique, it should not be necessary to rely on anticoagulants to obtain good results from vascular procedures. Use of anticoagulants is discussed later in this chapter.

Experience has shown that it is generally unwise to attribute poor results to arterial spasm. When the results of reconstructive procedures are poor and pulses do not return as expected, thrombosis is a more likely explanation than is severe arterial spasm.

It is essential at the end of a surgical procedure to be certain that the blood vessels are open distally. Arteriograms at the end of an operation are frequently helpful and permit a prompt correction.

Other helpful measures to evaluate operative results at the time of surgery are arteriography with the aid of a portable image amplifier, if available; flowmeters of the square wave variety that can be applied to the trunk of the exposed vessel; and the routine use of Fogarty catheters and irrigation distally with heparinized saline before final suture. Fig. 1-1 shows a continuous irrigating device that is extremely useful and can save a good deal of time. It is possible to develop some judgment about the distal outflow tract by sensing the pressure necessary to inject heparinized saline distally.

If circulation was previously poor, distal pulses are not a good guide unless known to be present before surgery. Warmth of the limb can be used as a guide, but both warmth and color may not return soon to a limb that previously had poor circulation.

If the suspicion of spasm still lingers, irrigation with a small amount of lidocaine local anesthetic solution or with papaverine, 60 mg. in 100 ml. of sterile heparin in saline solution, may be useful. Peripheral vasoconstriction due to shock must be treated by quick and appropriate treatment of the shock itself; usually this requires adequate fluid and blood replacement. It should not be forgotten that peripheral vasoconstriction may also occur because of a low body temperature; this is secondary to cooling under anesthesia. The danger is greater in operations in which large exposed areas are involved.

Perivascular dissection

Perivascular dissection is a basic technique in vascular surgery. The easiest and clearest plane of dissection is close to the blood vessel. The procedure is begun by picking up the perivascular tissue with fine forceps and cutting it. The plane along the vessel is developed by sharp and blunt dissection with Metzenbaum scissors. Curved Metzenbaum scissors modified by grinding the points to resemble the Stevens tenotomy scissors are very useful.

Small rolls of umbilical tape held in a hemostat are used to dissect about the complete circumference of a thin-walled vessel. They can be employed in pairs, one to hold the vessel aside and the other to roll the perivascular areolar tissue away. The same method may be used to dissect longitudinally along the blood vessel.

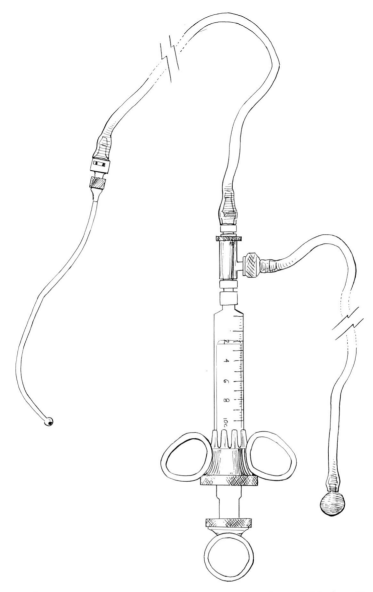

Fig. 1-1. Device for continuous irrigation. (All component parts available from Becton, Dickinson & Co., Rutherford, N. J.)

When dissecting longitudinally, all dissection and application of tension should follow the long axis of the vessel. Tapes under the vessel aid in handling and in exposure and are relatively atraumatic. Experience teaches the amounts of tension that are necessary and safe. However, intimal tears with consequent thrombosis are produced by overstretching thin blood vessels.

Anastomosis of small vessels requires meticulous techniques. At the site of anastomosis, even the finest shreds of adventitia should be trimmed from the edge. After transection, retraction of the tissues will often produce new shreds of tissue that should be removed. Removal of the loose adventitia facilitates anastomosis of small vessels, for if this is not excised, the mobility of the outer layer can leave the operator in some doubt about piercing the intima of the vessel with each stitch. When large

9

vessels are sutured, adventitia is needed for a secure closure. In small vessels, however, an overly thick adventitial layer will slide back and forth, making each passage of the needle a problem in visualization. Fragments of adventitial tissue falling into the suture line or being carried into the lumen of the vessel by the suture increase the danger of postoperative thrombosis. In diseased vessels it may be impossible to distinguish the usual anatomical layers.

Suture techniques

The currently preferred suture material for vascular surgery is braided Dacron in sizes ranging from 3-0 to 7-0. This material is available commercially. Various manufacturers use different systems of lubrications for their suture material. Tevdek* is impregnated with Teflon; Ti-Cron† is lubricated with silicone oil instead of Teflon. Both of these are excellent suture materials and eliminate the need for any extra lubrication. In all cases, extra knots should be tied because the lubricated material does tend to be a little less secure than ordinary braided silk, and an ordinary surgeon's knot cannot be trusted to hold indefinitely as the suture must.

For vein grafts the least reactive materials are polyethylene and polypropylene.‡ This suture material stretches approximately 15% before breaking; it is quite strong for its size. It is extremely unlikely that it would be stretched that amount in actual use, but in a large artery with high pressure the possibility must be kept in mind.

It is well for the vascular surgeon to acquaint himself with these materials by handling them, stretching them, tying knots, and pulling on the knots so that he can appreciate the moderate differences between vascular suture materials and black braided silk.

Dacron maintains its strength in the tissues throughout years of implantation. Since no true healing occurs between prosthetic implants and the host artery, such a material is essential to prevent disruption at the suture line between the prosthesis and the artery.

These suture materials are supplied with swaged-on atraumatic needles. Previously, in the direct suture of blood vessels, lubrication of the suture material has been employed, primarily as an anticoagulation measure. Lubrication also makes passage of the suture material through atherosclerotic blood vessel walls easier and prevents the suture from sawing the arterial wall. Silicone oil and mineral oil are excellent lubricants. However, Teflon-coated Dacron may be used as supplied without further lubrication.

We now prefer polyethylene and polypropylene suture material for all vein grafts. These materials slip through the thin vein wall easily and with mimimum trauma. They will not catch the adventitia by friction, pulling it into the lumen; this is a minor but significant advantage, since the presence of adventitia stimulates thrombosis. If there is a little spring to the suture, extra knots should be used to give the security needed when tying. The previously mentioned 15% stretch factor of polypropylene is not brought into play when doing vein grafts, so that in practical application this is not a consideration.

---

*Supplied by Deknatal, Inc., Queens Village, N.Y.
†Supplied by Davis & Geck, American Cyanamid Co., Pearl River, N.Y.
‡Polypropylene available as Prolene from Ethicon, Inc., Somerville, N.J.

When using finer sutures or working in a difficult location, the surgeon can advantageously employ double-armed sutures. Then if a suture breaks or a fine needle is bent, a spare needle and suture are already in place, and he can put them to use without taking down and reconstructing an entire anastomosis.

In medium-sized vessels the sutures are placed about 1 mm. apart and about 1 mm. back from the edge of the vessel. This distance should be lessened for small vessels and when 7-0 silk is used. When aneurysms of the aorta are sutured, sutures

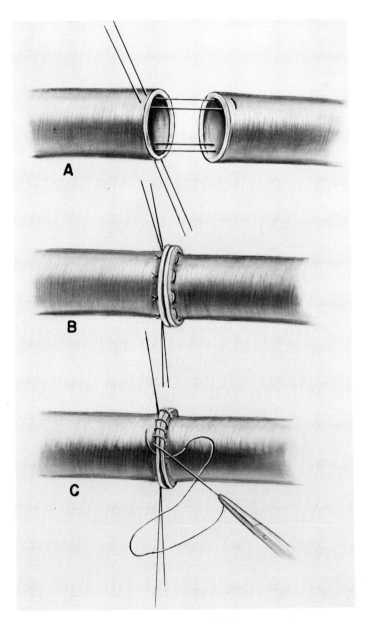

Fig. 1-2. Anastomosis of a moderate-sized artery. **A,** Placement of mattress sutures to begin anastomosis. **B,** Completion of end-to-end anastomosis with interrupted mattress sutures. **C,** Completion of end-to-end anastomosis with continuous everting suture. (Adapted from Linton, R. R.: Surgery **38:**817, 1955.)

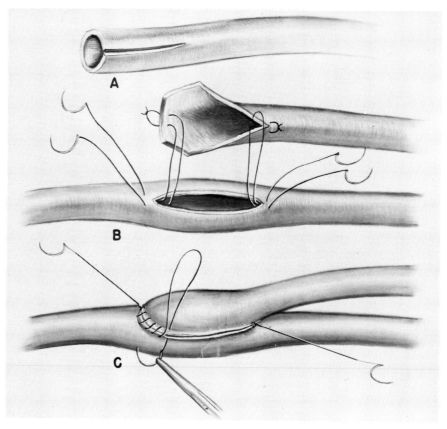

Fig. 1-3. End-to-side arterial anastomosis. **A,** End of blood vessel slit and shaped. **B,** Two everting mattress-type sutures inserted to begin closure. **C,** Closure completed with over-and-over technique. (Adapted from Linton, R. R.: Surgery **38:**817, 1955.)

may be widely spaced (that is, 2 or 3 mm. apart) without leakage. The physical properties of the arterial wall may make accurate placement of sutures difficult. Sutures can be guided into place and the edge of the vessel everted with a long right-angle nerve hook or a sharp-pointed skin hook.

A number of techniques of anastomosis are illustrated throughout this book. Veins are most efficiently handled by the technique of triangulation of the ends of the vessels with three separate stay sutures that are used to steady the vessel while end-to-end approximation with a continuous simple suture through all layers is accomplished. For larger vessels it is more secure to evert a cuff of artery (Fig. 1-2, *A* and *B*); this will allow intima-to-intima approximation with less suture material exposed to the bloodstream. Such suture lines eliminate leakage, but they have the disadvantages of requiring slightly more artery and of producing moderate constriction. Mattress sutures, therefore, should be avoided in small blood vessels. End-to-side anastomosis is illustrated in Fig. 1-3.

The technique of suture depends on the age of the patient. In children, growth is expected; therefore, a continuous suture should not be used. Such a suture will first straighten out with growth and subsequently migrate through the wall of the vessel toward the intima. Dissection occurs with an internal constricting septum.

The septum becomes fenestrated and the suture, now on the inside of the artery, sloughs internally with a thrombus attached. In growing children, therefore, interrupted mattress sutures should be used instead of a continuous suture (Fig. 1-2, B), or the continous suture may be used for one-half the circumference of the anastomosis and interrupted mattress sutures for the remainder.

Studies of early suture line strength, that is, up to fourteen days, show that anastomotic strength usually exceeds the bursting strength of canine blood vessels and that this in turn is also somewhat independent of the suture size in the ranges studied from 3-0 to 6-0 or nominal strengths of 4 to $^1/_2$ pound breaking strength for the suture material. Also experimentally, the continuous over-and-over suture is as strong or stronger than interrupted, interrupted horizontal mattress, continuous mattress, and more significantly, complicated back sutures.

A well-constructed suture line will leak very little after the vascular clamps are released. Some leakage usually will be observed as the tensions of continuous suture lines readjust to the intervascular pressure. Small openings will close spontaneously. It is wise first to remove the distal clamp, exposing the anastomosis to an initially lower pressure. Experience will teach the surgeon which leaks are self-sealing and which require correction. In aortic anastomoses, some small leaks are repaired by sutures through the adventitia only. Blood flow should be shut off momentarily when an extra suture is to be placed. Sutures placed in an artery carrying blood under pressure or under full tension can only be placed in the cuff of the anastomosis. Otherwise more bleeding results from the new hole in the vessel. Tears may result when a needle is passed through a pulsating vessel. Patched anastomoses are less satisfactory. There is little substitute for precision and perfection of technique in anastomosis of small vessels. Suture lines in diseased or large arteries require sturdy wide cuffs and tight approximation of the edges.

Microsuture and microsurgical techniques

Microsuture techniques have been developed by Jacobson, employing a binocular dissecting microscope with magnifications of from 6× to 40×. An essential for this work is an objective lens of long working distance—8 to 12 inches. A rest is used to stabilize the hands and the blood vessels being operated on. The instruments are modifications of those devised for ophthalmic surgery, and suture materials are very fine (7-0) silk or ultrafine monofilament nylon with a diameter of 0.001 inch.

Attempts to reconstruct arterial vessels and veins less than 4 mm. in diameter have been compicated by a high rate of thrombosis. The work of Jacobson and associates has illustrated that the basic principles of surgical technique necessary for successful primary vascular surgery are entirely applicable to small vessels. Using microscopic techniques, anastomoses can be accomplished in vessels as small as 1 mm. Sutures are placed much more closely than for larger work.

To date, the insertion of small prostheses has not proved practical because of the lining that forms within the prosthesis.

Those interested in further study are referred to the monograph *Micro-vascular Surgery* by Donaghy and Yaşargil.

When microsurgical methods are perfected, there may be practical applications, particularly in the field of organ transplantation. Under ordinary circumstances the surgeon may not have immediate access to the instruments and equipment necessary for microsurgical procedures. In dealing with smaller vessels in the 4 mm. to 6 mm.

range, there should be no hesitancy to employ the long-focus binocular loupe used for ophthalmic surgery, which is usually readily available.

Nonsuture techniques

Various nonsuture techniques of vascular repair have been used recently. Perhaps the most familiar of these employs stapling instruments, a number of which are now available. With the exception of the Japanese (Nakayama) stapler, all are confined to use for end-to-end anastomoses. The Nakayama stapler, with which we have had considerable laboratory experience, may be used for both end-to-end and end-to-side anastomoses, as illustrated on pp. 269 and 270. All these instruments promise to be useful in the union of small vessels in the 2 to 4 mm. range. In general, however, there is not yet any wide clinical application. The instruments have long handles and are awkward to manipulate. A length of normal blood vessel is necessary to thread within the cuffs and anvils of their machinery, and atherosclerotic blood vessels cannot be handled easily. We do not, therefore, anticipate that such instruments will replace ordinary suture methods for large or diseased blood vessels. Indeed, with the help of a binocular operating microscope of long working distance, the human hand can probably surpass these instruments in precision, if not in speed.

A small self-loading stapling device available in a hemostatic forceps design and in a thumb forceps design is available for the insertion of small staples one at a time and more or less under the operator's control.* This device is occasionally useful when exposure is limited.

Recently, rapid-setting amide-glue materials (methyl 2-cyanoacrylate) have been proposed to repair skin, bronchus, and blood vessels without the aid of sutures. Circumferential union of both arteries and veins have been accomplished with these materials, but with a high incidence of early thrombosis and late aneurysm formation. This technique of vascular repair continues to be experimental, and, like the stapling technique, does not possess the dependability, versatility, or precision of suture techniques.

Prevention of thromboses

Thrombosis after anastomosis in large arteries results mainly from turbulence or distal obstruction. In small vessels, however, other factors are also important, and refined techniques become more necessary. The clotting process is catalytic and is initiated by release of thromboplastin from injured intimal or other cells. In large arteries a thin layer of clot forms on the internal raw surface after removal of the intima by endarterectomy or after insertion of a prosthesis. There is no obstructive thrombosis if flow is rapid and if there is no narrowing or turbulence. The mechanical problems and also the release of thromboplastin initiated by injury are more troublesome in smaller vessels. Blood vessels should not be overstretched, and the intima should be disturbed or handled as little as possible. Occluding arterial clamps should be noncrushing. Guide sutures are helpful during anastomosis to hold vessels together with a minimum of instrumental handling. Cuffed types of anastomoses expose less suture material to the bloodstream than do those that have no cuff everted. Well-placed sutures are not significant causes of thrombosis.

Disruption and infection of suture lines are less and less of a problem as technical

---

* Manufactured by Codman & Shurtleff, Inc., Randolph, Mass.

abilities grow and the suture materials become better. Thrombosis at the suture line has been a problem in blood vessel surgery since its inception. It is in the situation of low flow, low distal runoff, handling of small blood vessels, endarterectomy, and carotid endarterectomy that the problem of thrombotic occlusion is at its worst. In such operations, liberal irrigation with heparin in saline solution (50 mg. per 500 ml.), heparinization at surgery, and postoperative heparinization are most often used.

Successful suture of small arteries requires atraumatic technique, lubrication of sutures, or the use of nonwetting sutures such as Teflon-coated Dacron or monofilament polyethylene, along with exclusion of adventitial tissue from the suture line. These techniques minimize the release of thromboplastin and thus the initiation of clotting. When a vessel is first opened, all blood should be immediately washed out with physiological saline solution. Washing out the blood before it clots minimizes the production of thrombin. Instillation of heparin solution into the vessel proximal and distal to the occluding clamps is advisable. Another hazard is formation of fibrin clot in areas of turbulent blood flow through rough or constricting anastomoses. These faulty anastomoses are always undesirable.

When a fabric prosthesis has been inserted, there is no intima, and it is necessary to depend on the clotting mechanism to seal the prosthesis and on rapid, unobstructed, smooth blood flow to prevent thrombosis on the interior of the prosthetic graft. The thin layer of fibrin is slowly replaced by flat lining tissue that resembles intima.

Ligation of major blood vessels

Sacrifice of major blood vessels produces disabling symptoms. Occasionally after a large artery has been ligated, gangrene does not develop, but arterial insufficiency may be disabling. The symptoms of such insufficiency are coldness, claudication, atrophy of the skin and muscles, pain, decrease in strength, sensory and motor disturbances, edema, and chronic cyanosis. All these unfavorable sequelae of ligation of major vessels can be avoided by restoration of vascular continuity. The aims of vascular surgery are to preserve and to restore blood flow when possible.

When ligation of a major blood vessel is unavoidable, selection of the best site is important. In general, ligation between proximal and distal collateral channels minimizes disability and the occurrence of gangrene. Ligation of certain arteries is known from experience to be relatively safe. The external carotid, the internal iliac and the profunda femoris are examples of vessels that are ligated with impunity. Usually ligation of such vessels as the axillary, the external iliac, or the femoral artery below the exit of the profunda femoris artery is severely disabling but is not accompanied by gangrene. Ligation of the subclavian artery, the femoral artery above the exit of the profunda femoris artery or in the adductor canal, the internal carotid artery, or the common iliac artery is frequently catastrophic.

The surgical principles for ligation of major arteries are as follows:
1. Arteries should be divided and not ligated in continuity.
2. A transfixion ligature distal to the tie is advisable on large blood vessels to prevent dislodgment of the ligature by arterial pulastions.
3. Tensile strength and size of ligatures and suture ligatures must be sufficient so that there is little danger of breakage.
4. The ligatures should be tied squarely across the vessel with a secure square knot. Several extra "throws" are desirable for the utmost in security.

15

5. Ligatures should be tied close to the vessel wall, without including any surrounding tissue. Failure to isolate the vessel and the inclusion of perivascular areolar tissue and fat allow the ligature to slip off easily.

When large arteries are atherosclerotic, encircling ligatures may fragment and tear the brittle and calcific wall. It is sometimes better to close the vessel with a continuous everting suture over the open end. If the wall of the vessel is extremely hard, an endarterectomy may be necessary before closure can be accomplished. This suture technique also preserves collateral vessels that arise just proximal to the site of proposed ligation and that would otherwise be sacrificed to have sufficient cuff distal to the ligature.

Back bleeding from the distal portion of the ligated vessel is evidence of good collateral flow. In no case should distal ligature of the artery be omitted. It is not necessary to ligate veins accompanying arteries, as once suggested. Venous ligation increases the possibility of venous insufficiency and will not improve the arterial blood flow in the involved extremity.

Preoperative, operative, and postoperative use of anticoagulants

The coumarin group of drugs, heparin, dextran, and aspirin (for depressing platelet adhesiveness) are the drugs to be considered in this section.

In the period before, during, and after surgery the coumarin group is best avoided. There are a number of reasons for this, the most meaningful being the longer time necessary for onset of action and for termination of action. Occasionally we must operate on a patient receiving anticoagulants, and we have even successfully resected ruptured aortic aneurysms in patients receiving coumarin; but it is certainly not an optimal situation for survival. Another disadvantage of the coumarin anticoagulants is incomplete action once a clot has begun to form. In a suitable patient with superficial saphenous vein phlebitis ascending the leg, one can occasionally observe the progression of phlebitis even when prothrombin times are prolonged to over double the control times. The explanation is that the antiprothrombin drugs although depressing the level of several clotting factors besides prothrombin, actually leave enough of them to interact with the excess of thromboplastin at the site of injury or where a thrombus formation has already commenced. Even the traces of thrombin that result act as a catalyst for the further production of thrombin and clot. Heparin, however, blocks the action of thrombin. Finally, the antiprothrombin drugs have many drug interactions that make treatment difficult. Their action is inhibited by many hypnotics and by corticosteroids and potentiated by phenylbutazone, salicylates, quinidine, aspirin, and others; furthermore, the antiprothrombin drugs themselves may potentiate the actions of other drugs such as diphenylhydantoin and tolbutamide. The list given is short, and reported interactions are much more extensive than indicated.

Dextran, particularly low–molecular weight dextran, may at times be useful, particularly when microcirculation seems deficient. Its use has been suggested for prevention of thrombosis in almost every situation in which this may or has occurred. We seldom use it therapeutically; occasionally a small amount is permissible in case of shock, but if arterial surgery is contemplated, the use of more than two units within a short period of time can produce an annoying bleeding tendency. Massive replacement with either type of dextran results in bleeding that is very difficult to control, and it should therefore not be used to replace blood or plasma. Reconstruction procedures vary so much that it is difficult to produce a series in which one would, say, use low–molecular weight dextran daily postoperatively in one set of patients and not use it in another. Experimental evidence suggests that dextran of either high or low molecular weight will increase backflow from a proximally clamped limb artery. Studies of blood viscosity and regional blood flow show that viscosity is almost an exponential function of hematocrit value over limited ranges. Low–molecular weight dextran can decrease viscosity of the blood, and some of this decrease is probably due to hemodilution. The effects, nevertheless, seem to last longer than the similar effects of balanced electrolyte solutions. Dextran may be used to advantage in situations in which there is low regional blood flow such as in marginal or incipient gangrene and also during uncomplicated surgery on the blood vessels in the extremity, but never in large amounts at one time.

Aspirin does not directly change the prothrombin time, but thrombus formation time is prolonged in vitro. This effect, in turn, appears to be mediated through some effect on the blood platelets, preventing platelet aggregation of "white" thrombi. Salzman and associates (1971) compared warfarin, dipyridamole, aspirin, and dextran and their efficacy in reducing thromboembolism after hip arthroplasty. They found that, except for dipyridamole, these drugs reduced the incidence of thromboembolism postoperatively and that all had about the same incidence of hemorrhagic complications, with perhaps some quantitative differences.

A more elegant double-blind study using heparin as the prophylactic agent was reported by Kakkar and associates in 1972. Their clinical material was major surgery and hip fractures. The heparin dosage was 5,000 units given subcutaneously two hours before surgery and every twelve hours for the next seven days. The evidence of deep thrombosis was 42% in a control group versus 8% in the treated group as determined by ^{125}I-labeled human fibrinogen detection. Results were poorer in the emergency surgery of fractured hips, considered by many to be the highest-risk group.

Heparin remains the best choice for the vascular surgeon during the period just before, during, and after surgery. As a rule, the use of anticoagulants is unnecessary and unwise at this time, but there are outstanding exceptions, such as situations in which there is low outflow in the leg, extensive endarterectomy, a patient whose blood is known to be or suspected of being hypercoagulable, thrombectomy for extensive ileofemoral thrombosis, pulmonary embolism, and carotid endarterectomy.

Heparin may be given before the surgical wound is closed, particularly if the wound is drained. During surgery, heparin is used regionally by injecting a small quantity, 1,000 units (10 mg.), into the distal portion of an artery just before clamping. This gives some, but not total, insurance against thrombosis distally. Collateral circulation may carry the heparin away, but such good collateral circulation may also protect against thrombosis. The terminal use of a Fogarty catheter and rinsing with heparin in saline solution gives further insurance against distal thrombus formation and is particularly useful when working in the leg or just prior to opening the limb of an aortic replacement.

Systemic heparinization can be used more freely in operations confined to the leg or to the neck; for there hemorrhage is at once apparent, and a drain may remove extravasated blood with fair efficiency.

A basic heparinization routine consists of the initial administration of 5,000 units (50 mg.) introvenously with a reseal needle. Intramuscularly or subcutaneously given heparin produces almost the same results; however, the onset of action is delayed.

17

The dose should be repeated and adjusted regardless of the route of administration about every six hours initially and, later, every twenty-four to seventy-two hours. The first test of clotting time should be done after about five and one-half hours or just before the next scheduled dose of heparin. At this time the action of heparin is diminishing, and clotting time of fifteen to thirty minutes is adequate. If the determination is too low, the dosage schedule should be changed to every four hours and, after that, as indicated by clotting times. Thus after ten hours, adequate anticoagulation with laboratory control can be achieved. Clotting times are accurate only when determined with meticulous care and technique, and parctically all the errors tend to produce a lower rather than a higher time. When the clinical picture and the laboratory picture disagree, this must be taken into consideration.

Occasionally the problem of intraoperative or postoperative bleeding occurs in a heparinized patient; if the bleeding is from a localized area or from a suture line, it can sometimes be controlled by the application of very dilute topical thrombin solution. *This must not be injected.* When this procedure is followed, heparinization can be maintained with careful postoperative care.

Leveen (1965) has shown experimentally that clot deposition and lysis proceed simultaneously in the wounded canine vena cava and that ϵ-aminocaproic acid stabilizes the thrombi, sealing the wound while not otherwise interfering with the action of heparin. The result is that established clots remain attached better and hemorrhage is prevented. These findings have not been clinically confirmed or exploited, but they may be the answer to the problem of preventing further embolism once thrombosis has occurred. The same property of heparin that makes it useful for pulmonary embolism may also pose a danger in, for instance, an ileofemoral vein segment where clots are known to exist and heparin must be used to prevent extension.

Thrombolysis with urokinase and streptokinase enzymes is still under trial and has yet to show safe, dependable, and reproducible results. The search for an in vitro thrombolysis system that will not result in otherwise uncontrollable hemorrhage and that is dependable should be continued. Occasionally heparin is said to be thrombolytic, but we doubt this. Another valid point of view is that a clot, say in the pulmonary vasculature, has its own thrombolytic mechanism that is furthered by the addition of an antithrombin agent, so that the effect is present but indirect.

Another problem that arises in patients receiving anticoagulants is whether or not to use a Teflon or a woven prosthesis that would leak a good deal less than the standard knitted Dacron materials. The choice of Teflon can usually be avoided by spending a little time and effort preclotting the Dacron graft. Sufficient blood is withdrawn from the patient's aorta or from any other source to saturate the graft, which is then stretched several times. If this is done as early as possible, the efficiency of preclotting is as good with heparinized blood as with normal whole blood, even though it may take somewhat longer. The manufacturers of the Weavenit material suggest a second preclotting after the proximal anastomosis is performed. The many long-term complications of Teflon, even in high-flow situations, are discussed later.

INSTRUMENTATION

From the earliest days it has been known that meticulous and atraumatic technique is necessary to avoid thrombosis at the site of an arterial anastomosis or other blood vessel suture. From time to time in working with arteriosclerotic vessels and with cloth prostheses, it would seem that this is not important; indeed, there may be less opportunity to observe all the technical details, particularly when one depends on blood clot and fibrin linings in cloth tubes to initially seal them and prevent leakage.

Early operators used bulldog clamps with smooth jaws or rubber-covered clamps. The original Carrel clamps resembled a short thumb forceps and were tightened with a screw. One of the jaws was made with a lip to prevent the vessel from slipping out the end. Many new and special-purpose clamps and other vascular instruments have since been devised; however, there is little data available concerning the traumatic potentialities of these instruments.

Henson and Rob (1956) studied the subject by applying various types of clamps for fifteen minutes to the gastroepiploic artery, which was then excised and examined microscopically. As a rule, gross damage was found. The least traumatic forms of occlusion occurred with rubber-covered blades and smooth bulldog clamps, as might have been expected from older experiences. These studies included some of the vascular clamps of the day and form a model that should be repeated with the clamps available currently.

A more recent but somewhat different approach was taken by Nickell (1969), who demostrated lessened or minimal intimal damage with the soft Hydragrip* clamps; however, these have the disadvantage of slipping easily. Although we can get an aortic clamp made to these specifications, we would not have the courage

*Manufactured by Edwards Laboratories, Santa Ana, Calif.

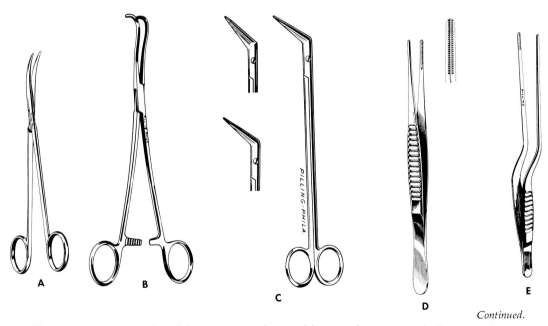

Continued.

Fig. 1-4. Assortment of useful instruments designed for vascular surgery. **A,** Jamison scissors. **B,** Curved dissecting clamp. **C,** Potts-Smith type of scissors. **D** and **E,** DeBakey vascular thumb forceps. **F,** Double-curved clamp for occluding aorta. **G** and **H,** Multipurpose straight clamps frequently referred to as coarctation clamps. **I,** Small curved peripheral vascular clamp. **J,** Henley subclavian artery clamp. **K,** Tangential partial occlusion or Satinsky clamp. **L,** DeBakey multipurpose angle clamps. These are only a small selection from an extensive catalog of specialized instruments. (Courtesy Pilling Co., Ft. Washington, Pa.)

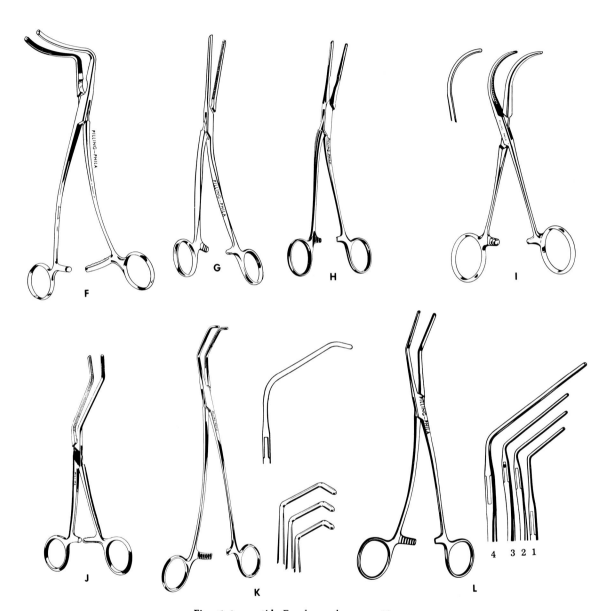

Fig. 1-4, cont'd. For legend see p. 19.

to use it routinely. Therefore, to occlude larger vessels and for special purposes when it is necessary to turn or deliver blood vessels into the surgical field, clamps with a surer grip having some type of tooth are necessary.

The teeth of the Cooley, DeBakey, Potts, and Burford clamps showed either an imprint on the intima or slight perforation without disruption. It is important that intimal disruption and damage be avoided. To this end most of these clamps have now been modified by the Pilling Company so that the former three to five steps in closure are now increased to seven. It is therefore more possible to use light tension and to select lightweight clamps when applicable. Currently there are a large variety of instruments available from the Pilling Company. Some of the more useful ones are illustrated in Fig. 1-4. Occlusion clamps may be improvised, as in the past, from rubber-shod forceps, but the usual problem with these is insecurity. Tying a vessel over a small section of rubber tubing is also atraumatic but tends to be awkward.

In 1966 Polin and Hershey developed a partial occlusion technique for minimizing the occlusion time when closing carotid endarterectomies. We found that the clamps available were bulky and left little lumen for flow during closure. As a consequence, we sought 1 mm. jaws, and they were carefully made by the Pilling Company. These have now been developed as their pediatric clamps (Fig. 1-5) and are suitable for peripheral use in adults as well.

Curved Metzenbaum scissors with the tips ground down to resemble the Stevens tenotomy scissors are now widely available as Jamison scissors. Fine scissors and needle holders with carbide inserts that will firmly hold small needles are available from many suppliers.*

ENDARTERECTOMY TECHNIQUE

Endarterectomy reopens an occluded artery through removal of the occlusive contents, which hopefully, are only loosely attached thrombotic material and athero-sclerotic plaques. At times a very short area of arteriosclerotic occlusion, such as one frequently sees at the bifurcation of the common carotid artery, can be removed very easily, leaving a smooth muscularis behind. At other times calcification and inflammatory reaction bind the "core" to the adventitia of the artery, and a good cleavage plane cannot be found.

There is no way to know in advance whether or not a particular proposed endarterectomy will be feasible in the superficial femoral artery. The ideal situation for endarterectomy is a localized occlusion or stenosis, such as is found in the distal common carotid and at its bifurcation or in the common femoral artery and the profunda femoris artery. Endarterectomy of the superficial femoral artery, particularly throughout its length, is rarely indicated, and the long-term follow-up is disappointing. The preferable operation in this situation is a bypass using the reversed saphenous vein. It is an excellent policy when proposing endarterectomy, particularly in the superficial femoral artery, to be prepared to switch to another technique or to use the vein bypass technique as a primary operation.

Even a short-segment endarterectomy can be very difficult, if not impossible, in the superficial femoral artery. However, not to exclude this technique completely,

*Those that should be known to the vascular surgeon include the Pilling Co., Ft. Washington, Pa.; Edwards Laboratories, Santa Ana, Calif.; Snowden-Pencer, Los Gatos, Calif.; Storz Instrument Co., St. Louis, Mo., whose eye instruments are occasionally useful; and the Sparta Instrument Co., Fairfield, N. J., also specializing in micro and finer instruments.

BOTH SIZES AVAILABLE IN <u>3 HANDLE SHAPES</u>

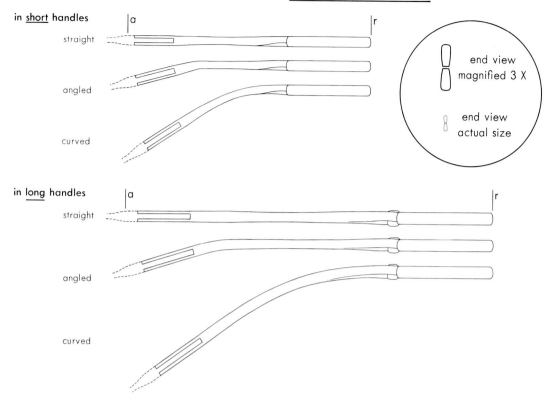

in <u>short</u> handles

straight

angled

curved

end view
magnified 3 X

end view
actual size

in <u>long</u> handles

straight

angled

curved

AND FOR EACH LENGTH AND SHAPE OF HANDLE <u>9 BLADE SHAPES</u>

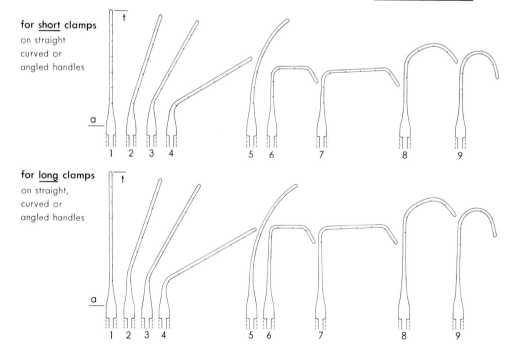

for <u>short</u> clamps
on straight
curved or
angled handles

1 2 3 4   5 6   7   8   9

for <u>long</u> clamps
on straight,
curved or
angled handles

1 2 3 4   5 6   7   8   9

Fig. 1-5. Pediatric clamp and handle combinations available from Pilling Co. with 1 mm. jaws. Useful in surgery on adults as well as children.

we have observed cases of stable occlusions existing over a period of five to seven years, confirmed by old and recent arteriograms, in which endarterectomy proved to be relatively easy.

The usual technique is to expose the artery where necessary and to make a short incision. Small separating instruments of various sizes are available from surgical supply companies. These are used to develop the plane of cleavage between adventitia and the inner occlusive core of the artery. Specially made sets of loops, wire loops, or circles are available; they should be placed around the core once it is loosened and then moved up and down to remove the inner contents. This process is usually best started distally rather than proximally. With reference to the superficial femoral artery, it is often necessary to expose the entire adductor canal and to open the artery in several places in order to complete an endarterectomy. Such a long endarterectomy is usually an indication that a bypass would have been a better technique to employ, particularly if a suitable saphenous vein is available. The endarterectomy process is technically easier in the carotid artery, since only a short length of artery is usually involved. The same is true in the case of subclavian occlusion and some distal aortic and iliac occlusions. As a rule, the surgeon must be versatile and adaptable and have an alternative plan in mind. No single reconstructive routine seems to work out consistently well in all places and in all patients.

A new method of endarterectomy uses carbon dioxide gas. This is obtained from a standard cylinder with the pressure reduced. The gas is then conveyed into the wall of the artery through a 22-gauge short-bevel needle and very quickly and gently defines the plane of dissection. This method does not separate the inner occlusive core from the adventitia in places where it may be tightly bound down, so that although it is a gentle and rapid technique, it does not increase the number of cases in which endarterectomy can be done successfully. Sets of spatulas with small holes in them designed for carbon dioxide gas endarterectomy are obtainable on special order.* It is claimed that the gas endarterectomy method opens the branches of the endarterectomized artery rather than leaving them closed; however, we have not been able to achieve this. As a rule, the postoperative x-ray film of an endarterectomy shows, particularly in the superficial femoral artery, a straight tube without any branching collateral vessels.

Rapid flow is necessary for maintenance of patency after endarterectomy. Since the procedure is traumatic and does not leave an intimal lining, it is probably best to heparinize these patients before they leave the operating room and keep them heparinized for four or five days after surgery. Some operators continue anticoagulation therapy, particularly when a low-flow situation in the leg is involved. Others claim that pseudointima formation is hastened by heparinization, and they continue to use it for this reason, particularly in carotid endarterectomy, in which the formation of small thrombi and distal embolization can be a distinct postoperative problem. Our own practice is to start with heparin in both cases, that is, carotid endarterectomy and superficial femoral endarterectomy, and to switch to coumarin anticoagulants provided that there are no problems with these drugs.

As more and more experience has been gained with endarterectomy, it has become obvious that the best place to do this operation is at the carotid bifurcation and perhaps the worst place to do it is throughout the length of the superficial femoral artery.

---

*Obtainable from Becton, Dickinson & Co., Rutherford, N. J.

Endarterectomies that have a short length are more likely to be successful than the long ones. Endarterectomy in the aorta and iliac arteries is also more successful than long-segment endarterectomy in the superficial femoral artery.

During the healing process, the interior of the endarterectomized vessel develops a thick, glistening, almost fibrous hypertrophic lining. This lining is thick enough that occlusion of a small superficial femoral artery may take place on this basis alone. A somewhat similar process may be seen in saphenous vein bypasses both in the leg and from the aorta to the coronary arteries. A process that is apparently identical has been observed experimentally for many years in transplantation of venous segments into the arterial system.

In the leg the saphenous vein transplant is definitely superior to endarterectomy in terms of eventual occlusion by the process just described and in terms of long-term functioning without any other occlusive accidents such as thrombosis in a low-flow or low-runoff situation.

LAWS OF FLUID FLOW AND THEIR APPLICATION TO VASCULAR SURGERY

Liquids flowing through conduits such as the vascular system flow in two fashions: laminar flow or turbulent flow.

Laminar flow

In laminar or streamline flow (Fig. 1-6, *A*) the liquid may be visualized as moving in infinitesimally thin and concentric cylindrical layers, parallel to the wall of the containing vessel. The basic law of laminar fluid flow is that of Poiseuille, a physician whose interest in the circulation of the blood led him to study and quantitate the dynamics of fluid flow. His findings can be expressed mathematically as follows:

$$P = \frac{8\,L}{\pi\,R^4}\,V\,Q \qquad (1)$$

P = Pressure difference (dynes/cm.^{2})
L = Length of tube in centimeters
R = Radius of tube in centimeters
V = A constant, the coefficient of viscosity, in poises
Q = Volume rate of flow (ml./sec.)

It can be seen from the equation that the change in pressure necessary to deliver a constant quantity of fluid varies directly with the length of the tube and inversely with the *fourth power* of the radius.

Laminar flow and a rigid straight tube are basic assumptions in deriving Poiseuille's law, either experimentally or theoretically. The law is not strictly applicable to (1) conditions of turbulent flow, (2) colloidal or particulate suspensions, or (3) elastic tubes.

With regard to the physiological systems, Poiseuille's law does indeed apply experimentally to viscous fluids in the blood vascular system, and hindrance in such systems remains constant through a wide range of pressures. Pulsatile instead of steady pressure does not alter the results. It is possible that the vessels both elongate and dilate to produce this result. At any rate, the behavior is analogous to a rigid

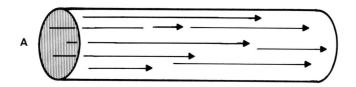

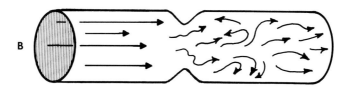

Fig. 1-6. **A,** Laminar flow. **B,** Turbulent flow.

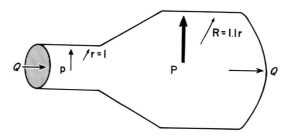

Fig. 1-7. Bernoulli's theorem, illustrating change in pressure with change in radius. Q = Q. R = 1.1 r (radius). P = 1.16 p (pressure).

system. Blood, however, is not a strictly viscous fluid but a pseudoplastic liquid that flows disproportionately faster as the propelling forces are increased. It is generally assumed that flow in the human arterial system is of the laminar nature when there is no deformity or disease.

Recently Weale developed a theory of blood flow that assumes two distinct layers: an outer layer and an inner core that may be turbulent. This mechanism is proposed as an explanation for those cases in which the Poiseuille formula cannot be applied or comfirmed.

The vascular system contains only very short stretches of uniform artery, flow is pulsatile, vessel walls have differing degrees of elasticity, flow divides into branches at various angles, and the blood flow itself is not homogeneous. A substitute formula for volume blood flow has been suggested as follows:

$$Q = a\ P^n \tag{2}$$

Q = Volume
a = A constant
P = Pressure or pressure differential
n = An exponent from 1 to 5

It is freely admitted that such a formula is only an approximation, with the exponent being fitted to the circumstances.

Application of Bernoulli's theorem demonstrating pressure change when there is a change in tubular size with constant flow is graphically illustrated in Fig. 1-7. As shown, application of this theorem yields for P a figure of 1.16 p for the small increase of 0.1 unit in radius (exaggerated in Fig. 1-7). Such considerations have been used to explain, for instance, poststenotic dilatation of a blood vessel. It is probable, however, that in poststenotic dilatation, at least three influences are at work: (1) conversion of kinetic energy of motion into static energy available for lateral pressure on, and elastic deformation of, the blood vessel wall (Fig. 1-7); (2) conversion of kinetic energy of laminar or streamlined flow into static pressure as the result of turbulence just distal to the stenotic area in the blood vessel; and (3) fatigue phenomena that allow gradual weakening of the arterial walls where they are subjected to increased lateral pressure. In poststenotic areas where turbulent flow has been created, small fibrin thrombi can be precipitated from the blood as the result of the localized area of turbulence, this being analogous to the familiar process of defibrinating blood by agitation with a wire stirring device.

Turbulent flow

Turbulent flow is the other major form of internal motion in moving fluids. In contrast to laminar flow, the fluid particles move in irregular paths at different angles to the main direction of motion (Fig. 1-6, *B*). Such flow is not so efficient as laminar flow. When turbulence is created in a streamlined system, pressure decreases secondary to the inceased dissipation of energy in the form of internal frictional losses.

Conditions for turbulent flow can be determined from the following equation:

$$\text{Re} = \frac{2\ \text{VRP}}{\text{vis}} \tag{3}$$

$$
\begin{aligned}
\text{Re} &= \text{Reynold's number (a dimensionless number)} \\
\text{V} &= \text{Average velocity} \\
\text{R} &= \text{Radius of conduit} \\
\text{P} &= \text{Density} \\
\text{vis} &= \text{Viscosity}
\end{aligned}
$$

When the right side of the equation exceeds the Reynold number for the fluid in question, streamlined flow becomes turbulent.

For human blood the Reynold number is approximately 970. If the constants of viscosity, density, and the number 2 are eliminated, it will be seen that flow velocity and the radius of the blood vessel determine the conditions necessary for turbulent flow and that turbulence would be difficult with a small velocity or in a vessel of very small radius. Turbulence can also be influenced or created by (1) change in size of tube, (2) change in direction of tube, (3) irregularity of inner surface of tube, and (4) a branching system of tubes. Turbulence is more likely to be created by sudden changes in the diameter or direction of a tube or by sudden changes in flow velocities than by gradual changes in these factors. The points in the vascular system where such changes occur seem to be more susceptible to formation of arteriosclerotic plaques than the remainder of the vascular system.

Application

Vascular reconstruction, although bridging anatomical defects, does not necessarily produce an adequate physiological or functional conduit for the blood. It has been demonstrated at times that even though a pulse is present where none was present before, total blood flow may not be materially increased.

Szilagyi and associates (1960) have made extensive studies of grafting procedures and their effects on blood flow. The experiments were conducted with a bubble flowmeter inserted into each femoral blood vessel of the experimental animal, with one side serving as a control. End-to-end anastomoses of a blood vessel reduced flow to 87% of control values. Replacement of a segment of vessel reduced blood flow to approximately 82% of control values. Comparison of a bypass graft with a linearly inserted graft as a control revealed a 20% reduction in flow through the bypass.

Increasing the internal diameter of bypass grafts allows an increase in blood flow until the graft has reached a diameter almost double that of the control vessel. After this there is again a decrease in flow, with further increases in size of the bypass graft. This phenomenon is possibly the result of the creation of turbulence as the product of V and R increases in equation 3.

When various plastic prosthetic materials are compared to intima-lined homografts, flow is found to be 10% or 20% less through the prosthetic devices. This is a result of the internal surface irregularities of the prosthetic materials.

Practical applications resulting from consideration of the laws of fluid flow and from experimental measurements are as follows:

1. Avoid constricting anastomoses.
2. Optimum size for a prosthesis is somewhat larger, that is, 1.4 to 1.6 the diameter of the host vessel.
3. End-to-side anastomoses should be made bell mouthed when possible (Fig. 1-3).
4. Bypass prostheses should take off and enter the parent artery at oblique angles, simulating normal arterial bifurcations.

Critical stenosis

Recently a great deal of attention has been focused on the question of the factors influencing flow through a stenotic area in an artery. When measurements are made, it is at once apparent that a large diminution in arterial cross section is necessary before a significant reduction in flow can be observed. Obviously in such experiments, adjustment in the totality of the circulation must also be considered. The results have clinical significance in two separate situations: (1) in determining if an observed narrowing is the cause of symptoms and (2) if an asymptomatic stenosis exists, in determining the effect of hypotension on flow through it.

In experimental work, the results in those experiments in which the usual peripheral resistance of a perfused limb or brain is retained are different from the results in those in which blood is shunted into an adjacent vein. The former type of experiment has tended to demonstrate that a stenosis of as much as 80% may be necessary before flow is decreased. Such a stenosis is analogous to narrowing of a vessel by a localized plaque and not similar to the long rough area of stenosis in advanced atherosclerosis. When peripheral resistance is decreased by work, sympathectomy, or direct shunting to the venous system, less stenosis will produce a reduction in flow. Peripheral pedal pulses may even disappear under the vasodilating influence of leg exercise. The notion of a necessary "critical stenosis" elaborated by work of this type indicates some caution in attributing symptoms to relatively small alterations in the diameter of blood vessels, particularly in the carotid system.

An almost necessary corollary is that ischemic symptoms such as stroke or myocardial infarct may be produced by a "critical combination" of stenosis, perfusion pressure reduction, and decreasing peripheral resistance.

ESTIMATION AND MEASUREMENT OF BLOOD FLOW

An extensive clinical history taken with the symptoms of vascular disease being considered and the examination of all palpable pulses constitute the initial approach to estimating arterial insufficiency. This is supplemented by the patient's history of color changes or by the inducement and observation of color changes. Gross temperature changes, particularly in the lower extremities, are usually readily apparent. Occult pulsation in the extremities can be detected and quantitated by the Collen's oscillometer. The surgeon should seek pulsation in the temporal artery when examining the carotid artery; it is not always detectable, and this may be normal in some patients. The same is true of the ulnar artery, which can be palpated at the wrist with the wrist extended. If the ulnar artery is not palpable, both ulnar and radial arteries at the wrist should be occluded with firm digital pressure. The patient should clench and release his hand several times until it is blanched. If color returns on releasing the ulnar side, the artery is considered patent (Allen's test).

A bruit over a major artery indicates turbulence and possibly, but not necessarily, constriction. A bruit can be found over the carotid bifurcation, for instance, without any demonstrable occlusion. In addition, as flow becomes greatly restricted, a bruit may disappear, signaling imminent or completed occlusion. Recent thrombosis in a large artery, such as the femoral, can continue for a short time to transmit pulsation through the jellylike clot, without any flow at all.

Temperature changes are most helpful in diagnosing arterial insufficiency in the lower extremities; detection of these changes can be refined by the use of simple thermometers, thermocouple thermometers, or thermistors. We prefer the thermocouple type, since thermistors are more sensitive to ambient temperature changes. Infrared thermography is not universally available, but may in the future be a screening and diagnostic method of wide acceptability. Radiometry using exquisitely sensitive thermocouples is a fast, accurate, and noninvasive method free from ambient interference, but we know of no current source of the instrument (Hardy dermal radiometer).

Accurate measurement of the cerebral circulation is accomplished by the technique of Kety and Schmidt, using nitrous oxide inhalation. Since this measures the cerebral distribution of the gas, it is essentially a clearance technique. Too cumbersome to use routinely, it is usually supplanted at the time of surgery by measuring oxygen tension of the jugular venous return from the brain.

A crude clearance method used in the past was to observe the rate of disappearance of a subcuticular wheal made with a small amount of saline solution. Normal disappearance time is about thirty seconds, and disappearance is prolonged if the local circulation is impaired. This method, although never satisfactory, has been improved by using ^{233}Xe as the injection material. Since this is radioactive, disappearance locally and excretion from the lungs can be continuously observed, quantitated, and integrated.

28

Oxygen electrodes were used by Davies and Brink for the measurement of local oxygen tension in the brain as early as 1942. This technique has been quite unexploited in vascular surgery, but small needle electrodes are commercially available and may be used to monitor oxygen tension in almost any tissue. The disadvantages are, of course, that actual blood flow is only a derivative of the oxygen tension and that interfering potentials from other sources can cause aberration of the results. The same indirectness is, however, true of many other systems employing deep or superficial temperatures, Doppler detection, and strain-gauge and photoelectric plethysmography. The oxygen microelectrodes are small, and the possibility of loss in the tissues is real enough to limit routine use and require reasonable care to prevent loss or to retrieve broken needles.

A number of ultrasonic instruments operating on the Doppler principle are offered on the market. The detected parameter is velocity of blood motion, and not volume flow. High amplification is used, and extrinsic noise is a problem. Occasionally an artery is pulsatile and patent and can be detected by this method and not by ordinary palpation. In most of these cases an ordinary oscillometer would accomplish the same end and measure pressure as well. We remain unconvinced that venous flow can be estimated by the Doppler method.

Plethysmography should, strictly speaking, measure volume change and volume flow. Excluding flowmeters, only venous-occlusion plethysmography accomplishes this, and the method requires a good deal of expert management to extract meaningful results. These results, in turn, are only somewhat quantitative and then only for a short period of time. Strain-gauge and photoelectric types of plethysmography actually attempt to derive an estimation of volume flow from pulse monitoring. Unfortunately, it is in exactly those situations in which blood flow is minimal and in which pulses are absent that a quantitative estimate of the amounts of blood available to the tissues is most important.

One of the most useful items to have available is an electromagnetic square-wave flowmeter that can be used to measure volume flow at the time of surgery. The instrumentation is reasonably accurate but requires open exposure of an artery or prosthesis and must be carefully applied. It is therefore invasive but not as disruptive and difficult as, for instance, a bubble flowmeter.

Calorimetry, that is, the careful observation of the ability of the circulation in a limb to radiate or absorb heat under controlled conditions, seems to be the only way in which to quantitate blood flow in a pulseless extremity. The method is time consuming but should be developed and explored, since this is the common clinical situation in which information is desired.

On the venous side of the circulation there are no clinical quantitative methods. The incorporation of ^{125}I-labeled human fibrinogen into a clot is rapidly becoming recognized as a sensitive diagnostic method for the detection of early thrombophlebitis (and is in active use in every civilized country with the exception of the United States, where government regulation as of 1972 limits wider application).

Impedance plethysmography is a method of measuring volume changes in the limb and deriving from this an estimation about whether or not there is obstruction in the large deep veins of the limb. The impedance changes detected are minute; however, it is hoped that this can be used as a noninvasive screening procedure for the detection of phlebitis in the future.

Angiography, discussed in the next chapter, is, of course, one of the vascular surgeon's greatest assets in locating obstructive disease and evaluating the circulation. Arteriosclerosis can be visualized and diagnosed, even though pulses are present. Angiography is invaluable in the detection of multiple lesions that may be unsuspected on clinical examination alone. At times collateral circulation can be visualized and its effect estimated from the angiographic examination.

Some of the limitations of angiography are that it is a completely anatomical picture. The status of the blood vessels may change; there is limitation of information to the area viewed; and at times the density of the contrast medium can be misleading by rendering a sharp outline in one plane when actually only a thin layer is present. Simultaneous biplane films with a rapid changer can overcome this difficulty, but they are usually unavailable when needed.

Nevertheless, angiography distinguishes normal arteries from diseased ones. Clots and atherosclerotic obstructions can be accurately located, and an approach can be made to flow rates by using rapid film-changing devices and comparing both sides. In arteriectasis the very slow progression of the arterial stream is well brought out by angiography, which may reveal a delay of a minute or more in the progress of the dye column from the femoral triangle to the popliteal area. In the case illustrated in Fig. 2-5, the anatomical diagnosis is that of a large patent artery, but perfusion of the limb was slow and nutrition was poor, resulting in amputation.

SYNTHETIC ARTERIAL GRAFTS

Cloth fabrics both as woven and as knitted materials were introduced in the 1950's as substitute tubes for the conduction of blood, and since then there has been extensive study of various materials used for this purpose. A great deal of this work has been carried out and extended by Wesolowski and Sauvage. From among the many materials studied, high-porosity knitted Dacron has emerged as the best substitute.

It has been obvious from both experience and from many experimental studies that low-porosity materials do not heal within and have a high index of calcification and degeneration. Although the fabric wall remains intact, the inner capsule can degenerate, sequestrate, calcify, and become thick and contracted so that the lumen is nonfunctional. All these processes are more rapid and pronounced in tightly woven fabrics and in nonwettable fabrics such as Teflon or nylon. Woven fabrics, moreover, ravel at the end and cause an unending technical problem. Aneurysm formation, rupture, and dilatation are more prone to take place in woven fabrics than in knitted fabrics. Teflon materials account for a great deal of the postoperative mortality and morbidity when they are used, the woven type being the worst in this respect. Boyd and Midell in 1971 summarized a recent poor experience along these lines, but the problem is not at all new.

The original knitted Dacron grafts knitted with twenty-two or thirty needles per inch were quite crude compared to those available today. Some of these are still being sold and used, the large gaps and porousness of the material being remedied by the use of texturized yarn. Currently nontexturized knitted Dacron* has proved to be an almost ideal material. It has all the characteristics laid down by Wesolowski (1962) for an ideal material. It is nontoxic and nonallergenic; it is mechanically strong and durable; and the individual pores are small so that clotting is rapid but total porosity is high. Such grafts are finely knitted, with forty or even fifty needles to

---

*Supplied by Golaski Laboratories, Inc., Philadelphia, Pa.

the inch, and can be used and clotted even in a heparinized patient. At the same time, the porosity of the fabric is such that the graft is soon incorporated into the surrounding soft tissues in a minimum of time, depending on the experimental subject and on the fineness of the material. In the past, such superior knitted material was sold under the name of Weavenit.* Although the trade name has been retained, the supplier apparently no longer furnishes the surgeon with the original material (Wesolowski, 1972). Since undoubtedly there will never be enough homografts or other similar materials available and since Dacron knit is the material on which a great deal of reliance is being placed now and for the future, it is important to use the currently optimal material that exhibits the minimum of early and late postoperative complications and to continue the search for better materials.

A Dacron knit that is in all respects identical to the material formerly known as Weavenit and that offers a combination of lightness, strength, porosity, fine crimping, easy handling, freedom from raveling, and conformability at the anastomotic lines is now obtainable under the name of Microknit.† A new material named Milliknit† is similar but supplies finer interstices, and a thinner wall is now available. In the past it was next to impossible to use a 6 mm. Dacron prosthetic bypass in the leg; however, this newer, lighter material again offers the possibility of a suitable prosthesis to use in the superficial femoral artery. Even though extremely porous, such materials are somewhat easier to clot than it may appear at first acquaintance. If they are wetted with blood and stretched a few times, they usually seal well and are almost watertight. Not only can they be sealed quite easily, but also their pliability and handling qualities should greatly appeal to anyone using them. Since a single thread is used for knitting, it is never necessary to double the ends or to reinforce the ends in order to keep needles from pulling out, nor is it at all difficult to drive an ordinary needle through the prosthesis; these difficulties have been found with some of the closely woven materials.

Since no true healing takes place at the host artery–prosthesis junction, suture material must remain strong, and disruption at the edge of the prosthesis must not occur. Materials known to be stable over long periods when implanted are Dacron, Teflon, and polyethylene. Dacron in one form or another is the preferred suture material; it will keep its strength indefinitely after implantation.

The weak point of the artery-prosthesis junction is not the prosthetic side, nor is it the suture. It is the weak arterial side that has become aneurysmal or perhaps has been endarterectomized. We cannot improve this substance that is given us to work with. We are in the custom of reinforcing this junction either by forming a snap-tight cuff of the prosthetic graft material (described fully later) or by sewing a small cuff of the fabric material around this important junction where pulsation may cause a sawing motion that will weaken the suture line on the arterial side and allow the suture material literally to saw or cut through the weakened arterial wall.

A knitted Dacron arterial prosthesis once implanted becomes lined with a thin layer of fibrin, which also permeates the pores in the prosthesis and prevents leakage. It becomes surrounded by a fibrous tissue capsule, and from this, fibroblasts grow into the prosthesis through the interstices and its wall. Eventually there is a replacement of the fibrin lining by fibrous tissue. This process apparently takes place only

*Supplied by Meadox Medicals, Inc., Oakland, N. J.
†Obtainable from Golaski Laboratories, Inc., Philadelphia, Pa.

poorly when Teflon is used as the graft material; the result is that the lining is poorly attached and is liable to detachment and distal embolization.

This process of neointima formation, which may take place in a short period of time, perhaps about three weeks in a normal growing pig and six to eight weeks in a normal adult dog, can be slow or even incomplete in human beings with arteriosclerosis. Since it is a function to some extent of the thickness of the materials used, the thinnest and most porous materials compatible with practical use, currently Milliknit and Microknit, should be employed.

As implantation time lengthens, atheroma and calcification may develop in synthetic fabric grafts just as in diseased arteries, autografts, and homografts.

If a graft material lacks porosity, the fibrin lining detaches with some ease, leading to septum formation and thrombosis with ultimate occlusion. Because of the lack of adherence to surrounding tissues, hematoma, serum collections, and infections dissect along low-porosity and nonwettable materials more easily. Secure and rapid healing is therefore facilitated by using a material with some porosity and by covering it with living tissue as a source of fibroblasts.

Several factors are involved in the prevention of thromboses in prosthetic materials. In addition to the firm attachment of the fibrinous lining of the graft, as detailed previously, desirable factors are (1) rapid blood flow through the prosthetic segment, (2) lack of distal obstruction so that rapid flow through the prosthesis is possible, and (3) avoidance of constricting or irregular anastomoses on which fibrin thrombi can form secondary to turbulent blood flow.

Because of the healing process within the lumen of prosthetic arterial grafts, the irregularities of the interior of the tube are soon smoothed over. Also, because the fibrin lining may thicken before healing occurs, the use of prostheses smaller than 8 mm. in diameter are inadvisable, and the incidence of immediate and late occlusion rises when prostheses of smaller diameters are used. Vein grafts have many advantages for long-term replacement of small arteries.

Infected arterial prostheses

Sepsis occuring in or about synthetic arterial prostheses is a dreaded complication. Arterial thrombosis and hemorrhage are the usual sequels when infection involves a host artery–prosthesis suture line. In these cases the prostheses must be removed and blood flow rerouted through new prostheses implanted in uncontaminated areas, bypassing the infected area completely.

When a host artery–prosthesis anastomosis is not involved, infected areas may be opened, drained, irrigated with antibiotics, and closed secondarily with some degree of success and without interruption of blood flow through the prosthesis. Consistent, intense, and long-continued use of antibiotics adjusted to the sensitivities of the infecting organisms is essential for success by this method.

When infection involves an anastomosis between a prosthesis and the host artery, disruption of the suture line and hemorrhage are inevitable if the infection is neglected. It is necessary to remove the prosthesis and ligate the host artery. The arterial tissue at the infected anastomosis will be friable.

Once an infected prosthesis has been removed and the danger of bleeding from the host artery has been eliminated, the question of further reconstruction arises. Individualized solutions are obviously necessary in these cases. However, the general solution is that of operating with great care and inserting a longer bypass through tissue that has not been invaded by infection. In the femoral area, iliofemoral bypass may be accomplished from the terminal aorta or iliac artery using the obturator foramen as a passageway for the new prosthesis. Bypasses have been accomplished from as far distant as the axillary artery for infected aortic bifurcation prostheses, and bypass from the opposite iliac or femoral artery is possible when infection is confined to the iliac region.

GRAFTS OF LIVING TISSUE: AUTOGRAFTS, HETEROGRAFTS, AND HOMOGRAFTS

Early workers with fabric grafts, particularly of the nonwetting type such as Teflon or nylon, were occasionally tempted to pull them loose, since they slid away easily from the tube that had formed about the prosthesis. This procedure resulted in almost immediate aneurysm formation and showed that such fibrous tissue structures would not withstand the pressure of blood in the arterial system.

The first autograft and homograft insertions were done quite a while ago. Wesolowski in 1972 cited Gluck's 1894 replacement of a vein graft in a carotid artery. Homograft arteries were mentioned by Yamanouchi in 1911. Jackson in 1972 reviewed approximately fifty cases of homologous saphenous veins used in arterial reconstruction. Very little experience has been gathered with homologous vein grafts, the general feeling being that if homologous tissue is to be used, it is just as easy to substitute an artery for an artery. It has been believed and from time to time observed that vein grafts will not withstand the pressure of the arterial system. This is not entirely true and certainly has not been true of the saphenous vein in the leg, where vein autografts have their greatest utility.

Unfortunately, autograft material is not always available, and one must rely on the homograft to take its place. This subject was experimentally investigated in the very early days of vascular surgery by Guthrie and others, who after suceeding in transplanting vein segments from animal to animal, proceeded to investigate various methods of long-term preservation.

The early workers had some small success with cooling the vein segments and also with preserving them in dilute formalin. The total experience, however, has been that methods of preservation that are essentially cytotoxic, such as treating with formalin, slow freezing, treating with alcohol, and boiling, lead to disintegration or disruption of the homograft. Good early results were obtained by Gross and associates (1949) using human material taken under sterile conditions from young recently dead persons and then simply preserved for a short period of time at low but not freezing temperatures.

Particularly in the large muscular arteries such as the aorta or the iliac arteries, there appears to be enough elastic tissue preserved that a human homograft will function without failure for a long time, and we know of homografts implanted for over ten years without deterioration.

In the early 1950's frozen and freeze-dried artery homografts were prepared by Hershey (1958) and others on a large scale. Electron irradiation was found to be a good method of sterilization and a better one than the previously used treatment with ethylene oxide. The greatest danger to the effectiveness of this type of artery homograft is ice-crystal formation in the arterial wall, and viability can be increased, as has been shown by Luyet (1938), by very rapid freezing and also by partial dehydration with glycerin as a preliminary preparation. Recent advances in low-temperature preservation suggest that dimethyl sulfoxide (DMSO) may be more effective than glycerin in protecting viability during freezing.

Early homografts showed their most striking success in abdominal aortic aneurysm (Oudot, 1951) and in the treatment of coarctation. Homografts were rapidly succeeded, however, by cloth prostheses, and the full development of homograft technology has therefore never been reached. The use of homografts is, of course, hampered by the lack of fresh sterile material, and the demand for artery replacements far exceeds the amount available.

Newer developments in this field that have not had a great deal of exposure or experience are artery grafts of bovine origin and mandril-grown Dacron-reinforced homograft tubes. The bovine arteries have, in some cases, been observed for ten years after ficin digestion and implantation and remain patent without aneurysm formation. This is in sharp contrast to the rapid and early aneurysm formation noted in untreated equine heterografts.

The heterograft arteries that are currently available commercially are subjected to a digestive process, after which they are tanned and stored in alcohol and propylene oxide. Keshishian and associates in 1971 reported the use of a large number of these without early deterioration and with generally satisfactory function. Nevertheless, the advantage over a cloth prosthesis or over autogenous vein grafts is not obviously apparent.

It would seem that the ultimate development along these lines would be the suitable preparation of giraffe carotid arteries, notable at least for their length.

An alternative and somewhat promising approach has been to grow collagen tubes in the patient's own body. This approach is suggested both by the pseudointima that forms within a cloth prosthesis and the very smooth intima-like lining that one can see about the plastic covering of electronic pacemakers. Benjamin and associates (1963) showed the feasibility of this by growing collagenous tubes around nylon obturators implanted in the subcutaneous tissue of dogs. They also found that this obturator could be placed close to the femoral artery and that the tube so formed substituted for the artery after two or three weeks. These tubes apparently were strong enough to be used as aortic replacement in dogs; however, we are skeptical about the idea that they would have enduring strength. More recently Sparks (1970, 1972) used a flexible silicone rubber mandril covered with two layers of knitted Dacron to form an endothelialized tube for future grafting. Ordinarily the mandril and its surrounding Dacron fabric are implanted near the vessel to be bypassed for about six weeks. Then the mandril is withdrawn, and the in situ autogenous graft is cut, trimmed, and anastomosed as a bypass to the occluded artery.

Of course the best alternative is an autograft of a suitable vein. The vein used with greatest success today is the greater saphenous vein, although as early as 1906 Goyanes substituted the superficial femoral vein for the superficial femoral artery. Perhaps the greatest advantage of the vein graft lies in the anticoagulant properties of the vein wall. This can be easily observed in an operation such as neck dissection, in which after both ends of the jugular vein are tied, the blood remains liquid not only throughout the surgery in the operating room but also frequently until the pathologist receives the specimen.

Long-term complications after arterial grafting

Almost any disease that can occur in a normal artery can occur in any type of tissue or cloth replacement. Calcification, aneurysm formation, and rupture have all been reported. In the past, false aneurysm formation at the suture line was a common long-term complication and still may be if silk is used as the suture material. The reason for this is that a cloth prosthesis is never truly incorporated into normal tissues. It is particularly poorly incorporated if it is made of a nonwettable material such as Teflon.

We have seen a striking case of this last type of complication in an elderly gentleman who had undergone an aortofemoral bypass operation six or seven years previously. He was observed with occlusion of the bypass on one side and a small aneurysm at the prosthesis–common femoral artery suture line on the other. If anything preserved his feet from gangrene, it was not the reconstructive surgery, but sympathectomy. While he was receiving anticoagulants, a small aneurysm developed at the site of the suture line between the prosthetic limb from the aorta and his common femoral artery. This disappeared when he was not receiving anticoagulants and reappeared when they were again used. The small false aneurysm was repaired; only a stitch or two were required to obliterate it. We do not believe that this phenomenon would have been observed with a wettable material that was better incorporated into the surrounding tissues.

Such complications should disappear for the most part with the use of Dacron suture material and Dacron prostheses. Most of the cases have been seen with end-to-side anastomoses, usually at the common femoral or popliteal level. In our experience it has been impossible to tell whether the nonwettable cloth prosthesis or the atherosclerotic arterial wall is more deficient. Undoubtedly the use of silk sutures has been, at least in the past, a leading or originating cause.

When the original anastomosis has been an end-to-side type and a simple reapproximation of the disrupted ends appears to be ineffective, then the best reconstruction is conversion of the anastomosis to an end-to-end type. This must be done carefully in the groin area so that flow into the profunda femoris artery is maintained.

Woven prostheses that become aneurysmal must simply be replaced.

Current obstruction and calcific degeneration of grafts is best treated by replacement, since these complications usually indicate a fault in the original prosthetic material. Clotting and septum formation in prosthetic materials are found when the prosthesis has been placed in an area having a poor outflow tract. In these cases replacement with a similar prosthesis cannot be successful and a vein graft should be substituted. Sympathectomy may also be advisable if it has not already been done.

In other cases, obstruction occurs where a cloth prosthesis crosses a joint level and can be attributed to the trauma of repeated flexing of the joint. If at all possible, a suitable autogenous vein should be sought to take the place of the cloth tube or should be used originally.

When complications occur, it is incumbent on the vascular surgeon to accurately evaluate the patient's disability. We have frequently found that physiological incapacity does not necessarily parallel anatomical occlusion. We have observed many patients who have been operated on seven to ten years ago who are now in their seventh decade of life and do not have a great number of symptoms. In perhaps half of these cases, if it had not already been done, sympathectomy improved the circulation enough for the patient to carry out his daily routine of living.

Only once have we seen infection develop in a prosthetic graft originating from within and similar to endocarditis. This event, obviously rare, must be included in the list of long-term complications.

ARTERIOSCLEROSIS AND THE PREDISPOSITION TO ARTERIOSCLEROSIS

The cause of arteriosclerosis is basically unknown. The parameters of the Framington study are elevated serum cholesterol, blood pressure elevation, cigarette smoking, glucose intolerence, and electrocardiographic evidence of left ventricular hypertrophy. Patients should be screened for abnormalities of lipoprotein metabolism when there is premature arteriosclerosis. In our experience, cigarette smoking is an outstanding finding in women in the fifth and sixth decades of life with severe and extensive iliofemoral disease. The latest report of this study, now sixteen years old, showed that all factors play a part in intermittent claudication and that arteriosclerotic brain infarct is more clearly related to arterial hypertension. The same risk for women that we have noted clinically is also found statistically, that is, that cigarette smoking carries a significant risk of claudication in women.

Surgeons usually see these patients after some symptomatic event has taken place; if there has been no prior intensive medical effort to evaluate the extent of arteriosclerotic disease, it may conveniently be done at this time.

Another very important clinical observation is that there is a high correlation between probable disease of the coronary arteries and the disappearance of pedal pulses in men. Therefore, the patient who presents himself with symptomatic arteriosclerotic disease of the lower extremities must also be regarded as having an increased potential for cardiac complications if, indeed, he is not already known to have clinical cardiac disease.

C.H.C.

References

Arnulf, G.: Chirurgie Artérielle, Paris, 1950, Masson & Cie, Editeurs.

Ballance, A., and Edmunds, W.: The ligation of the larger arteries in their continuity. An experimental inquiry, Med. Chir. Tr. 69:443-472, 1886.

Bauer, F. V.: Fall von Embolus aortae abdominalis, Operation, Heilung, Zentralb. Chir. 51: 1945-46, 1913.

Bazy, L., et al.: Technique des "Endarteriectomies" pour artérites obliterantes chroniques des membres inferieurs, des iliaques et de l'aorte abdominale inferieure, J. Chir. (Paris.) 65: 196-210, 1949.

Beck, C. S.: Revascularization of the heart, Ann. Surg. 128:854-864, 1948.

Beck, C. S., et al.: Revascularization of the brain through the establishment of a cervical arteriovenous fistula, J. Pediatr. 35:317-329, 1949.

Benjamin, H. B., Becker, A. B., and Pawlowski, E. J.: New approach to peripheral vascular deficit. Collagen deposition—new blood vessels for old, Angiology 14:390-393, 1963.

Bernheim, B. M.: Arteriovenous anastomosis; reversal of the circulation as a preventative of gangrene of the extremities; review of the literature and report of six additional cases, Ann. Surg. 55:195-207, 1912.

Bernheim, B. M.: Surgery of the vascular system, Philadelphia, 1913, J. B. Lippincott Co.

Bernheim, B. M.: Blood-vessel surgery in the war, Surg. Gynecol. Obstet. 30:564-567, 1920.

Bernheim, B. M.: Arteriovenous anastomosis, follow-up after eighteen years of "successful reversal of the circulation in all four extremities of the same individual," J.A.M.A. 96:1296-1297, 1931.

Bloch, M. H.: Proposal to repair wounds of the heart, Verh. Dtsch. Ges. Chir. part 1, pp. 108, 109, 1882.

Borst and Enderlen: Ueber transplantation von Gefässen und ganzen Organen, Dtsch. Zeit. Chir. 99(1-2):54-163, 1909.

Boyd, D. P., and Midell, A. I.: Woven Teflon aortic grafts, an unsatisfactory prosthesis, Vasc. Surg. 5:148-153, 1971.

Brooks, B.: Intra-arterial injection of sodium iodide; preliminary report, J.A.M.A. 82:1016-1019, 1924.

Cannon, J. A., et al.: Successful management of obstructive femoral arteriosclerosis by endarterectomy, Surgery 38:48-60, 1955.

Carrel, A.: La technique opératoire des anastomoses vasculaires et la transplantation des viscéres, Lyon Med. 98:859-864, 1902.

Carrel, A.: The surgery of the blood vessels, etc., Bull. Johns Hopkins Hosp. 190:18-28, Jan. 1907.

Carrel, A.: Latent life of arteries, J. Exp. Med. 12:460-486, 1910.

Carrel, A., and Guthrie, C. C.: Uniterminal and biterminal venous transplantations, Surg. Gynecol. Obstet. 2:266-286, 1906.

Carrel, A., et al.: The reversal of the circulation in a limb, Ann. Surg. 43:203-215, 1906.

Coelho, H. M., et al.: Arteriosclerotic occlusion of the terminal aorta and common iliac arteries treated by thromboendarterectomy, Surgery 37:105-114, 1955.

Crafoord, C., and Nylin, G.: Congenital coarctation of the aorta and its surgical treatment, J. Thorac. Surg. 14:347-361, 1945.

Cutter, B. C., et al.: The surgical treatment of mitral stenosis. Experimental and clinical studies, Arch. Surg. 9:689-748, 1924.

Davies, H. M.: The value of arteriovenous anastomosis in gangrene of the lower limb, Ann. Surg. 60:864–876, 1912.

Davies, P. W., and Brink, F.: Micro-electrodes for measuring local oxygen tension in animal tissues, Rev. Sci. Instrum. 13:524-533, 1942.

DeBakey, M. E., Creech, O., Jr., and Cooley, D. A.: Occlusive disease of the aorta and its treatment by resection and homograft replacement, Ann. Surg. 140:290-310, 1954.

Donaghy, R. M. P., and Yaşargil, M. G.: Micro-vascular surgery, St. Louis, 1967, The C. V. Mosby Co.

Dörfler: Ueber Arteriennaht, Beitr. Klin. Chir. 25:781, 1899.

Dorrence, G. M.: An experimental study of the suture of arteries with a description of a new suture, Ann. Surg. 44:409-424, 1906.

dos Santos, J. C.: Sur la désobstruction des thromboses artérielles anciennes, Mem. Acad. Chir. 73:409-411, 1947.

Dubost, C., Allary, M., and Oeconomos, N.: Resection of an aneurysm of the abdominal aorta; reestablishment of continuity by preserved human arterial graft, with result after 5 months, Arch. Sug. 64:405-408, 1952.

Dubost, C., et al.: A propos du traitement des anévrysmes de l'aorte. Ablation de l'anévrysme. Rétablissment de la continuité par greffe d'aorte humaine conservée, Mem. Acad. Chir. 77:381-383, 1951.

Dubost, C., et al.: Les greffes vasculaires. Étude expérimentale. Application chez l'homme, Rev. Chir. Orthop. p. 167, May-June 1952.

Eastcott, H. H. G.: Arterial grafting for the ischaemic lower limb, Ann R. Coll. Surg. Engl. 13:177-198, 1953.

Eck, N. V.: On the question of ligature of the portal vein, Voyenno Med. J. 130:1-2, 1877. (Available translated in Surg. Gynecol. Obstet. 96:375-376, 1953.)

Farina, G.: A wound of the heart repaired, Zentralbl. Klin. Chir. 23:1224, 1896.

Frey, M. von, and Gruber, M.: Untersuchungen über den Stoffwechsel isolierter organe. Ein respirations-apparat für isolierte organe, Virchows Arch. Physiol. 9:519-532, 1885. Cited by Galletti, P.M., and Brecher, G.A.: Heart-lung bypass; principles and techiques of extra-corporeal circulation, New York, 1962, Grune & Stratton, Inc.

Garrison, F. H.: An introduction to the history of medicine, Philadelphia, 1913, W. B. Saunders Co.

Gibbon, J. H., Jr.: Application of a mechanical heart and lung apparatus to cardiac surgery, Minn. Med. **37:**171-180, 1954.

Gluck, T.: Die moderne Chirurgie des circulation apparates, Berlin Klinic **70:**1, 1898.

Golaski, W. M.: Engineering design factor in the construction and evaluation of knitted arterial prosthesis. Symposium on Bio-Chemical Engineering Materials, Part II, Materials Conference, Philadelphia, 1968. (Reprints available from American Institute of Chemical Engineers, 345 E. 47th St., New York, N. Y. 10017.)

Goodman, C.: Arteriovenous anastomosis of the femoral vessels for impending gangrene, Ann. Surg. **60:**62-87, 1914.

Gordon, T., and Kannel, W. B.: Predisposition to atherosclerosis in the head, heart, and legs. The Framingham study, J.A.M.A. **221:**661-666, 1972.

Goyanes, J.: Nuevos trabajos de cirugía vascular, Siglo Med. **53:**546-549, 1906.

Gross, R. E.: Surgical correction for coarctation of the aorta, Surgery **18:**673-678, 1945.

Gross, R. E., Bill, A. H., Jr., and Peirce, E. C., II: Methods of preservation and transplantation of arterial grafts; observations on arterial grafts in dogs; report of transplantation of preserved arterial grafts in nine human cases, Surg. Gynecol. Obstet. **88:**689-701, 1949.

Gross, R. E., and Hubbard, J. P.: Surgical ligation of patent ductus arteriosus; report of first successful case, J.A.M.A. **112:**729-731, 1939.

Guthrie, C. C.: Transplantation of formaldehyde-fixed blood vessels, Science **27:**473, 1908.

Guthrie, C. C.: Blood vessel surgery and its applications, New York, 1912, Longmans, Green & Co. Reprinted in Harrison, S. P., and Fisher, B.: The contributions of Dr. C. C. Guthrie to vascular surgery, Pittsburg, 1959, University of Pittsburg Press. The reprint contains most of the original work, together with annotations, biographic and bibliographic material, and a bibliography of other work to the time of publication.

Hardy, J. D.: Radiation of heat from the human body; (1) instrument for measuring radiation and surface temperature of the skin, J. Clin. Invest. **13:**593, 1934.

Hardy, J. D.: Radiation of heat from the human body; (2) comparison of some methods of measurement, J. Clin. Invest. **13:**605-614, 1934.

Harvey W.: Anatomical studies of the motion of the heart and blood, 1628. Modern English translation with annotations by C. D. Leake, Springfield, 1941, Charles C Thomas, Publisher.

Henson, G. F., and Rob, C. G.: A comparative study of the effects of different arterial clamps on the vessel wall, Br. J. Surg. **43:**561-564, 1956.

Hershey, F. B., et al.: Electron-irradiated and freeze-dried arterial homografts, Ann. Surg. **147:**562-570, 1958.

Holman, E.: Surgery of large arteries with report of case of ligation of innominate artery for varicose aneurism of subclavian vessels, Ann. Surg. **85:**173-184, 1927.

Hopfner, E.: Ueber Gefässnaht, Gefässtransplantationen and Replantation von amputirten Extremitäten, Arch. Klin. Chir. **70:**417-471, 1903.

Horsley, J. S.: Operative treatment for threatened gangrene of the foot, with special reference to reversal of the circulation, J.A.M.A. **67:**492-499, 1916.

Horsley, J. S.: Suturing blood vessels, J.A.M.A. **77:**117-121, 1921.

Jaboulay and Briau: Recherches experimentales sur la greffe artérielle, Lyon Med. **81:**97, 1896.

Jackson, D. R.: The homologous saphenous vein in arterial reconstruction, Vasc. Surg. **6:**85-92, 1972.

Jacobson, J. H.: The development of microsurgical technique. In Donaghy, R. M. P., and Yaşargil, M. G.: Micro-vascular surgery, St. Louis, 1967, The C. V. Mosby Co.

Jacobson, J. H.: Microsurgery. In Current problems in surgery, Chicago, 1971, Year Book Medical Publishers, Inc.

Jassinowski: Die Arteriennaht. Inaugural dissertation, Dorpat (Tartu, U.S.S.R.), 1899 (unobtainable).

Julian, O. C., Grove, W. J., and Norberg, C. A.: Techniques in arterial surgery, Surgery **36:**161-170, 1954.

Julian, O. C., et al.: Direct surgery of arteriosclerosis; resection of abdominal aorta with homologous aortic graft replacement, Ann. Surg. 138:387-399, 1953.

Kakkar, V. V., et. al.: Efficacy of low doses of heparin in prevention of deep vein thrombosis after major surgery, Lancet 2:101-106, 1972.

Keshishian, J. M., et al.: Surgical techniques using the bovine arterial graft, Surg. Gynecol. Obstet. 133:268-272, 1971.

Key, E.: Embolectomy in the treatment of circulatory distrubances in the extremities, Surg. Gynecol. Obstet. 36:309-316,1923. Gives earlier history.

Kirchner, W. C. G.: Treatment of wounds of the heart, Ann. Surg. 52:96-110, 1910.

Kocher, T.: Text book of operative surgery. Third English translation, London, 1911, Adam & Charles Black.

Lam, C. R., et al.: Resection of the descending thoracic aorta for aneurysm, Ann. Surg. 134:743, 1951.

Lambert: Letter to Dr. Hunter. In Medical observations and inquiries, Vol. II, p. 360, London, 1762.

Lancisi, G. M.: De aneurysmatibus, opus post-humum. Aneurysms, the Latin text of Rome, 1745. Revised with translation and notes by W. C. Wright, New York, 1952, The Macmillan Co.

Leriche, R.: Des obliterations artérielles hautes (oblitération de la termination de l'aorte) comme causes des insuffisances circulatoires des membres inférieurs, Bull. Mem. Soc. Chir. Paris 49:1404-1406, 1923.

Leriche, R.: De la résection du carrefour aortico-iliaque avec double sympathectomie lombaire pour thrombose artéritique de l'aorte; le syndrome de l'oblitération termino-aortique par artérite, Presse Med. 48:601-604, 1940.

Leriche, R., and Morel, A.: The syndrome of thrombotic obliteration of the aortic bifurcation, Ann. Surg. 127:193-206, 1948.

LeVeen, H. H., et al.: Prevention of wound hemorrhage and embolism during heparin therapy, Arch. Surg. 91:817-822, 1965.

Lexer, E.: Cases reported during Einundrierzigster Congress. Deutschen Gesellschaft fur Chirurgie, Berlin, April 1912, pp. 131-135, Hirshwald Verlag, 1912.

Lowenberg, E. L.: Aneurysm of the abdominal aorta; report of two cases treated by "cutis grafting," Angiology 1:396-404, 1950.

Luyet, B. J., and Thoennes, G.: The revival of muscle fibers vitrified in liquid air, C. R. Acad. Sci. 207:1256-1257, 1938.

Makins, G.: On the vascular lesions produced by gunshot injuries and their results, Br. J. Surg. 5:353-421, 1916.

Makins, G.: Gunshot injuries to the blood vessels, Bristol, England, 1919, John Wright & Sons.

Matas, R.: Traumatic aneurism of the left brachial artery. Failure of direct and indirect pressure; ligation of the artery immediately above tumor; return of pulsation on the tenth day; ligation immediately below tumor; failure to arrest pulsation; incision and partial excision of sac; recovery, Medical News (Philadelphia) 53:462-466, 1888.

Matas, R.: An operation for the radical cure of aneurism, based upon arteriorrhaphy, Ann. Surg. 37:161-196, 1903.

Murphy, J. B.: Resection of arteries and veins injured in continuity-end-to-end suture—experimental and clinical research, Med. Rec. 51:73-88, 1897.

Neff, J. M.: Blood vessel suture, Surg. Gynecol. Obstet. 33:657-669, 1921.

Newton, W. T., et al.: Equine arterial heterografts altered by controlled enzymatic digestion; preliminary report, Arch. Surg. 73:432-439, 1956.

Nickell, W. B., Bartley, T. D., et al.: Arteries and anastomoses. Some basic controversies settled, Ann. Thorac. Surg. 7:221-230, 1969.

Oudot, J.: Deux cas de greffe de la bifurcation aortique pour syndrome de Leriche par thrombose artéritique, Mem. Acad. Chir. 77:636, 642, 644, 1951.

Oudot, J., et al: Thrombosis of aortic bifurcation treated by resection and homograft replacement: report of five cases, Arch. Surg. **66**:365-374, 1953.

Polin, S. G., and Hershey, F. B.: Technic of shunt removal from the carotid artery without interruption of blood flow, Am. J. Surg. **111**:296-297, 1966.

Reboul, H.: L'artériographie des membres et de l'aorte abdominale; étude critique, Paris, 1935, Masson & Cie, Editeurs. Numerous excellent reproductions of arteriograms.

Rehn, L.: Repair of stab wound of right ventricle, Arch. Klin. Chir. **60**:315-329, 1897.

Salzman, E. W., Harris, W. H., and De Sanctis, R. W.: Reduction in venous thromboembolism by agents affecting platelet function, N. Engl. J. Med. **284**:1287-1292, 1971.

Satrustegui, San Martin y: La chirurgie de l'appareil circulatoire, Sem. Med. pp. 395-396, 1902.

Sauvage, L. R.: Growth of vascular anastomosis; an experimental study of the influence of suture type and suture method with a note on certain mechanical factors involved, Bull. Johns Hopkins Hosp. **91**:276-297, 1952.

Sauvage, L. R., et al.: An experimental study of the effects of preservation on the fate of aortic and vena-caval homografts in the growing pig, Ann. Surg. **136**:439-458, 1952.

Sauvage, L. R., et al.: Freeze-dry process for arteries, Surgery **37**:585-601, 1955.

Sauvage, L. R., et al.: The healing and fate of arterial grafts, Surgery **38**:1090-1131, 1955.

Sauvage, L. R., et al.: A very thin, porous, knitted arterial prosthesis; experimental data and early clinical assessment, Surgery **65**:78-88, 1969.

Sicard, J. A., and Forestier, J.: Injection intra-vasculaire de Lipiodol sous contrôle radiologique, Bull. Biol. p. 1200, May 1923.

Sparks, C. H.: Die-grown reinforced arterial grafts, Ann. Surg. **172**:787-794, 1970.

Sparks, C. H.: Silicone mandril method of femoropopliteal artery by-pass, Am. J. Surg. **124**:244-249, 1972.

Swan, H. C., et al.: Arterial homografts; resection of thoracic aortic aneurysm using a stored human arterial transplant, Arch. Surg. **61**:732-737, 1950.

Szilagyi, D. E., et al.: Resectional surgery of the abodominal aorta; problems of case selection and operative technique, Arch. Surg. **71**:491-511, 1955.

Szilagyi, D. E., et al.: The clinical use of an elastic Dacron prosthesis, Arch. Surg. **77**:538-551, 1958.

Szilagyi, D. E., et al.: The laws of fluid flow and arterial grafting, Surgery **47**:55-61, 1960.

Terrier, F., and Raymond, E.: Chirurgie de la plévre et du poumon, Paris, 1899, Alcon.

Ullmann, E.: Experimentelle Nierentransplantation, Wien. Klin. Wochenschr. **281**:707, 1902.

Watts, S. H.: The suture of blood vessels; implantation and transplantation of vessels and organs; an historical and experimental study, Bull. Johns Hopkins Hosp. **18**:153-179, 1907.

Weale, F. E.: An Introduction to surgical hemodynamics, Chicago, 1967, Year Book Medical Publishers, Inc.

Wesolowski, S. A.: Evaluation of tissue and prosthetic vascular grafts, Springfield, Ill., 1962, Charles C Thomas, Publisher.

Wesolowski, S. A.: Performance of materials as prosthetic blood vessels, Bull. N. Y. Acad. Med. **48**:331-356, 1972.

Wesolowski, S. A., et al.: Factors contributing to long-term failures in human vascular prosthetic grafts, J. Cardiovasc. Surg. **5**:544-567, 1964.

Wylie, E. J., An experimental study of regional heparinization, Surgey **28**:29-36, 1950.

Yamanouchi, H.: Über die zirkulären Gefässnähte und Arterienvenenanastomosen, sowie über die Gefässtransplantationen, Dtsch. Z. Chir. **112**:1-118, 1911.

2
Arteriography

INTRODUCTION AND GENERAL COMMENTS

Progress in vascular surgery has been dependent in many instances on the development and improvement of angiographic techniques. Such techniques provide essential pathological and anatomical information prior to operation. Opacification of blood vessels for radiographic study was first performed only eleven weeks after Roentgen's discovery. However, refinements in equipment and techniques and improvement in the opacity and safety of contrast media have greatly advanced the clinical application of angiography.

Techniques suitable for visualizing the carotid, subclavian, vertebral, and femoral arteries and their branches, as well as the thoracic and abdominal aorta, are described. It is not unusual that special modifications to meet special circumstances must be devised and employed. Incorrect arterial puncture is the commonest cause of failure of angiographic techniques. When an area is inaccessible to arterial puncture or when it is advisable to make repeated x-ray films or to move the patient, retrograde catheterization is a useful technique.

In recent years contrast media for arteriography have been significantly improved. Meglumine iothalamate (Conray) has proved to have relatively low nephrotoxicity and neurotoxicity, both of which had previously been problems, particularly in direct translumbar aortography. Also, with its use there has been an acceptably low incidence of irritation to blood vessels, although it can cause some discomfort in unanesthetized patients. Several concentrations are available, and viscosity is low in the less concentrated solutions. The most concentrated solutions may be advantageously warmed to body temperature before injection.

When angiography is done with the use of local anesthesia, patients always experience momentary pain in the area perfused by the radiopaque medium, with the sensation of heat, prickling, or burning. A transient flush may be observed, particularly in the extremities, and may last for several minutes. The combination of sensations may be extremely unpleasant, and the patients should be warned and reassured prior to injection. Children and patients who are unable to cooperate will need general anesthesia to prevent motion during exposure of the films.

Roentgenograms of quality adequate for diagnosis can usually be obtained with a single injection of contrast medium. A rapid cassette changer is essential to obtain the finer details of filling and flow. To some extent, these details may also be obtained by using relatively long exposures on a single film. In femoral arteriography a single film will adequately delineate the common femoral artery and its branches, but a second injection and sequential films may be necessary to delineate the details of popliteal filling.

A simple apparatus such as the Amplatz injector is a very useful adjunct for the rapid pressure injection of contrast media and is quite essential for transbrachial arch aortography and angiocardiography. For femoral arteriograms, adequate pressure through an 18-gauge needle may be obtained with a hand-held syringe, a 20 ml. syringe with finger grips being particularly effective. For translumbar aortograms, the medium can be rapidly injected using a large syringe with a 12-gauge outlet (Robb syringe) and a finger-grip attachment. When the material is injected by hand and a single film is used, a long exposure (one second) should be employed.

In the search for ever more detailed arteriograms, to delineate tumors and locate sites of bleeding, selective arteriography with the Seldinger technique of retrograde catheterization is commonly used. This has some complications and difficulties, which are mentioned later. One problem, however, is a tendency to inject more and more contrast medium. Ordinarily no harm comes from a total dosage of 2 to 3 ml. of medium per kilogram of body weight, and in some cases this dosage has been far exceeded. Selective catheterization, however, also selectively exposes a particular area to high concentrations of medium, so that the general rule may not apply. Dosage can be minimized by using small short injections, separating them, and by using a cine recording device so that the maximum of information is obtained. The specialized monographs of Curry and Howland (1966), Sutton (1962), and Hanafee (1972) supply more details.

All vascular surgeons must be acquainted with the necessary diagnostic angiography, and many prefer to perform it. The surgeon will know better than the radiologist if the films are satisfactory for his purpose and if they demostrate the pathological condition well. Technique can be adjusted, and unsatisfactory films can be repeated without delay. Of course, the surgeon *reviews the films himself* and compares them with the operative findings.

CEREBRAL ARTERIOGRAPHY
Indications

Both the internal carotid and the vertebral arteries may be sites of obliterative lesions that cause cerebral arterial insufficiency. Symptoms of basilar artery insufficiency require radiographic examination of the vertebral arteries. Techniques employed for detection of extracranial obliterative lesions are not identical to those used for detection of intracranial disease.

An almost complete examination of the cerebral circulation is accomplished by percutaneous right transbrachial-cerebral arteriography combined with left percutaneous common carotid arteriography. The common carotid arteries and their bifurcations, the internal carotid arteries, and the anterior and middle cerebral vessels should be visualized. When occlusive disease in the neck is suspected of being present, lateral views are possibly more revealing than anteroposterior projections, but anteroposterior and Towne projections should be utilized to adequately visualize intracranial circulation, and particularly any intracranial crossover.

There are some advocates of four-vessel angiography. This is excellent, complete, and reassuring if well done; but this technique usually requires retrograde catheterization, prolongs the procedure, and requires larger quantities of contrast medium. When the technique is done routinely, the extra yield does not justify the extra risks. The only compelling reason for using this method is to visualize occlusions or stenoses known or suspected of being at the aortic arch level. If necessary, the left vertebral artery can be visualized by left retrograde brachial injection.

Preoperative care

Cerebral arteriography may be done with the use of local anesthesia in cooperative patients. We frequently use general anesthesia for prolonged procedures that can become a trial for the patient. Preoperative medication should be generous, including an anticonvulsant barbiturate. Practically, this limits the choice to phenobarbital. When local anesthesia is used, convulsion may occur; therefore, the equipment to establish an airway and treat aspiration should be on hand. Hemiparesis due to thrombosis or dislodgment of atheromatous material may also complicate cerebral angiography. This is quickly evident in patients operated on with the use of local anesthesia. Patients operated on with general anesthesia should be observed carefully in the recovery room. Rarely, a needle and injection in the carotid artery may create an intimal flap and thrombosis that is correctable before permanent brain damage occurs.

Percutaneous transbrachial-cerebral arteriography

The use of percutaneous brachial artery puncture, together with pressure injection, is currently the best routine method of visualizing the proximal aortic arch, the right vertebral and common carotid arteries and their branches, and the innominate artery. Slightly delayed films will show the descending thoracic aorta and even the abdominal aorta. As a rule, the left carotid and left vertebral arteries are not well visualized, and to complete examination of the cerebral circulation an arteriogram of the left carotid artery must also be done. It is not necessary to visualize both vertebral arteries if there is adequate flow in one of them and no symptoms of basilar artery insufficiency. As a rule, therefore, transbrachial-cerebral angiography is performed on the right side in combination with a percutaneous arteriogram of the left common carotid artery. When it is necessary to visualize the basilar circulation on the left in more detail, transbrachial-cerebral arteriograms may be made from the left side.

Occasionally, brachial puncture as described on p. 44, may be used for simple visualization of the brachial artery, particularly for follow-up of procedures for occlusive disease, congenital malformations, embolism, or injury suspected of involving the brachial artery, the forearm, or the hand. In such cases, a tourniquet, digital pressure, or a blood pressure cuff over the proximal end of the brachial artery will assure distal injection, and a pressure injector is not necessary.

Procedure—percutaneous right transbrachial-cerebral arteriography

1. Place the patient in the supine position, with the upper portion of the chest, the neck, and the head positioned over the automatic cassette-changing device. The Sanchez-Perez automatic seriograph that takes a sequence of six to twelve films at intervals of one-half to one second is quite satisfactory. Several views may be necessary. If available, simultaneous biplane x-ray films with two seriographic machines are desirable.

In those patients in whom buckling, tortuosity, or compression by osteophytes or by the transverse processes of the vertebras is suspected, cineradiography with rotation of the head and neck during injection may be necessary to demonstrate the suspected difficulty.

Place the right arm on a long arm board that will stabilize the entire arm, shoulder, and wrist. Place a pad about 1 1/2 inches thick beneath the right elbow to secure hyperextension.

COMMENT: *Correct position of the arm is essential for safe and easy percutaneous puncture. Hyperextension at the elbow makes the brachial artery more superficial and prevents it from rolling. At times a small incision over the brachial artery may be needed. The best position of the wrist is variable. In some patients the brachial artery is more readily palpable with the hand in full supination or pronation. If the brachial artery is not palpable in this position, rotate the arm, turning the wrist so that the thumb points upward, and again seek the brachial pulse by palpation before making an incision.*

2. Prepare and drape the antecubital region. Inject a small amount of local anesthetic just distal to the most prominent pulsation of the brachial artery.

3. Transfix the brachial artery with a quick vertical thrust of a Seldinger No. 160 or similar type of arterial needle. During the puncture, compress and hold the artery with the opposite hand.

4. Remove the obturator from the arterial cannula and withdraw it slowly until a strong jet of arterial blood appears. Advance the cannula its full length or as far as possible into the lumen of the artery, tape it into position, and again insert the obturator.

5. Prepare the contrast medium. Remove the obturator from the arterial needle, and connect the needle securely to the pressure tubing filled with saline solution or contrast medium. Tape the tubing securely to the forearm.

6. Connect the pressure tubing to the automatic pressure injector, warn the patient regarding the sensations that he may soon feel, and rapidly inject about 60 ml. of Conray 60%.* The automatic cassette changer may be started either manually or by the automatic contacts built into some types of pressure injectors. No more than three injections should be made. Do not exceed a total dose of 150 ml. of Conray 60%.

7. Irrigate the needle and maintain it in position until the films have been checked. On withdrawal, maintain light pressure over the puncture site for a few minutes with an alcohol sponge.

COMMENT: *If pressure injection equipment is not available or fails, this examination can be completed by manual pressure. A plastic disposable syringe with a Luer-Lok tip should be used to avoid the leaking and breakage of glass multifit syringes under maximum pressure.*

Left transbrachial-vertebral arteriography

The technique for left transbrachial-vertebral arteriography is the same as that described for right transbrachial-cerebral arteriography except that the left arm is used. An injection of 30 ml. of radiographic contrast medium is sufficient to show the left subclavian and vertebral arteries.

Left transbrachial aortography

Left transbrachial aortography may be used to visualize the descending thoracic aorta and occasionally the abdominal aorta. Use of the transbrachial route eliminates catheterization. A relatively large quantity of radiopaque material (about 100 ml. of Conray 60%) should be used. Otherwise, the only modifications of technique are in the positioning of the patient, the film, and the x-ray tube.

---

*Recently we have observed that Conray 400 is equally satisfactory for most purposes.

The descending aorta is best visualized in the left anterior oblique view. Since timing may be somewhat difficult in abdominal aortography, a rapid cassette changer is necessary. In general, the translumbar route is superior for visualization of the abdominal aorta, but this approach is contraindicated in patients with aneurysms.

Procedure—percutaneous carotid arteriography

1. Hyperextend the patient's head by placing a rolled towel or sandbag between the shoulders (Fig. 2-1, *A*). Excessive hyperextension is undersirable.

2. Make a wheal with a local anesthetic over the carotid pulsation at the anterior edge of sternocleidomastoid muscle and at about the level of the lower border of the thyroid cartilage, which marks the carotid bifurcation. Infiltrate the subcutaneous tissues with the anesthetic agent.

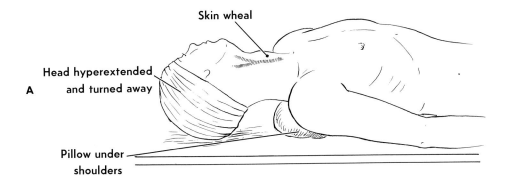

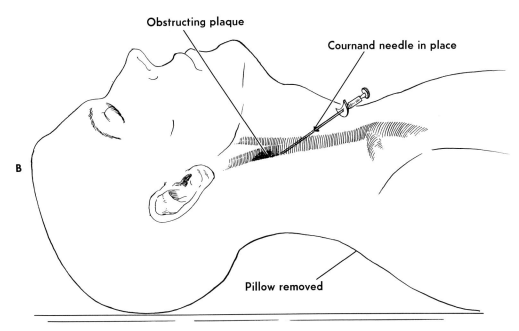

Fig. 2-1. Position and landmarks for carotid arteriography. **A,** Position of head, neck, and shoulders for puncture. **B,** Position during exposure of arteriograms.

3. Turn the patient's head slightly away from the side of injection to stretch the artery and move it medial to the sternocleidomastoid. Insert a No. 18 Cournand needle almost vertically over the arterial pulsation, and when it is against the artery, transfix it quickly. Withdraw the obturator. Lower the hub of the needle, and withdraw the needle slowly. As the needle is withdrawn into the artery, a pulsatile stream of bright red blood will spurt from it. Now advance the needle about 1 cm. into the lumen of the vessel, depressing the hub to do so (Fig. 2-1, *B*). Connect plastic tubing and a syringe of saline solution. Inject saline solution slowly to keep the needle open.

COMMENT: *A quick technique is to use a disposable 18-gauge short-bevel needle for the puncture and to connect it to a plastic tubing and disposable syringe. We use the Venotube,* available in various lengths. The connections are all of the plastic-to-plastic type instead of metal-to-glass or metal-to-metal types and remain intact under moderate pressure. The method is quick and convenient and assures one of a sharp needle at all times. See the same technique illustrated for the femoral artery in Fig. 2-2.*

4. For lateral views, straighten the head, remove the towels or other support from beneath the shoulders, and prepare a large 14-by-17-inch grid-front cassette to visualize both the head and neck. Allow blood to fill the tubing and drive out any bubbles. Connect a syringe containing Hypaque 50% or Conray 60%. Caution the patient, and then rapidly inject 8 to 10 ml. of contrast medium, exposing the film toward the end of the injection. The needle may now be connected to a syringe filled with saline solution or be plugged with the obturator until the films are developed and inspected.

The Towne view with the axial ray 20 to 30 degrees from the vertical will show the intracranial portion of the internal carotid artery projected away from the base of the skull. A rapid cassette changer, set to take four large (11-by-14-inch) films at one-second intervals, is desirable. Both carotid arteries may be examined on the same day. However, no more than two injections are advisable on each side.

Postoperative care

Gentle pressure should be kept over the puncture site for a few minutes, and a small bandage should be applied. An ice collar and mild analgesics are usually sufficient to control pain.

FEMORAL ARTERIOGRAPHY
Introduction

Examination of the arteries in the lower extremities via the femoral artery is one of the most frequently employed angiographic procedures. The indication for such examinations is usually arterial insufficiency associated with atherosclerotic occlusive disease. Careful evaluation is essential to choose the proper position of the leg and appropriate injection rates and exposure timing.

If disease of the iliac artery is suspected of being present, the iliac arteries can be visualized by rapid injection into the common femoral artery in a retrograde fashion as described on p. 59. When a hand-held syringe is used, increased pressure for injection may be obtained by using a 20 ml. syringe with finger grips or by using

---

*Available from Abbott Laboratories, North Chicago, Ill.

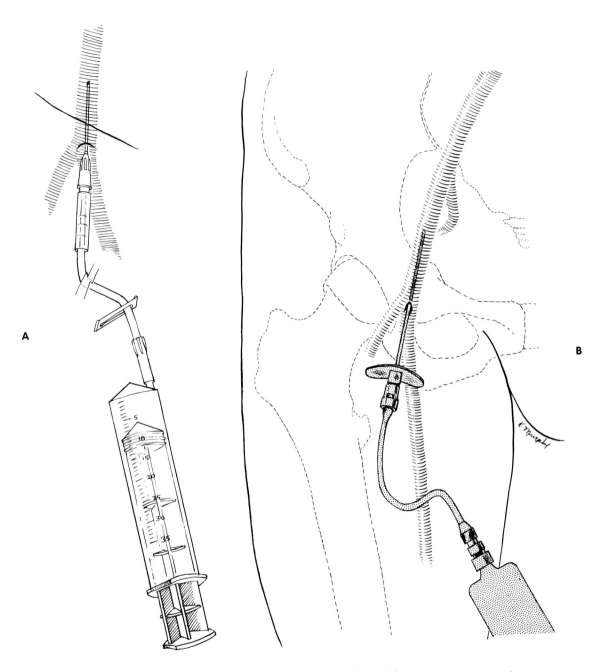

Fig. 2-2. Femoral arteriography. **A,** Technique using disposable equipment. **B,** Technique using Seldinger arterial needle.

the now widely available plastic syringes. We prefer syringes with an eccentric tip and a conical bubble trap at the end (see Fig. 2-2). The ipsilateral iliac artery and the aortic bifurcation and runoff into the opposite iliac and femoral arteries frequently can be visualized with a single injection.

In the presence of obstruction in the superficial femoral artery, popliteal filling from collateral vessels is a most significant preoperative finding. When searching for such information, it is most desirable, if not essential, to use sequential films produced by a rapid cassette changer, to catch the short but delayed filling phase.

Bilateral examination is advised unless there is a contralateral amputation or unless the contralateral femoral pulse is absent. Frequently, comparison of both sides, particularly in the runoff films, yields helpful information. For instance, in Fig. 2-4 the runoff films show severe disease on one side, but the patient's symptoms were due to a more proximal obstruction. Usually both legs can be examined simultaneously on the same film.

Anatomy

The femoral artery is most superficial immediately distal to the inguinal ligament. Puncture at this level is techically easy, since the pulse is readily palpable and the vessel can be kept from rolling.

Procedure

1. Place the patient in the supine position. The entire leg is positioned over a specially constructed tunnel or over separate films, using separate x-ray machines.

2. Prepare and drape the inguinal region. Infiltrate the skin just over the femoral pulsation and just below the inguinal ligament with local anesthetic.

3. Place a finger on either side of the femoral pulsation to prevent the artery from moving (Fig. 2-2). Insert a small (No. 160) Seldinger, Cournand, or similar (disposable, 18-gauge, short-bevel) needle at an angle of about 45 degrees to the skin. Direct the needle along the course of the femoral artery, roughly toward the umbilicus. Advance the needle until the arterial pulsation can be felt. Now penetrate the artery quickly, transfixing it if necessary. Withdraw the obturator and inner needle. Withdraw the cannula slowly until a pulsatile flow of bright red blood appears. Now depress the hub of the cannula toward the skin. Advance the cannula within the artery for about 1 to 2 cm. Connect plastic tubing and a syringe filled with saline solution (Fig. 2-2, *B*).

4. Details of position, needle size, volume of injection, concentration of medium, and exposure may vary according to the indications for angiography (Table 1).

Two or three exposures may be made on the same 14-by-34-inch film in a specially constructed tunnel (Fig. 2-6). With this device the cassette is held in a tunnel that shields the remainder of the film. The radiolucent portion of the cover is moved sidewise at appropriate intervals for consecutive exposures. For arteriovenous fistula, a rapid cassette changer positioned below the fistula should be employed because of the rapid circulation time.

When a special long cassette is not available, make a single 14-by-17-inch exposure covering the groin and thigh area. This will usually give sufficient initial information to plan the more distal investigation of runoff. After examining the upper film, arrange the popliteal area over a rapid cassette changer, to view the runoff bilaterally. We usually set the apparatus for about ten films at one-second to two-sec-

48

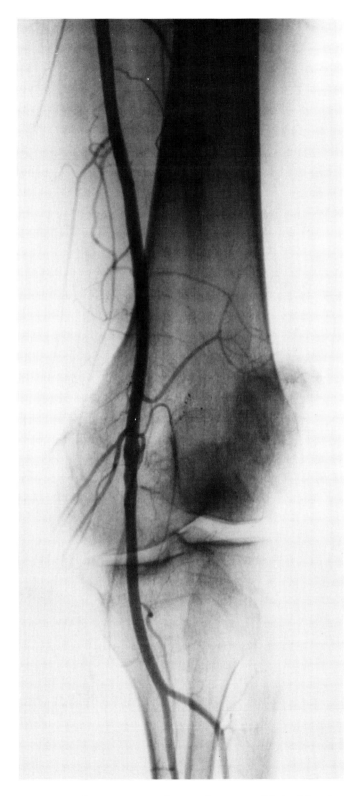

Fig. 2-3. Smooth appearance of normal arteries. Medical-legal case.

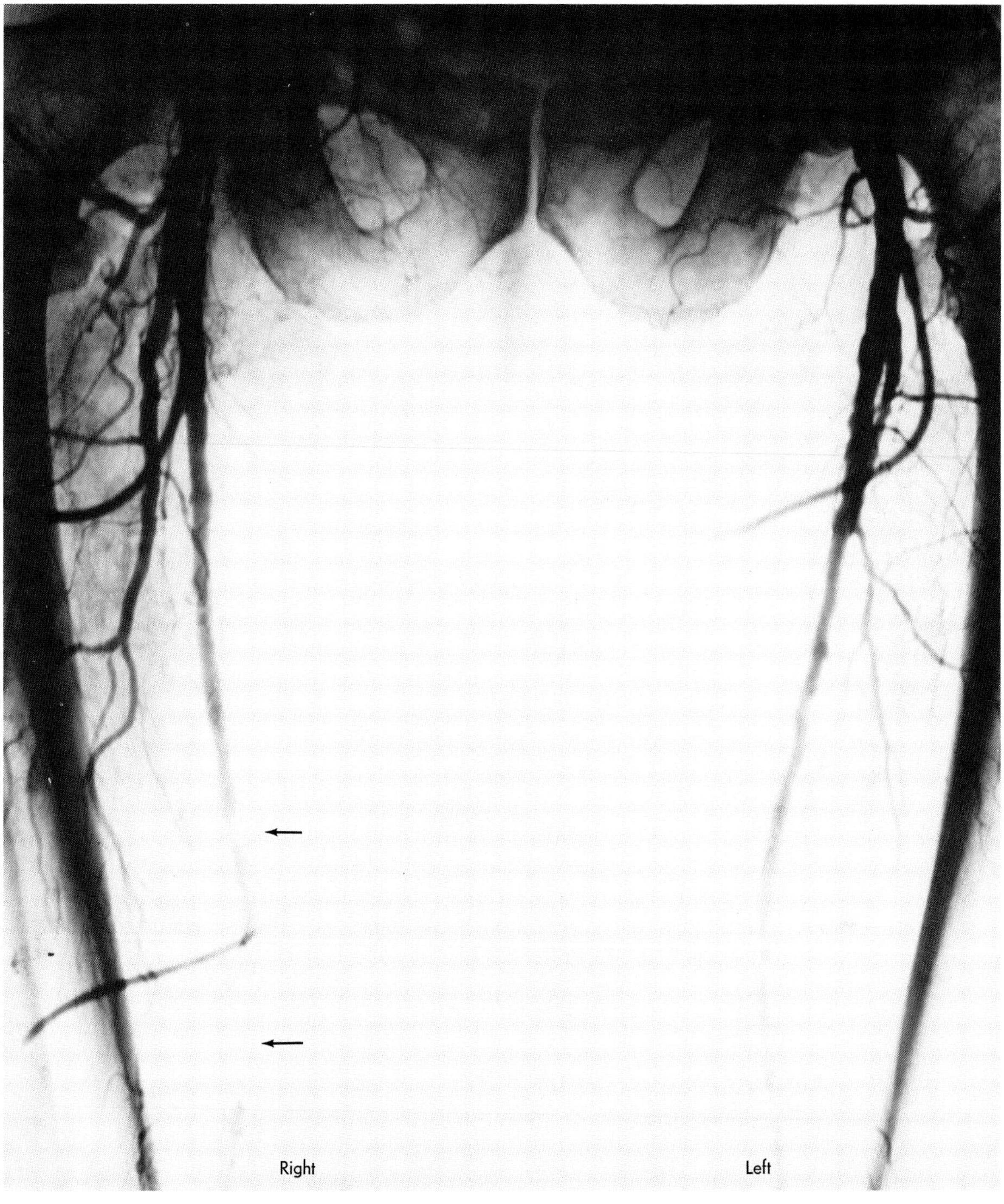

Fig. 2-4. A, Bilateral femoral arteriogram. Slow filling on right. Original films show only a slight opening on the right (*arrow*). Right side severely symptomatic.

Right   Left

50

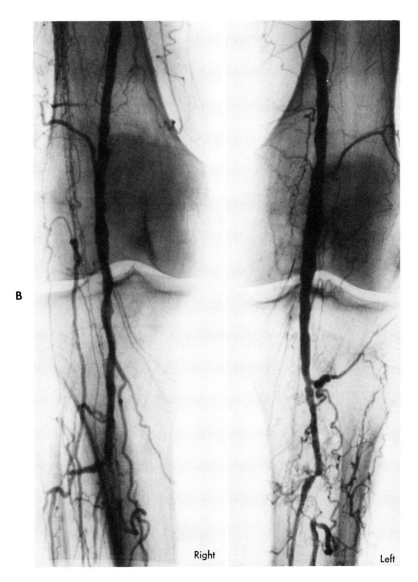

B

Right   Left

Fig. 2-4, cont'd. B, Runoff film from bilateral femoral arteriograms. There is more distal disease on the left side, but the right side is symptomatic. Symptoms are determined by the more proximal obstruction.

Table 1. Techniques of femoral arteriography

Indication	Position	Needle	Injection time (sec.)	Repeat films	Comment
1. Unilateral occlusive disease of leg					
(a) Mild arterial insufficiency (intermittent claudication)	Anteroposterior with internal rotation of foot	18-gauge or 160	5-10	1 or 2	Prolonged injection avoids reflux of dye up into pelvis; bilateral films for comparison advisable
(b) Moderate arterial insufficiency	Anteroposterior with internal rotation of foot	18-gauge or 160	12	1 or 2	To see block and outflow
(c) Severe femoral block (rest pain, gangrene)	Anteroposterior with internal rotation of foot	18-gauge or 160	15	Several films at 3-sec. to 5-sec. intervals	Circulation time to calf is slow and variable
(d) Popliteal artery not open, proximal branches not visualized—search for open arteries in leg, particularly posterior tibial	Anteroposterior with internal rotation of foot	18-gauge or 160	10-15	Delay first exposure; then get about 10 films at 1-sec. intervals	Slow perfusion requires judgment in delaying the first film and programming multiple films so that small open distal arteries are not missed
2. Bilateral occlusive disease of legs and one iliac artery	Anteroposterior with internal rotation of foot	17-gauge, thin-wall, or 205	5	Several films at 3-sec. to 5-sec. intervals	Visualize iliac arteries and terminal aorta by retrograde reflux; use 14″ × 34″ cassette first, then 14″ × 17″ films
3. Visualization of popliteal artery	Maximum internal rotation of foot	17-gauge, thin-wall, or 205	5	Use multiple films in cassette changer	This position widens interosseous space and outflow can be seen without overlying bone
(a) Outflow					
(b) Popliteal aneurysm	Lateral				
4. Visualization of calf or fine details of thigh					

(a) Arteriovenous fistula	According to location	17-gauge, thin-wall, or 205	5	6 films at 0.5-sec. intervals	Rapid circulation time and rapid dilution of dye require rapid injection
(b) Congenital anomalies	According to location	17-gauge, thin-wall, or 205		6 films at 0.5-sec. intervals	To visualize small vessels in capillary and venous phases
(c) Tumors of bone or soft tissue	According to location	17-gauge, thin-wall, or 205	5	6 films at 0.5-sec. intervals	To visualize small vessels in capillary and venous phases
(d) Arterial injuries	According to location	17-gauge, thin-wall, or 205		6 films at 0.5-sec. intervals	Techniques according to findings in 1, 2, or 3 under Indications

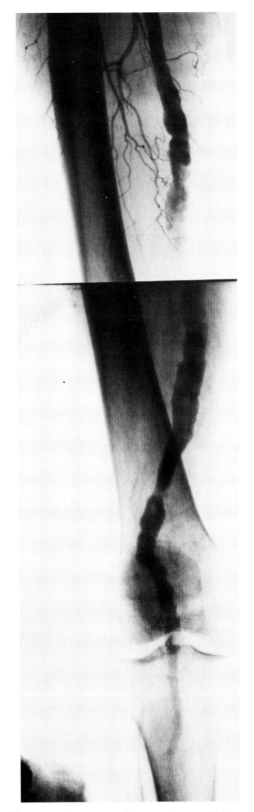

Fig. 2-5. An unusual exception to Table 1. Composite upper and lower femoral arteriograms showing diffuse arteriectasis. Both films taken over a minute after injection.

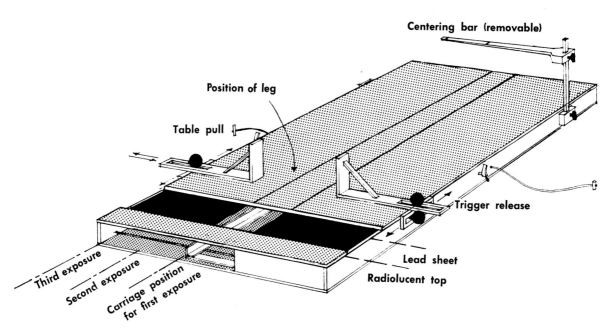

Centering bar (removable)

Position of leg

Table pull

Trigger release

Lead sheet

Radiolucent top

Third exposure

Second exposure

Carriage position for first exposure

Fig. 2-6. Radiographic tunnel for multiple exposures of entire leg. (Courtesy Dr. Noah Susman, St. Louis, Mo.)

ond intervals. Distal runoff is essential in femoral-popliteal reconstruction; if there is none, arterial reconstruction will fail. If the proximal popliteal runoff is poor, attempt to locate the distal tibial artery and/or peroneal artery. Bypass to these vessels will salvage some legs (p. 192). We do a complete examination bilaterally when the first femoral arteriograms are done.

Retrograde aortogram and bilateral femoral arteriogram

If one femoral pulse is palpable, the terminal aorta and both iliac and femoral arteries may be visualized by the percutaneous femoral route, by injecting the medium up and around by forceful hand injection. This technique can replace a translumbar aortogram and retrograde catheterization in those cases in which information about the arteries to a little above the aortic bifurcation is all that is desired.

Procedure

1. Anesthesia, preparation, and draping are identical with those for angiography of the leg by the femoral route. Have the patient practice the Valsalva maneuver with your command to "shoot" on the count of 10.

2. Make the femoral puncture with a large (No. 205) Seldinger needle. Connect to a 50 ml. syringe of 60% contrast medium in a large-bore (Robb) syringe or to a syringe-pressure injector mechanism.

3. Position the patient over a large film to show the terminal aorta. After injection, expose several 14-by-17-inch films beneath the thigh and leg to demonstrate the pattern of flow through the extremities. Inject contrast medium as rapidly as possible after the Valsalva maneuver has been held for ten seconds. Expose the abdominal film, using a long exposure time (one second) just before the completion of the injection.

Postoperative care

The operator should withdraw the needle after inspecting the films. Firm pressure should be held over the puncture site for five minutes. When a large-bore needle is used, compression for ten minutes may be necessary. Pain is usually minimal, and complications are rare.

Discussion

A complete map of the arteries from the terminal aorta to the midcalf area may be obtained by the percutaneous femoral route. Thorough investigation is mandatory prior to any elective operation, since one of the more common causes of failure to restore blood flow after operation is unrecognized and uncorrected narrowing of vessels proximal or distal to the site of surgery. Retrograde catheterization of the iliac arteries may be difficult if the patient has occlusive disease and unnecessary if reflux injection via the cannula is successful. If neither femoral pulse is palpable, the retrograde method cannot be employed and translumbar aortography becomes necessary.

TRANSLUMBAR AORTOGRAPHY

Translumbar aortography is performed to investigate occlusive disease of the abdominal aorta, the aortic visceral branches, the iliac arteries, and the proximal portion of the common femoral arteries. It is unwise to use this method for the investigation of possible aneurysm of the abdominal aorta. For lateral views of the renal, superior mesenteric, and celiac arteries, a long needle with a Teflon cannula fitted over it may be employed, the patient being turned after withdrawal of the metallic portion of the needle.

Contraindications to the use of translumbar aortography are hemorrhagic disease, severe hypertension, renal disease, and suspected aneurysm of the abdominal aorta. In aneurysm a central channel surrounded by atheromatous material may give a false picture of the pathological condition. If translumbar aortography is necessary to demonstrate, for instance, a meandering aorta, the aortic puncture should be sufficiently high that the aneurysm is not entered. Puncture of an aneurysm can precipitate an emergency situation. The x-ray film of a meandering aorta in Fig. 3-1 illustrates the high placement of the needle. Alternative techniques for visualization of the aorta and its branches are intravenous aortography and selective retrograde catheterization of the aorta and its branches. The latter technique is described later in this chapter.

Adequate hydration should be maintained. When impaired renal function may be due to vascular insufficiency and this is the reason for aortography, the translumbar aortogram should be performed during mannitol diuresis induced by the infusion of 500 ml. of 5% to 10% mannitol solution (Osmitrol).

Anesthesia

Either local or general anesthesia is satisfactory. Local anesthesia is preferred unless the patient is extremely apprehensive and restless.

Position

Place the patient in the prone position (Fig. 2-7, *A*). A pillow may be placed under the shoulders and upper chest but not under the abdomen. A pillow under the abdomen places the aorta at a greater distance from the skin.

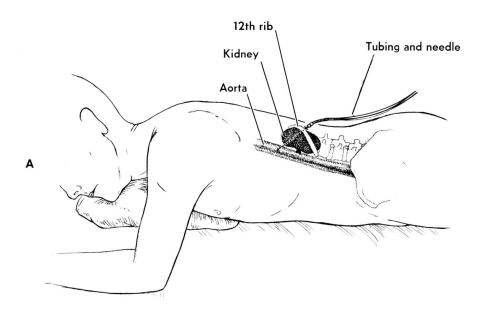

A

12th rib

Kidney

Aorta

Tubing and needle

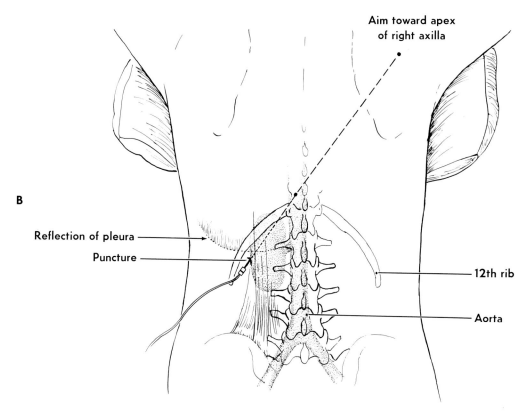

B

Aim toward apex
of right axilla

Reflection of pleura

Puncture

12th rib

Aorta

Fig. 2-7. Translumbar aortogram. **A,** Position. **B,** Landmarks.

Procedure

1. Administer an intravenous dose of contrast medium to test sensitivity, using 4 or 5 ml.

2. Prepare and drape the skin of the back on the left side. The site of injection is 2 cm. below the twelfth rib on the left and 5 or 6 cm. to the left of the midline (Fig. 2-7, B). Infiltrate the site of injection with local anesthetic. Advance the needle along the line that will be followed by the long aortographic needle, and infiltrate the sacrospinalis muscle mass with a small amount of anesthetic agent.

3. Make a small stab wound in the skin at the anesthetized site. Introduce a 17-gauge 7-inch Touhy thin-wall needle, directing it toward the apex of the right axilla. The side of the vertebral body is usually encountered. When this happens, withdraw the needle slightly and redirect it at a somewhat more acute angle with the midsagittal plane. Note that a 7-inch needle is necessary. Shorter needles often fail, particularly when a high injection is needed. Sharp needles are essential. The conscientious surgeon may keep his own needle and sharpen it himself.

4. A brisk pulsating stream of bright red blood will spurt out when the needle has punctured the aorta. Test the patency of the connection with a small amount of saline solution. Flow should be without significant resistance and without pain if the patient is awake. Do not inject contrast medium if the flow of blood is slow, if it is dark in color, or if it is not definitely pulsatile. When the needle is introduced, the tip should lie within the abdominal aorta, at the level of the eleventh or twelfth thoracic vertebra, and well above the visceral branches of the aorta.

5. Connect the needle to a syringe filled with Conray (60%) and to plastic connecting tubing. Rapidly inject 10 ml. of contrast medium and immediately expose the first film. The film will confirm that the needle is properly placed and is not opposite or in the orifice of the renal artery or other vital visceral branches. Keep the needle open with small injections of saline solution until the test film has been developed. When all is satisfactory, inject 30 to 50 ml. of contrast medium by pressure injection. Either mechanical injectors or hand pressure can be used. When injecting by hand, use plastic syringes that do not break in your hand. Expose the abdominal film immediately. A second exposure may be arranged at a lower level to show the femoral arteries.

6. Withdraw the needle. If the initial films are unsuccessful, do not make another attempt at translumbar aortography on the same day. Second injections have proved to be dangerous.

Complications

Complications are rare when suitable precautions are taken and safe routines enforced.

Retroperitoneal extravasation

Retroperitoneal extravasation of contrast medium usually causes no ill effects. X-ray films show the contrast medium spreading along the vertebral column. Temporary back pain and warmth in the left leg due to increased blood flow rapidly subside.

Hemorrhage

Minor leakage from the puncture site causes no difficulty. Aortography is contraindicated for patients with hemorrhagic diathesis and for those receiving anticoagulant therapy. The Touhy needle makes a smaller puncture wound than needles with conventionally tapered points. Multiple punctures should be avoided, and translumbar aortography should not be employed if there is any suspicion of aortic aneurysm.

Renal damage

Renal damage is a frequent serious complication of translumbar aortography. Significant renal disease is consequently a contraindication unless stenosis or occlusion of a renal artery is suspected. Trial arteriograms after injection of 10 ml. of contrast medium are recommended to avoid accidental injection of large amounts of contrast medium directly into the renal arteries. Normally, the tip of the aortographic needle will lie well above the origin of the renal arteries and the trial dose will be delivered directly into the aorta. The volume of contrast medium injected at any day's examination should be limited to about 50 ml. Multiple and repeated injections must be avoided even though the contrast material is not directed exclusively into the renal arteries. Patients should be well hydrated at the time of examination. Mannitol diuresis is advisable during renal arteriograms if renal function is borderline.

Intramural dissection of aorta

Dissection of the aortic wall by contrast medium has been observed without harmful effects. However, it causes pain and discomfort. This complication is avoided by not injecting contrast medium unless there is a free pulsatile flow of blood and by testing the position of the needle with a small trial injection of 10 ml. of contrast medium. Intramural dissection occurs if the tip of the needle lies partly in the aortic wall during the injection of contrast medium. Such dissection might tear or occlude the orgins of small branches, causing ischemia of the spinal cord or other organs.

Paraplegia

Paraplegia is one of the rarer but most feared complications of translumbar aortography. The incidence of paraplegia is reduced by using less toxic contrast media, by employing smaller amounts of medium, and by insisting on correct placement of the needle. The toxicity of contrast agents increases with repeated injections, and more than half of the patients with paraplegia received more than one injection during the same examination.

The blood supply to the spinal cord is segmental in the embryo. In adults, however, two larger arteries predominate and supply the cord. In about 15% of adults the major artery is at the level of the fifth to the eighth thoracic vertebras. In the remaining 85% the major supply to the cord is a moderately large artery that accompanies the left second lumbar nerve root and enters the cord at the level of the ninth thoracic to the second lumbar vertebras. In anatomical literature this artery is named the artery of Adamkiewicz and Kadyi, the artery of the lumbar enlargement, or the great anterior medullary artery.

It is probably occlusion of the lower artery that causes or contributes to the rare cases of paraplegia after lumbar aortography or surgery of the abdominal aorta. The rare instances of paraplegia after operations on the thoracic aorta probably result from occlusion of the less frequent fifth to eighth thoracic vertebral origin of the blood supply. The whole subject needs to be studied further. If the orifice of the artery were known, possibly it could be perfused during surgery and then reimplanted by severing a cuff of the aorta at the orifice of the vessel. (See Fig. 6-10.)

This tragic complication is fortunately rare, the incidence being estimated at 0.2%. Fear of the complication has encouraged more frequent employment of other methods to visualize the aorta and its branches, such as intravenous aortography and percutaneous retrograde catheterization of the aorta.

SELECTIVE PERCUTANEOUS RETROGRADE AORTIC CATHETERIZATION

Selective retrograde catheterization is a valuable and rather universally applicable technique for visualization of many portions of the arterial tree. Selective retrograde techniques employing long catheters have been extended to visualize the renal, coronary, and bronchial arterial circulations in detail in combination with cinefluoroscopic roentgenographic techniques.

Retrograde aortography has several advantages over the translumbar method, including better visualization, greater scope in visualization, and freedom in positioning the patient. The method described may also be employed in conjunction with retrograde pyelography. Intravenous aortography is employed when iliac vessels are occluded or when aneurysms of the aorta preclude safe and accurate passage of retrograde catheters.

Selective retrograde aortography can usually be performed by the cutaneous route, via the femoral vessels in adults. Open operation is preferable for the brachial artery and also for the small femoral vessel in infants and children.

The most versatile material for special aortic catheters to visualize particular locations, such as mesenteric, renal, or hepatic vessels, is the soft but relatively firm and thick-walled x-ray-opaque polyethylene (Ödman-Leden*) tubing. Special tips may be formed by heating the material at relatively low temperatures, facilitating catheterization of various branches of the aorta. This soft material has the disadvantage of requiring cold sterilization in bactericidal solution or by gas. When retrograde aortography is to be done, catheters of proper length and with whatever curved tips may be necessary should be designed and carefully prepared in advance. Recently, special steerable and proximally controlled catheters have been developed.

During a long procedure, a modification of the continuous irrigating apparatus is used to flush the vessel intermittently with heparin in saline solution. The side arm of this apparatus can be conveniently connected by a Y-shaped connector to a flask of contrast medium and a flask of irrigation solution. These are alternated at the surgeon's request (Fig. 2-8, I).

A portable image amplifier with cine capability greatly shortens the procedure and allows later review and rerun of the tape.

Anesthesia

General anesthesia may be employed. However, local infiltration with adequate preoperative medication, including a barbiturate, is quite satisfactory.

Seldinger technique

Retrograde aortography was originally performed by introducing a needle into the femoral artery and passing a small polyethylene catheter through it. Hematomas occurred frequently because the hole in the artery was considerably larger than the catheter within it. With the Seldinger technique larger catheters can be passed through small punctures by using a flexible metal guide.

*Similar materials are now available from Becton, Dickinson & Co., Rutherford, N. J.

The Seldinger technique employs three basic pieces of apparatus: a thin-walled pointed needle, a blunt outer cannula that cannot injure the arterial wall (Fig. 2-8, *B*), and a flexible metal guide. The cannula is introduced into the artery with the pointed needle within it. The needle is withdrawn to permit introduction of a flexible guide through the cannula instead of the needle. The cannula is withdrawn, leaving the guide in the artery. Finally, the angiographic catheter is threaded over the guide and thence into the artery. Positioning is done fluoroscopically, after which the guide is withdrawn to permit the injection of contrast medium.

Procedure

The skin of the groin has been previously shaved and prepared. The catheters used in this procedure may be several feet long and must not touch an unsterile field. Consequently, the operators should wear sterile gowns, and the operative area should be draped widely.

1. Infiltrate the area overlying the femoral pulse and just below the inguinal ligament with a local anesthetic. Make a small vertical 1/4-inch incision through the skin. (See Fig. 2-8, *A*.)

2. Introduce a Seldinger needle slowly until the arterial pulsation is felt. Pierce the arterial wall with a quick motion. The artery is usually transfixed. (See Fig. 2-8, *B*.)

3. Remove the stylet. If the artery has been transfixed, withdraw the needle slowly. When the tip is in the artery, there will be a pulsatile flow of bright red blood from the needle. (See Fig. 2-8, *C*.)

4. Remove the sharp inner needle, leaving the blunt cannula in the artery. Advance the blunt cannula proximally for 1 to 2 cm. (See Fig. 2-8, *D*.)

5. Insert the flexible wire guide (Fig. 2-8, *E*). Guides are available in several lengths, and the length of the guide is chosen to reach the site for radiological examination. When the flexible guide has been introduced several centimeters beyond the tip of the needle, withdraw the blunt cannula.

6. Now pass the catheter over the guide (Fig. 2-8, *F*). This catheter must be of known length and always shorter than the total length of the guide.

When the catheter reaches the skin, advance it and the arterial guide together until the catheter is several inches within the artery. Withdraw the flexible guide partially until it protrudes only slightly from the plastic tubing. This is determined by measurement of both prior to insertion. Now advance the guide and catheter together to the desired injection site.

7. Scout films, fluoroscopy, or image intensification fluoroscopy is employed to check the location of the catheter. The flexible metal guide shoudd be retained within the catheter during the introduction in order to prevent bending or kinking of the tubing. (See Fig. 2-8, *G*.)

8. When the position of the catheter is satisfactory, withdraw the guide. Connect the plastic tubing to the coupling and the combination of syringes and three-way stopcock illustrated (Fig. 2-8, *H*). The arrangement of syringes makes a convenient handle and allows considerable pressure to be placed on the injecting syringe. Inject the contrast medium by hand under as much pressure as possible or, preferably, in one-half to one and one-half seconds with a mechanical injector. The amount and other details vary somewhat, depending on the area to be visualized (Table 2). A small trial injection of 10 ml. of contrast medium is usually advisable to check the position of the catheter.

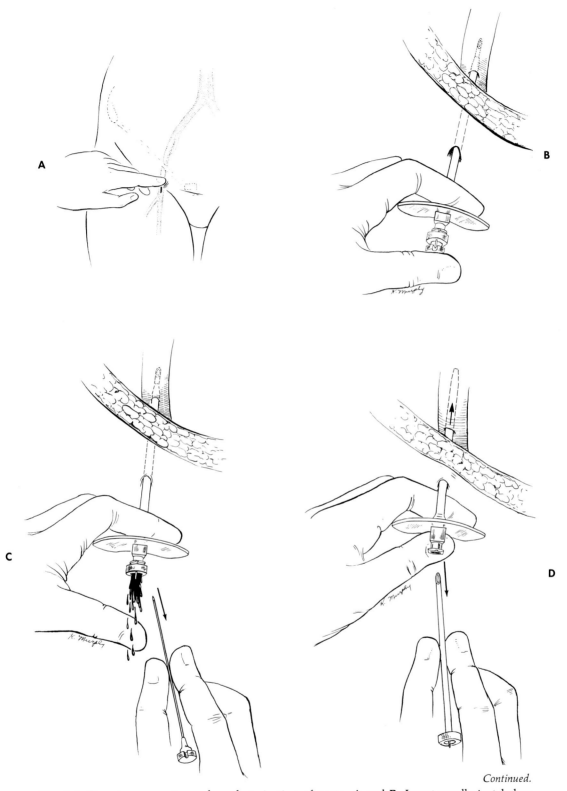

Continued.

Fig. 2-8. Percutaneous retrograde catheterization of aorta. **A** and **B,** Insert needle just below inguinal ligament. **C,** Withdraw stylet and observe pulsatile bleeding. **D,** Withdraw sharp obturator and advance cannula.

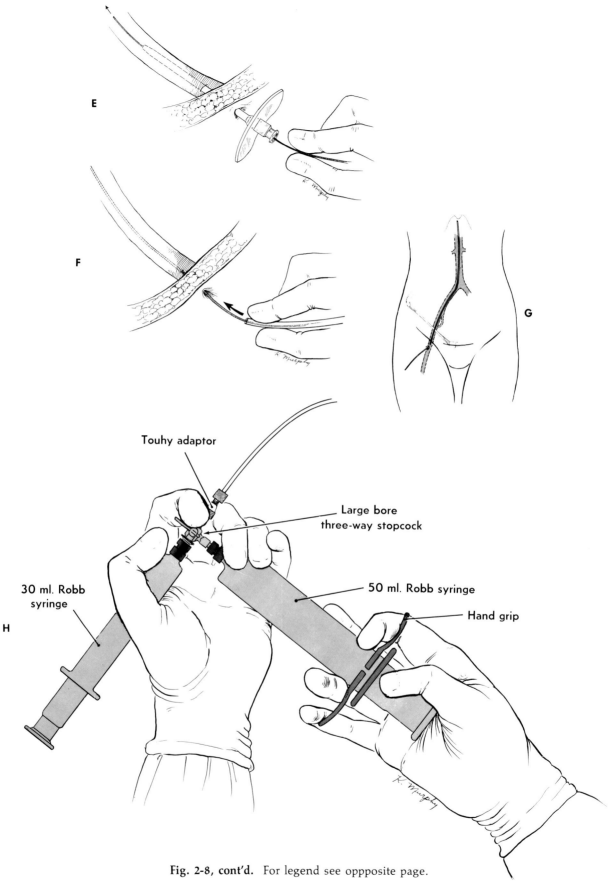

E

F

G

Touhy adaptor

Large bore
three-way stopcock

30 ml. Robb
syringe

50 ml. Robb syringe

Hand grip

H

Fig. 2-8, cont'd. For legend see oppposite page.

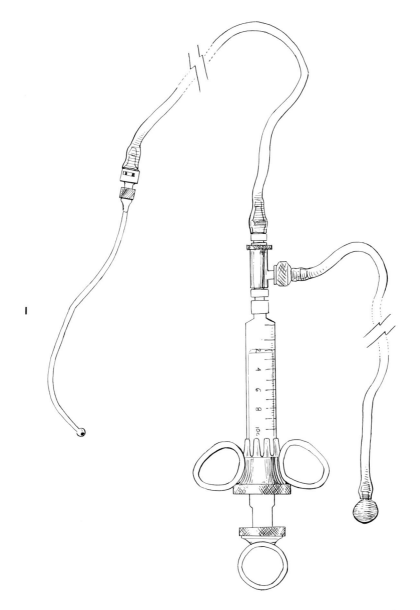

Fig. 2-8, cont'd. Percutaneous retrograde catheterization of aorta. **E,** Insert flexible metal guide and then remove cannula. **F,** Thread catheter over metal guide. **G,** Advance both to desired location in artery. **H,** Arrangement of equipment for rapid injection by hand. **I,** Device for continuous irrigation. (All component parts available from Becton, Dickinson & Co., Rutherford, N. J.)

Table 2. Retrograde catheterization of the aorta

Purpose	Puncture	Seldinger needle	Position of catheter	Volume	Films and position
Aortic arch arteriogram	Femoral	No. 205	Arch of aorta	100 ml. mechanically	Biplane changer with careful carotid compression
Aortic-renal arteriogram	Femoral	No. 160 or 205	Twelfth thoracic vertebral level	10-30 ml.	Supine; changer, single film, or cine films
Superior mesenteric arteriogram	Femoral	No. 205	Twelfth thoracic vertebral level	50 ml.	Supine and lateral; single films or cine films
Teminal aorta and bilateral femoral arteriogram	Femoral	No. 205	Catheter usually unnecessary	50 ml.	Supine; single film, changer, or cine films

Special catheters are available for special purposes. Tips are sometimes bent to go around the arch or into selected orifices. Radiopaque catheters have thick walls and small lumens. Side holes at the tips prevent recoil of the tip during brisk injection.

COMMENT: *Know and set up all the apparatus in advance. Do not depend on other people to help unless they are thoroughly familiar with the method and with your own procedures. Portable image amplification is an important adjunct as is cinefluoroscopy. Have sharp needles. We find that the Swedish-made Seldinger needles are the best because they are precision made and require only infrequent sharpening. One of the main causes of difficulty is a dull needle. Be prepared to sharpen your own.*

When retrograde catheterization via the femoral artery is done in elderly people, the iliac artery may be too tortuous, and the procedure should then be abandoned in favor of a translumbar approach.

There is a small incidence of aneurysm after the retrograde procedure, particularly when the larger No. 205 needle is used.

OPERATIVE ARTERIOGRAMS

Emergency situations occasionally arise wherein arteriograms must be obtained on the operating room table. Such situations most frequently arise when operative findings in patients with traumatic injuries or embolism suggest distal arteriosclerosis, thrombosis, or distal embolism that was unsuspected before operation.

In vascular operations on an extremity it is always wise to prepare and drape the entire limb, since this will facilitate distal exploration or arteriography when necessary.

The x-ray grid-front cassette is placed in a sterile pillowcase and positioned under the limb or other part to be investigated. The artery, vein, or prosthesis is then punctured for injection of contrast medium. Alternatively, a small or tapered catheter may be held in place by a Javid clamp for the arteriogram. From 10 to 30 ml. of contrast medium is then injected in the same way as for any other arteriographic procedure, using relatively long exposures and injection times. Immediately afterward, the artery should be flushed with about 100 ml. of dilute heparin solution in normal saline solution to prevent excessive arterial irritation and possible spasm.

Operative arteriography or survey with the portable image amplifier should be used freely after reconstructive procedures in the lower extremity. This is particularly true when operative findings, including measurement of blood flow, suggest that some distal obstruction may remain and that such remaining outflow obstruction might compromise the result of the primary surgical operation. After a bypass operation, the distal anastomosis can be checked and also the anatomical outflow tract. A distal obstruction or other problems can be evaluated at this time. There is no better time to correct technical defects and errors than at the time of the initial operation.

C.H.C.

References

Abrams, H. L.: Angiography, ed. 2, Boston, 1971, Little, Brown and Co.

Curry, J. L., and Howland W. J.: Arteriography; principles and techniques, emphasizing its application in community hospital practice, Philadelphia, 1966, W. B. Saunders Co.

Doppman, J. L., Di Chiro, G., and Ommaya, A. K.: Selective arteriography of the spinal cord, St. Louis, 1969, Warren H. Green, Inc.

Hanafee, W. N., editor: Selective angiography. In Robbins, L. L., editor: Golden's Diagnostic Radiology, Baltimore, 1972, The Williams & Wilkins Co.

Sutton, D.: Arteriography, Edinburgh, 1962, E. & S. Livingstone Ltd.

Toole, J. F., chairman, et al.: Cerebral vascular diseases—seventh conference, New York, 1971, Grune & Stratton, Inc.

3

Aneurysms of the abdominal aorta

INTRODUCTION

Aneurysm, localized disease, and embolic disease are conditions of the abdominal aorta that are correctable by surgical operation with highly satisfactory results and moderate risks, particularly for elective excision of abdominal aneurysms. DeWeese, Blaisdell, and Foster in 1972 in the study for the Intersociety Commission for Heart Disease reported recent mortality of elective resection of abdominal aorta aneurysm ranging from 2.7% to 7%. Survivors have the same life expectancy as other patients with comparable arteriosclerosis elsewhere.

There is naturally some difference in the selection of cases by various individuals or teams, and occasionally for medical reasons, we reject or postpone an elective operation. When this is done, serial lateral abdominal films to observe the size or change in size of the aneurysm are advisable. Usually the slight calcification of the aneurysm wall can be observed best in lateral x-ray films, and the vertebras can be used as fixed points for comparison of the size. If there is rapid enlargement, surgery is required, even in the face of other medical problems, whereas stability permits delay of surgery.

Survivors of surgery have more or less the same life expectancy for their age and arteriosclerosis as do other patients with comparable arteriosclerotic disease, provided that correct technique avoids late complications. In our experience such complications are quite rare.

Diagnosis

The diagnosis is usually obvious, but it is sometimes difficult to evaluate the size of the aneurysm by palpation, particularly in an obese patient. Associated iliac aneurysms are frequently unsuspected.

Aortograms are not employed in diagnosis because as a rule the aneurysm is filled with atherosclerotic material and it will not be filled by the contrast medium. We use aortography only in those cases in which palpation reveals a pulsatile mass off to one side, usually the right. Frequently these cases are meandering aortas rather than aneurysms (Fig. 3-1).

Diagnosis of ruptured aneurysm may be difficult. Severe, constant abdominal or back pain and shock are the usual clinical signs and symptoms. Peritoneal tap is useless, since the hemorrhage is retroperitoneal. Hemorrhage may take place so rapidly that there is no initial decrease in hemoglobin or hematocrit value. At times rupture can be confused with ureteral colic, and rupture of an iliac aneurysm producing severe low pelvic pain can be confusing.

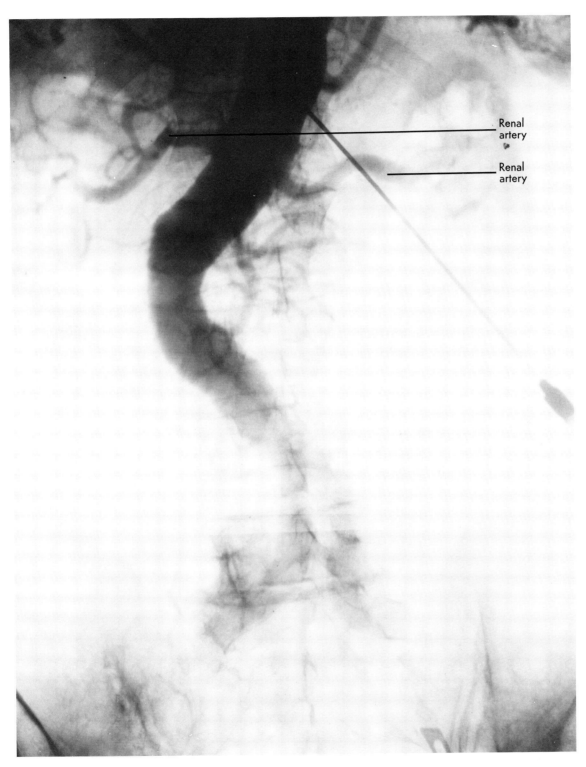

Renal
artery

Renal
artery

Fig. 3-1. Meandering aorta originally diagnosed as an aneurysm.

Surgical anatomy and physiology

The infrarenal portion of the aorta and the iliac arteries are readily uncovered by incisions in the posterior parietal peritoneum and dissection in an avascular retroperitoneal plane. The duodenum, small bowel, and sigmoid colon may be readily mobilized. The only important structures overlying the lower portion of the abdominal aorta are the sigmoid colon and its mesentery and, retroperitoneally, the ureters. Lymphatic vessels appear anterior to the aorta as fibrous bands and are divided without danger. Aneurysms of the aorta are frequently adherent to the vena cava or to the iliac veins, especially the right, and may make dissection difficult and dangerous in their vicinity.

Although most of the pathological conditions of the abdominal aorta are centered below the renal arteries, the visceral branches of the upper abdominal aorta may develop aneurysmal or atherosclerotic disease that can be surgically corrected. Details for exposure of these vessels are presented in Chapter 11.

The exposure most frequently used is a long vertical midline incision. A paramedian incision, as illustrated in Fig. 3-2, may also be used. Through either of these incisions, the inferior vena cava below the renal veins can also be approached for ligation, for repair of injuries, or for external partial occlusion with a plastic clip. Both transverse abdominal and retroperitoneal left flank incisions have been used to approach the abdominal aorta and repair abdominal aortic aneurysms; however, these exposures may be inadequate and are not advisable.

Occlusion time is not especially critical when the aorta is clamped below the renal arteries. However, prolonged occlusion should be avoided. Flow through the aorta and one leg can usually be reestablished within forty-five minutes to one hour. Prolonged cross clamping leads to complications and may result in poor renal function after aortic surgery. Experimental evidence regarding noxious reflexes arising from clamping the aorta is conflicting, but complications from embolism by atherosclerotic sludge and from prolonged hypotension are more frequent. Methods that avoid such complications are described in this chapter.

Surgical exploration

1. Make an incision from the xiphoid process to the pubis (Fig. 3-2, A). Shorter incisions usually prove to be inadequate, and the long incision is necessary even though only the lower aorta is to be explored. The paramedian route is illustrated, but midline incisions are now preferred.

2. Retract the small intestine to the right. Incise the posterior parietal peritoneum overlying the aorta. This is medial to the mesentery of the small bowel. The incision is expedited by delicately elevating the peritoneum alone, sliding the dissecting scissors underneath it, and then dividing the isolated leaflet of peritoneum. Fig. 3-2, B, shows this incision extended to mobilize the ascending colon, a procedure that may be necessary in obese persons (Fig. 3-2, C). Further upward exposure of the aorta is obtained by upward extension of the peritoneal incision, division of the ligament of Treitz, and retraction of the third portion of the duodenum to the right.

3. When delivery of the small intestine and ascending colon outside the abdomen is necessary, the intestine should be protected with pads soaked in warm saline solution and enclosed in a Lahey bag or plastic sheet. Thus protected, the entire intestine supplied by the superior mesenteric arery may be delivered from the abdomen. Helpful adjuncts in obtaining adequate exposure are oversized retractors made in extra depths (5 inches and 7 inches) and similar widths.

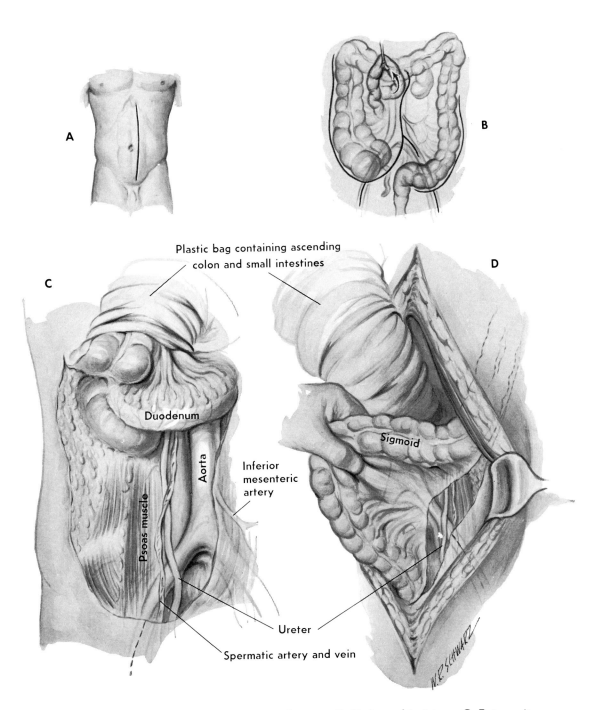

Labels within figure:

A

B

C

Plastic bag containing ascending
colon and small intestines

D

Duodenum

Aorta

Psoas muscle

Inferior
mesenteric
artery

Sigmoid

Ureter

Spermatic artery and vein

W.P.SCHWARZ

Fig. 3-2. Exploration of abdominal aorta. **A,** Incision. **B,** Peritoneal incisions. **C,** Retroperitoneal structures on right side after delivery of ascending colon and small bowel outside abdomen. **D,** Exposure of left external iliac artery by reflection of sigmoid colon.

69

4. For access to the left iliac artery, extend the incision over the aorta downward along the left iliac artery and make an additional incision in the posterior parietal peritoneum lateral to the lower portion of the descending colon and the upper sigmoid colon (Fig. 3-2, *B*). Elevate the sigmoid colon (Fig. 3-2, *D*). The left ureter can be identified readily to the left of the sigmoid mesentery and may be allowed to remain in situ. Isolation and retraction of the ureter with a tape is usually unnecessary.

RESECTION OF ANEURYSMS OF ABDOMINAL AORTA
Introduction

Resection of aneurysms of the abdominal aorta can be performed with reasonable risk but requires more than average surgical skill. Resection of the entire sac is unnecessary and frequently hazardous. Therefore, we leave some of the sac and use it to cover the prosthesis. Surgery is almost always advisable because arteriosclerotic aneurysms that cause symptoms usually continue to enlarge and rupture within a year. Operation is advisable for patients with large aneurysms, aneurysms observed to increase in size, and aneurysms that cause symptoms. Because of the magnitude of the procedure, operation is contraindicated in patients with serious medical diseases who already have a poor prognosis. Operation is not advisable for extremely elderly patients or those who present an excessively high surgical risk. Such patients are poor risks, and complications are usually catastrophic. However, in experienced hands, the mortality of elective resection must not exceed 10%.

Preoperative preparation and anesthesia

Aortograms, particularly lumbar aortograms, are unnecessary and may even be dangerous. Aneurysmal sacs are filled with laminated clot, so that the channel may appear to be normal on the arteriograms. The only certain way to determine operability, size, and location of the aneurysm is surgical exploration.

We advise prophylactic digitalization for this and all other major arterial surgery in elderly patients. Bowel preparation by enemas and cathartics is essential. The patient should practice and be familiar with the intermittent-positive-pressure-breathing apparatus before the operation.

Other preoperative preparations in the operating room include setting up a cardiac monitor and central venous pressure measuring apparatus and inserting several large needles or transfusion cannulas so that rapid transfusion can be carried out if and when required.

Light general and endotracheal anesthesia should be supplemented with muscle relaxants when necessary. An infusion of 1 liter of 10% mannitol solution* should be started in patients with large aneurysms or with borderline renal function. The anesthesiologist must prevent hypotension by proper blood and fluid replacement. Usually 2 or 3 pints of blood will be required, but at least 6 units should be on hand before the operation. Before the aortic clamp is released, blood must be running at a rapid rate in a large vein. Rapid transfusion requires the use of a cannula, and if necessary, surgical cutdown is performed before the operation is begun and a central venous pressure catheter is inserted. Declamping shock is seldom observed when

---

*Solutions of mannitol are commerically available (Osmitrol), or 12.5 or 25 Gm. may be added to 800 ml. of 5% dextrose solution in water.

adequate lactated Ringer's solution is given during surgery. The average patient receives 3,000 ml. of lactated Ringer's solution in addition to blood.

Procedure

1. Place the patient in the supine position. Palpate and mark the pedal pulses for future reference. Insert a urethral catheter for measurement of urine output during and after surgery. Prepare and drape the groins as well as the abdomen so that this area will be accessible if necessary.

2. Make a long midline or paramedian incision extending from the xiphoid process to the pubis (Fig. 3-3). Explore the abdominal cavity for evidence of other disease. Retract the small intestine to the right, uncovering the aorta. If necessary,

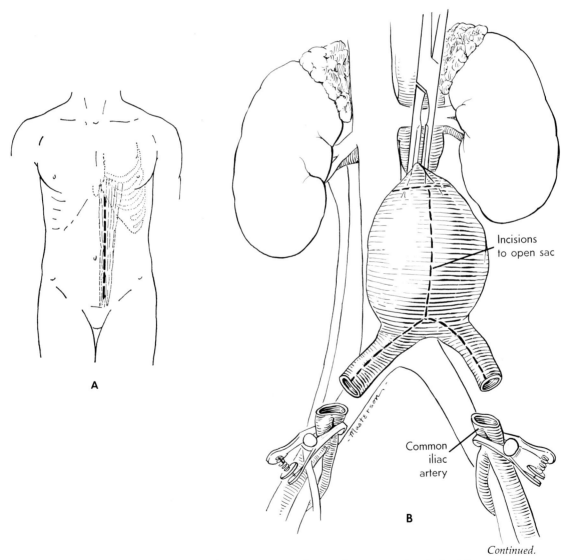

Continued.

Fig. 3-3. Resection of abdominal aneurysm—end-to-end anastomosis. **A,** Incision. **B,** Open sac after obtaining proximal and distal control.

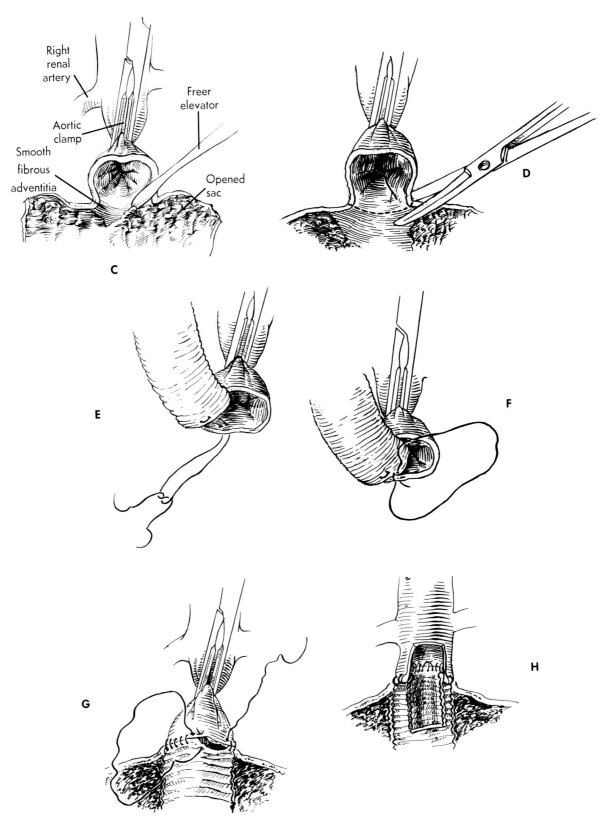

Labels in figure C:
- Right renal artery
- Aortic clamp
- Smooth fibrous adventitia
- Freer elevator
- Opened sac

Fig. 3-3, cont'd. Resection of abdominal aneurysm—end-to-end anastomosis. **C,** Endarterectomy at cuff of aorta. **D,** Divide posterior wall or proceed to anastomosis as in Fig. 3-9 if posterior wall is adherent. **E,** Start anastomosis posteriorly. **F,** Sew over and over from graft to aorta. **G,** Complete anastomosis in front. **H,** Cutaway view.

the small intestine may be displaced from the abdomen. Incise the peritoneum at the left side of the mesentery of the small bowel, and divide the ligament of Treitz to permit retraction of the duodenum and small bowel farther to the right. Incise the peritoneum over the left common iliac artery, and retract the mesentery of the sigmoid colon to the left to uncover the left common iliac artery to its bifurcation. Usually the left ureter cannot be seen from the medial side. To retract the mesentery of the sigmoid colon farther to the left, ligate and divide the inferior mesenteric artery at its origin from the aorta. Do not disturb the connection between the left colic and sigmoid branches. If the inferior mesenteric artery is not clearly visible, wait and ligate it inside the sac.

COMMENT: *Good exposure and thorough exploration are essential for safety. The incision must be long, and the small bowel must be retracted well out of the way. We have never regretted delivery of the small intestine outside the abdomen. Keep the intestine moist, covered, and warm; this is accomplished by protecting the bowel with a large piece of gauze moistened with saline solution and covering it with a piece of plastic sheet or a Lahey bag. (See p. 68 for more details regarding exploration of the aorta.)*

3. Determine the operability of the lesion as follows: Identify the left renal vein as it crosses the aorta. Find the inferior mesenteric vein in the edge of the left mesocolon, crossing the aneurysm and vanishing beneath the pancreas to join the splenic vein. Dissect around the sides of the aorta at the level of the left renal vein. The aorta is most likely to be free from the inferior vena cava at this level.

COMMENT: *The neck of the aneurysm always appears to be wide and anterior in position. Dissection posteriorly reveals that the aneurysmal sac has lifted the posterior wall of the proximal portion of the aorta forward, leaving a triangular space between the proximal portion of the aorta and the spine. There is 1 inch or more of relatively normal aorta between the left renal artery and the aneurysm. The availability of a variety of prostheses permits reconstruction even though the diameter of the aorta at this level may exceed 25 mm. Almost all abdominal aneurysms have been operable since appropriate sizes of prostheses have been available and since we have learned to find the "free angle" between the proximal portion of the aorta and the spine.*

4. Obtain control of the aorta proximally above the aneurysm. It is usually unnecessary to dissect around the back of the aorta. Make maximum use of the free space already mentioned between the posterior aortic wall and the spine just proximal to the aneurysmal sac. It is unwise to lift, roll, or retract the aneurysm. These movements may dislodge emboli from the clotted contents of the aneurysmal sac. Select an aortic clamp of appropriate size and angulation. Usually a Craaford or coarctation clamp is applied vertically, or a double-curved aortic clamp fits well transversely.

COMMENT: *When the sides of the aorta are free proximal to the neck of the aneurysm, it is unnecessary to dissect around the back of the aorta. Frequently there are troublesome veins there, and the anastomosis can be performed without dividing the posterior wall of the aorta. (See Figs. 3-8 and 3-9.)*

5. Obtain control of the iliac arteries distal to the aneurysm. Free the iliac arteries from the underlying veins distal to the aneurysm. You can clamp them vertically later without always freeing them completely from the underlying vein. This assures distal control of the aneurysm. Avoid the ureters.

COMMENT: *Secondary aneurysms can be present in one or both common iliac arteries. Save at least one hypogastric artery for blood supply to the pelvic organs. Coincidental occlusive disease may be present and may require local endarterectomy. Long occlusions may be bypassed by connecting the end of the graft to the side of the iliac artery distal to the occlusion.*

6. Control is now assured proximally and distally. With the aortic clamp in position but with the jaws open, rapidly inject into the aorta through a No. 18 needle, 3,000 units (30 mg.) of heparin in 30 ml. of saline solution. Close the aortic clamp immediately. Clamp the iliac arteries with toothed bulldog or other suitable clamps.

Opening of aneurysm and preparation for anastomosis

1. Incise the sac longitudinally as diagrammed in Fig. 3-3, *B* and scoop out the contents.

2. Ligate orifices of bleeding vessels that enter the sac. Usually several pairs of lumbar arteries and the inferior mesenteric artery will bleed briskly. Figure-of-eight-stitch ligatures may not close the orifice until rigid plaque is peeled away.

3. Cut transversely at the neck of the aneurysm, leaving a cuff of the sac. When the posterior wall is free from the spine, it is safely divided and end-to-end anastomosis is performed.

4. Leave a generous cuff distal to the aortic clamp (Fig. 3-3, *D*). The proximal part of the anastomosis can be performed inside the cuff of the proximal portion of the aorta.

Aortic anastomosis

1. Select a prosthesis with a proximal diameter matching that of the severed aorta. Shorten the prosthesis proximally so that the bifurcation will be at the same or at a higher level than that of the excised aorta. Do not cut the iliac ends of the graft at this time.

2. Begin the anastomosis of the aorta and graft with a mattress suture (Fig. 3-3, *E*). On thick-walled aneurysms, use 3-0 Dacron suture (Ti-Cron, Tevdek) with a large needle. These large needle and suture holes will not leak in thick-walled structures, and the sutures can be pulled so that they are very snug. Sutures are placed first through the prosthesis and then through the proximal portion of the aorta. Suspend the graft superiorly. Sew the posterior edges together with an everting continuous over-and-over stitch, with the sutures placed 1.5 to 2 mm. apart and 3 to 5 mm. from the edge of the aorta. To prevent leakage, pull each stitch until it is snug. It is preferable to sew from the prosthesis toward the aorta.

Lower the prosthesis into the abdomen and complete the anterior row of sutures in the same fashion (Fig 3-3, *G*).

COMMENT: *Occasionally the aortic cuff is quite large and requires a large prosthesis. Double layers of stitches are useless if the artery is very fragile, and a single layer of continuous over-and-over sutures holds the edges well when placed 3 mm. or more from the edge of the artery. The aortic anastomosis may be disrupted when the wall has been weakened by removal of a calcific plaque. This problem is met by covering the aortic anastomosis and proximal part of the aorta with a sleeve of prosthetic material from the remainder of the graft (Fig. 3-10).*

3. Preclot the prosthesis under pressure as follows: Pinch the ends of the prosthesis with the fingers. Momentarily release the aortic clamp in order to flush out the aorta and to force blood through the pores under pressure. Aspirate excess blood and blood clots from the prosthesis, and then cover it with gauze soaked in bacitracin solution. When the correct preclotting procedure is used, there is little leakage from the DeBakey Dacron prosthesis.

COMMENT: *The newer grafts with greater porosity leak more under pressure and should be preclotted under pressure several times.*

Iliac anastomosis

COMMENT: *This technique of iliac anastomosis may be adapted to the aorta, popliteal artery, or other vessels. The vertical end-to-end anastomosis described below is the most widely applicable type. Special situations will be discussed later. Avoid the common error of leaving the prosthesis too long, and allow for about 10% lengthening when it is filled under normal blood pressure. If this is not anticipated, the prosthesis may lengthen and bow anteriorly as it is stretched by the pressure of the restored blood flow. If local endarterectomy of calcified plaque has weakened the artery wall, slip a loose sleeve of the graft over this limb of the prosthesis. This will be slipped down over the completed anastomosis (Fig. 3-10, C).*

1. Shorten the iliac limb of the prosthesis. Clamp the iliac limb of the prosthesis vertically, and stretch it to meet the divided iliac artery. Replace the bulldog clamp on the iliac artery with a long-handled arterial clamp also applied vertically, so that the tip of the clamp is at the middle of the posterior wall. The assistant holds the ends of the prosthesis and the artery together with the clamps while the anastomosis is begun.

COMMENT: *Other techniques are needed for dilated, narrowed, or occluded iliac arteries as discussed later and illustrated in Fig. 3-11.*

Place a double-armed suture of 4-0 Dacron from the prosthesis to the iliac artery, starting at the tips of the clamps posteriorly (Fig. 3-4, A). Tie the suture while the assistant holds the ends in approximation with the clamps. Rotate the clamps sufficiently, about 90 degrees, to gain access to the sutures and begin the medial row (Fig. 3-4, B).

2. Suture the medial side of the prosthesis and the artery together with a continuous over-and-over stitch using one of the needles. Sew from the prosthesis toward the artery. Place the sutures 2 mm. apart and 2 mm. from the edge of the vessels and pull them until they are snug.

3. Rotate the arterial clamps to gain access to the lateral side (Fig. 3-4, C) and perform the anastomosis in the same fashion as on the medial side (Fig. 3-4, D). Release the distal clamp to check back bleeding before completing the anastomosis. Join the medial and lateral sutures anteriorly and tie them with a secure knot.

Restoration of blood flow to first leg

1. Flush the completed iliac anastomosis in a retrograde direction by briefly releasing the clamp on the iliac artery (Fig. 3-4, E).

2. Flush the proximal portion of the aorta through the uncompleted iliac end as follows: Apply an arterial clamp near the bifurcation on the finished side, and release the aortic clamp briefly to flush possible clots from the prosthesis (Fig. 3-4, F).

3. Open flow to the first leg as follows. Quickly reapply the clamp to the open limb of the graft. Slowly remove the clamp on the aorta to establish blood flow to the first limb (Fig. 3-4, G).

COMMENT: *Hypotension may result unless the aortic clamp is released very slowly over a five-minute period. Blood should be running rapidly at this time. Ample intravenous infusion of saline or lactated Ringer's solution in the amounts of 3 to 6 liters may be necessary during the operation to prevent declamping shock. Central venous pressure is monitored to prevent overloading of the circulation.*

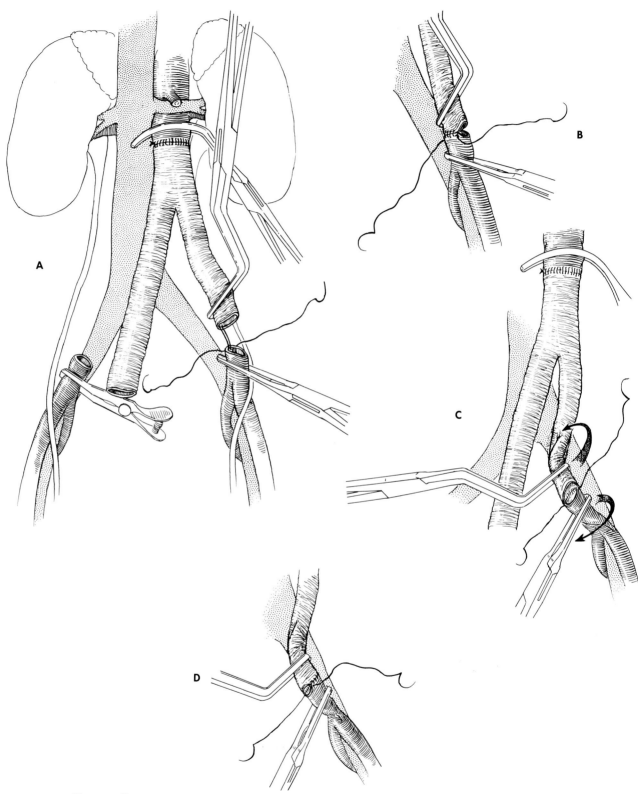

Fig. 3-4. Iliac anastomoses. **A** to **D**, First iliac anastomosis. **A**, Placement of mattress suture. **B**, Medial row. **C**, Medial row completed. Rotation for lateral row. **D**, Lateral row.

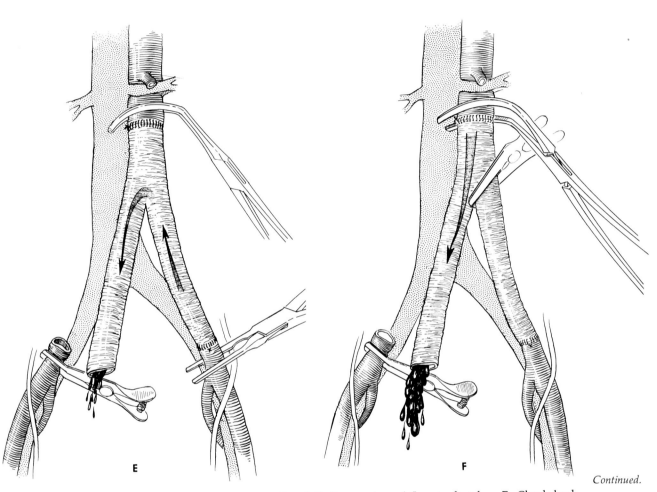

E

F

Continued.

Fig. 3-4, cont'd. Iliac anastomoses. **E** and **F**, Restoration of flow to first leg. **E**, Check back bleeding. **F**, Flush proximal aorta.

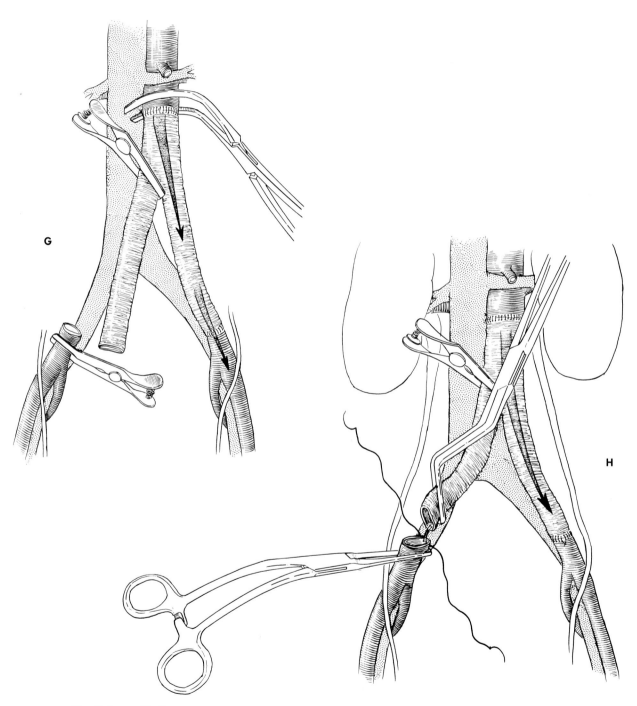

Fig. 3-4, cont'd. Iliac anastomoses. **G,** Clamp open limb of graft. Release aortic clamp slowly to restore flow to first leg. **H,** Begin remaining iliac anastomosis.

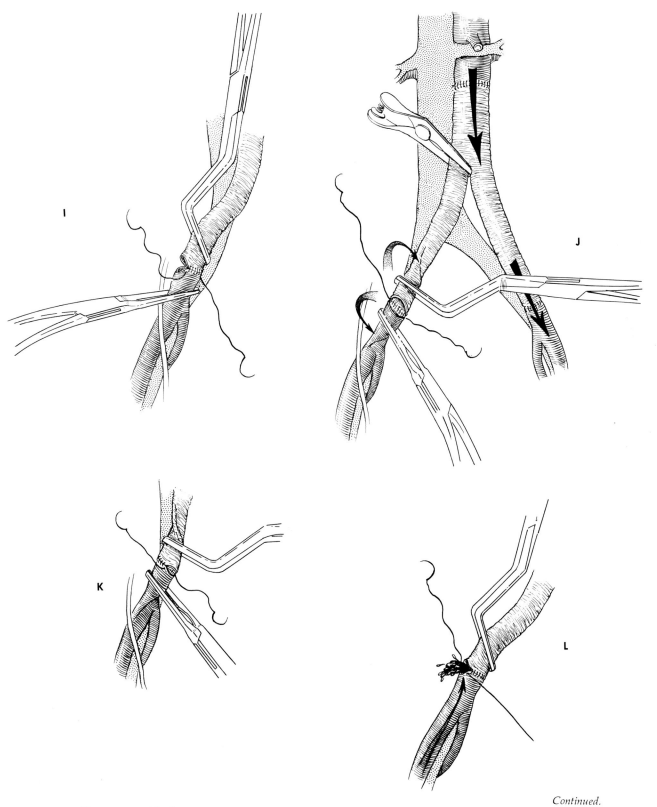

Continued.

Fig. 3-4, cont'd. Iliac anastomoses. **I** to **L,** Second iliac anastomosis. **I,** Medial row completed.
J, Rotation of clamps for access to lateral row. **K,** Lateral row of sutures partially completed.
L, Check back bleeding from leg by release of distal clamp.

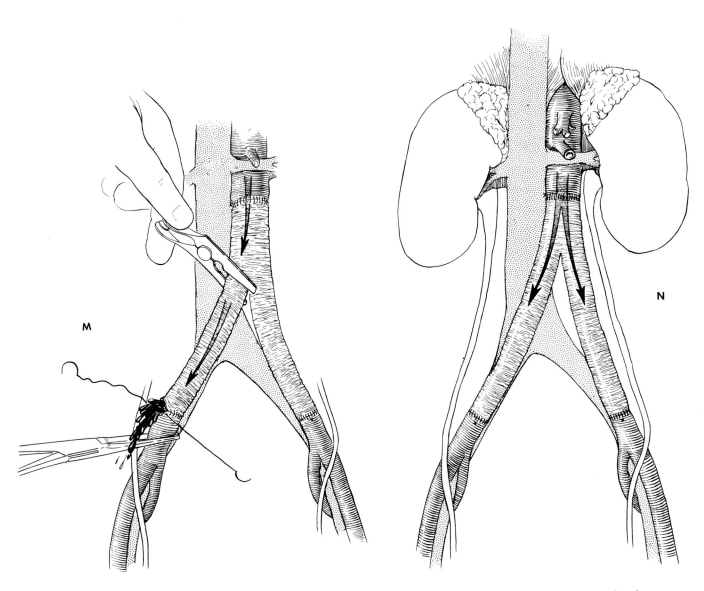

Fig. 3-4, cont'd. Iliac anastomoses. **M,** Flushing proximal aorta. **N,** Anastomosis completed and flow restored.

Second iliac anastomosis

1. Cut the remaining iliac limb of the prosthesis to the correct length. Clamp the vessels in a vertical direction. Have the assistant approximate the vessels. Place the mattress suture and tie it securely (Fig. 3-4, *H*).

2. Suture the medial side of the prosthesis and artery with a continuous over-and-over stitch, repeating step 2 under iliac anastomosis (Fig. 3-4, *I*).

3. Rotate the arterial clamps (Fig. 3-4, *J*), and suture the lateral side of the anastomosis in the same fashion as the medial side, repeating step 3 under iliac anastomosis (Fig. 3-4, *K*). Leave 1 cm. of the front of the anastomosis unfinished until the following flushing procedure is performed.

Restoration of blood flow to second leg

   1. Check back bleeding by removing the clamp from the iliac artery (Fig. 3-4, *L*). Then reapply the clamp.

   2. Briefly release the proximal iliac clamp on the second side and flush out the second iliac limb of the prosthesis (Fig. 3-4, *M*). Reapply this clamp proximally for a few moments to allow completion of the anastomosis. Now remove the distal clamp and allow the empty artery and prothesis to be filled with blood. Tie the suture to complete the anastomosis. (See Fig. 3-4, *N*.)

   3. Remove the proximal clamp slowly to restore pulsatile blood through the new anastomosis and into the second leg. Cover the prostheses and anastomoses with gauze soaked in bacitracin. To prevent hypotension at this point, it may be advisable to transfuse rapidly a unit or more of blood.

   COMMENT: *The flushing technique should be done carefully, since it is essential to remove atheromatous debris, clots, and sludge proximal to the aortic clamp. If occlusion time has been prolonged, clots can also form distally, and these must be detected and removed. Back bleeding is encouraged by brisk pressure or massage over the femoral triangle. Distal embolism or thrombosis is prevented by the routine use of Fogarty catheters placed down the iliac and femoral arteries and withdrawn immediately before closure. Flushing out the air in the graft prevents air embolism so that pulses in the feet are restored promptly. Leaking pores are covered with Gelfoam temporarily.*

Closure

   The prosthesis must be covered with living tissue and must not be permitted to lie against the jejunum or the duodenum. Remnants of the posterior portion of the aneurysm sac, peritoneum, preaortic areolar tissue, and mesentery of the descending colon are available for suturing over the graft. Omentum is rarely needed but may be applied on top of the graft. If the omentum is short, it may be drawn through a hole in the transverse mesocolon. Coverage of the prosthetic graft with soft tissue is necessary to prevent accumulations of serum or blood and to allow fibroblasts to invade the meshwork and anchor the new intima or pseudointima in place. The ligament of Treitz has been divided, and the duodenum and upper jejunum lie to the right of the graft and should be separated from the prosthesis by preaortic tissues and omentum. Otherwise, aortoenteric fistulas from the anastomosis to the duodenum may form. We know of one iliocecal fistula. The interposition of soft tissue will prevent this complication.

   A tube gastrostomy with a Foley or Hurwitt triple-lumen gastrostomy catheter may be employed to avoid postoperative distension.

Postoperative care

   1. Do not use anticoagulants.

   2. Observe and chart extremity pulses hourly during the first twenty-four hours.

   3. Replace fluids and electrolytes and blood after careful consideration of cardiac status and renal status. Usually 3 liters of electrolyte solution such as lactated Ringer's solution are needed during surgery in addition to blood.

   4. Maintain prophylactic digitalization.

   5. Give antibiotics for five days to prevent pulmonary infections.

   6. Employ gastric suction for several days to prevent abdominal distension.

   7. Reoperate immediately if femoral pulses disappear.

   8. Prescribe intermittent-positive-pressure-breathing treatments.

Complications

Hemorrhage and embolism are almost always avoidable. Oliguria occurs infrequently unless the aorta has been occluded for long periods or hypotension occurs during the operation. Multiple small renal emboli and infarcts have been reported in patients with fatal oliguria. We have found pulmonary complications and abdominal distension infrequently since we abandoned the use of the nasogastric tube and substituted gastrostomy for gastrointestinal decompression.

Cardiac and cerebrovascular complications are the most common causes of postoperative deaths.

Lack of pedal pulses after an aortoiliac graft is also disturbing but may occur from peripheral vasoconstriction, in a stout patient, or from hypotension. In the past when in doubt, we opened the groin and uncovered the common femoral artery. Now the transcutaneous Doppler ultrasound technique makes exploration unnecessary in most cases by demonstrating adequate flow and pressure or the need for reexploration without further observation and delay.

Occlusion of one limb of the graft occurs if an anastomosis is not properly constructed or if the anastomosis was made to a stenotic artery with poor outflow. You may avoid reopening the abdomen in a critically ill patient and bypass the occlusion with a femorofemoral graft accross the pubis. (See Chapter 5.)

Interference with the blood supply of the colon, particularly the combination of ligation of the inferior mesenteric and both hypogastric arteries, may result in ischemia or gangrene of the sigmoid colon. Mucosal ulceration of the rectosigmoid produces a bloody diarrhea. The severity of this complication is lessened by preparation of the bowel. Fortunately, the collateral blood supply to the colon from the superior mesenteric artery via the marginal artery and the left colic-sigmoid arterial anastomoses as well as from the hemorrhoidal arteries via one hypogastric artery is almost always sufficient. Sigmoid ischemia not sufficient to produce necrosis or ulceration may be manifested as bloating, cramping, and diarrhea. Sigmoidoscopic examination reveals a change from normal pink mucosa to dusky cyanotic mucosa at or just above the rectosigmoid junction. (See pp. 98 and 99 for prevention and treatment.)

VARIATIONS IN ANEURYSMS OF ABDOMINAL AORTA

Fig. 3-5 shows some of the variations in abdominal aneurysms that may be encountered.

Aneurysms involving renal arteries

When the dilatation is moderate, resection is not needed. The method of external reinforcement described by Robicsek and associates makes anastomosis unnecessary. This is illustrated in Fig. 3-5, A to C. The reinforcing sleeve must fit well and be sutured so that it is snug. It requires circumferential mobilization of the aora. The sleeve of prosthesis will be a tube of Dacron 30 to 35 mm. in diameter, such as is used to replace thoracic aneurysms. If mural thrombosis extends up to the level of the renal arteries, then the aorta must be cross-clamped above them during the endarterectomy. (See Fig. 4-3, D.)

If the left renal vein is in the way of these maneuvers, bring the end of the aorta anterior to the left renal vein (Fig. 4-2, E), or it can be divided and ligated. As long as the tributaries are preserved, they provide sufficient outflow. If there is doubt, the divided renal vein may be resutured.

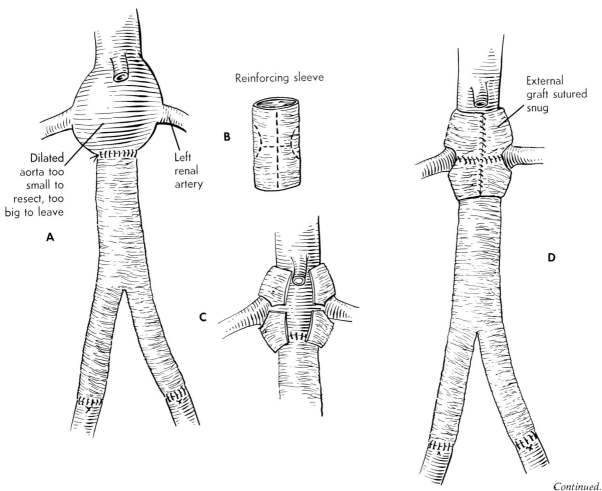

Fig. 3-5. A to D, External grafting of dilated aorta. A, Dilated aorta proximal to bifurcation graft. B, Reinforcing sleeve. Dotted lines show cut. C, Reinforcing sleeve applied and tailored well. D, Reinforcing sleeve sutured snugly.

Continued.

Tube grafts

Bifurcation grafts are not always necessary for abdominal aneurysms. In some cases the operation can be simplified by inserting a tube prosthesis of appropriate diameter into the distal and proximal cuff of the aneurysm. This is illustrated in Fig. 3-5, *E* to *H*. This simplifies the operation since only two anastomoses are needed instead of three, the aneurysm need not be dissected off the inferior vena cava, and the prosthesis is covered, padded, and separated from the duodenum by use of the sac. After control is accomplished proximally and distally, the aneurysm is opened boldly and the contents of the sac removed. The sac is trimmed at the sides and sutured over the prosthesis after debris and lining of the sac are curetted away. The orifices of the lumbar arteries and also the orifice of the inferior mesenteric artery are sutured if they bleed.

End-to-end anastomosis in presence of iliac aneurysm

At times aneurysmal dilatation of an iliac artery (Fig. 3-5, *K* and *L*) may require division of the artery near the junction of the internal and external iliac arteries.

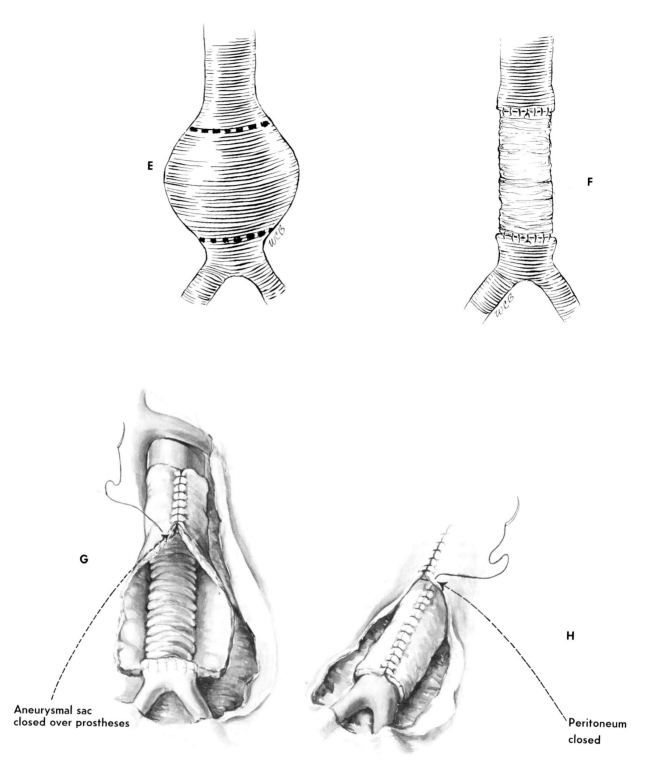

Aneurysmal sac
closed over prostheses

Peritoneum
closed

Fig. 3-5, cont'd. E, Small abdominal aneurysm. **F,** Tube graft for small abdominal aneurysm. **G,** Closure of aneurysm sac over prosthesis. It seldom needs to be trimmed. **H,** Closure of other tissue over sac need not be meticulous. (**A** to **F** redrawn from Robicsek, F., Daugherty, H. K., Mullen, D. C., Harbold, N. B., Jr., and Masters, T. N.: Is there a place for wall reinforcement in modern aortic surgery, Arch. Surg. **105:**824-829, 1972.)

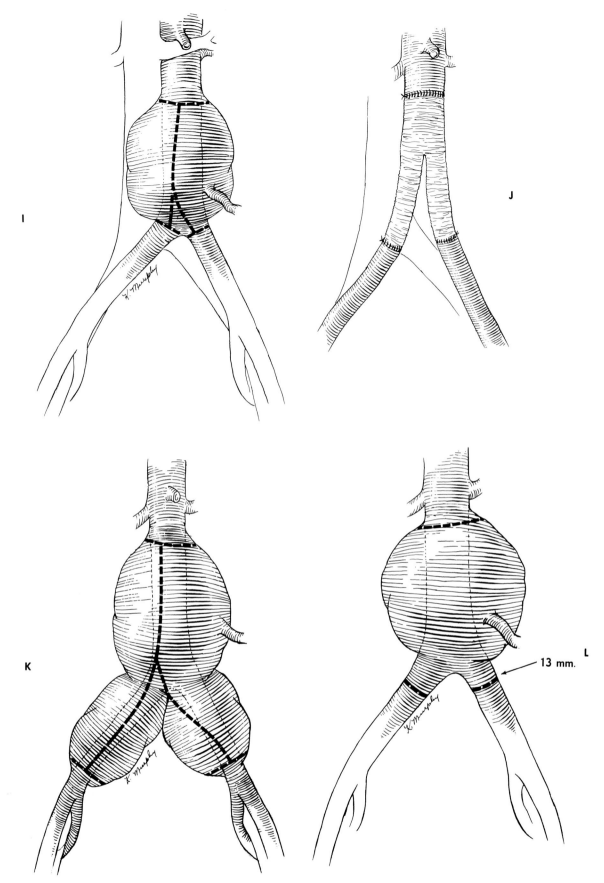

Fig. 3-5, cont'd. I to L, Alternative methods of anastomosis. I and J, Higher bifurcation making iliac anastomoses easier. K and L, Dilated iliac arteries.

Division of both hypogastric arteries should be avoided. The iliac arteries cannot be rotated a full 180 degrees. Therefore, the iliac clamps should be applied vertically and anastomosis begun posteriorly and carried forward on either side. Because this technique of anastomosis is so convenient, we prefer it to all other techniques and use it most frequently. (See Fig. 3-4, *A* to *D*.)

At least one hypogastric artery should be saved to avoid ischemia of the colon. Flow to both hypogastric arteries should be restored whenever possible. It is unnecessary to resect the large iliac sacs. The end of the bifurcation graft is sutured into the cuff of the distal end of the iliac artery. After the clot and lining of the aneurysms have been removed, the sac can be trimmed and sutured over the prosthesis.

COMMENT: *The details of suturing are less important than snug coaptation of the edges through sturdy tissue. During completion of the anastomoses, the clamps are released following the maneuvers already detailed to flush out any debris or accumulated clots proximal and distal to the anastomotic sites. (See Fig. 3-4, E, F, and L.)*

BLEEDING ANEURYSMS OF ABDOMINAL AORTA
Introduction

The usual terminal event of abdominal aortic aneurysm is bleeding. Once leakage of blood has commenced, further disruption of the wall of the aneurysm, hemorrhage, irreversible shock, and death may be expected. In some instances the rupture and hemorrhage progress slowly. There may be a few hours or even days before death, and in this interval accurate diagnosis and early surgery offer some hope of survival for these patients.

When it is suspected that an aneurysm has ruptured, the patient should be taken to the operating room immediately and resuscitation begun there while other preparations are under way. The operation differs from the elective operation because of the need to stop hemorrhage quickly by clamping the aorta above the aneurysm. Isolation of the aorta below the renal arteries by the method described earlier is usually feasible, but at times proximal control of the bleeding may be obtained only by the transthoracic route. Manual compression of the neck of the aneurysm below the renal arteries is unsatisfactory during dissection of that region. Although the transabdominal route is more accessible, the transthoracic route may be necessary when a large amount of intra-abdominal bleeding has occurred.

Operation should not be denied to any patient who is a reasonable risk, since the outlook is hopeless without surgery. Patients who are poor risks for elective resection of an aneurysm are usually beyond any surgical help following rupture.

Diagnosis

A pulsating abdominal mass is usually obvious. Back pain is an early sign of bleeding in some patients. Signs of blood loss may not occur for several hours or until the aneurysm ruptures into the free peritoneal cavity. As a rule, the pulsating hematoma is confined to the retroperitoneal tissues and is more prominent on the left side. Although the aneurysm most often ruptures at the point where it is thinned out by contact with the vertebras, we have observed rupture into the duodenum, and rupture into the inferior vena cava has been reported.

Anesthesia

General anesthesia is essential. Induction should be accomplished rapidly and without straining. Rapid blood replacement as indicated should accompany the anesthetic. It is sometimes necessary to use type-specific uncrossmatched blood.

Normal blood pressure may not be obtainable until control of the proximal portion of the aorta has been achieved.

Procedure

Proximal control of aorta just below diaphragm

A hematoma, a very high sac, or an anterior sac that covers the left renal vein may prevent a safe approach to the aorta below the renal vein and the renal arteries until proximal control can be obtained at a higher level. In thin patients, the aorta may be identified and clamped as it emerges beneath the diaphragm. In obese patients or when bleeding is very active, transthoracic control is safer and faster.

1. Extend the abdominal incision as high as possible, and excise the xiphoid process (Fig. 3-6, A).
2. Elevate the left lobe of the liver with Weinberg or Harrington retractors.
3. Divide the gastrohepatic omentum high, near the esophagus and above the left gastric artery.
4. Push the esophagus to the left with your fingers (Fig. 3-6, B).
5. Palpate the aorta lying between the crura of the diaphragm.
6. Apply a long straight arterial clamp vertically to occlude the aorta (Fig. 3-6, C).
7. Release the clamp when control of the aorta has been obtained above the aneurysm and below the renal arteries.

Transthoracic supradiaphragmatic control of aorta

1. Make an anterolateral submammary incision in the sixth or seventh interspace (Fig. 3-7, A). Tilt the operating table so that the left side of the chest is anterior.
2. Insert the rib spreader, retract the lung upward, and identify the pulsating aorta. For immediate control of bleeding, press the aorta against the vertebras.
3. Retract the diaphragm downward, open the pleural reflection over the aorta, and dissect about it with your fingers.
4. Apply the Crafoord clamp or another suitable clamp to the aorta (Fig. 3-7, B).
5. Begin the abdominal operation, and obtain control of the abdominal aorta below the renal arteries as soon as possible.
6. Release the aortic clamp in the chest when the abdominal aorta has been clamped above the aneurysm and below the renal arteries.

Resection of bleeding aneurysms

The technique of resection of a bleeding aneurysm resembles that of the elective operation except that the presence of a hematoma requires technical modifications: first, rapid proximal control of the neck of the aneurysm and, later, the intrasaccular anastomosis and reconstruction. The hematoma obscures the usual landmarks.

1. Make a midline incision speedily (Fig. 3-8, A). Divide the ligament of Treitz immediately. The hematoma usually will obscure all other landmarks. Retract the duodenum and small bowel mesentery to the right. Incise the peritoneum over the neck of the sac (Fig. 3-8, B).

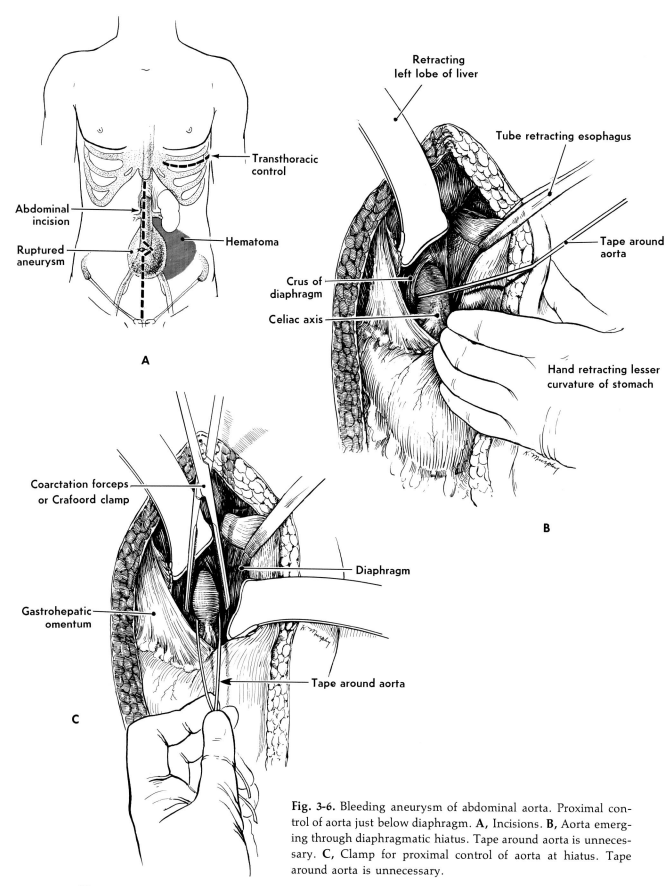

Fig. 3-6. Bleeding aneurysm of abdominal aorta. Proximal control of aorta just below diaphragm. **A,** Incisions. **B,** Aorta emerging through diaphragmatic hiatus. Tape around aorta is unnecessary. **C,** Clamp for proximal control of aorta at hiatus. Tape around aorta is unnecessary.

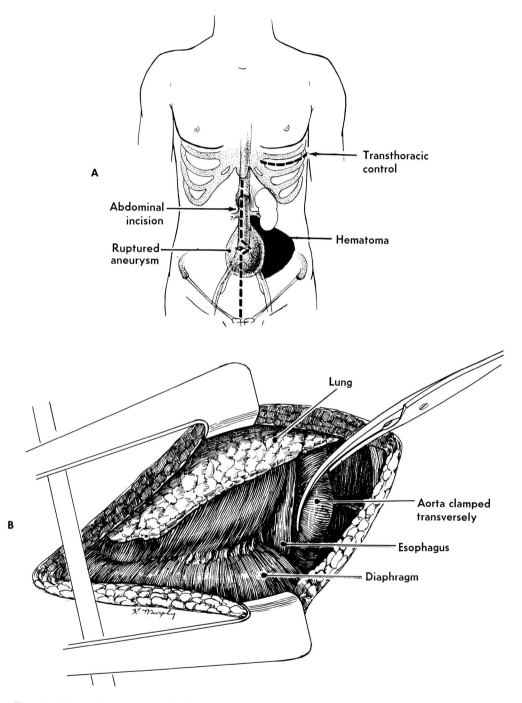

Fig. 3-7. Transthoracic control of aorta for bleeding abdominal aneurysm. **A,** Intercostal incision, supine view. **B,** Anterolateral view of aorta and adjacent structures through sixth or seventh rib intercostal incision. Operating table tilted to right.

89

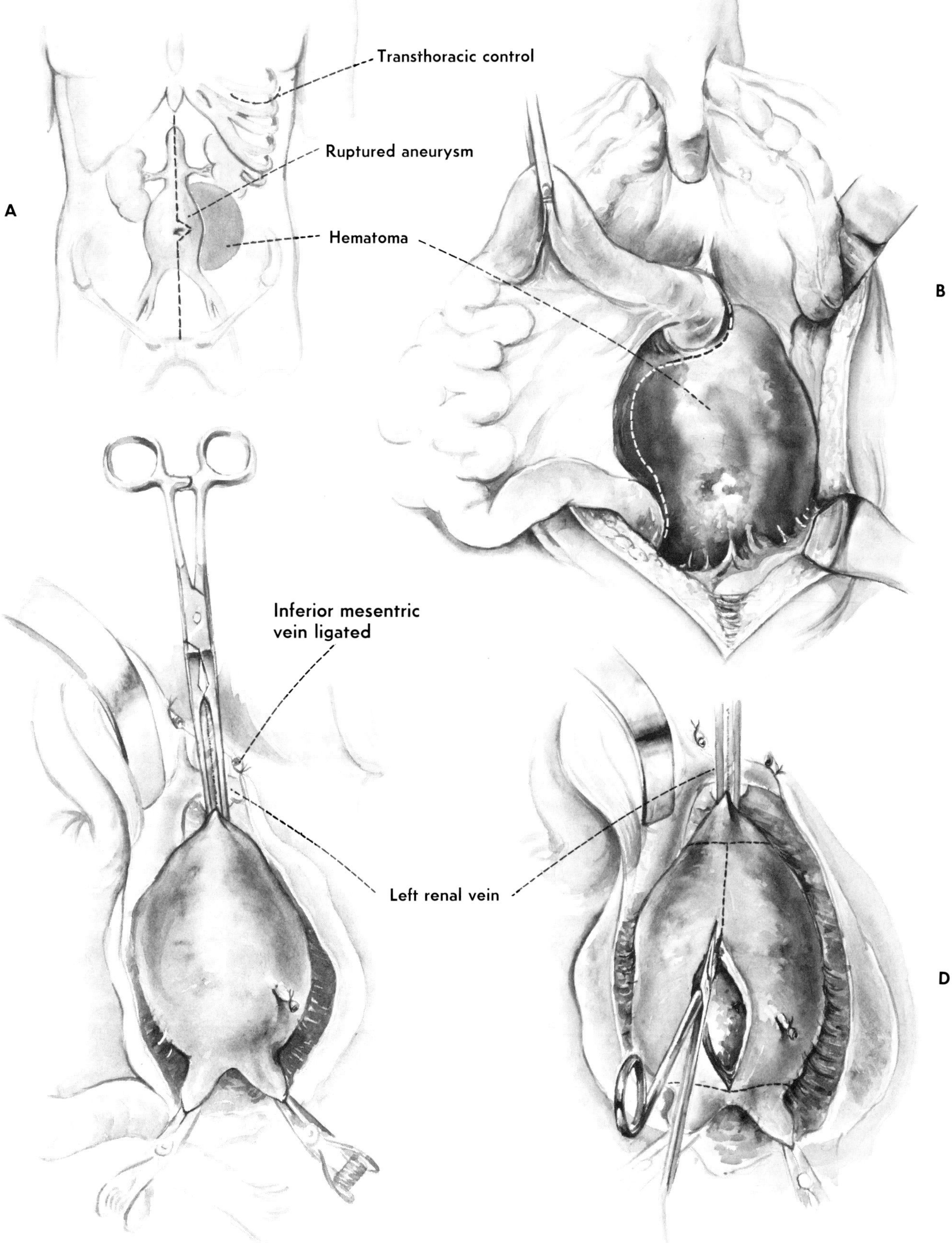
Transthoracic control
Ruptured aneurysm
Hematoma
A
B
Inferior mesentric vein ligated
Left renal vein
C
D

Fig. 3-8. Resection of bleeding aneurysm. **A,** Incision. **B,** Peritoneal incision over hematoma. **C,** Proximal control of aorta below renal arteries. **D,** Open aneurysmal sac.

2. Dissect with the fingertips alongside the neck of the aneurysm down to the spine and apply a large clamp vertically at the inferior border of the pancreas (Fig. 3-8, C).

COMMENT: *When the hematoma obscures the landmarks, it has already begun the dissection for you. Worry about the left renal vein and the renal arteries after the clamp is on and the bleeding is stopped.*

3. Boldly open the aneurysm hematoma and sac and evacuate its contents (Fig. 3-8, D). Now you have room to work and can more easily identify and cross-clamp the iliac arteries.

4. Isolate and clamp the iliac arteries at any convenient site. Beware of ureters concealed by hematoma.

5. Lumbar arteries may continue to bleed into the sac. These are easily sutured inside the sac.

6. Inspect the neck of the sac inside and out. Look for orifices of renal arteries, which will usually ooze and bleed. Sometimes it is advisable to replace the clamp slightly higher or lower. On the outside of the cuff, identify the left renal vein. It can be ligated or repaired if damaged. The inferior mesenteric vein must be ligated if torn.

7. Trim the cuff of the sac and perform the anastomosis up in the neck of the sac close to the vertical aortic clamp.

Aortic anastomosis—intrasaccular

It is unnecessary to divide the posterior wall of the sac, and frequently it is unwise to attempt to do so. When the sac is adherent to the spine, a troublesome plexus of veins is encountered between the spine and the aorta.

1. Peel and scrape intima from the posterior wall at the site of the anastomosis, leaving the flexible, tough fibrous tissue, which will be gathered into the suture line (Fig. 3-9, A).

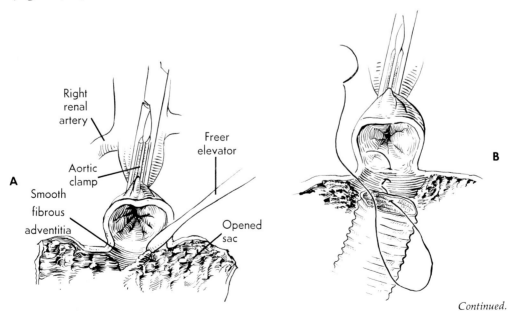

Continued.

Fig. 3-9. Resection of abdominal aneurysm—intrasaccular anastomosis. **A,** Endarterectomy at distal edge of posterior wall. **B,** Gather wide cuff of fibrous tissue with first suture.

91

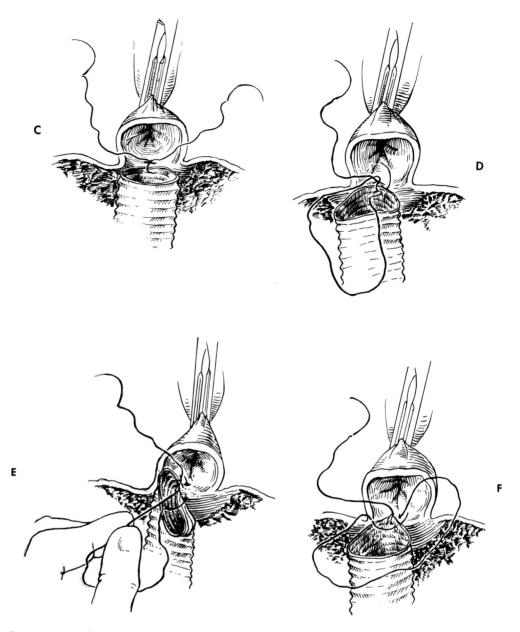

Fig. 3-9, cont'd. Resection of abdominal aneurysm—intrasaccular anastomosis. **C,** Tie knot in lumen. **D,** Pass needle close to end of prosthesis. **E,** Pull suture so that it holds edge of prosthesis back while needle gathers wide cuff of fibrous tissue. **F,** Repeat **D.**

COMMENT: *Cautery is useful to stop bleeding from the edge of the sac.*

2. Select a Dacron bifurcation graft of suitable size. The woven type does not leak and needs no preclotting, and it may be preferable for ruptured aneurysms. The type that is 19 or 22 mm. in diameter fits in almost all cases.

3. Begin the anastomosis with a sturdy wide bite of the fibrous sac, and tie the knot inside the lumen (Fig. 3-9, *B* and *C*). Use 3-0 Dacron sutures with a large T-5 needle.

92

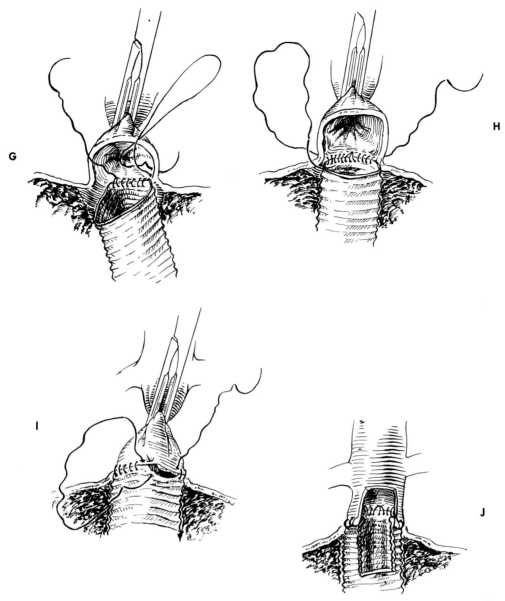

Fig. 3-9, cont'd. Resection of abdominal aneurysm—intrasaccular anastomosis. **G,** Complete left posterior row inside lumen and pass needle outside of aorta. **H,** Complete posterior row and bring both needles outside of aorta ready to sew from graft to aorta. **I,** Sew anteriorly from graft to aorta and tie together in front. **J,** Cutaway view of anastomosis.

4. Pass the needle through close to the edge of the prosthesis (Fig. 3-9, *D*); then pull the suture so that it holds the edge of the prosthesis back out of the way while the needle is inserted through the flexible posterior bare fibrous wall, 1 cm. from the intimal edge (Fig. 3-9, *E*).

5. Complete the posterior part of the anastomosis inside the sac in this fashion until you reach the corner (Fig. 3-9, *F*).

6. At the corner (Fig. 3-9, *G*), pass the needle outside on the cuff of the aorta

and then continue to sew over and over from the graft to the aorta (Fig. 3-9, *I*) with a narrow edge of the woven prosthesis and a deep cuff of the aorta.

7. Tie the sutures together where they join in the front. The edge of the prosthesis is up inside a sturdy wide cuff (Fig. 3-9, *J*).

8. Flush the graft momentarily and test the suture line by pinching the ends of the prosthesis and releasing the aortic clamp momentarily. Do not waste blood. Empty the graft by suction or by milking.

Distal anastomosis to iliac arteries

Perform the distal anastomosis by the same method, using wide, deep, secure bites with sturdy 3-0 or 4-0 suture. Review Fig. 3-4.

Closure

Closure is the same as that in elective cases. Irrigate with bacitracin solution. Cover the prosthesis with the sac sutured loosely in place. There will be abundant oozing from the raw areas of the hematoma. A tube gastrostomy is essential to avoid abdominal distension.

Postoperative care

The most serious complication is oliguria. Prolonged hypotension, multiple transfusions, temporary cross clamping of the aorta above the renal arteries, and preexisting renal disease may all contribute to renal failure. Hourly observation of the urine volume and of the hematocrit value is advisable during the period immediately after surgery. The central venous pressure is the best guide for blood and fluid replacement. Several liters of balanced electrolyte solution and blood should be supplied as needed to keep central venous pressure less than 10 cm. and to maintain adequate urinary output. Other postoperative measures are identical with those for elective resection. Mannitol is also indicated for diagnosis and treatment of oliguria.

COMBINATIONS OF ANEURYSMS OF ABDOMINAL AORTA AND OCCLUSIVE DISEASE
Endarterectomy of proximal portion of aorta and reinforcement of suture line

Aneurysm, occlusive disease, and calcific disease of the arterial walls fairly commonly occur in combinations, so that modifications of technique are required. The usual location of the calcific plaque is on the posterior wall of the proximal part of the aorta or along the posterior walls of the iliac arteries. Calcific plaques frequently cannot be removed or sutured without weakening the aortic wall or the suture line. If possible, resection through such plaques should be avoided.

If the arterial wall near the suture line has been weakened by calcific plaques and higher resection is not feasible, it is wise to reinforce the area with a sleeve of the unused prosthetic material. The need for this is best anticipated before the iliac anastomosis is made. Then the snap-tight cuff can be slipped over the anastomosis, as shown in Fig. 3-10, *B*. When an anastomosis must be reinforced after flow is restored, cut open the remaining cylinder of the prosthesis (Fig. 3-10, *D*), pass it under the anastomosis, and suture it snugly with a continuous everting mattress suture (Fig. 3-10, *E*). Trim off any extra prosthesis, leaving a 2 mm. cuff (Fig. 3-10, *F*).

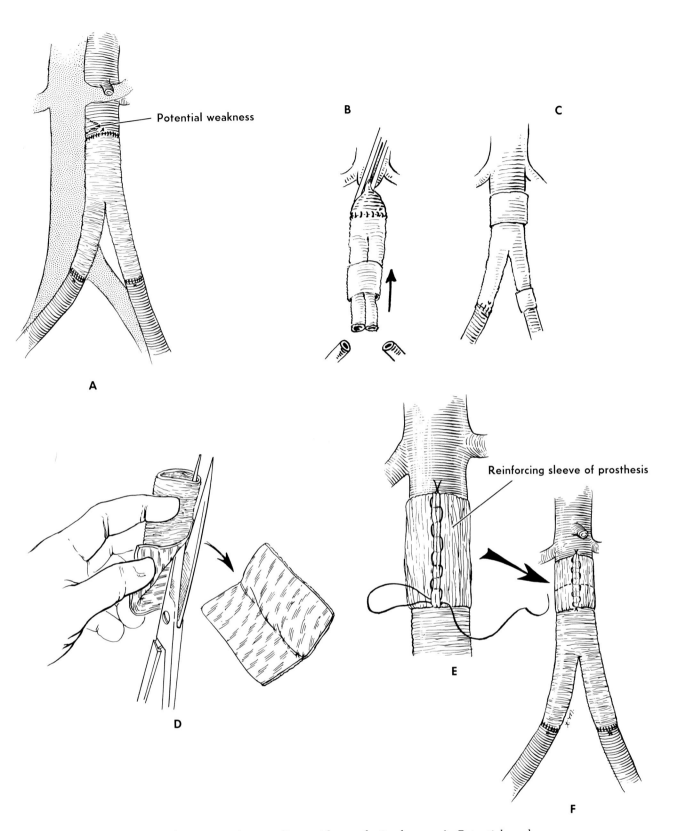

Fig. 3-10. Reinforcement of suture lines with prosthetic sleeves. **A,** Potential weakness near aortic suture line. **B,** Prosthetic sleeve slipped up to reinforce. **C,** Prosthetic sleeve in place: snap-tight reinforcement. **D** to **F,** Prosthetic sleeve sutured over anastomosis. (**B** and **C** redrawn from Sapirstein, W.: Surgery **70**:744-745, 1971.)

Endarterectomy of iliac arteries

Occasionally the iliac arteries must be transected through atherosclerotic plaques (Fig. 3-11, *A*). The atherosclerotic plaques are usually on the posterior wall and may extend far down into the internal and external iliac vessels. After endarterectomy is done, the end of the prosthetic tube is anastomosed to the end of the artery. The snap-tight cuff reinforcement is very helpful after endarterectomy like this.

The intimal plaque is detached from the media by blunt dissection with a small periosteal elevator (Freer). The plane of cleavage between the intima and media is usually obvious (Fig. 3-11, *B*).

Cut the edge of the plaque from the normal intima with a small scissors (Fig. 3-11, *C*). Evert the artery if necessary to permit more accurate dissection (Fig. 3-11, *D* and *E*). The long thin extension on the posterior arterial wall need not be totally excised and may be transected, beveled, and attached by suture.

Suture the remaining intima to the media of the artery (Fig. 3-11, *F*). Arterial sutures, 4-0 or 5-0, with needles at both ends are useful for this procedure. Pass the needles from within outward, pushing the intima toward the media and tying the suture outside the artery.

COMMENT: *Extensive iliac endarterectomy is unnecessary. If the calcific plaque on the posterior wall of the iliac artery is extensive, endarterectomy may be unsafe. In such instances, close the common iliac artery proximally and join the iliac limb of the prosthesis to the soft anterior surface of the artery at a more distal point.*

Bypass operations

The bypass procedure (Fig. 3-11, *H*) avoids extensive endarterectomy and avoids sacrifice of the hypogastric artery. As a rule, the proximal end of the iliac artery would be oversewn rather than simply ligated, as shown in the drawings. The bypass procedures described in Chapter 4, that is, aortoiliac and aortofemoral, may be needed when stenosis accompanies aneurysms.

COMPLICATIONS OF ABDOMINAL AORTIC GRAFTS
Ischemia and necrosis of bowel

Ischemia of the left colon is a rare but frequently catastrophic complication of abdominal aortic grafting. It can occur after any type of abdominal aortic grafting but is most common with ruptured aneurysms. Fortunately, it is rare even with those and occurs in less than 2% of all cases of aortic grafts in large vascular surgical centers. In abdominal aortic grafting, the inferior mesenteric artery is always ligated and usually the inferior mesenteric vein is also. As in most complications, the best treatment is prevention, and the following precautions should be taken:

1. The inferior mesenteric artery must be ligated proximal to the left colic branch, and in aneurysms, it generally must be ligated inside the sac.

2. One or both hypogastric arteries must be preserved and must be perfused either from a graft attached proximally in the common iliac or retrograde by a graft attached in the external iliac or common femoral arteries.

Ischemia of the colon, however, may occur in spite of these precautions, with ruptured aneurysms, because of the hematoma in the mesentery, retraction of the mesentery of the sigmoid colon, or further damage during the dissection obscured by the hematoma. Hypotension also is a predisposing factor or etiological factor. Undue retraction of the left colon mesentery is best avoided by implanting the end

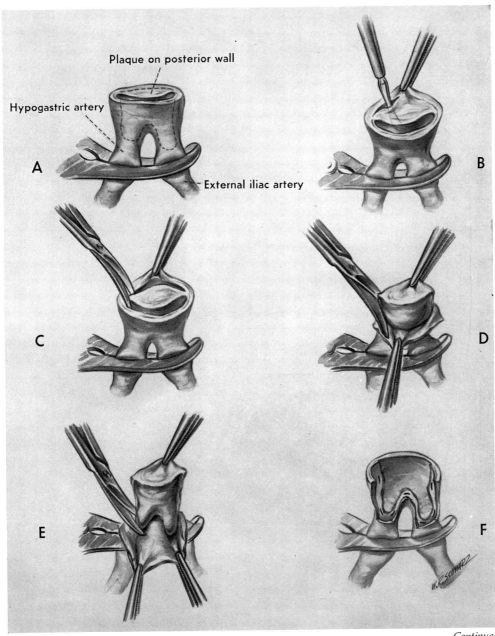

Fig. 3-11. **A** to **F**, Local endarterectomy of iliac artery bifurcation. **A**, Plaque extends distally. **B**, Develop cleavage plane between plaque and media. **C**, Cut attachment of plaque to normal intima. **D** and **E**, Evert artery if necessary to visualize plaque and its distal extensions. **F**, Cutaway view to show mattress sutures reattaching distal intimal edge.

Continued.

97

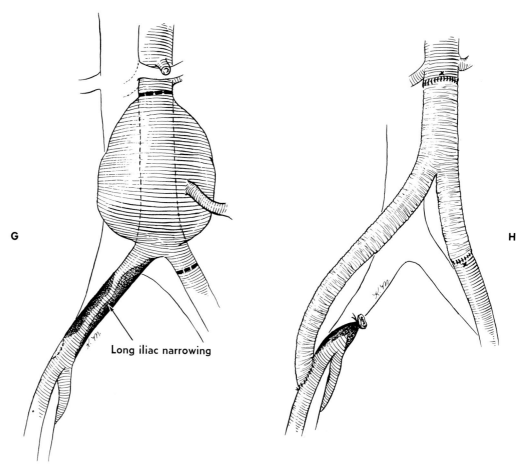

G

H

Long iliac narrowing

Fig. 3-11, cont'd. G, Combination of aneurysm and distal occlusive disease. H, Resection and bypass for extensive atherosclerosis of iliac artery distal to aneurysm.

of the bifurcation graft in the external iliac and suturing over the common iliac artery. The external iliac artery is much more accessible than the common iliac artery, particularly in the presence of hematomas. Embolism from sludge in the proximal clamp and embolism from thrombi loosened by dissection or manipulation of the sac before cross clamping of the neck of the ruptured aneurysm are also contributory in some cases.

Ischemia of the left colon is avoidable by reimplanting the inferior mesenteric artery when it is recognized that it is needed for collateral circulation. Anastomosis of the small artery is greatly facilitated by preserving a button of the aortic wall at its entrance. This button, which should be more than 1 cm. in diameter, is easily sutured to a slit in the prosthesis, and there is no narrowing of the artery itself by any sutures. Signs that reimplantation may be needed include (1) enlargement of the diameter of the inferior mesenteric artery to more than 3 mm., (2) poor back bleeding from the ostium of the inferior mesenteric artery when the aneurysm is open, and (3) a meandering mesenteric artery visible on the preoperative aortogram. Any of these signs signify that the inferior mesenteric artery is necessary for collateral circulation and should be reimplanted.

Ischemia of the colon may be of the following types: (1) ischemia involving only the mucosa, (2) ischemia leading to stricture that occurs when the deeper layers are damaged, and (3) early gangrene and perforation resulting when the full thickness of the colon has been deprived of its blood supply. The signs and symptoms vary, of course, with the degree of ischemia, its extent and location, and time of onset. The diagnosis early in the postoperative period is quite difficult because of the many other usual abdominal findings in the patient postoperatively. Diarrhea with or without blood should lead one to suspect the presence of colon ischemia. Sigmoidoscopy may show cyanosis early, or it may show friability of a mucous membrane and diffuse ulceration later. Other details are described in a recent paper by Ottinger and associates (1972).

Early closure of graft

Thrombosis or occlusion of one limb of an aortic graft may occur as a result of a technical error or because poor inflow or poor outflow was not corrected at the time of surgery. If the patient's condition was operable at the first try, the cause is probably still correctable provided that reoperation is performed promptly. Early in the postoperative period, pulses may be poor and the skin pale as the result of various problems, including hypovolemia due to insufficient fluid or blood replacement. Some vasoconstriction is seen occasionally also when prolonged operation with exposed bowel leads to hypothermia. The patient's temperature can drop several degrees as a result of the heat loss from the evaporation from bowel exposed more than an hour and a half. This hypothermia leads to vasoconstriction and poor pulses. Femoral pulses are normally palpable unless the patient is very stout, but the presence of peripheral pulses may be equivocal. In such a situation, the Doppler instrument has been a great help; it may demonstrate pulsatile flow that is reassuring and thus avoid an unnecessary exploration.

If femoral pulses are absent, however, and the leg appears to be in peril, exploration of the groin is clearly preferable to reopening the abdomen; exploration of the groin will permit thrombectomy and restoration of flow. Thrombectomy of the graft alone is not sufficient if an underlying basic cause is left uncorrected. In such an exploration, if the graft extends to the groin, the procedure of reopening the skin and making an incision in the prosthesis permits the use of the Fogarty catheters proximally and distally. If the prosthesis ends more proximally, an arteriotomy in the common femoral artery overlying the orifice of the profunda femoris artery permits the use of Fogarty catheters proximally up the external iliac, possibly into the graft itself, and distally down the superficial femoral and into the profunda femoris artery.

If flow cannot be restored through a proximal prosthesis, femorofemoral bypass grafting from the opposite femoral artery across the pubis through a subcutaneous tunnel will restore flow without the necessity of reopening the abdomen. Full details of this technique are described in Chapter 5.

Hemorrhage—disruption of anastomosis

Arterial anastomoses are subject to high pressures, and one bad stitch can cause massive hemorrhage. A loose stitch or a pucker or gap may cause leakage sometime later. Any leakage at the time of operation is readily detected and corrected. Calcific deposits in the arterial wall and rigidity of the arterial wall may prevent coaptation of the edges. Friability of thin, diseased arteries permits stitch holes sometimes to become slits or "buttonholes," causing leakage.

As always, prevention is preferable. Arterial stitches should be placed far from the edge and drawn until they are snug and placed in relatively sturdy arteries. Anastomoses may be reinforced with sleeves of prosthesis or by the snap-tight closure. This is particularly useful when endarterectomy of the artery adjacent to the anastomosis has been necessary and the remaining wall is thin and friable (Fig. 3-10, *A* to *C*).

Embolism or distal thrombosis

Embolism or distal thrombosis when recognized is easily corrected during the operation. It is best prevented by avoiding prolonged arterial occlusion. Injecting 3,000 units of heparin before cross-clamping the aorta is sufficient for one and one-half hours of occlusion time, which should be sufficient for most aortic grafting procedures. Thrombosis in the iliac or femoral arteries while the clamps are applied and anastomoses are performed may be detected at the operating table by testing the back bleeding. While the aorta is clamped, back bleeding from iliac arteries will be poor. Normally, thrombosis will not occur in any reasonable occlusion time. If there is doubt, however, the Fogarty catheters can easily be inserted distally before the iliac anastomosis is completed. The Fogarty catheters should be picked out and be in the operating room ready for use, but not necessarily on the operating table. After flow is restored to one iliac and hypogastric artery, back bleeding is much more profuse; but if for any reason, occlusion time has been prolonged, a passage of the Fogarty catheter gives assurance that thrombi did not form distally. Judgment of back bleeding even by experts is frequently fallacious, since it is subject to so many variables.

Embolism from the proximal part of the aorta may result from thrombi or cholesterol sludge churned up during the cross clamping of the aorta. Aortas in some patients have the appearance of tree bark, and ulcerated areas shed sludge that may cause renal emboli and renal failure. Complications from this are avoided by keeping the aortic occlusion time short and by flushing the aorta after the aortic and iliac anastomoses.

Postischemic swelling of extremities—fasciotomy

Prolonged ischemia may be followed by swelling of the muscles, which because it is confined beneath the sturdy deep fascia, results in compression of capillaries and venules and, ultimately, obliteration even of pedal pulses. This is discussed in more detail in Chapter 10. It occurs occasionally after restoration of flow when embolectomy has been delayed, but it is also occasionally seen after arterial grafting in cases of advanced occlusive disease. Some patients cannot tolerate even one and one-half hours of occlusion of the aorta and profunda femoris arteries without postischemic swelling. Such patients will have advanced stenosis or occlusion of the iliac as well as the common and superficial femoral and popliteal arteries.

Postischemic swelling has a latent period of three to six hours. The pulses that were present after the restoration of arterial flow begin to fade, and the normal color and venous filling gradually are replaced by signs and symptoms of ischemia, namely, pallor, numbness, coldness, and loss of pulses. The telltale sign, however, is the firmness of the calf muscle caused by the swelling. No swelling of the skin or subcutaneous tissue of the extremity is evident at this early stage.

The diagnosis is made by incision of the skin and fascia with the use of local anesthesia. Arteriograms are unnecessary and wasteful and cause only further delay. The diagnostic incision a few inches long can be made at the bedside with sterile technique; if pale muscle bulges through the fascial incision, the diagnosis is confirmed.

To relieve the pressure, lengthen the fascial incision by pushing the long scissors beneath the skin proximally and distally. This is called subcutaneous fasciotomy because the skin incision is only a few inches long. If you are in doubt about the adequacy of the small incision, make another small incision distally and push the scissors proximally and distally again.

All three muscle compartments must be opened. Vertical incisions a few inches long are made in the upper third of the leg, over the anterior tibial muscle and over the medial side and lateral side of the calf. In severe cases, it may be advisable to open the deep compartment containing the soleus muscle.

Occasionally, the edema and pressure are so severe that the skin is tight. These are usually cases of popliteal artery injuries with venous damage, trauma to the muscle, and postischemic swelling. In any type of case in which the skin is tight, the skin incisions are also lengthened as far as necessary. This is the so-called decompression dermotomy.

F.B.H.

References

Ottinger, L. W., Darling, R. C., Nathan, M. J., and Linton, R. R.: Left colon ischemia complicating aorto-iliac reconstruction, Arch. Surg. **105:**841-846, 1972.

Robicsek, F., Daugherty, H. K., Mullen, D. C., Harbold, N. B., Jr., and Masters, T. N.: Is there a place for wall reinforcement in modern aortic surgery, Arch. Surg. **105:**824-829, 1972.

4

Aortoiliac occlusive disease

INTRODUCTION

Signs and symptoms

The surgeon who undertakes vascular procedures must realize that the basic pathological process of arteriosclerosis is diffuse. When occlusion is segmental, surgical replacement or bypass procedures are applicable. Many elderly persons have extensive occlusive disease, particularly in the lower extremities, but live out their lives without acquiring gangrene because collateral circulation is adequate to maintain viability of the limbs. Patients without symptoms or with nonprogressive symptoms, particularly those in whom intermittent claudication is the sole symptom, may develop collateral circulation and do not require surgery unless symptoms become severe or progressive.

Atherosclerotic disease affecting the legs is usually most pronounced and is most likely to be segmental at the aortic bifurcation or nearby iliac artery, in the upper femoral artery near the origin of the profunda femoris branch, in the superficial femoral artery as it passes through the adductor canal, and in the distal end of the popliteal artery at the branching of the anterior tibial or posterior tibial arteries.

Symptoms of occlusive disease depend on the pattern, on the degree of narrowing or occlusion, and on the adequacy of collateral circulation. When blood flow is insufficient during exercise, fatigue or pain results; and this intermittent claudication is usually the first and perhaps the only symptom. Occlusion in the iliac artery produces claudication in the hip or thigh. If the bifurcation of the aorta is involved (Leriche's syndrome), the patient complains of claudication in both hips and thighs. Occlusion in the superficial femoral artery usually results in claudication in the calf. If occlusions are multiple, there may be insufficient blood flow at all times. Atrophy of skin and muscle develops, and ischemic neuritis causes pain even when the limb is at rest. Nonhealing ulcers develop after trivial trauma or injections. Sometimes occlusion involves the most important collateral vessels as well as the major artery. A frequent example of this is occlusive disease in the superficial femoral artery, with narrowing at the orifice of the profunda femoris branch.

In the general spectrum of occlusive arterial vascular disease amenable to surgical correction, however, aortoiliac occlusion is the area in which surgical operation is most successful.

Frequently the patients are relatively young (that is, under 60 years of age), and their atherosclerosis is localized to the terminal portion of the aorta and the common iliac vessels. On exploration, the vessel is found to be plugged with atheromatous debris of a soft rubbery consistency that is rather easily removed. There is very little secondary calcification, and intimectomy is sufficient to relieve the obstruction.

Contraindications to elective surgery

We do not operate on patients with minimal disease, and poor-risk patients or patients with a short life expectancy from other diseases should not be operated on. Patients with recent coronary occlusion, angina pectoris, or poor cardiac reserve in general are not surgical candidates unless the reasons for surgery are exceedingly compelling. Other degenerative diseases are common in this age group. Borderline renal function and obstructive pulmonary disease increase the risks of surgery considerably. The "pink puffer" may be carried through major surgery, but the "blue bloater" is an extremely poor risk. Blood gas determinations are useful. The surgeon has two important tasks: to evaluate these patients very carefully and to prevent and treat complications that may result from these associated diseases.

The most noteworthy failures in arterial reconstructive surgery in the lower limb occur in those patients in whom the popliteal artery and its branches are completely occluded at the time of operation. At times this information cannot be obtained preoperatively, or information obtained from preoperative angiography may prove to be unreliable. Operative angiography of the popliteal artery annd lower leg is helpful in such cases.

Summary

Successful vascular reconstruction requires adequate inflow and outflow. When the proper operation is performed and there are no technical errors, the long-term result will depend mainly on future progression or lack of progression of stenoses and occlusions. Fortunately, many patients do very well, but they remain at risk from cerebral, cardiac, and renal complications of the arteriosclerosis.

We are conservative in our treatment of patients who have partial or complete aortic occlusion and obvious widespread atherosclerosis. The extent of this disease is estimated by taking into account the patient's age, any history of previous vascular accidents, and a thorough physical examination directed toward vascular disease. Most of these patients have claudication, but this is not sufficient indication for major surgery. Patients with ulceration, gangrene, intermittent numbness, and severe pain on rest are in danger of acquiring gangrene and must have angiograms and arterial reconstruction by bypass or endarterectomy whenever feasible. Extensive reconstructive procedures (that is, those extending from the aorta to the popliteal artery) are seldom needed and should be staged.

AORTOILIAC ENDARTERECTOMY
Introduction

Open endarterectomy is the simplest and most effective surgical procedure for localized occlusive disease in the terminal portion of the aorta and in the common iliac arteries. The occluding atheromatous material almost always is found in both iliac arteries. Occlusive disease that extends down the iliac arteries past the hypogastric arteries may be better treated by the bypass technique than by endarterectomy.

The purpose of endarterectomy is to remove intraluminal atheromatous obstructions and to restore arterial flow to the extremities through the artery. In the terminal portion of the aorta and the proximal end of the iliac artery, atheromatous debris, a soft putty- or rubber-like material, can be removed in many instances by establishing a subintimal cleavage plane. The media and adventitia are effective conduits for blood after endarterectomy. The "peel" frequently includes media, and tags of media must not be left in the lining after endarterectomy.

The usual indication is disabling intermittent claudication. In addition to the usual general systemic contraindications in poor-risk patients and patients with cancer or other terminal disease, endarterectomy should not be attempted when there is calcification of the arteriosclerotic plaques or of the media of the artery. It is also usually unwise to pursue endarterectomy far into the iliac vessels.

Preoperative care

Preoperative arteriograms reveal the site and degree of obstruction. The terminal portion of the aorta and iliac arteries are visualized by percutaneous retrograde arteriography via a femoral artery if a femoral pulse is palpable or by translumbar aortic injection. Preoperative digitalization and bowel preparation are recommended.

Procedure
Exploration and evaluation

1. Place the patient in the supine position. Prepare and drape the entire abdomen, thighs, and legs.

2. Make a long midline incision from the xiphoid process to the pubis. As in other surgical procedures involving the aorta and the iliac arteries, wide exposure is essential. Expose and explore the aorta and the iliac arteries by incisions of the peritonium, mobilization and retraction of the small bowel, retraction of the sigmoid colon, and division of the ligament of Treitz as illustrated (Fig. 3-2) and described previously.

COMMENT: *Careful palpation of the aorta and iliac arteries will reveal the extent of disease. The occlusions are usually worse than anticipated from preoperative evaluation of angiograms. Widespread endarterectomy is usually unwise. The bifurcation prostheses should be sterile and immediately available in the event aortoiliac or aortofemoral bypass operation is preferable. A long, thin atherosclerotic plaque usually occupies the posterior wall of the iliac artery. This need not be followed distally but may be cut across as detailed later in this chapter.*

Proximal and distal control

1. Pass umbilical tapes about the aorta proximal to the occlusive process.

2. Pass umbilical tapes about the external iliac and hypogastric arteries distal to all palpable atherosclerotic plaques.

3. Select appropriate clamps to apply at the proximal and distal limits of the operation. Complete circumferential exposure of the aorta is unnecessary.

4. Dissect along the left side of the aorta and apply a bulldog clamp to the inferior mesenteric artery. This vessel may be divided if occlusive disease is high and if retraction of the sigmoid mesocolon is necessary for satisfactory exposure of the lumbar arteries.

5. Dissect behind the aorta, isolate and identify the paired lumbar vessels, and occlude them with bulldog clamps or with large *temporary* silk ligatures secured by a single knot.

104

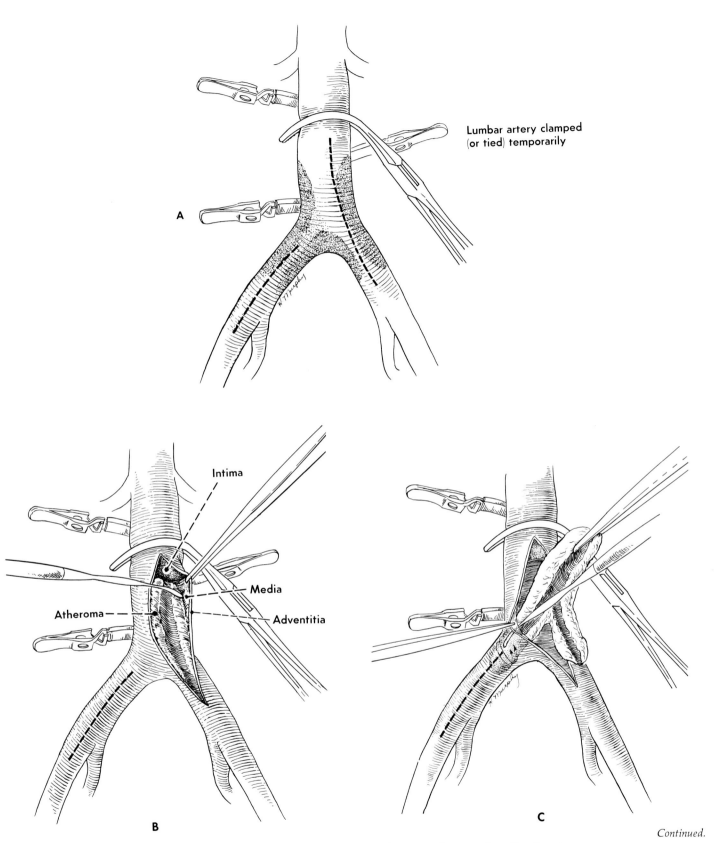

Lumbar artery clamped (or tied) temporarily

A

Intima

Media

Atheroma

Adventitia

B

C

Continued.

Fig. 4-1. Aortoiliac endarterectomy. A, Incisions. B, Plane between plaque and media of aorta. C, Free up plaque from other iliac artery from above.

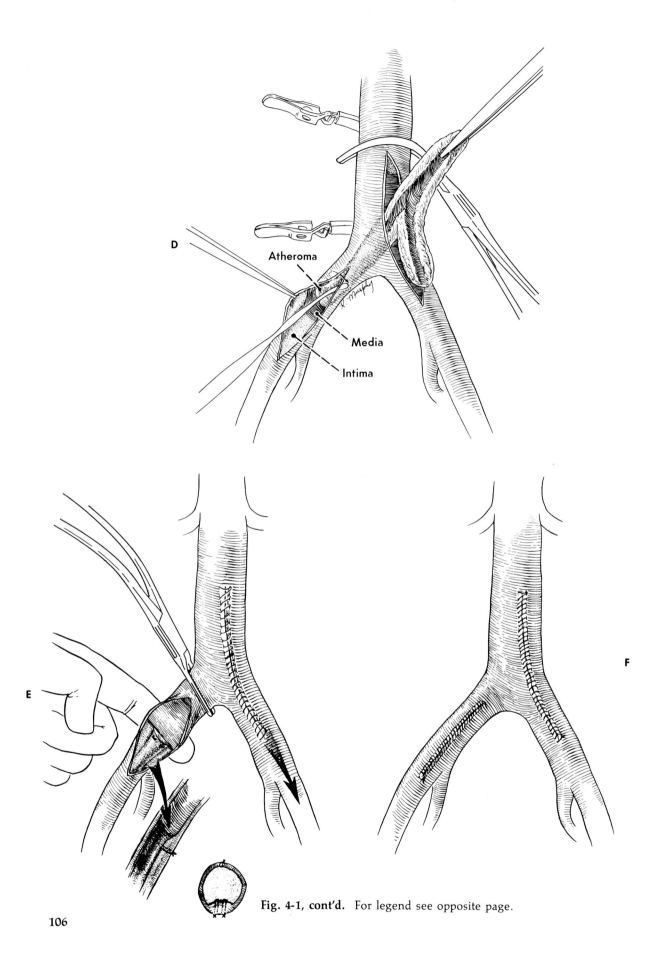

D

Atheroma

Media

Intima

E

F

Fig. 4-1, cont'd. For legend see opposite page.

Arteriotomies

1. Place the aortic clamp across the aorta superiorly. Before closing the clamp, inject 3,000 units (30 mg.) of heparin rapidly into the aorta just below the clamp and then immediately tighten the clamp. If occlusion time is over one hour, another supplementary dose of 20 to 30 mg. of heparin should be given intravenously. Apply clamps to iliac arteries distally. These are not shown in Fig. 4-1 in order to simplify the drawings.

COMMENT: *If aortic occlusion time exceeds ninety minutes, the atherosclerotic process was too extensive for endarterectomy and a bypass procedure would have been preferable.*

2. Incise the aorta vertically in the midline and extend the incision downward into the iliac artery on the side with the most extensive occlusion (Fig. 4-1, A).

3. Incise the other iliac artery (Fig. 4-1, A).

COMMENT: *The two incisions described should not join. An incision at the aortic bifurcation in the shape of an inverted Y is most undesirable. The two incisions are not joined so that a clamp may be applied between them on the proximal end of the iliac artery, and the long incision extending into the aorta may then be closed to restore flow to one leg during completion of the operation on the opposite iliac artery. The aortic incision should not extend too high, usually stopping within 3 cm. of the renal artery. Plaques and atheromas above this level can be removed from below. When disease does extend to the level of the renal arteries, additional exposure is necessary. In such an instance, the left renal vein must be dissected so that it is free and lifted from the anterior surface of the aorta. The origins of both renal arteries and the superior mesenteric artery must be exposed and temporarily occluded to prevent embolization of atherosclerotic debris loosened during the blind proximal endarterectomy.*

If it is discovered that endarterectomy must continue down to the groin, an incision should be made over the common femoral artery. Even though staged procedures are to be performed, it is desirable that the first operation restore flow as far distal as the profunda femoris artery. This vessel is seldom involved in the arteriosclerotic process except at its origin from the common femoral artery. Restoration of pulsatile blood flow into the profunda femoris artery is sufficient to preserve the leg.

Endarterectomy between the distal part of the iliac artery and the bifurcation of the common femoral artery is done with a wire loop or a Wylie or Leveen endarterectomy instrument passed between the femoral and iliac arteriotomies. It is tedious and unnecessary to open the full length of these arteries for open endarterectomy.

Endarterectomy

1. If occlusion is extensive and a groin incision has been made, endarterectomize the common femoral and iliac arteries by passing the endarterectomy loop upward from a longitudinal arteriotomy in the common femoral artery. At this point, remove

---

Fig. 4-1, cont'd. Aortoiliac endarterectomy. **D,** Dissect plaque from right iliac artery. **E,** Distal intima beveled and attached with suture. Insets show side view and cross section of plaque sutured in place. **F,** Arteriotomies sutured.

only easily accessible atheromatous material from the superficial femoral artery, and concentrate on restoring blood flow to the bifurcation of the common femoral artery and the profunda femoris artery.

2. Through the incision in the aorta, dissect the mass of atheromatous material extending down into the iliac artery (Fig. 4-1, B). In dissecting the mass, place traction on the inside atheroma, not on the arterial wall. The subintimal plane of cleavage is recognized by the appearance of the circular fibers of the muscularis. A Freer elevator is a useful dissector for this procedure. Frequently the mass can be dissected from both iliac arteries and the aorta in one piece (Fig. 4-1, C and D). The area between the two incisions is gradually freed by working first from below and then from above (Fig. 4-1, D).

3. Visualize the distal end of the plaque, and cut the plaque from the normal intima with a scissors.

Restoration of blood flow to first leg

1. Irrigate the interior of the aorta with saline or heparin-saline solution.

2. Using an over-and-over suture, close the longer arteriotomy in the aorta and one iliac artery first, beginning at the aortic end and continuning to within 1 cm. of the distal end of the incision.

3. Clamp the opposite iliac artery proximally.

4. Release the proximal aortic clamp for a few seconds to flush out sludge and clots that may have accumulated proximally.

5. Close any distal arteriotomy in the common femoral artery, and fill the vessel with heparin-saline solution.

6. Release the distal iliac clamp on that side momentarily to back-flush any clots. Quickly reapply the clamp.

7. Quickly finish the suture line. Release the distal clamp to fill the artery with blood and force out air before the last suture is tied.

8. Release the proximal aortic clamp slowly.

COMMENT: *When a thin atherosclerotic plaque continues down the posterior aspect of the iliac artery (Fig. 4-1, E), bevel the distal plaque and prevent further dissection by suturing the remaining intima and plaque to the arterial wall with several interrupted mattress sutures.*

Suture of iliac arteriotomy

Suture the iliac arteriotomy in the same fashion as the longer arteriotomy. Check back bleeding prior to completion of the closure, and force out air before completion of the suture line as described. Slowly release the proximal clamp (Fig. 4-1, F.)

Closure

The peritoneum is loosely approximated over the arteries. As a rule, no drainage is necessary. The abdominal incision is closed. A tube gastrostomy prevents postoperative distension.

Postoperative care

1. Anticoagulant treatment after aortoiliac endarterectomy is elective. Heparin should probably be used if the endarterectomy has been extensive, particularly if it has extended into the femoral regions. We begin heparinization before closing

the abdomen so that all pulses can be checked at this time. If endarterectomy has been limited to the aortic bifurcation, anticoagulation is probably unnecessary. The dose should be conservative and should not exceed 2,500 to 5,000 units every four to six hours.

2. Femoral and/or pedal pulses are observed hourly for the first forty-eight hours. Immediate reoperation is essential if the pulses disappear.

COMMENT: *Prolonged occlusion time should be avoided by choosing the correct operation. Endarterectomy should not be attempted when the procedure would involve extensive dissection. In such cases, a bypass procedure should be elected. Disruption of the aortic suture lines is prevented by avoiding a Y-shaped incision. Also, in suturing the aortic arteriotomy, at least 1 mm. of aortic wall should be included in the bites. Double layers of sutures are ineffective if the adventitia is not utilized in closure and are unnecessary when it is. When weakness of the aortic wall appears to be a distinct problem, the aorta may be reinforced by a sleeve of prosthesis. High endarterectomy that is close to the renal vessels should not be attempted without control of the aorta proximally by a suitable cross clamp. Digital compression of the aorta is not safe, because when this method is used, the hand and fingers are in the operator's field.*

AORTOILIAC BYPASS OPERATION
Introduction

When aortoiliac occlusions are extensive, a bypass operation is used to restore pulsatile flow into the iliac or the femoral arteries. Extensive endarterectomy is not as safe or satisfactory as the bypass procedure. Before a bypass operation is done, patency of the outflow at the profunda femoris artery and at the popliteal arteries should be demonstrated by angiography. If one femoral pulse is palpable at the groin, retrograde aortography is the safest method to demonstrate the extent of occlusive disease. Poor outflow at the hypogastric artery or at the profunda femoris artery must be recognized.

The diagrams in Fig. 4-2 show the types of bypass procedures for more extensive occlusions. The end of the bifurcation graft may be anastomosed to either the common femoral or the external iliac artery (Fig. 4-2, A).

Note that the aorta is not resected in this illustration. Now, however, we divide the aorta and oversew the distal end in most cases. There is less turbulence and less likelihood of aneurysm formation at the anastomosis, and there is ample retrograde filling of the hypogastric arteries so that the division of the aorta need cause no concern for viability of the colon.

Severe occlusive disease is so commonly bilateral that bypass grafts from the aorta to one side are not shown. Plaques on the posterior wall of the iliac artery are thick before any narrowing is visible in the anteroposterior view of the arteriogram.

Even if one common iliac artery is open, the proximal end of the bifurcation bypass prosthesis is usually attached to the end of the divided aorta (Fig. 4-2, D). An occluded aorta may present proximal localized thinning and early formation of aneurysm anteriorly (Fig. 4-2, C). In such cases, the thin portion of the aorta is resected, and end-to-end anastomosis is made between the graft and the proximal end of the aorta. The distal part of the aorta is closed securely.

When the aorta must be transected high and close to the renal vessels, transposition of the divided aorta in front of the left renal vein facilitates the anastomosis

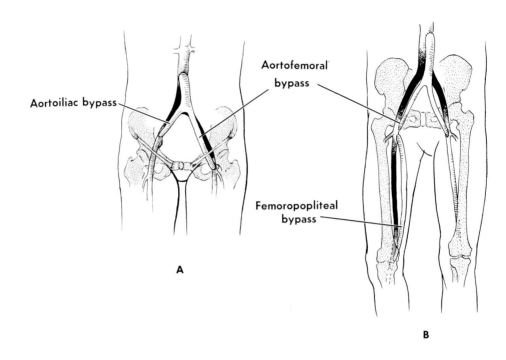

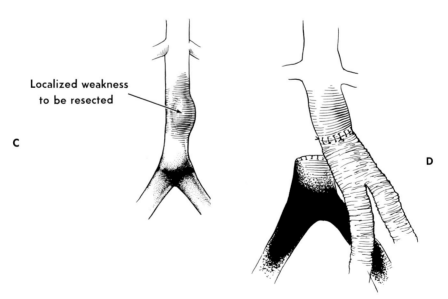

Fig. 4-2. A to **D,** Types of bypass for aortoiliac occlusion. Type in **C** is best treated by dividing aorta. Do not resect only the "blister." It is preferable in most cases to divide the aorta and to suture the aorta and prosthesis end to end.

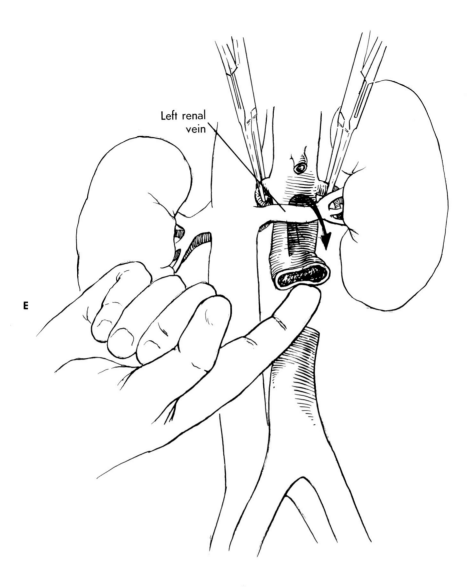

Left renal
vein

E

Fig. 4-2, cont'd. E, Transposition of divided aorta anterior to left renal vein.

and endarterectomy of the proximal end of the aorta. This is described in more detail in Chapter 12 (Fig. 12-3).

Combinations of both aortoiliac and femoropopliteal stenoses are difficult problems. If the leg is in danger, aortoiliac or aortofemoral bypasses must be done to reestablish abundant pulsatile flow into the profunda femoris artery. When this is accomplished, few patients will need femoropopliteal reconstructions.

Preparation

Preparation of the patient is the same as for other major surgery on the abdominal aorta. The large intestine should be prepared preoperatively.

Procedure

Exposure and exploration

1. Place the patient in the supine position. Prepare and drape the entire abdomen, groins, and legs to below the knee.

2. Make a long midline abdominal incision from the xiphoid process to the pubis. Expose and explore the aorta (see Chapter 3) by incising the peritoneum to the left of the small bowel, dividing the ligament of Treitz, and mobilizing the duodenum to the right of the aorta. Select the proximal aortic site for attachment of the bypass.

Palpate the iliac arteries. Compare the findings with the preoperative angiograms. Select the sites of the distal anastomoses. Incise the peritoneum over the iliac arteries at the proposed sites of the iliac arteriotomies, and palpate the patency of the vessels at these points.

COMMENT: *Since resection is not intended and the lumbar arteries need not be isolated, the peritoneal incisions for exposure of the aorta and iliac arteries are necessary only for exploration and for choosing the sites for anastomoses. In the average patient the small bowel and the ascending colon may be retracted to the right. In obese patients these must be lifted from the abdomen and enclosed in a plastic wrap or a Lahey bag. Incisions for this procedure are detailed in Fig. 3-2.*

Proximal control of aorta

1. Divide and ligate the inferior mesenteric artery to permit retraction of the sigmoid mesocolon to the left. Avoid the inferior mesenteric vein, or divide it.

2. Dissect around the aorta, clearing approximately 1 cm. of vessel below the renal arteries and above the occlusive disease.

3. Free the distal portion of the aorta by dissecting anteriorly from the bifurcation up to the previously placed tape. The lumbar arteries need not be visualized, since they are controlled by the Crafoord clamp.

4. Select the prosthesis, and soak it in blood drawn from the aorta or inferior vena cava.

COMMENT: *The 16-by-8-mm. knitted DeBakey Dacron prosthesis fits in almost all bypass cases.*

5. Rapidly inject 3,000 units (30 mg.) of heparin in 30 ml. of saline solution into the aorta below the tape. Quickly apply the aortic cross clamp proximally. A vertically applied clamp fits best.

6. Apply the Crafoord clamp, pinching the distal end of the aorta vertically (Fig. 4-3, *A*) as shown in the side view (Fig. 4-3, *B*). The tip of the S-curved clamp is posterior, close to the upper clamp, and temporarily occludes the lumbar arteries.

COMMENT: *Satisfactory control of the aorta for the bypass operation is obtained with only enough dissection for the proximal clamp and the distal Crafoord clamp or DeBakey aneurysm clamp that controls the lumbar arteries without individual dissection and identification. Endarterectomy of the aorta above and below the site of the anastomosis may be necessary, and the surgeon may find that this must be done before the clamp can be securely closed distally.*

Early formation of aneurysm can accompany occlusive disease. If the operator observes weakening and bulging of the anterior aortic wall proximal to the occlusive disease, the area should be excluded by division of the aorta (Fig. 4-2, B).

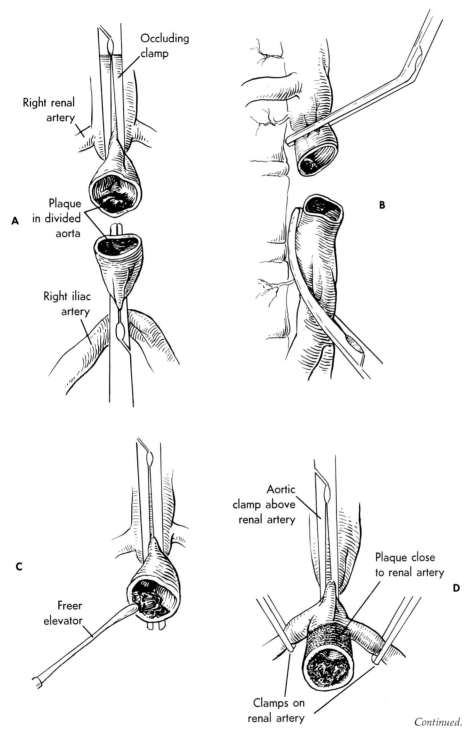

Fig. 4-3. Aortic bypass prosthesis—end-to-end anastomosis. **A,** Anterior view of divided aorta. **B,** Side view of divided aorta. **C,** Endarterectomy of proximal aorta. **D,** Cross clamping of renal arteries and upper aorta during endarterectomy close to renal arteries.

Continued.

113

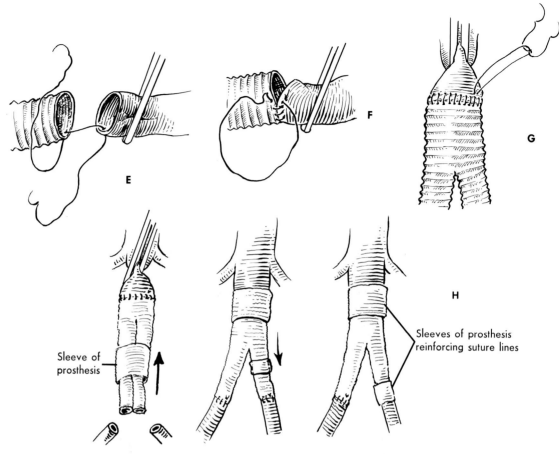

Fig. 4-3, cont'd. Aortic bypass prosthesis—end-to-end anastomosis. E and F, Side views of anastomosis. G, Anteroposterior view: completion of anastomosis. H, Reinforcement of aortic and left iliac anastomosis with snap-tight sleeve. (H redrawn from Sapirstein, W.: Surgery 70:744-745, 1971.)

Aortic anastomosis—end-to-end graft to proximal portion of aorta

End-to-end graft to the proximal portion of the aorta is the preferred aortic bypass procedure, even when the common iliac arteries are not completely occluded. The end-to-end anastomosis causes less turbulence, and progression of atherosclerosis in the distal end of the aorta causes no complications. The anastomosis is readily reinforced when necessary. As long as one hypogastric artery is perfused retrograde from the distal iliac or femoral anastomosis, the colon is viable.

1. Divide the aorta transversely as close to the proximal clamp as is convenient for anastomosis (Fig. 4-3, *A*).

2. Suture the distal end of the aorta crudely and securely before doing the proximal anastomosis. A 1 to 3 cm. section of it is unplugged so that it is flexible. Use 3-0 Dacron thread on the large T-5 needle to make several rows of overlapping continuous sutures. Use a cuff at least 1 cm. wide for the first row, and fold this over in the second row.

COMMENT: *Fig. 4-3, D, illustrates the maneuvers for performing endarterectomy close to the renal arteries. Replace the aortic clamp above the renal arteries for a few minutes and clamp each renal artery temporarily so that no sludge can become renal emboli.*

114

3. Flush away sludge and tease out thick or ulcerated atheromas that are frequently present on the posterior wall (Fig. 4-3, C).

4. Cut the prosthesis at least 1.5 to 2 cm. above its bifurcation.

5. Start the anastomosis posteriorly with 4-0 Ti-Cron on the T-5 needle (Fig 4-3, E). Larger needle and suture holes leak excessively in thin vessels, especially after endarterectomy.

6. Suture from the prosthesis to the aorta. The needle can be passed through close to the end of the prosthesis but should pass at least 3 mm. from the edge of the aorta.

7. If the aorta seems slightly too small to fit the prosthesis, a vertical incision anteriorly on the aorta enlarges the opening.

8. Complete the anastomosis, tying the sutures anteriorly (Fig. 4-3, G).

9. Slip a reinforcing sleeve over the ends of the prosthesis whenever you are concerned about the anastomosis, particularly after removal of plaques in the proximal end of the aorta (Fig. 4-3, H). This is described in the next section.

10. Preclot the graft and flush out the proximal end of the aorta by releasing the proximal aortic clamp momentarily. Pinch the iliac end of the graft to fill the graft under pressure so that all the pores are filled and any leaks revealed.

11. Reapply the aortic clamp and inspect the suture line. Empty the prosthesis and slide the reinforcing sleeve up over the anastomosis (Fig. 4-3, H).

Snap-tight cuff reinforcement for prosthetic arterial anastomoses (Fig. 4-3, H)*

Reinforcement of anastomoses between a fragile arteriosclerotic artery, usually the abdominal aorta, and a cloth prosthesis continues to be the major technical problem. The snap-tight cuff reinforcement technique is an easy method by which to reinforce suture lines or the rare prosthesis that has a leak because of a defect in the knitting.

Secure anastomosis requires a sturdy relatively normal artery or thick-walled aneurysm with a sturdy adventitia. Regrettably, this is sometimes weakened by disease, particularly in the aorta. Endarterectomy of calcified plaques or stenotic plaques adjacent to the intended suture line may leave only a fragile adventitial layer for the anastomosis. Various types of reinforcements and techniques have been proposed.[†]

Sometimes a cuff of the aneurysm can be used to surround the anastomosis, but this is not always suitable.

Thin needles and 4-0 Dacron suture are best for anastomoses after endarterectomy. The needle and thread holes should be small, and 4-0 Dacron is sufficiently strong; silk gradually loses its strength after implantation and permits disruption and development of false aneurysms.

It has been proposed that a stronger anastomosis may be obtained by doubling back the end of the prosthesis. This is incorrect because the weakest link is not the prosthesis, but the artery and the suture line between the artery and the prosthesis.

The earlier editions of this atlas illustrated reinforcement of undependable anasto-

---

*This section prepared by Carl H. Calman.
†I have used the snap-tight sleeve or cuff method since 1968. It has been published by Sapirstein, W.: A method of reinforcing vascular prosthetic anastomosis, Surgery **70**:744-745, 1971. (c.h.c.)

mosis with a strip of the prosthesis material, which was wrapped around the suture line. The ends were sutured anteriorly. This method may still be needed if the artery is much larger than the graft.

The present method of snap-tight cuff reinforcement covers and reinforces the usual end-to-end anastomosis in a more rapid and simple manner. It is well to practice this a few times in cases in which it seems unnecessary. It can be used for all anastomoses of a bifurcation graft provided that a 1 to 2 cm. section of the artery is freed posteriorly from adjacent veins or other structures. After the proximal anastomosis has been done take a small portion of the excess preclotted prosthetic tube, approximately 3/4 to 1 inch long, and slide it from below over the entire graft and carefully bring it up to and over the proximal suture line.

COMMENT: *There should not be much difference in the size of the prosthesis and the artery, or the earlier method will be needed.*

Test the primary suture line for major leaks before the final fitting. The snap-tight method seals minor leaks more quickly than they would be sealed by clotting mechanisms alone.

To reinforce a distal anastomosis, slide the rings either onto the limbs of the bifurcation graft or onto the main tube if a tube graft is used before beginning the inferior anastomosis. When pulsatile blood flow is restored through the prosthesis, the internal pressure automatically snaps the prosthesis and the anastomosis tight against the outer ring of prosthetic material, and no further adjustment or suturing is necessary except for perhaps a slight positional adjustment of the ring or collar to place it properly.

COMMENT: *This method is no substitute for good technique. It is, however, an easy method of reinforcement; the reinforcement cuff extends both above and below the anastomosis, restricts pulsatile motion at the anastomotic junction, and thereby diminishes the sawing or cutting action of the suture material along the anastomosis. Furthermore, this cuff reinforces a thin or weak segment of artery adjacent to the anastomosis. It will be needed after endarterectomy, particularly of calcified plaques, which frequently involve the adventitia and weaken it.*

Aortic anastomosis—end of graft to front of aorta

Division of the aorta and end-to-end anastomosis of the prosthesis and the proximal end of the aorta is preferable in most cases, as discussed earlier. However, the older procedure of suturing the end of the prosthesis to the front of the aorta is still useful when there is extensive calcification or when difficulties are encountered in dissecting posterior to the aorta. The aperture on the front of the aorta can be made at the most suitable and accessible spot, not necessarily midline or vertical.

1. Incise the aorta longitudinally. Flush out any atheromatous debris at the site of the original incision. For the end-to-side anastomosis, lengthen the incision to about one and one-half times the diameter of the aorta (Fig. 4-4, *A.*)

2. Select a bifurcation prosthesis of the same size as the aorta. Measure the prosthesis so that the bifurcation will be no lower than the diseased aortic bifurcation. Cut the superior margin of the prosthesis (Fig. 4-4, *B*).

3. Begin the anastomosis with a mattress suture of 4-0 Dacron at the inferior end of the arteriotomy, using a double-armed suture (Fig. 4-4, *B*).

4. Suture one side of the anastomosis with a continuous over-and-over stitch, passing the needle from the prosthesis side to the aortic side (Fig. 4-4, *C*).

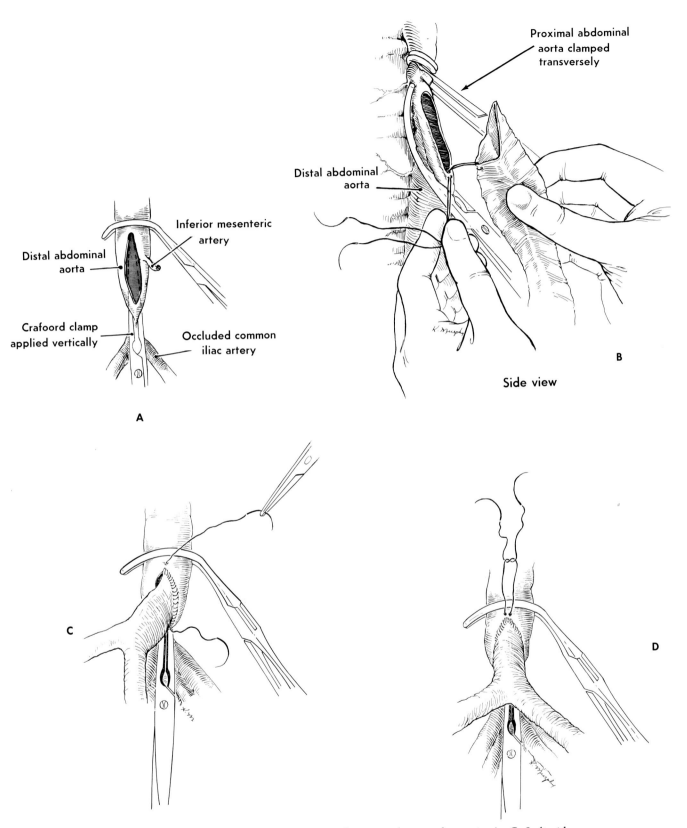

Fig. 4-4. Aortoiliac bypass. **A,** Front view. **B,** Side view of aorta shown in **A. C,** Left side of anastomosis completed. **D,** Completed anastomosis.

5. End the first side at the superior end of the aortotomy, with the needle emerging from the aorta (Fig. 4-4, *C*). Occasionally it may be necessary to lengthen the aortotomy superiorly or trim the tip of the prosthesis.

6. Suture the opposite side of the prosthesis to the aorta in an identical fashion. End the suture line with the needle emerging from the aorta, and tie the sutures together at the superior end of the anastomosis (Fig. 4-4, *D*).

COMMENT: *The best outflow through the prosthesis will be obtained by constructing apertures and anastomoses that conform to the shape of the normal arterial bifurcation. The longitudinal arteriotomy will gap sufficiently; rarely some of the aortic wall must be removed to secure an adequate opening. Anastomosis should be begun at the inferior end of the prosthesis. The tip of the obliquely cut prosthesis is drawn up so that it is taut, and the corrugations are smoothed out as it is sewn to the aorta superiorly. This ensures that the completed anastomosis will branch obliquely from the aorta when it is filled with blood under pressure.*

7. Preclot the graft and flush out the proximal portion of the aorta by releasing the proximal clamp momentarily to fill the prosthesis and its porous wall with blood under pressure. Quickly reapply the clamp and empty the prosthesis.

COMMENT: *This maneuver removes sludge and clots that may have accumulated proximal to the clamp. Woven prostheses have extremely small mesh, so that preclotting may be omitted. However, woven prostheses are generally undesirable. If one iliac artery is still patent, flush out the aorta and iliac artery and then clamp the prosthesis and release the aortic clamp to restore flow to the corresponding leg.*

Iliac artery anastomosis

Select the site for distal anastomosis where good outflow is assured and where the artery is normal and easily accessible. The iliac plaques are not always symmetrical, and one limb of the bypass may be attached to the common femoral artery as discussed in the section on aortofemoral bypass.

1. Draw the limbs of the prosthesis beneath the peritoneum on the right and beneath the peritoneum and the sigmoid colon on the left. Take care not to twist the limbs of the graft.

2. Apply a sidewise clamp to the iliac artery as it is elevated by forceps or by two encircling tapes.

COMMENT: *A single sidewise clamp on the iliac artery at the site of anastomosis is preferable to bulldog clamps, since the handle can be used to steady the artery and the prosthesis and to turn the artery from side to side while the anastomosis is being completed. Choose a clamp of appropriate shape and apply it so that the handle is out of the way. The DeBakey tangential occlusion clamp or the Cooley, Beck, or small Satinsky clamp may be employed.*

3. Make a longitudinal arteriotomy in the iliac artery. Place stay sutures to hold the edges apart.

COMMENT: *It is unnecessary to trim the edges.*

4. Draw the prosthesis downward, determine the correct length, and cut the end obliquely. Hold the prosthesis in position for anastomosis with an arterial clamp applied vertically about 1 cm. from the cut end (Fig. 4-5, *A*).

COMMENT: *It is essential to have a blunt tip on any prosthesis or other graft used for end-to-side anastomosis or for patch angioplasties. A good method of cutting the prosthesis is shown in Fig. 4-8, C.*

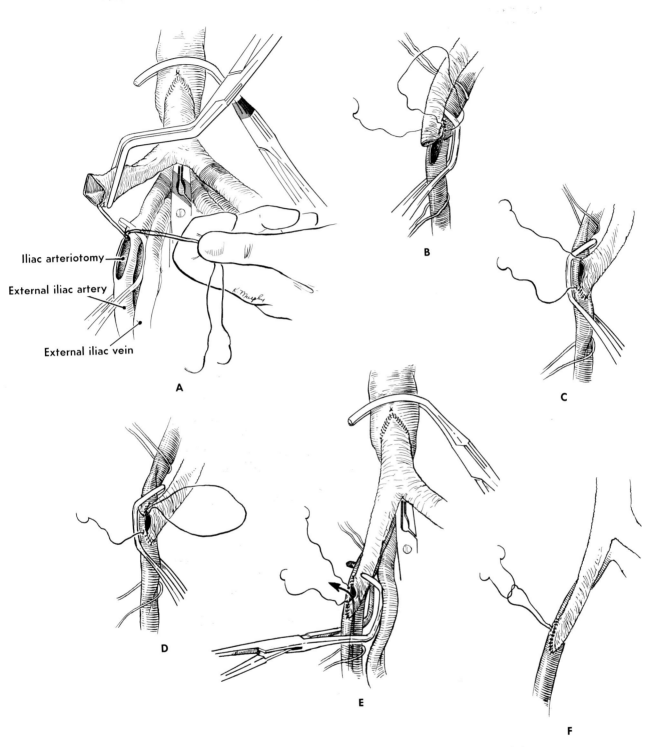

Iliac arteriotomy

External iliac artery

External iliac vein

A

B

C

D

E

F

Fig. 4-5. Aortoiliac bypass. **A,** Start end-to-side anastomosis of prosthesis and iliac artery. **B,** Medial row of sutures. **C,** Continue medial suture around tip of prosthesis and rotate clamp to gain access to lateral side. **D,** Begin lateral row of sutures at oblique proximal angle. **E,** Check back bleeding. **F,** Complete anastomosis.

5. Hold the clamp so that the artery and the prosthesis are in the correct position for anastomosis. Begin the anastomosis with a suture at the proximal end (Fig. 4-5, A). Tie the knot outside, and pass one needle under the graft for use on the other side of the anastomosis.

6. Sew from the graft to the artery; but on this proximal end, that is, the acute angle of the anastomosis, after passing the needle through the graft, lift the suture to retract the edge of the graft in order to pass the needle through the edge of the artery very accurately.

COMMENT: *In the proximal part, that is, the acute angle of the anastomosis, approximate the edges of the prosthesis and of the artery without attempting eversion of the edge of the prosthesis. Pass the sutures at least 2 mm. from the edges. The mattress suture as illustrated is no longer used.*

7. At the sides of the anastomosis, eversion is feasible and desirable. Sew from the graft to the artery at least 2 mm. from the edge.

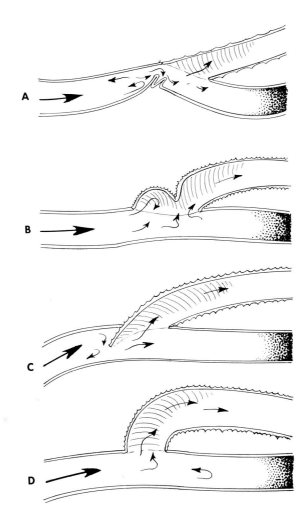

Fig. 4-6. Common errors in adjusting and completing an anastomosis. A, Excessive tension. B, Insufficient tension. C, Careless anastomosis. D, Right-angle exit not sufficiently oblique.

8. Continue the suture around the tip of the prosthesis and the distal end of the arteriotomy (Fig. 4-5, *C*). Stretch the tip distally, and if necessary, lengthen the arteriotomy distally to ensure an oblique attachment of the prosthesis to the artery.

9. Begin suture of the proximal end of the lateral portion of the anastomosis with the remaining end of the first mattress suture (Fig. 4-5, *D*).

10. Release the iliac clamp momentarily to check the back bleeding and reapply the clamp (Fig. 4-5, *E*), and rapidly complete the anastomosis (Fig. 4-5, *F*).

COMMENT: *Correct fit of the graft is essential. Some technical causes of narrowing and failure in end-to-side anastomosis are shown in Fig. 4-6.*

Restoration of flow to first leg

1. Begin to transfuse a pint of blood rapidly. Release the iliac clamp to permit back bleeding as high as the bifurcation and thereby extrude any air.

2. Apply an occluding clamp to the completed side at the bifurcation of the prosthesis.

3. Release the aortic clamps briefly to flush clots and debris from the open limb of the graft.

4. Reapply the proximal aortic clamp momentarily.

5. Release the clamp from the completed side and reapply it to the open side at the bifurcation.

6. Release the proximal aortic clamp slowly, restoring flow to the leg through the completed anastomosis. Slow down the blood transfusion when bleeding stops and flow is restored to the first leg.

COMMENT: *The light-weight porous prostheses will bleed briskly through the pores unless preclotted under pressure at least twice. However, Gelfoam held in place for five minutes with firm pressure by moist gauze will control this.*

Second iliac anastomosis

Commonly only one external iliac artery is suitable for anastomosis, and one side of the prosthesis is extended under the inguinal ligament (pp. 122-126).

1. Select an appropriate sidewise clamp, or use two angle clamps if they fit better.

2. Pass tape about the iliac artery at the site of anastomosis.

3. Inject 1,000 units of heparin in 10 ml. of saline solution distally; then close the clamps.

4. Make a longitudinal arteriotomy and loosen the clamp briefly to observe back bleeding. Reapply the clamps. Insert guide sutures on either side to hold the edges of the arteriotomy apart.

5. Proceed with fitting and anastomosis of the graft as described for the first side.

6. Remove the iliac clamp briefly before completion of the anastomosis to check back bleeding. Open the bifurcation clamp to flush out any clots and fill the graft with blood. Quickly close the proximal clamp, complete the anastomosis, and release the distal iliac clamp. Slowly release the proximal clamp.

7. Lumbar sympathectomy through the abdominal incision may be performed before closure (Fig. 4-9).

8. The iliac limbs of the bypass prosthesis are drawn beneath the peritoneum over the common iliac arteries so that closure over the distal anastomoses is simpli-

121

fied. Draw the mesocolon and mesentery of the small bowel together over the aorta anteriorly, covering the proximal portion of the prosthesis. Review closure on p. 81.

AORTOFEMORAL BYPASS
Importance of profunda femoris artery

Prolongation of aortic grafts into the leg may be necessary to assure satisfactory outflow when the external iliac artery is narrowed. However, atherosclerosis of the external iliac artery commonly extends distally into the common femoral artery, and most of the patients also have associated narrowing or occlusions of the superficial femoral artery.

The deep femoral artery (profunda femoris) is the most important collateral artery in the leg, and in any operation on the arteries of the leg, normal pulsatile flow through the profunda femoris artery must be assured. Some of the various maneuvers performed on the profunda femoris artery are illustrated in Fig. 4-8.

The profunda femoris artery is so important that restoration of pulsatile flow in it may save a leg even though the superficial femoral and popliteal arteries are both narrowed and inoperable. Aortofemoral bypass revascularization of the profunda femoris artery may not be ideal but may be all that is feasible. The amount of outflow and collateral circulation via the profunda femoris artery is large. In many patients the femoropopliteal outflow is too poor for femoral endarterectomy or femoral bypass procedures. Other patients are poor risks, and the combined operation from the abdominal aorta to the popliteal arteries is too formidable even in two stages. The surgeon must be absolutely certain that in patients in whom the superficial femoral artery is also occluded, the profunda artery outflow is satisfactory.

When serving as collateral circulation, the profunda femoris artery may dilate tremendously. Its abundant large muscular branches provide a superb "runoff," and in some patients, pedal pulses return after aortoprofunda bypass even though the superficial femoral artery is occluded.

The orifice or the proximal centimeter of the profunda femoris artery is frequently narrowed by atherosclerotic plaques, particularly in those patients who need the profunda femoris artery outflow most (that is, those with aortoiliac atherosclerosis extending down into the femoral artery). This is usually overlooked in the routine anteroposterior arteriograms because the shadow of the common femoral artery overlies the origin of the profunda femoris artery from the posterior side of the common femoral artery. The distal portion of the deep femoral artery is usually free of atherosclerosis.

Procedure

The aortic portion of the operation has already been illustrated (Fig. 4-3) and described.

Exposure of common femoral and profunda femoris arteries

1. Make a vertical incision over the common femoral artery, and avoid dissection near the more medially placed lymphatic vessels and the femoral vein (Fig. 4-7, *A*).
2. Dissect out and isolate with umbilical tapes the profunda femoris, common femoral, and superficial femoral arteries. Palpate the vessels, and note localized plaques that may require endarterectomy. The arteriotomy should be made over the

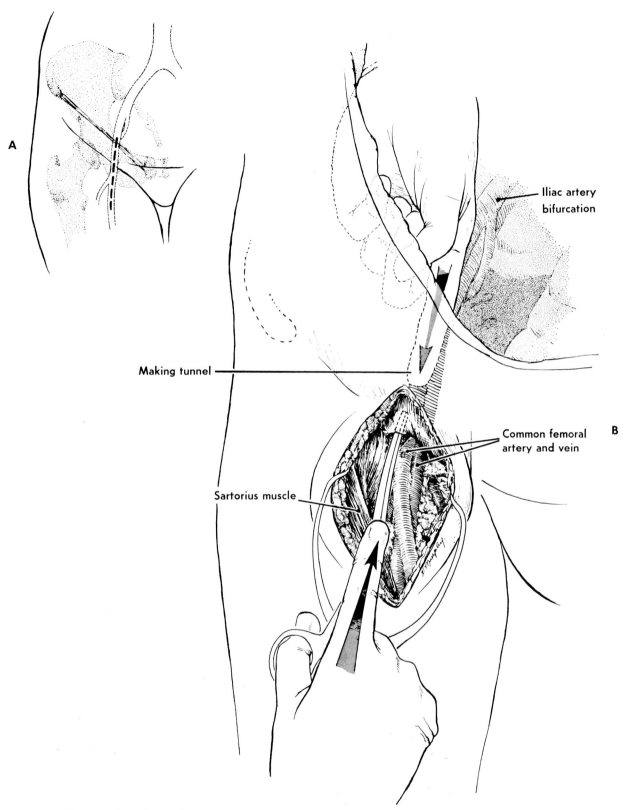

A

B

Iliac artery
bifurcation

Making tunnel

Common femoral
artery and vein

Sartorius muscle

Fig. 4-7. Aortofemoral bypass. **A,** Incision for exposure of common femoral artery. **B,** Make a tunnel beneath inguinal ligament. (See also Fig. 4-8.)

123

orifice of the profunda femoris artery so that it can be inspected. This is frequently narrowed by plaques that must be removed to ensure adequate outflow.

COMMENT: *Inspection of the orifice of the profunda femoris artery should be part of all revascularization operations if (1) the proximal superficial femoral artery is occluded, (2) the leg is in peril, or (3) palpation reveals significant plaque on the posterior wall of the common femoral artery. In such cases the probability of narrowing of the profunda femoris artery is great, and the need for an adequate outflow from the profunda femoris artery is crucial. The arteriogram does not visualize the origin of the profunda femoris artery, where the narrowing occurs. A notch or slight narrowing on the arteriogram of the common femoral artery, signifying plaque on the side of the artery, always means that there is thicker plaque on the posterior wall of the artery.*

3. Incise the inguinal ligament and the external oblique and transverse fascia so that there will be ample room for your finger anterior to the artery. Lift the conjoined tendon anteriorly with an Army-Navy retractor and spread the retroperitoneal tissue anterior to the artery and vein. Tributaries of the vein are easily torn.

COMMENT: *No hernia has yet occurred alongside the graft. Dividing the fascia permits safer blunt dissection of the tunnel and prevents compression of the graft during flexion of the thigh.*

4. Make a tunnel anterior and medial to the iliac artery by blunt dissection carried upward under the inguinal ligament and retroperitoneally to the common iliac artery or the aorta (Fig. 4-7, *B*).

5. Draw the prosthesis through this tunnel without kinks or twists. Adjust the length and apply an arterial clamp about 1 cm. from the proposed anastomosis. Trim the end of the prosthesis, leaving some excess.

COMMENT: *The correct length of the prosthesis must be carefully adjusted later, since incorrect tension will disturb the flow at the anastomotic site (Fig. 4-6), and excessive tension leads to disruption and development of false aneurysms.*

Arteriotomy and inspection of profunda femoris artery

1. Make a longitudinal arteriotomy in the common femoral artery. Do not extend the arteriotomy distally past the orifice of the profunda femoris artery until you have determined the need for doing so. It may be necessary to extend the incision into the profunda femoris artery (Fig. 4-8, *A* and *E*) after your inspection of the inside of the artery.

COMMENT: *Dilation of the orifice of the profunda femoris artery (Fig. 4-8, B) is sometimes necessary because the fascial hiatus limits the dilation of the artery. Since the distal portion of the profunda femoris artery is invisible behind the fascia, the Fogarty catheter is useful for exploring and calibrating the artery.*

2. Complete the arteriotomy. Fig. 4-8 shows how the tip of the prosthesis can be extended to widen the superficial femoral or the profunda femoris artery when stenosis makes this advisable. Other maneuvers used when more extensive narrowing or plaques are found in the common femoral or profunda femoris artery are discussed in Chapter 5.

3. Cut the prosthesis to the correct length. Cut it as shown in Fig. 4-8, *C,* so that the ends are blunt. Avoid excessive tension, especially at the most proximal end of the anastomosis.

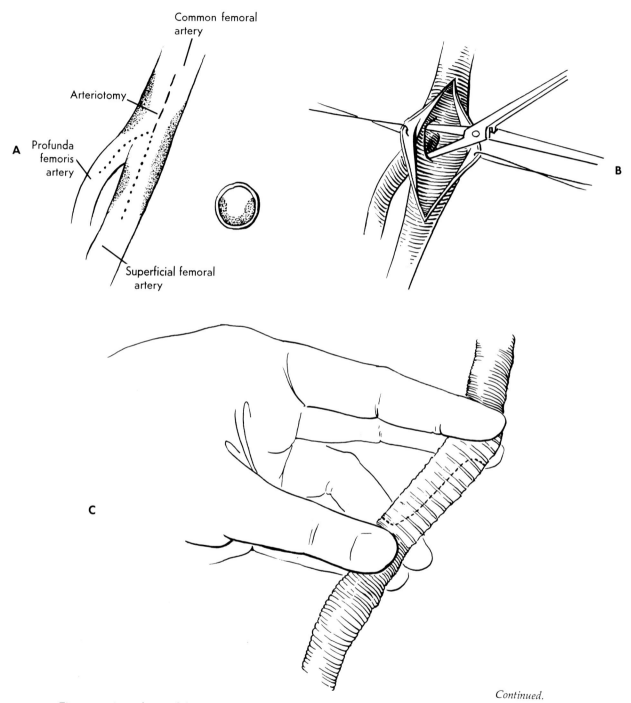

Continued.

Fig. 4-8. Aortofemoral bypass. **A,** Make incision to inspect orifice of profunda femoris artery and then extend the incision distally if necessary onto either the superficial femoral or the profunda femoris artery as indicated by the dotted lines. **B,** Dilate orifice of profunda femoris artery. **C,** Cut prosthesis so that ends are blunt.

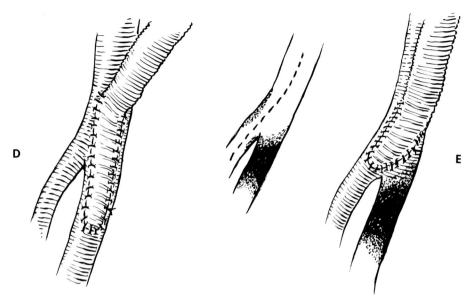

Fig. 4-8, cont'd. Aortofemoral bypass. **D,** Extend tip of prosthesis to widen superficial femoral artery. **E,** Extend tip of prosthesis to widen profunda femoris artery.

Anastomosis of prosthesis to common femoral artery

1. Use the malleable laryngeal cannula to rapidly inject 10 ml. of irrigating heparin into the profunda femoris and common femoral arteries, and apply appropriate arterial occluding clamps. Separate angled clamps are convenient for clamping the three arteries individually.

2. Begin the anastomosis with a double-armed suture placed at the acute angle between the graft and the arteriotomy. Continue as described for the end-to-side iliac anastomosis. Sew with an over-and-over stitch down each side of the arteriotomy, lengthening it if necessary. Review pp. 118-119 and Fig. 4-5.

3. Check back bleeding from the distal end of the femoral artery. Flush clots from the prosthesis by releasing the proximal clamp before completing the anastomosis.

4. Finish the last portion of the anastomosis, and tie the sutures after releasing the distal clamp to extrude air from the femoral artery.

5. Restore flow to the leg by removing the proximal clamp slowly.

COMMENT: *Delayed disruption and false aneurysms are more common in these anastomoses than elsewhere, probably due to motion of the prosthesis with flexion and the more common serum and lymph collections that prevent adherence and incorporation of the prosthesis and suture line into healthy tissue. Arterial silk loses its tensile strength after prolonged implantation, and Dacron, Tevdek, polyethylene, or polypropylene sutures are necessary for these as for other host artery–prosthesis anastomoses.*

Closure and postoperative care of groin incisions

Closure and postoperative care of groin incisions merit special attention in order to avoid the problems so frequently reported. The problems and complications so commonly reported in groin incisions are easily avoided. The longitudinal incision directly over the artery gives the best exposure of the entire length of the common femoral artery, proximal end of the profunda femoris artery, and proximal end of the superficial femoral artery. This incision is easily extended when the profunda femoris artery originates low or when it must be explored or revascularized. Notwithstanding other opinions, we always use, and have never regretted using, the longitudinal incision directly over the common femoral artery. It divides no arteries or veins and few lymphatic vessels and gives the best exposure. Occasionally the skin is incised across the crease of the groin. Grafts passing beneath the inguinal ligament need a roomy tunnel; therefore, the inguinal ligament should not be sutured. Hernias have not developed in the tunnels or along the prostheses. The wound should be irrigated with bacitracin solution.

The incision should be closed so that lymph, serum, or hematomas cannot accumulate around the prosthesis. Several layers of interrupted silk will cover the prosthesis with living tissue and avoid dead space. Superficial layers may be closed with continuous sutures of catgut. The skin edges should be carefully approximated with continuous monofilament nylon sutures.

The use of anticoagulants is hazardous and unnecessary. Prevention of venous thrombosis with the "mini-heparin" regimen proposed by Kakkar has caused no problems as yet; the dose, 5,000 units given deep subcutaneously twice daily, does not produce a marked bleeding tendency.

Antibiotics are given before, during, and for five days after operation whenever prostheses are implanted.

Acute flexion of the thighs should be avoided for seven to ten days.

When the saphenous vein has been removed for use as a graft or if edema of the leg appears, rest and elevate the leg in order to reduce lymph flow and avoid edema and lymph accumulations in the incisions.

Beware of edema of the leg. It may signify phlebitis, but it is usually due to disruption of lymphatic vessels. Elastic wrappings and stockings assist venous and lymphatic return. The external resistance of the elastic wrapping helps the leg muscles to compress and propel venous blood and lymph proximally.

Other maneuvers and variations

The arteriotomy for aortofemoral or aortoprofunda bypass described in detail earlier should be extended onto the profunda femoris artery as illustrated in Fig. 4-8, A, if inspection through the common femoral arteriotomy reveals a plaque causing narrowing of the orifice of the profunda femoris artery.

The orifice of the profunda femoris artery can be widened whenever necessary by inserting the tip of the aortofemoral prosthesis (Fig. 4-8, E). When aortoiliac endarterectomy must be extended into the femoral and profunda femoris arteries, patch angioplasty is the best closure, since it widens the profunda femoris artery and wide secure stitches can be used for closure without narrowing the arterial lumen.

Local endarterectomy (that is, removal of the plaque) is performed in the profunda femoris artery only when the plaque is localized to the proximal centimeter and is thick or ulcerated. When an atherosclerotic plaque in a small artery has a smooth normal intima or extends a considerable distance, it is preferable to widen the lumen by patch angioplasty rather than by removal of the plaque.

Extended exposure of the profunda femoris artery is readily accomplished by incision of the fascia overlying it. Tributaries of the femoral vein cross in front of it and may be troublesome. The profunda femoris artery gives off many branches posteriorly. To temporarily occlude these, either loosely applied removable silver neurosurgical clips or a loop of 2-0 suture is used. Bulldog clamps are too bulky for this location.

BILATERAL ABDOMINAL SYMPATHECTOMY

Bilateral abdominal lumbar sympathectomy should be used frequently as an adjunct to either endarterectomy or bypass operations for aortoiliac occlusive disease. The lumbar sympathetic ganglia are removed from about the second or third lumbar segment to the pelvic brim. It is not possible to get as high on the chain of ganglia as during lumbar sympathectomy through a lateral retroperitoneal approach. However, the lumbar sympathetic chains are easily accessible at the time the aorta is exposed and may be removed either before or after the primary procedure.

Procedure
Technique—right side

1. Dissect the fat and lymphatic tissue from the right side of the inferior vena cava. Retract this tissue and the spermatic or ovarian vessels laterally.

2. Roll the inferior vena cava medially with a sponge stick, and palpate the anterior aspects of the fourth and fifth lumbar vertebras to locate the sympathetic chain. The chain is unique and may be identified by the small nodular ganglia.

3. Roll the nerve against the vertebral bodies. Lift the chain with a nerve hook, and dissect it from the groove between the psoas muscle and the vertebral bodies. Carry the dissection inferiorly to the right iliac vein. Divide the rami only, leaving the chain intact. The lumbar veins ordinarily are posterior to the sympathetic chain. However, care must be taken to visualize and to avoid injury of these vessels (Fig. 4-9, A). If necessary, divide lumbar veins before they are injured. Silver clips are useful for hemostasis.

4. The kidney is not displaced forward with the anterior approach. Follow the sympathetic chain upward, posteriorly, and somewhat deeper, until the right renal pedicle limits further dissection. Use a narrow Deaver retractor to expose the upper possible limit of dissection. Dissection may be extended slightly by using one's finger or a small "peanut" sponge to dissect a little farther up the sympathetic chain. Clip the upper end of the sympathetic chain with several silver clips and divide it.

Technique—left side

Sympathectomy on the left may be more difficult than on the right, particularly if there is much inflammatory or fibrotic reaction about the terminal part of the aorta.

If exposure is difficult by the following method, the sigmoid colon may be reflected superiorly and medially and the sympathetic chain approached retroperitoneally after a posterior peritoneal incision is made.

1. Divide the inferior mesenteric artery, and retract the descending colon and its mesentery to the left. Retract the lymphatic and fatty tissues and gonadal vessels laterally. The sympathetic chain lies in the groove between the psoas muscle and the vertebral bodies and is located by palpation as a firm nodular cord.

2. Lift the sympathetic chain with a nerve hook. Dissect inferiorly, and apply silver clips at the pelvic brim. Divide the terminal rami of the lumbar sympathetic

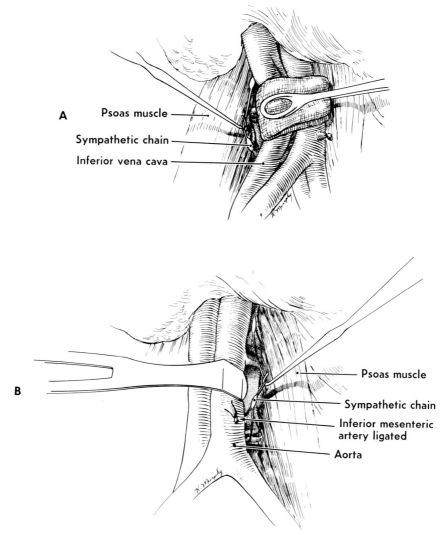

A

Psoas muscle
Sympathetic chain
Inferior vena cava

B

Psoas muscle
Sympathetic chain
Inferior mesenteric
artery ligated
Aorta

Fig. 4-9. Technique of bilateral abdominal sympathectomy. **A,** Right side. **B,** Left side.

chain here, seize the chain with a hemostat, and dissect upward as described for the right side, dividing the rami of the sympathetic chain in the process. Apply silver clips to the superior limit of the dissection and divide the chain to remove it.

COMPLICATIONS OF AORTOFEMORAL PROSTHESES

General principles are reviewed in Chapter 1.

The diagnosis of acute occlusion of an aortofemoral graft is easily made because the pulse in the prosthesis is superficial. Its disappearance is obvious.

Early thrombosis

Early thrombosis can usually be treated without opening the abdomen unless there is reason to suspect that the proximal anastomosis at the aorta is at fault. The cause will almost always be found to be previously unrecognized poor outflow. The

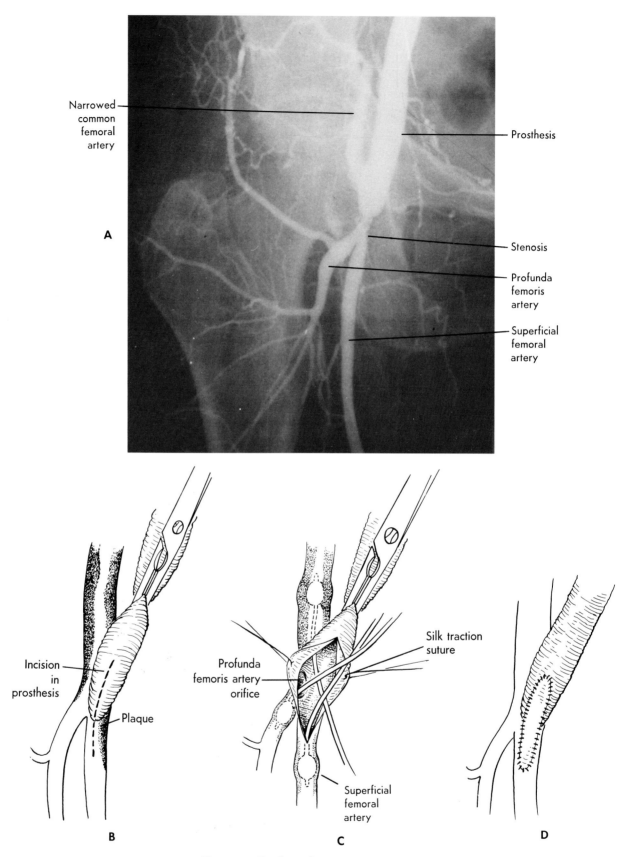

Fig. 4-10. For legend see opposite page.

procedure of reopening the groin incision and making an incision into the end of the graft permits embolectomy of the proximal end of the graft and distal branches of the artery with the Fogarty catheter. Arteriograms will be needed during the operation if the cause of the thrombosis is not immediately obvious through the incision. Profundaplasty or distal extension of the arteriotomy and the graft may be needed. See Chapter 6 (Figs. 6-5, 6-6, and 6-7).

Reoperation for outflow stenosis

Recurrence of ischemic symptoms months or years after aortofemoral prostheses are implanted may be due to various developments, and arteriograms will probably reveal the cause. A new or louder bruit may signify new stenosis such as illustrated in Fig. 4-10, A. Stenosis is soon followed by thrombosis and requires emergency operation if severe ischemia develops.

Fig. 4-10 illustrates the operation to correct stenosis caused by a new plaque near the tip of the prosthesis. During reoperation in the groin months or years after a bypass graft is implanted, certain maneuvers avoid unnecessary dissection in the scar and fibrosis around the prosthesis and the blood vessels. When still pulsating, the prosthesis is an obvious landmark. It is superficially located. Reopen the old incision and cut through scar down to the prosthesis with light strokes of a sharp knife. The prosthesis is sturdy and soon visible. Scrape or peel away the dense scar close to the prosthesis and apply a clamp vertically for proximal control (Fig. 4-10, B). Do not dissect behind the prosthesis, where the vein and artery may be very adherent. Uncover the anterior part of the prosthesis down to the tip. Make the arteriotomy in the prosthesis first. You may obtain distal control by the use of intraluminal balloon catheters. This avoids tedious and hazardous dissection in the previous scar around the vessels, and even if the profunda femoris artery must be dissected later for profundaplasty, you have located its orifice. See Chapter 6 (Figs. 6-5, 6-6, and 6-7) for more details about local endarterectomy, profundaplasty, and patch angioplasty in case they are needed.

Late occlusion

Late occlusion of aortofemoral bypasses can also be treated successfully without reopening the abdomen in many cases. Late occlusion may be signalled by recurrence of claudication or by severe pain at rest and ischemia requiring emergency operation.

Reopen the inguinal incision, and expose the distal part of the thrombosed graft and the bifurcation of the common femoral artery. Inject heparin, cross-clamp the graft, open the graft, and perform thrombectomy of the graft and femoral outflow arteries with Fogarty catheters. Fogarty or Noon balloon catheters can also be inflated in the outflow arteries to prevent back bleeding (Fig. 4-10, C). Scarring may make dissection around the profunda femoris artery difficult. The possibility of occurrence of embolism down the other side of the graft during passage of the Fogarty catheter

Fig. 4-10. Reoperation for stenosis at tip of bypass prosthesis. A, Arteriogram. B, Sketch of A with clamp on prosthesis. C, View through incision in prosthesis and artery. Balloon catheters in outflow arteries control back bleeding during local endarterectomy. D, Gusset patch widens profunda femoris artery.

upstream is worrisome. Cohn, Moore, and Hall compress the opposite side of the graft and femoral artery with the palm of their hand. Stopping flow to the good side should help fragments to wash out the side that was operated on, as the catheter is withdrawn.

Late occlusions resulting from poor outflow are frequently preceded by accumulation of a thick neointimal lining in the prosthesis, and this may be somewhat adherent. Pass the catheter several times until no more fragments appear and good inflow is obtained. Obtain an arteriogram; if residual neointima is seen, pass the wire-basket endarterectomy instrument or the endarterectomy loops and follow with the catheter again. The Dormia wire-basket catheter is useful for this.

When thick neointima is found, you can be sure that outflow stenosis is present and must be corrected. This usually means that profundaplasty or extension of the graft more distally must be done. (See Chapter 6.)

If after thrombectomy is done, the inflow or outflow cannot be restored by reoperation through the previous incision, *other types of bypasses* should be considered. These are discussed in Chapter 5.

Infected aortofemoral prostheses

Infected aortofemoral prostheses are also discussed in Chapter 5 because their treatment usually requires a new bypass through an uncontaminated operative field.

Anastomotic aneurysms

Anastomotic aneurysms are discussed in Chapter 6 because, although they are rare, they are more common in the common femoral artery than elsewhere.

F.B.H.

5
Other bypass operations to the groin

Aortofemoral bypass operations are described in Chapter 4.

When a limb is endangered by occlusion of the iliac artery or abdominal aorta, the direct approach to these major intra-abdominal vessels may be contraindicated because of recent surgery, intra-abdominal sepsis, age, or severe heart, lung, or renal disease. In such cases, it is safer to restore flow to an ischemic leg with a bypass attached to the artery in the opposite leg or to the axillary artery. Prostheses need not follow the normal anatomic pathways of blood vessels. Furthermore, it has been shown clinically and experimentally that a bypass will not rob the limb from which it originates. Unless there is a proximal stenosis, the flow in an axillary or iliofemoral artery may double in order to perfuse the bypass as well as its own normal outflow.

FEMOROFEMORAL BYPASS

Femorofemoral bypass is performed for unilateral iliac artery obstructions. This operation was first devised to bypass acute occlusions of one limb of an aortic graft without reentering the abdomen. In such cases—after resection of an abdominal aneurysm, for example—the arteries are wide open except for the occluded side of the bifurcation graft. Femorofemoral bypass is a safe and relatively simple operation requiring only local or light general anesthesia for the two groin incisions and a subcutaneous tunnel across the pubis (Fig. 5-1).

In occasional elective cases, iliac occlusion is unilateral and the iliac artery on the opposite side is sufficiently normal to serve as inflow for both legs. The inevitable plaques do not always narrow the inflow, and a murmur in the opposite groin need not contraindicate this procedure. Occasionally, supplementary maneuvers are needed to assure adequate inflow and outflow, such as local endarterectomy and widening of inflow or outflow with extensions of the tip of the prosthetic tube, as illustrated (Fig. 5-3) and described later. An open profunda femoris artery provides sufficient outflow to maintain patency of the graft. The entire iliofemoral arterial trunk is sometimes occluded; but if the leg is viable, the profunda femoris artery is open and may be occluded only at the ostium (Fig. 6-5). The long-term patency rate is higher than expected, and failure is rare when there is adequate outflow.

The sharp angulation of the proximal end of the graft (Fig. 5-2) causes turbulence but no complications, and atherosclerosis in the donor artery is not accelerated. Vetto believes that atherosclerosis in the donor iliac artery is slowed because the bypass increases linear flow and decreases lateral wall tension. There have been no long-term

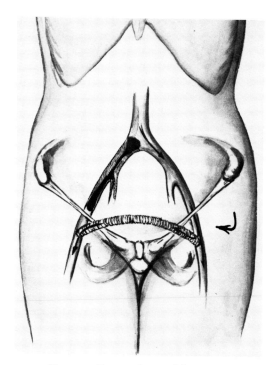

Fig. 5-1. Femorofemoral bypass.

deleterious effects on the donor limb. It is not a common operation but should be in the repertoire of all vascular surgeons. Many series of cases have been reported.*

Arteriography

Arteriograms are essential in elective cases and help the surgeon to plan the procedure. The aorta and both iliac and femoral arteries are demonstrated.

1. Insert a No. 160 Seldinger needle into the open femoral artery in the opposite groin.

2. Inject 60 ml. of Conray 60 at a pressure of 300 to 400 pounds per square inch. This should empty the syringe in three seconds and reflux the dye into the abdominal aorta.

3. Take a series of films at intervals of one to two seconds.

COMMENT: *A second injection and more delayed films are frequently needed for the dye to cross and percolate through the collateral vessels to fill the profunda femoris artery and vessels to the knee.*

If you are in doubt about the adequacy of the donor artery, measure the pressure before you withdraw the needle. The pressure should be the same as or slightly less than the arm pressure.

---

*See references by Blaisdell and associates (1970), Ehrenfeld and associates (1968), Foley and associates (1969), Parsonnet and associates (1970), and Vetto (1966).

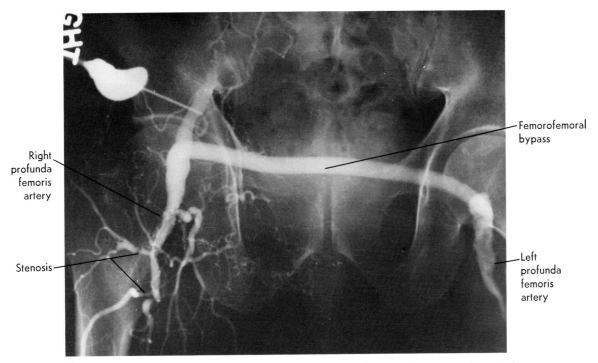

Right profunda femoris artery

Stenosis

Femorofemoral bypass

Left profunda femoris artery

Fig. 5-2. Postoperative arteriogram of femorofemoral prosthesis with poor outflow. Left profunda femoris outflow artery has no visible branches in its proximal portion. Graft relieved patient's ischemic pain and remained open until he died six months later. Both superficial femoral arteries are occluded. Profunda femoris artery of donor leg shows diffuse atherosclerosis with narrowing at origin of several branches and occlusion of the midportion of profunda femoris artery.

Procedure

The patient should be in the supine position. Prepare and drape the abdomen and both groins and upper thighs. If access to the profunda femoris artery in the midthigh may be needed, prepare the entire leg and review Fig. 6-8 and p. 160.

Two surgeons can work simultaneously in both groins.

Incision and exposure

1. Begin the vertical incisions at the inguinal ligament.
2. Dissect out the common femoral, the profunda femoris, and the proximal end of the superficial femoral vessels. Even though the femoral pulse is absent, the chronically occluded artery can be felt as a round firm cord slightly lateral to the foramen ovale where the saphenous vein joins the common femoral vein. This foramen is a distinct hollow that admits the fingertip and serves as a good landmark.
3. See the anatomy illustrated in Fig. 6-1.

Proximal anastomosis

1. Preclot the 8 mm. knitted Dacron tube. Spare the saphenous vein for use where it is indispensable. It offers no advantages here.
2. Inject 2,000 units of heparin into the common femoral artery, and vertically apply DeBakey angle clamps proximally and distally.

135

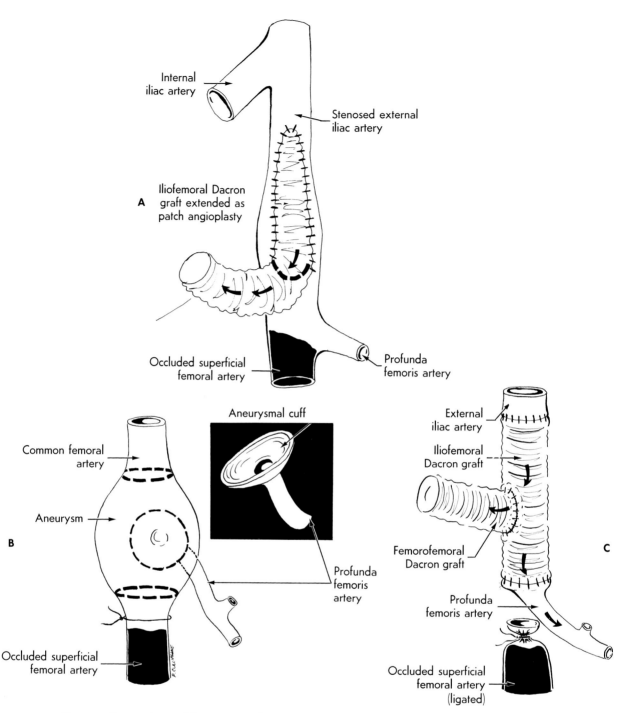

Fig. 5-3. Femorofemoral bypass prostheses—supplementary maneuvers for improving inflow and outflow. **A,** Dacron graft used as patch angioplasty over stenosed external iliac artery to provide adequate inflow for iliofemoral Dacron bypass. **B,** Aneurysm of common femoral artery resected. Occluded superficial femoral artery ligated. Origin of profunda femoris artery widened by including cuff of aneurysm around its origin. **C,** Resected aneurysm of common femoral artery repaired with Dacron graft, the side of which provides inflow to femorofemoral Dacron graft. Occluded superficial femoral artery ligated. (From Ayvazian, V. H., Auer, A. I., and Hershey, F. B.: Limb salvage by extended femorofemoral bypass, Surg. Gynecol. Obstet. **135:**737-741, 1972. By permission of Surgery, Gynecology & Obstetrics.)

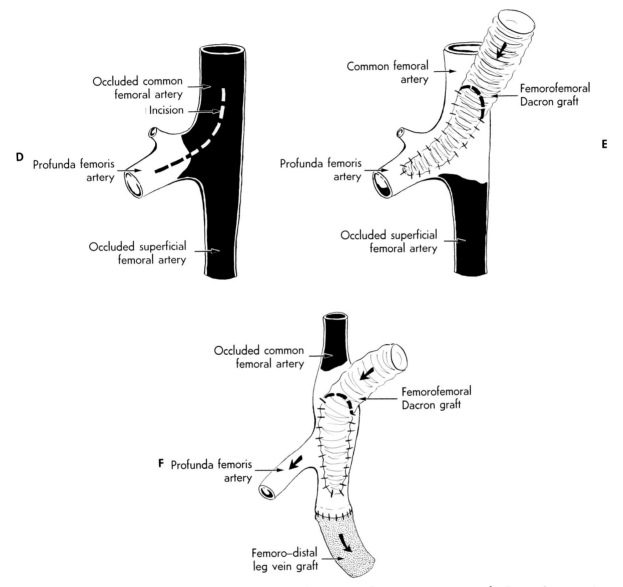

Fig. 5-3, cont'd. Femorofemoral bypass prostheses—supplementary maneuvers for improving inflow and outflow. **D,** Common and superficial femoral arteries occluded. Endarterectomy reopens the site of anastomosis. Incision extends from common femoral artery to profunda femoris artery, which provides sole outflow. **E,** Superficial femoral artery occluded. Femorofemoral Dacron graft attached to common femoral and profunda femoris arteries, usually after endarterectomy of proximal inch of profunda femoris artery. **F,** Femorofemoral graft revascularizes thigh. Femoral autogenous vein graft to distal part of leg is used to revascularize lower leg because of severe ischemia and extensive obliteration of popliteal artery and its outflow.

137

3. Make the arteriotomy 12 to 15 mm. long on the anteromedial aspect.

4. Cut the end of the prosthesis with a blunt tip and blunt heel (Fig. 4-8, C), and perform the anastomosis with 4-0 Dacron as described in Chapter 4, suturing the end of the prosthesis to the front of the common femoral artery.

5. Release the proximal clamp and fill the prosthesis under pressure to preclot it. Reapply the proximal clamp and release the distal clamp to back-bleed, flush, and fill the graft.

6. Clamp the graft close to the anastomosis; release the clamps on the artery and restore flow to the donor leg. Empty the graft and cover it with moist gauze.

COMMENT: *Other maneuvers may be needed as illustrated in Fig. 5-3, A, in which the inflow artery was widened to relieve a stenosis. The tip of the prosthesis could be extended inferiorly to widen the profunda femoris or superficial femoral artery when indicated. Fig. 5-3, B, shows the femorofemoral prosthesis originating from the tube graft replacing a femoral aneurysm.*

Making the tunnel

1. At the medial side of the upper end of the incision, bluntly dissect beneath the skin over the inguinal ligament, pushing the index finger superior to the pubic spine.

2. Do the same from the other incision until the fingertips touch. The tunnel must be roomy for the finger.

3. Pass a curved sponge-holding forceps through the tunnel. Orient the graft so that it may be drawn through the tunnel without a twist or kink.

COMMENT: *Tyson and Reichle in 1972 proposed the retropubic route through the space of Retzius as a more protected route. They dissect bluntly medial to the common femoral vein and beneath the inguinal ligament to enter the space behind the pubis and then dissect bluntly close to the pubis, posterior to the rectus muscles.*

Adequate outflow

For acute occlusions of the iliac artery or of one limb of a prosthesis replacing an aortic aneurysm, the common femoral artery and its bifurcation may be open or contain only fresh thrombus. In such cases, pass the Fogarty catheters distally into both branches of the common femoral artery to remove thrombus.

In chronic occlusions and elective cases, the common femoral and superficial femoral artery and ostium of the profunda femoris artery will most likely be occluded so that the profunda femoris artery will be the only outflow at this level (Fig. 5-3, D). Reopen enough of the common femoral artery to clear the ostium and extend the tip of the graft (Fig. 5-3, E). See the discussion of techniques of revascularizing the proximal end of the profunda femoris artery on p. 158 (Figs. 6-5 and 6-6).

Rarely, ischemia of the lower leg will be severe and the collateral circulation via the revascularized profunda femoris artery may be insufficient. Several times we have also performed vein graft bypasses to the lower leg (Fig. 5-3, F).

Distal anastomosis

1. Cut the prosthesis so that it has a blunt tip and blunt heel. Leave excess at the tip, to trim later.

2. Start the anastomosis at the acute angle. Avoid excessive tension on the prosthesis at the acute angle. The tip can be stretched and flattened as it is sutured. End the suture line at the side, not at the tip.

3. Check back bleeding by releasing the clamp on the profunda femoris artery. Flush the prosthesis and extrude air before tying the last stitch.

4. See the technique of end-to-side anastomosis described in Chapter 4 and illustrated in Figs. 4-5, 4-6, and 4-8.

AXILLOFEMORAL BYPASS

Axillofemoral bypass is a reasonable substitute for aortoiliac reconstruction in elderly poor-risk patients in whom both iliac arteries are diseased and inflow for a femorofemoral bypass would be insufficient. Axillofemoral bypass is essential when a previous aortoiliac prosthesis becomes infected and must be removed.

Because there are many complications and many late failures, the operation should not be performed unless the limb or life is in danger and the aortoiliac or aortofemoral bypass is too risky and femorofemoral bypass is not feasible.

One axillary artery can serve as donor to both legs if two grafts are joined at the groin and a femorofemoral bypass is performed to the other side.

The knitted Dacron prosthesis is convenient and effective, and the procurement of long veins would require extensive dissection. Good technique is necessary to avoid frequent early thromboses. We have had little experience with axillofemoral bypasses. Articles on this subject by other authors are very helpful.*

Procedure

Two surgeons can work simultaneously in the axilla and in the groin. Endotracheal general anesthesia is preferred and permits better control of oxygenation than local anesthesia. The patient should be in the supine position with the donor arm or arms extended on an arm board. The graft should be attached to the arm with the highest blood pressure and least murmur.

Prepare and drape the abdomen, chest, axilla, neck, and groins. Wrap and drape the arm so that it can be moved and the graft inspected in different positions.

Exposure of axillary artery

1. Incise the skin and split the fibers of the pectoralis major muscle two finger breadths below the clavicle. Gelpi retractors are very helpful.

2. Divide the tendon of the pectoralis minor muscle, and ligate the small artery it contains. Ligate and divide any tributaries of the axillary vein so that the vein can be safely retracted.

3. Trace the axillary artery up to the clavicle so that a 5 to 7 cm. length is exposed. Temporarily occlude branches with neurosurgical clips (they must all be accounted for prior to closure). Sometimes temporary ligatures looped around the branches help to steady the axillary artery.

4. Preclot a long knitted 8 mm. Dacron prosthesis. Use a 10 mm. graft if a branch will be attached for the other leg.

5. Inject 3,000 units of heparin.

6. The arteriotomy will be on the inferior aspect; therefore, apply the clamps so that they rotate the axillary artery about 45 degrees anteriorly.

---

*See references by Blaisdell and Hall (1963), Louw (1963), Mannick and Nasbeth, (1968), and Mannick and associates (1970).

Proximal anastomosis

1. The arteriotomy should be 12 to 15 mm. long. Cut the graft end so that it has a blunt tip and blunt heel (Fig. 4-8, *C*).

2. Make an oblique anastomosis, and do not try to evert the graft at the acute angle. Insert the needle 2 to 3 mm. from the edge of the arteriotomy. Start at the acute angle distally.

COMMENT: *This anastomosis is more prone to be disrupted than almost any other; therefore, make a sturdy suture line, and avoid tension on the graft when it is in the tunnel. An external graft can probably be devised to cover and reinforce the suture line, but we have not tried it yet. Remove the clamps to fill the graft under pressure and preclot it again. After flushing the graft, restore flow to the arm; and clamp the graft near the anastomosis, empty it, and cover it with moist gauze.*

Exposure of common femoral artery

Exposure of the common femoral artery proceeds simultaneously with the axillary exposure. It is described in full detail in Chapter 4 for aortofemoral bypasses and is illustrated in Fig. 6-1.

The outflow vessels are usually severely diseased, so that thromboendarterectomy in the common femoral and profunda femoris orifices will be necessary in most cases. This is described earlier for femorofemoral bypass and illustrated in Figs. 5-3, *D* and *E*, and 6-5.

Making the tunnel

1. Dissect bluntly beneath the pectoralis major muscle in an inferior direction toward the midaxillary line (Fig. 5-4). Make another incision in the midaxillary line midway between the axilla and the groin. The long DeBakey tunneler is useful here; otherwise another intervening incision may be needed.

2. Direct the tunnel anterior to the anterior, superior iliac spine and over the inguinal ligament onto the front of the common femoral artery.

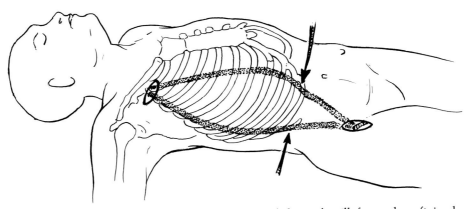

Fig. 5-4. A technical error that can result in early failure of axillofemoral graft is shown. If subcutaneous tunnel is placed too far anteriorly, graft will be kinked as it passes over costal margin when patient sits up. (Redrawn from Mannick, J. A., Williams, L. E., and Nasbeth, D. C.: The late results of axillofemoral grafts, Surgery **68:**1038-1043, 1970.)

3. Irrigate the tunnel with bacitracin solution. Before you draw the graft through the tunnel, release the clamp and fill the graft under pressure. The new porous grafts leak briskly unless they are preclotted thoroughly so that all the pores are filled with fibrin.

4. Empty the graft, fill it with a dilute heparin solution, and draw it through the tunnel without twist or kink and with no tension on the axillary anastomosis. Inspect the graft with the arm in different positions.

Distal anastomosis

Distal anastomosis is described and illustrated earlier in the chapter. Adequate outflow is absolutely essential. Good outflow is more crucial for prostheses than for vein grafts and seems to be particularly necessary for the long axillofemoral grafts.

Intraoperative arteriograms may be helpful before closure. Insert the needle in the graft and take a film beneath the groin and the thigh after injection of 30 ml. of Conray 60%.

When a branch is needed for the other groin also, attach an 8 mm. tube to the side of the 10 mm. tube wherever it is easily accessible in the groin incision; and make the subcutaneous suprapubic tunnel and anastomosis at the other groin as described in the femorofemoral bypass procedure. Mannick in 1970 reported good results in nine such cases.

REOPERATION FOR GRAFT THROMBOSIS AND OTHER COMPLICATIONS

Axillofemoral bypass prostheses appear to have a higher incidence of early and late closure than most other grafts. Thrombosis of the axillary artery occurs because of technical problems or complications at the proximal anastomosis. This rarely endangers the arm. However, many of the thromboses appear to be preventable or correctable by reoperation. The importance of correct position of the graft is emphasized by Mannick (1970), who also noted failures caused by tension and bowing of the axillary anastomosis. He reported that fourteen thrombectomies of axillofemoral prostheses were easily performed with local anesthesia, using Fogarty balloon catheters. Half of these were successful, but in some cases revision of the graft and/or outflow was required.

Poor outflow as a cause of late closure of these and other prostheses is manifested at reoperation by the thick neointimal lining. The finding of this lining should signal the need for local endarterectomy or other procedures to revascularize the profunda femoris artery. After thrombectomy of the prosthesis, intraoperative arteriogram may reveal a correctable cause.

As in most reoperations for poor outflow from a prosthesis, certain maneuvers avoid unnecessary dissection in the scar and fibrous tissue from the previous operation. A clamp is required on the reopened prosthesis for proximal control, but there is no need to remove the proximal clot unless or until the outflow problem has been corrected. Incision in the prosthesis close to the tip permits passage of Fogarty balloon catheters into the orifice of the profunda femoris artery and other orifices and removal of clots (Fig. 5-5). Then the catheters can remain inflated near the orifice in order to control back bleeding. Avoid dissecting these vessels in the surrounding scar. If operation on the profunda femoris artery is necessary, this maneuver reveals the orifice prior to dissection in the surrounding scar.

The midportion of the profunda femoris artery is least often involved by athero-

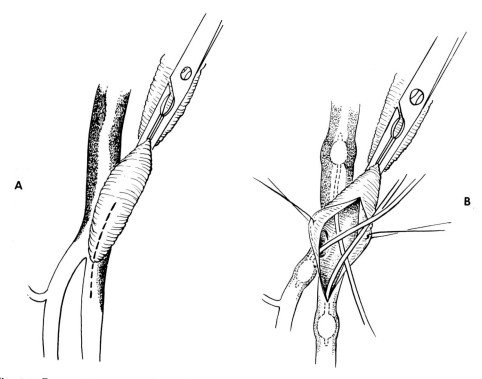

Fig. 5-5. Reoperation on aortofemoral anastomosis. **A,** Incision on prosthesis. **B,** Balloon catheters controlling back bleeding.

sclerosis; therefore, consider extending the bypass graft to the midportion as described in Chapter 6 and illustrated in Figs. 5-6 and 6-8. Long occlusions in the proximal end of the profunda femoris artery or occlusions of a previous proximal profundaplasty can more easily be bypassed than dissected and repaired.

CLOSURE AND POSTOPERATIVE CARE OF GROIN INCISIONS

Closure and postoperative care of groin incisions merit special attention in order to avoid the problems so frequently reported. The problems and complications so commonly reported in groin incisions are easily avoided. The longitudinal incision directly over the artery gives the best exposure of the entire length of the common femoral artery, the proximal end of the profunda femoris artery, and the proximal end of the superficial femoral artery. This incision is easily extended when the profunda femoris artery originates low or when it must be explored or revascularized. Notwithstanding other opinions, we always use, and have never regretted using, the longitudinal incision directly over the common femoral artery. It divides no arteries or veins and few lymphatic vessels and gives the best exposure. Occasionally the skin is incised across the crease of the groin. Grafts passing beneath the inguinal ligament need a roomy tunnel; therefore, the inguinal ligament is not sutured. Hernias have not developed in the tunnels or along the prostheses. Irrigate the wound with bacitracin solution.

The incision should be closed so that lymph, serum, or hematoma cannot accumulate around the prosthesis. Several layers of interrupted silk will cover the pros-

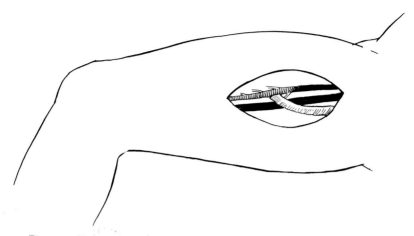

Fig. 5-6. Bypass prosthesis to profunda femoris artery in midthigh.

thesis with living tissue and avoid dead space. Superficial layers may be closed with continuous sutures of catgut. The skin edges should be carefully approximated with continuous sutures of monofilament nylon suture.

The use of anticoagulants is hazardous and unnecessary. Prevention of venous thrombosis with the "mini-heparin" regimen proposed by Kakkar has caused no problems as yet. The dose, 5,000 units given deep subcutaneously twice daily, does not affect the clotting or partial thromboplastin times.

Antibiotics are given before, during, and for five days after operation whenever prostheses are implanted.

Acute flexion of the thighs should be avoided for seven to ten days. When the saphenous vein has been removed for use as a graft or if edema of the leg appears, rest and elevation reduce lymph flow and avoid edema and lymph accumulations in the incisions.

Beware of edema of the leg. It may signify phlebitis, but it is usually due to disruption of lymphatic vessels. Elastic wrappings and stockings assist venous and lymphatic return. The external resistance of the elastic wrapping helps the leg muscles to compress and propel venous blood and lymph proximally.

OBTURATOR FORAMEN BYPASS

The obturator foramen is a useful route for a bypass prosthesis when sepsis in the groin causes complications in the common femoral artery or in a prosthesis attached there. These infections are grave complications that may lead to hemorrhage, high amputation, or even hip disarticulation or death. The principles of the treatment are simple and clear: (1) remove all infected plastic graft, and (2) restore arterial continuity. However, the application of these principles requires many choices and sound judgment. Articles on this technique by other authors are very helpful.*

There are occasional cases of radiation injury or trauma in which the occlusion or hemorrhage and infection involves only a short segment and there is no foreign-body vascular prosthesis present or only a small plastic patch angioplasty. A living

*See references by Dietrich and associates (1970), DePalma and Hubay (1968), Donahoe and associates (1967), Mahoney and Whelan (1966), and Shaw and Baue (1963).

143

arterial autograft as described by Stoney and Wylie (1970) can replace short infected diseased segments. The patient's own external iliac artery can be replaced with a Dacron tube, and the normal living artery will survive and heal when transplanted into the contaminated groin. Other autologous arteries, that is, segments of the hypogastric artery, need not be replaced. Occluded superficial femoral arteries are satisfactory after eversion endarterectomy.

Obturator foramen bypass will occasionally be needed because it avoids the infected groin when restoration of arterial continuity requires a new Dacron bypass through an uncontaminated operative field.

The proximal attachment for inflow can be to the axillary or opposite common femoral artery. The abdominal aortic prosthesis or proximal part of the aorta may also be a suitable takeoff for the new graft if infection arose in the groin after sufficient time for the intra-abdominal prosthesis to be surrounded and incorporated in the usual fibrous sheath (Dietrich and associates, 1970).

The distal anastomosis to restore circulation around the infected area may be done in one of several places, that is, the profunda femoris artery in the midthigh (Fig. 6-8, *C*) or the superficial femoral or popliteal artery if it is open and has sufficient outflow.

Early recognition and treatment of infected grafts before disruption and hemorrhage occur may permit elective removal of the infected graft at a separate operation.

Procedure

Preoperative preparation will include massive antibiotic coverage and adequate drainage.

The patient should be in the supine position. Prepare the area for proximal and distal attachment of the graft. Wall off the infected groin with plastic adherent drapes.

Proximal incision and exposure

1. Make a midline, suprapubic, or paramedian incision to expose the obturator foramen.

2. Peel the peritoneum and retract the bladder superiorly to uncover the pubic ramus. It is not necessary or advisable to enter the peritoneum if the proximal attachment of the graft will be extraperitoneal, that is, to the opposite femoral or axillary artery.

3. Incise the dense fascia medially near the pubic ramus, and extend the incision laterally from the edge of the obturator foramen. Cut away a circle of fascia at the foramen so that the opening admits a finger easily and loosely.

COMMENT: *An anomalous obturator foramen artery may arise from the inferior epigastric artery, and several small veins may be troublesome unless you start dissection medially.*

4. Palpate the neurovascular bundle; the artery and vein are inferior to the nerve. Note the vas deferens crossing the neurovascular bundle. If it is necessary to incise the fascia further, stay inferior to the neurovascular bundle.

5. Pass the tunneler through the foramen after you have started with the finger and have made the thigh incision.

Midthigh incision

The medial upper or midthigh approach gives access to either the profunda femoris or the superficial femoral artery for the distal anastomosis. See Fig. 6-8 and pp. 160 and 161 for full details.

1. Incise the skin and deep fascia and expose the artery at the site of intended anastomosis. During this maneuver, the thigh and knee must be flexed and the knee supported on folded sheets. This relaxes the rectus femoris and other anterior muscles so that they and their nerve supply can be retracted laterally.

2. Complete the tunnel when you are certain of the site of anastomosis. Unless the graft will continue down to the popliteal artery, the tunnel will come anteriorly through the adductor longus muscle to approach the superficial femoral or profunda femoris artery in the midthigh.

Proximal and distal anastomosis and closure of incisions

The principles, anatomy, and techniques are all illustrated and described elsewhere in this atlas (Figs. 4-5, 4-6, and 4-8).

Removal of infected graft

This is accomplished at this operation if necessary, but it is essential to keep the two operations separate even when they are done the same day. If the proximal anastomosis is at an uninfected area of the prosthesis in the abdomen, the old prosthesis must be divided through a clean area, and the distal end must be covered with clean peritoneum or living tissue so that the infected graft can be removed without contaminating the new graft.

F.B.H.

References

Blaisdell, F. W., and Hall, A. D.: Axillary-femoral artery bypass for lower extremity ischemia, Surgery 54:563-568, 1963.

Blaisdell, F. W., Hall, A. D., Lim, R. C., Jr., and Moore W. C.: Aorto-iliac arterial substitution utilizing subcutaneous grafts, Ann. Surg. 172:775-780, 1970.

DePalma, R. G., and Hubay, C. A.: Arterial bypass via the obturator foramen; an alternative in complicated vascular problems, Am. J. Surg. 115:323-328, 1968.

Dietrich, E. B., Noon, G. P., Liddicoat, J. E., and DeBakey, M. E.: Treatment of infected aorto-femoral arterial prosthesis, Surgery 68:1044-1052, 1970.

Donahoe, P. K., Froio, R. A., and Nabseth, D. C.: Obturator bypass graft in radical excision of inguinal neoplasm, Ann. Surg. 166:147-149, 1967.

Ehrenfeld, W. K., Harris, J. D., and Wylie, E. J.: Vascular "steal" phenomenon: an experimental study, Am. J. Surg. 116:192-197, 1968.

Foley, W. J., Dow, R. W., and Fry, W. J.: Crossover femoro-femoral bypass grafts, Arch. Surg. 99:83-87, 1969.

Gruda, P. N., and Moore, S. W.: Obturator bypass technique, Surg. Gynecol. Obstet. 128:1307-1316, 1969.

Louw, J. H.: Splenic-to-femoral and axillary-to-femoral bypass grafts in diffuse atherosclerotic occlusive disease, Lancet 1:1401-1402, 1963.

Mahoney, W. D., and Whelan, T. J.: Use of obturator foramen in iliofemoral artery grafting: case reports, Ann. Surg. 163:215-220, 1966.

Mannick, J. A., and Nabseth, D. C.: Axillofemoral bypass graft: a safe alternative to aortoiliac reconstruction, N. Engl. J. Med. 278:461-466, 1968.

Mannick, J. A, Williams, L. E., and Nabseth, D. C.: The late results of axillofemoral grafts, Surgery 68:1038-1043, 1970.

Parsonnet, V., Alpert, J., and Brief, D. K.: Femorofemoral and axillofemoral grafts—compromise or preference, Surgery 67:26-33, 1970.

Shaw, R. S., and Baue, A. E.: Management of sepsis complicating arterial reconstructive surgery, Surgery 53:75-86, 1963.

Stoney, R. J., and Wylie, E. J.: Arterial autografts, Surgery **67:**18-25, 1970.

Tyson, R. R., and Reichle, F. A.: Retropubic femoro-femoral bypass: a new route through the space of Retzius, Surgery **72:**401-403, 1972.

Vetto, R. M.: The femorofemoral shunt: an appraisal, Am. J. Surg. **112:**162-165, 1966.

6

Operations on the common femoral and profunda femoris arteries

INTRODUCTION

Reconstruction of the common femoral artery and revascularization of the profunda femoris artery is the preferred or sometimes the only operation feasible for many cases of femoropopliteal occlusions. Also, various maneuvers to restore flow in the common femoral and profunda femoris arteries are essential for the completion of aortic bypasses. These maneuvers may also be essential in operations such as femoropopliteal bypass that begin at the common femoral artery. All these procedures require a knowledge of the natural history and patterns of atherosclerotic disease as well as a knowledge of the normal anatomy.

In this chapter, various methods of reconstruction of the profunda femoris artery are described. These are sometimes the only feasible methods by which to revascularize ischemic limbs with advanced atherosclerotic occlusions; and although it rarely supplies sufficient flow to relieve pain with exercise, revascularization of the profunda femoris artery frequently salvages a limb, relieves ischemic pain at rest, and heals ischemic lesions or ischemic toes.

Natural history of occlusive disease in lower extremities

The superficial femoral artery is frequently the most vulnerable to atherosclerosis. Stenosis progressing to occlusion begins in the adductor canal and extends in stages proximally to the origin of the superficial femoral artery and extends distally into the popliteal artery. Sometimes stenosis begins at the origin of the superficial femoral artery from the common femoral artery. In the early stages, the only symptom is intermittent claudication, that is, ischemic pain with exercise. The arterial insufficiency is not severe because the profunda femoris artery is open and there are rich collateral connections to the lower leg. The atherosclerosis in the early stages begins with deposits on the posterior wall of the artery, and arteriograms of the lateral view are necessary to visualize the earliest stages. Arteriograms of the lateral view in the upper thigh, as reported by Martin, have shown plaques on the posterior wall of the common femoral artery and narrowing of the origin of the profunda femoris artery in 52.5% of patients whose only complaint was intermittent claudication.

Atherosclerosis in the profunda femoris artery is almost always localized to the ostium or the proximal segment. Martin reported from his arteriographic studies that three fourths of the plaques in the profunda femoris artery were found proximal to the first or second branch, and this is confirmed by operative observations by ourselves and many other surgeons. Only 10% of the patients have diffuse involvement of the profunda femoris artery, and even in some of these cases, it can be improved with correction of the ostial stenosis. Few surgeons have facilities for obtaining biplane arteriograms of the thigh and inguinal region, but recognition of these findings is important in the planning and conduct of all operations for ischemia of the leg.

Choice of operation

Arterial reconstruction for atherosclerosis below the inguinal ligament has been concerned mostly with restoring flow to the popliteal artery and its branches as described in Chapter 7. It must never be forgotten, however, that the profunda femoris artery is the lifeline of the lower limb, and we have already alluded to its importance as the outflow vessel after aortoiliac reconstruction. The following findings suggest the need to explore the common femoral artery, its bifurcation, and the profunda femoris artery in femoropopliteal reconstruction. When these findings are noted, narrowing of the profunda femoris artery and its origin are frequently found.

1. Occlusion of the superficial femoral artery at its origin or in its proximal segment.
2. Notching or beading of the superficial femoral artery by plaques in its upper portion as visualized in the usual anteroposterior arteriographic views. Femoropopliteal bypass must always begin at the common femoral artery whenever the atherosclerosis is so severe that femoropopliteal reconstruction is needed. In cases of popliteal aneurysm in which occlusive disease results only from distal embolism from the aneurysm, there will be a midportion of the superficial femoral artery satisfactory for the takeoff of the graft.
3. Combined aortoiliac and femoropopliteal disease.
4. Any notching of the common femoral artery visualized in the arteriograms of the anteroposterior view. This always means that there will be coincidental plaques on the posterior wall of the artery extending proximally and distally from the notching.

The common femoral artery is continuous with the external iliac artery above and divides promptly into two large branches: the superficial femoral artery, continuing down into the popliteal artery, and the profunda femoris artery, supplying the posterior part of the thigh. Atherosclerosis beginning above in the aortoiliac area or below in the femoropopliteal area frequently extends into the common femoral artery. The bifurcation of the common femoral artery, like arterial bifurcations elsewhere, such as at the aorta, the carotid artery, and iliac artery, is the site of early formation of atheromatous plaques. Such atheromas appear first most frequently and are thicker at bifurcations. The important exceptions are the atheromas at the adductor canal, and in this zone of the artery, the numerous muscular branches have plaques at their origin that are frequently close together and lead to early stenoses and occlusions in this zone. In certain metabolic abnormalities, such as certain cases of diabetes, the atheromatous deposits are widespread and diffuse.

The plaques appear first on the posterior wall of these arteries; this is highly significant, since arteriograms of the anteroposterior view, as customarily performed, do not show narrowing until the posterior plaque is so thick that it begins to encroach on the side of the artery. The arteriogram of the anteroposterior view of the ribbon appears as wide as a cylinder of the same diameter.

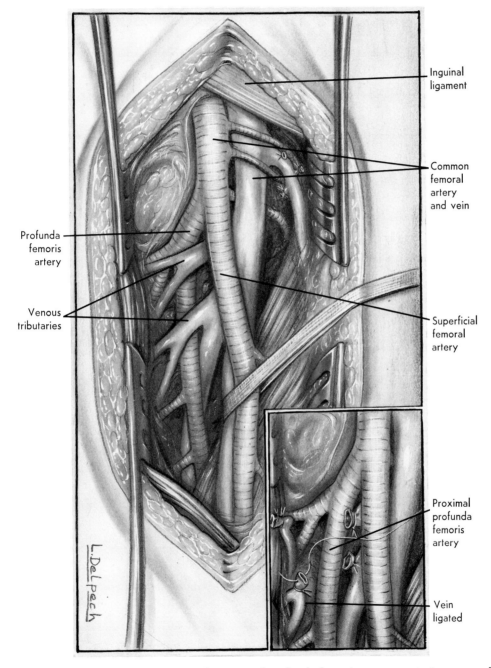

Inguinal ligament

Common femoral artery and vein

Profunda femoris artery

Venous tributaries

Superficial femoral artery

Proximal profunda femoris artery

Vein ligated

L.Delpech

Fig. 6-1. Surgical exposure of proximal portion of profunda femoris artery—anterior approach. Patient is in supine position, and the leg is extended. (Reproduced with permission from Cormier, J. M.: Chirurgie de l'artère fémorale profonde, 1970. Chapter from Techniques chirurgicales. Section in Encyclopédie médico-chirurgicale, Paris.)

SURGICAL ANATOMY OF COMMON FEMORAL ARTERY

The common femoral artery is the continuation of the external iliac artery beneath the inguinal ligament. It gives off small branches medially and laterally at that level and terminates 2 to 5 cm. distally by dividing into the superficial and the deep femoral (profunda femoris) arteries (Fig. 6-1). It is close beneath the skin and lies between the femoral vein medially and the femoral nerve laterally. This has been illustrated many times, since many vascular operations begin or end in this region.

SURGICAL ANATOMY OF PROFUNDA FEMORIS ARTERY

The upper 7 inches of the profunda femoris artery is accessible to the surgeon. For surgical purposes, the profunda femoris artery is composed of three portions. First, *the origin* of the artery and *the proximal* part of it, which is roughly 3 inches long, are accessible via the usual vertical incision beginning at the inguinal ligament (Fig. 6-1). Transverse groin incisions must not be used, since they cannot be extended when the profunda femoris artery takeoff point is low or when the reconstruction requires extension onto the profunda femoris artery. *The midportion* of the profunda femoris artery, which is 4 inches long, is approached by putting the leg in the position to relax the overlying rectus femoris and sartorius muscles. This is approached by the medial oblique incision. The lower 2 inches of the midportion of the artery lies behind the adductor longus muscle, but this is no serious obstacle (Fig. 6-8, *B*). The distal 5 inches of the profunda femoris artery pierces the adductor magnus muscle and lies in close proximity to the linea aspera femoris where it is covered by the dense attachments of the adductor muscles. This is inaccessible and of importance mainly because of its collateral connections with the muscular branches of the popliteal artery and the tibial recurrent arteries.

The profunda femoris artery arises from the back or from the outer side of the common femoral trunk within 2 to 5 cm. of the inguinal ligament. There are many variations in the origin and distribution of the profunda femoris artery (Fig. 6-2). It branches quickly, and one or both of the first branches—the medial and lateral femoral circumflex arteries—may arise from the common femoral artery instead of the profunda femoris artery. Fig. 6-3 shows the anterior view of the profunda femoris artery with the overlying muscles removed. The three perforating arteries pass backward close to the linea aspera femoris and form a double chain of connecting branches. One chain of anastomoses is in front of the linea aspera and one behind. The profunda femoris artery and its branches are usually very much enlarged when they serve as collateral pathways around an occluded superficial femoral artery, and arteriograms show large connections between the gluteal, obturator, and femoral circumflex arteries with the first perforating artery. The double arcade connects the perforating arteries' anastomoses distally with the important muscular branches of the popliteal and the recurrent tibial arteries. Surgical exposure and operations on the midportion of the profunda femoris artery are illustrated and discussed later.

EXPLORATION AND OPERATIONS FOR ATHEROSCLEROSIS OF COMMON FEMORAL ARTERY
Indications

Whenever an operation begins or terminates in the common femoral artery and whenever the common femoral artery is opened, it must be examined for plaques that are ulcerated or are obstructing the orifice of the profunda femoris or the superfi-

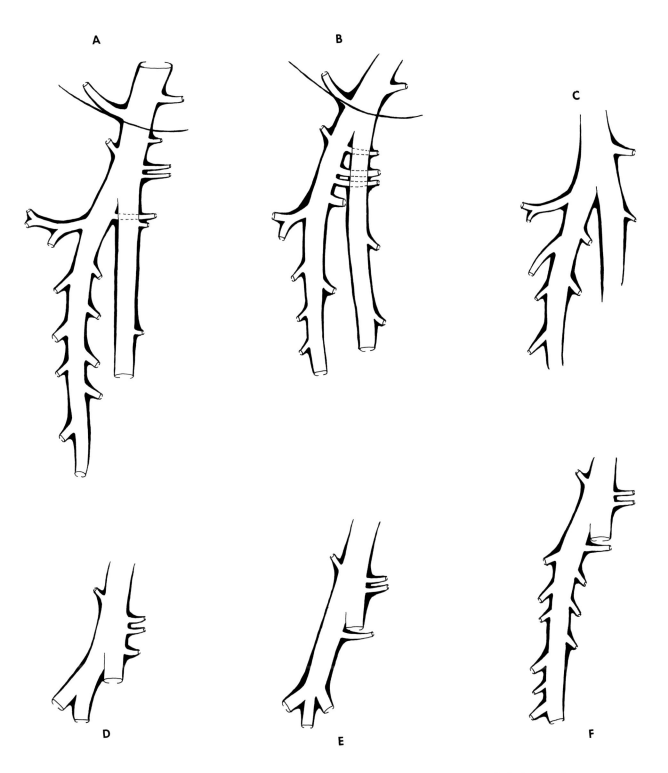

Fig. 6-2. Variations of common femoral and profunda femoris arteries and their branches. **A,** Usual arrangement. **B,** High takeoff of profunda femoris artery. **C** and **F,** Variations in branches of profunda femoris artery. **D** and **E,** Bifurcation and trifurcation of profunda femoris artery. (Adapted from Cormier, J. M.: Chirurgie de l'artère fémorale profonde, 1969. Chapter from Techniques chirurgicales. Section in Encyclopédie médico-chirurgicale, Paris.)

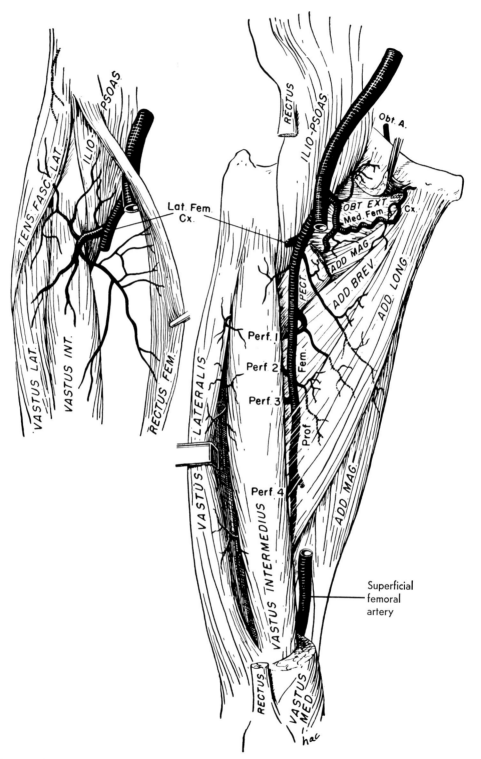

Fig. 6-3. Anterior view of profunda femoris artery. (From Edwards, E. A.: The anatomic basis for ischemia localized to certain muscles of lower limb, Surg. Gynecol. Obstet. **97**:87-94, 1953.)

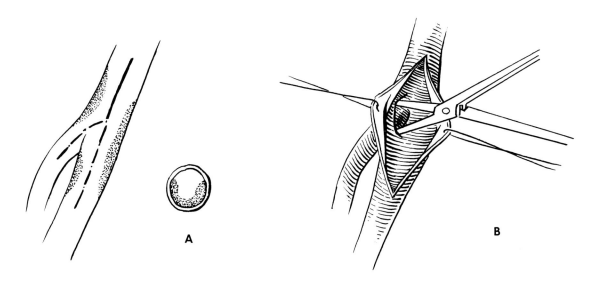

Fig. 6-4. A, Common femoral arteriotomy and possible choice of extension onto either branch. **B,** Dilation of orifice of profunda femoris artery.

cial femoral artery. These occur very frequently and are not visible in the routine anteroposterior view of the arteriograms.

Procedure
Incision and exposure

The vertical incision or hockey-stick incision beginning at the inguinal ligament is illustrated in Fig. 6-1.

Arteriotomy

1. Pass tapes about the profunda femoris as well as the superficial femoral and common femoral arteries for control proximally and distally. Smaller branches can be temporarily occluded with looped but untied ligatures. Inject heparin and apply clamps.

2. Open the common femoral artery longitudinally just proximal to the profunda femoris artery (Fig. 6-4).

COMMENT: *This arteriotomy can easily be extended onto either branch if necessary. Transverse arteriotomies are necessary or advisable only for small arteries.*

3. Inspect the back wall of the artery and the ostium of the profunda femoris artery.

4. Also inspect the back wall of the superficial femoral artery.

Dilation of ostium of profunda femoris artery

The fascial hiatus around the orifice of the profunda femoris artery sometimes restricts its dilation as collateral flow. The fascial hiatus is easily dilated through the arteriotomy of the common femoral artery before the aortofemoral or the femoropopliteal graft is attached. If the ostium seems small or if the back bleeding is poor, spread a hemostat to stretch the opening as illustrated in Fig. 6-4, *B.*

Local endarterectomy in common femoral artery

During arteriotomies for aortofemoral or femoropopliteal bypass, plaque is frequently noted. Occasionally, plaque on the posterior wall of the common femoral artery extends a short distance into the profunda femoris artery. Plaque is removed only if it is ulcerated, thick, or irregular.

Occasionally, complete occlusion of the common femoral artery occurs acutely by embolism or by hemorrhage under subintimal flap. Thrombectomy will be unsuccessful unless the underlying intimal flap or ulcerated plaque is recognized and removed as well as the thrombus.

The chronic complete occlusion of the common femoral artery will obstruct the orifice of the profunda femoris artery and will extend up into the iliac artery. Bypass from the aorta or opposite femoral artery may be needed for adequate inflow after disobliteration of the common femoral artery and the orifice of the profunda femoris artery. Bypasses are discussed later.

As the plaque in the orifice of the profunda femoris artery is teased away distally, the plaque usually tears away at its thin attachment, leaving no loose edge or flap (Fig. 6-5). When plaque extends down the posterior wall of the profunda femoris artery past the first or second branch, blind endarterectomy is always hazardous and we therefore extend arteriotomies several inches down the profunda femoris artery as discussed in the next section. When this tongue of plaque is less than 1 mm. thick, it seems unnecessary to trace it further. The curved endarterectomy scissors, which fits the curve of the lumen of the artery, will cut and bevel the distal edge. Whenever either in the profunda femoris or in the superficial femoral artery, the remaining thin edge of plaque seems loose, it must be sutured into place (Fig. 6-5, C); otherwise, pulsatile flow will loosen it further and curl it down like a trapdoor to obstruct the artery. These maneuvers are rarely needed except in diabetic patients in whom diffuse and soft loose atheroma extends everywhere up and down.

OPERATIONS ON PROXIMAL END OF PROFUNDA FEMORIS ARTERY

The upper portion (2 or 3 inches) of the profunda femoris artery is easily accessible with the leg extended and the patient in the usual supine position. The customary vertical groin incision is extended inferiorly; the table may be tilted slightly. The superficial femoral artery will always be occluded when significant atherosclerosis is found past the orifice of the profunda femoris artery. The superficial femoral artery can be retracted somewhat medially to reveal the profunda femoris artery more clearly.

There are several tributary veins that cross between the superficial femoral and the profunda femoris arteries and must be divided. These veins are short and should be ligated with sutures (Fig. 6-1).

PROFUNDAPLASTY FOR OCCLUSIVE DISEASE OF COMMON FEMORAL AND PROFUNDA FEMORIS ARTERIES

Various operations for profunda femoris artery reconstruction are diagrammed in Figs. 6-6 and 6-7. This procedure may be an essential part of bypass from above, in which case the surgeon may extend the tip of the prosthesis distally instead of using separate patch angioplasty; or during the femoropopliteal bypass operation, he would attach the vein graft to this arteriotomy after the endarterectomy. For long arteriotomies a separate patch as illustrated is sometimes preferred, and the bypass graft may be attached to the common femoral artery higher up.

154

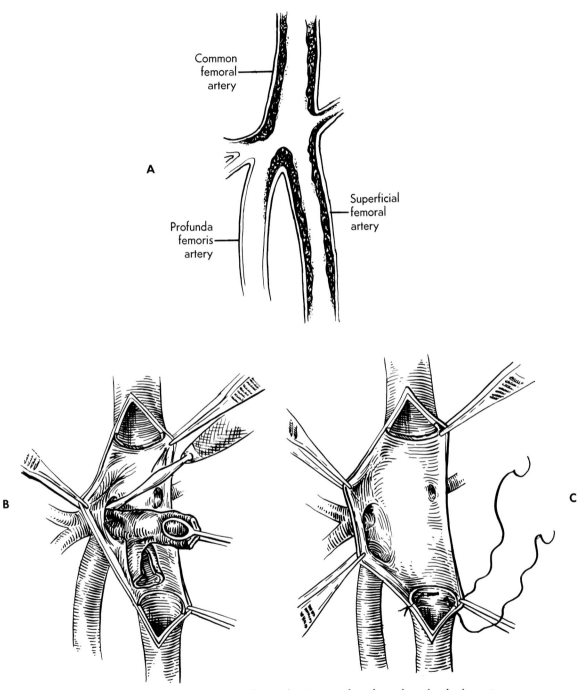

Fig. 6-5. Endarterectomy of common femoral artery and orifice of profunda femoris artery.
A, Diagram. **B,** Endarterectomy of orifice of profunda femoris artery. **C,** Suture of loose or
thick distal intima. (Adapted from Cormier, J. M.: Chirurgie de l'artère fémorale profonde,
1969. Chapter from Techniques chirurgicales. Section in Encyclopédie médico-chirurgicale,
Paris.)

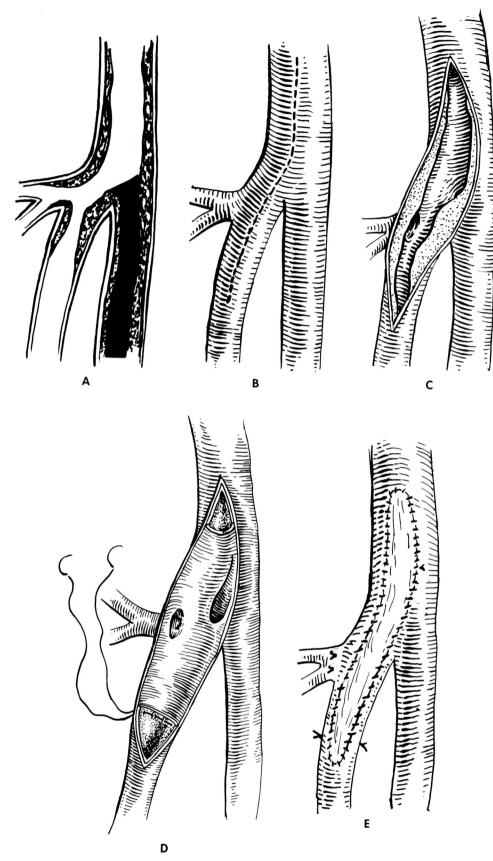

A   B   C

D   E

Fig. 6-6. For legend see opposite page.

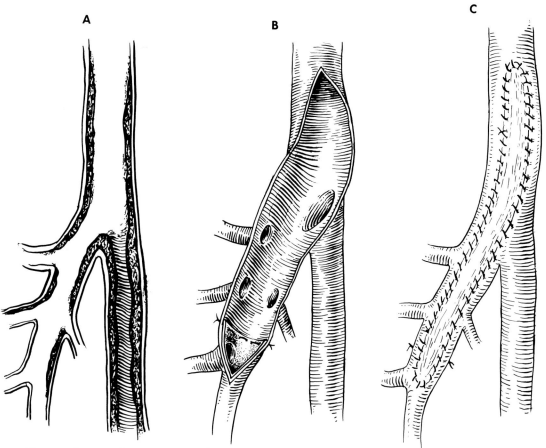

Fig. 6-7. Long endarterectomy and patch angioplasty of proximal portion of profunda femoris artery. **A,** Diagram. **B,** Completed thromboendarterectomy and suture of distal intima. **C,** Vein patch. (Adapted from Cormier, J. M.: Chirurgie de l'artère fémorale profonde, 1969. Chapter from Techniques chirurgicales. Section in Encyclopédie médico-chirurgicale, Paris.)

Fig. 6-6. Endarterectomy and patch angioplasty of profunda femoris artery. **A,** Diagram of stenotic profunda femoris and occluded superficial femoral arteries. **B,** Arteriotomy onto profunda femoris artery. **C,** View of plaque through arteriotomy. **D,** Suture of loose or thick distal intima in ostium of circumflex artery and in profunda femoris artery. **E,** Patch angioplasty. (Adapted from Cormier, J. M.: Chirurgie de l'artère fémorale profonde, 1969. Chapter from Techniques chirurgicales. Section in Encyclopédie médico-chirurgicale, Paris.)

Fig. 6-6 illustrates endarterectomy of the proximal end of the profunda femoris artery. The superficial femoral artery is occluded as is frequently the case. When the superficial femoral artery is occluded, stenosis of the profunda femoris artery is also frequently found. The distal intima is sutured whenever it is thick or loose.

Fig. 6-7 illustrates a longer profundaplasty down to the first perforating artery. *Following are the principles of patch angioplasty:*

1. The patch must not be so wide that it creates sacculations and turbulence.
2. It must end with a blunt tip. The suture is begun at one tip and is ended at the side.
3. It is usually preferable to end the patch at a large branch or bifurcation where the artery is already widened.
4. Vein is satisfactory for the patch material but not essential in the profunda femoris artery because, as in the carotid artery, the flow is large.
5. The thin DeBakey intracardiac Dacron patch material functions very well. This is easier to handle and more convenient than vein patches. We suspect that fibrosis or stricture is less likely to occur in a prosthetic patch than in the endarterectomized artery or a badly handled vein patch of doubtful viability.

In various ingenious maneuvers an endarterectomized superficial femoral artery is used as a tube or flap to bypass or to widen a narrow profunda femoris artery. This has not yet been necessary in our experience, but of course, the endarterectomized superficial femoral artery is autogenous tissue readily available if infection is suspected of being present. It might be useful as a short bypass already attached proximally to the common femoral artery if the proximal end of the profunda femoris artery has been damaged and the damage is irreparable.

OPERATIONS ON PROFUNDA FEMORIS ARTERY IN MIDTHIGH

Few operations have been done on the midsection of the profunda femoris artery, partly because it is deep and not easily accessible, partly because its importance has only recently been recognized, and also partly because it is seldom injured and seldom involved in atherosclerosis.

It is readily accessible for bypass or for repair by the medial oblique approach as described subsequently. Occasionally there is a long occlusion of the proximal end of the profunda femoris artery, failure of a previous proximal profundaplasty, or infection in a groin incision. In such situations, bypass to the midportion of the profunda femoris artery may save a leg. The profunda femoris artery enlarges when it serves as a collateral channel, and the three perforating arteries form a double arcade that connects distally with important muscular branches of the popliteal artery and the recurrent branches of the tibial arteries.

The proximal origin of the bypass will vary according to need and availability; it may be the aorta, occasionally the iliac or femoral artery, or even the opposite iliac or femoral artery. The bypass graft usually passes under the inguinal ligament in the usual fashion. The obturator foramen can be used to bypass an infected groin incision.

Surgical anatomy of profunda femoris artery in midthigh

The midsection of the femoral artery is deep and almost inaccessible until the leg is flexed and everted. The oblique medial approach with the leg in this position permits retraction of the overlying muscles and their accompanying nerve supply

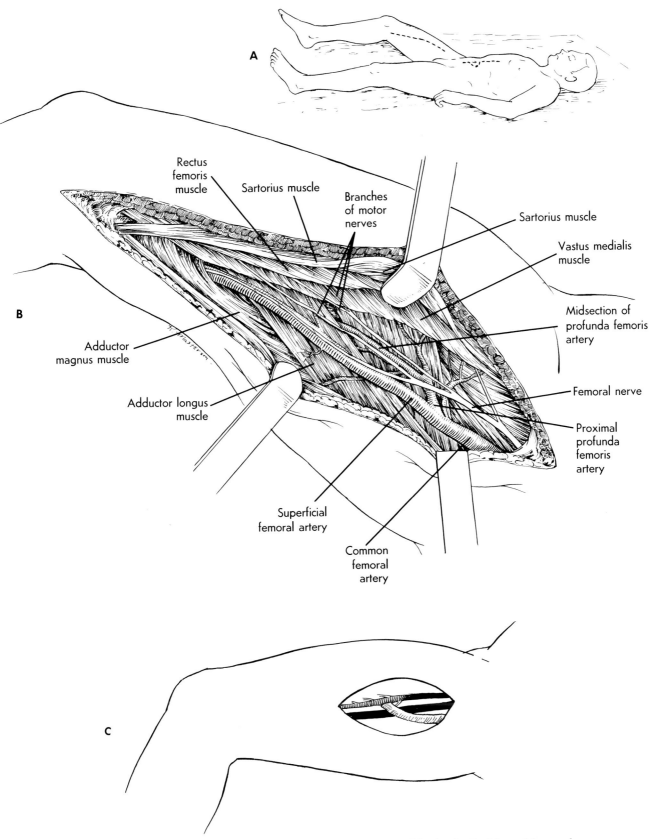

Fig. 6-8. Surgical exposure of profunda femoris artery in midthigh. **A,** Position of leg and incision. **B,** Anatomical dissection of proximal 7 inches of superficial femoral and profunda femoris arteries. Veins are omitted. **C,** Bypass prosthesis to profunda femoris artery in midthigh. (From Hershey, F. B.: Extended surgery applied to the profunda femoris artery, Surg. Gynecol. Obstet. In press.)

159

(Fig. 6-8, *A*). The nerves to the rectus femoris and the sartorius muscles cross the midportion of the profunda femoris artery but are drawn aside when the bellies of these muscles are relaxed and retracted outward. The saphenous nerve can be retracted medially or sacrificed with impunity. Fig. 6-8, *B* shows an anatomical dissection of the proximal 7 inches of the superficial and deep femoral vessels and illustrates their relationship. The profunda femoris artery is parallel close to the superficial femoral artery and is separated from the superficial femoral artery by the accompanying profunda femoris vein and the superficial femoral vein. The profunda femoris artery winds inferiorly in a loose half spiral until it lies posterior to the superficial femoral artery, but it is rarely more than 2 to 3 cm. separated from the superficial femoral artery. In the midthigh, the profunda femoris and superficial femoral arteries are deep, covered by thick muscles that can only be retracted when relaxed with the leg in the position illustrated in Fig. 6-8, *A*.

The midportion of the profunda femoris artery for 3 inches lies on the adductor brevis muscle, whose nerves are lateral and not too close to the artery. The artery then passes under the upper edge of the adductor longus muscle for about 2 inches before it dips posteriorly and becomes inaccessible. The fibers of the adductor longus muscles may be divided with impunity if further exposure is needed distally.

Bypass to midportion of profunda femoris artery

The purpose of bypass to the midportion of the profunda femoris artery is to restore flow to the profunda femoris artery when the proximal end of the profunda femoris artery is occluded or the groin is infected.

Proximally the bypass may be attached at whichever place is suitable: the aorta, iliac artery, or opposite femoral artery.

Preparation

The patient is placed in the supine position; the thigh and knee are flexed, and the thigh is externally rotated in order to relax the strong muscles in the anterior part of the thigh (Fig. 6-8, *A*).

COMMENT: *Prepare the entire leg. Cover the lower leg with a sterile stockinette so that it can be positioned for operation and later straightened to determine the correct length of the graft. Support the knee on a pile of folded sheets.*

Procedure
Incision

Begin the incision two finger breadths medial to the anterior superior spine and extend it inferiorly, aiming it toward the medial border of the patella. The incision should be 6 to 7 inches long.

COMMENT: *Obviously, if the groin is infected, the tunnel must be made through the obturator foramen and the infected groin is not entered. In such a case, approach the midportion of the profunda femoris artery via a shorter incision in the midthigh.*

Exposure

1. Divide the deep fascia and retract the inguinal glands medially from in front of the artery.

2. Mobilize the medial edge of the sartorius muscle and the medial edge of the rectus femoris muscle.

COMMENT: *Do not disturb the lateral femoral cutaneous artery, which originates several finger breadths below Poupart's ligament. Divide any fine threadlike nerves that cross the main arteries medially. Spare the important motor branches coursing laterally by retracting the sartorius and rectus femoris muscles laterally together with the accompanying motor nerves. Look for deeper nerves that are lateral to the superficial femoral artery and that may cross the medial aspect of the profunda femoris artery to supply the vastus muscles. Retract these nerves laterally also.*

3. Identify the occluded superficial femoral artery and vein medially, and pass over it without dissecting it or uncovering it.

COMMENT: *The relationship of femoral arteries and veins at this level from medial to lateral is as follows: The first medially and the most superficial is the superficial femoral artery. Adjacent and deep to this is the superficial femoral vein. Only 1 or 2 cm. deeper is the profunda femoris vein, which lies medial and somewhat anterior to its accompanying pulsating profunda femoris artery.*

4. Identify the profunda femoris vein medial to the profunda femoris artery. The artery is shifting laterally and no longer seems to go so deep and so far posterior.

COMMENT: *The deep femoral artery can now be palpated and traced distally to where it passes behind the upper edge of the adductor longus muscle, but it is only necessary to uncover sufficient length for the bypass anastomosis. When necessary, the upper edge of the adductor longus muscle can be mobilized to uncover another inch or two of the profunda femoris artery. This is seldom necessary.*

5. Uncover 1 or 2 inches of the profunda femoris artery for anastomosis. Divide any venous tributaries that cross the artery, and occlude the abundant muscular branches temporarily with tiny Schwartz clips or loop them with sturdy silk to lift and occlude them.

COMMENT: *The exposure of several inches of the profunda femoris artery in this fashion reveals soft artery that is as large or larger than the popliteal artery because of its increased collateral flow around the occlusions of the other femoral arteries. Tributaries of the vein crossing the artery at the part chosen for arteriotomy are divided, and a linear arteriotomy is made for attachment of the oblique end of the prosthesis.*

Making the tunnel

Make a tunnel under the skin of the upper thigh and under the inguinal ligament, and draw the end of the graft down through the tunnel, using a curved sponge-holding forceps or the DeBakey tunneler.

Anastomosis

1. Measure the correct length of graft, with the leg straightened.

2. Cut the graft with excess at the tip and little or no tension at the heel. Of course, the proximal portion of the graft must be straight so that there is no kink or curve at the origin.

3. Details of this type of anastomosis are described elsewhere and are identical with those of the technique used for end-to-side anastomosis to the iliac, femoral, or popliteal arteries (Figs. 4-5, 4-6, 4-8, and 7-9).

Closure

Before closure, check the position of the graft with the thigh flexed. Make sure that the tunnel under the inguinal ligament is roomy for one finger. Sutures of deep layers for closure must not confine the graft or cause angulation during flexion of the thigh.

FEMORAL ANEURYSMS

Femoral aneurysms are less common than popliteal aneurysms, but they present all the same problems, mainly embolism or thrombosis and, rarely, rupture. Compression of veins may cause edema and phlebitis.

The best operation is usually resection and grafting.

Femoral aneurysms may arise from degeneration of the artery wall, that is, true aneurysm, or from rupture of the wall, causing false aneurysm. False aneurysms may arise from slight disruption of an aortofemoral bypass anastomosis years after the operation. Prevention is discussed in Chapter 4. The main problems encountered with these are (1) fibrosis around the prosthesis; (2) occult infection as an unrecognized cause of the disruption; and (3) displacement of or adherence to femoral nerve and veins by the large aneurysm sac.

Primary arteriosclerotic aneurysms of the femoral artery are frequently accompanied by others in the abdomen or popliteal space and sometimes by generalized dilation or ectasia of many arteries. Therefore, the surgeon must look for other lesions and establish priorities of treatment. Some patients will not be candidates for any operation because of prohibitive risk of associated disease or generalized arterial ectasia.

Diagnosis

The diagnosis is easily made by palpation, but arteriograms are helpful. When distal pulses are poor, the arteriograms reveal the extent of associated stenosis or occlusions. Many patients have associated abdominal aneurysms, and plain films of the abdomen may be helpful also.

Indications for surgical treatment

Elective surgery is appropriate when the aneurysm is symptomatic, expanding, or of significant size. The outflow must be sufficient to maintain patency of the graft. The superficial femoral artery is frequently occluded at its origin, but revascularization of the profunda femoris artery is sufficient to maintain the leg. The chronic occlusions of the superficial femoral artery cannot be reopened.

Objectives of surgery

The objectives of surgery are to prevent complications by resection of the aneurysm and to preserve a functional extremity by restoring continuity and flow into the profunda femoris artery in all cases and into the superficial femoral artery when feasible.

Operation for aneurysm of common femoral artery

Anastomotic aneurysms are discussed later. The type of operation is adapted to the findings and needs. The aneurysm need not be excised completely, and it is advantageous to leave some of the back wall around the orifice of the profunda femoris artery. The use of an 8 to 10 mm. knitted Dacron prosthesis is preferable. Endarterectomy, thrombectomy, and plastic repair of the aneurysm sac are compromises that frequently fail.

Procedure

Incision and exposure

Since the first step is to obtain control proximally, the incision may extend well above the inguinal ligament.

1. Divide the inguinal ligament over the pulse.

2. Retract the peritoneum up off the external iliac artery, and pass a tape about it.

COMMENT: *If the aneurysm is in the way, divide the external oblique aponeurosis, and if necessary, split the internal oblique muscle and sweep the peritoneum upward to uncover the external iliac artery well above the aneurysm. Do not roll, squeeze, or manipulate the aneurysm sac, or emboli may be dislodged.*

3. Incise the skin over the aneurysm and distally to uncover the superficial femoral artery.

Proximal and distal control

Pick out and preclot the appropriate knitted Dacron prosthesis (usually 8 to 10 mm). You are now ready to cross-clamp the arteries, but the profunda femoris artery may still be concealed by the overlying aneurysm.

1. Inject 3,000 units of heparin, and clamp the external iliac and superficial femoral arteries. Temporarily occlude the small branches at the inguinal ligament if they are distal to your proximal clamp.

2. Boldly open the aneurysm, scoop out the contents, and place a fingertip over the briskly bleeding orifice of the profunda femoris artery. Small bleeding orifices may be ligated with figure-of-eight sutures inside the sac as illustrated in Fig. 8-3, C.

3. Now the profunda femoris artery may be accessible outside the empty aneurysm and can be dissected and clamped with the DeBakey peripheral vascular angle clamp, or the profunda femoris artery can be occluded inside the sac by inserting the tip of the No. 3 or 4 Fogarty balloon catheter and blowing up the balloon just inside the orifice.

COMMENT: *Noon has devised some short balloon catheters with various sizes of balloons that are excellent for this purpose.* However, balloons can cause damage if they are overinflated in a fragile artery.*

Resection of aneurysm

If the aneurysm is not too large or adherent, dissect it out, but save a 2 to 3 mm. cuff around the orifice of the profunda femoris artery. Divide the common femoral or external iliac artery proximal to the aneurysm.

COMMENT: *Most aneurysms stop at the inguinal ligament, and happily they never involve more than the proximal 1 to 2 cm. section of the profunda femoris artery.*

Suturing of prosthesis

Fig. 6-9 shows reconstruction that is done when the superficial femoral artery is occluded. However, there will be three anastomoses if the superficial femoral artery is still open (Fig. 6-10). It is not necessary to devise bifurcation prostheses.

1. Anastomose the profunda femoris artery first to a longitudinal incision in the prosthesis. The cuff saved at the orifice of the artery permits secure suturing without stricture or tension. Use 4-0 Dacron vascular sutures. Preclot the graft again when you flush the artery.

2. Trim the proximal end to the correct length, and suture the prosthesis and external iliac artery in the end-to-end position. Then perform the usual maneuvers: Flush the inflow vessel and reclamp it. Flush the profunda femoris artery and reclamp

---

*Made by U. S. Catheter and Instrument Corp., Glen Falls, N. Y.

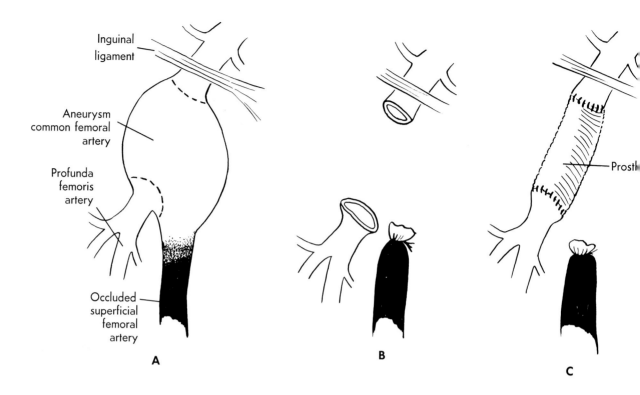

Inguinal ligament

Aneurysm common femoral artery

Profunda femoris artery

Occluded superficial femoral artery

A

B

C

Prosth

Fig. 6-9. Resection of femoral aneurysm. **A,** Aneurysm. Dotted line shows incision to save cuff around orifice of profunda femoris artery. **B,** Cuff of profunda femoris artery. Superficial femoral artery occluded. **C,** Prosthesis in place.

it. Clamp the graft just below the profunda femoris artery. Release the clamp on the profunda femoris artery, and cover any leaks with Gelfoam. Release the inflow to restore full pressure and flow into the profunda femoris artery.

3. Perform the distal anastomosis: Trim the end of the graft to the correct length. Flush the superficial femoral artery, and check back bleeding. Suture the distal end of the graft to the artery. Release the distal clamp briefly to flush and extrude air before tying the final suture. Release the distal clamp, and apply Gelfoam if it is needed. Release the proximal clamp.

Closure of incisions

Good hemostasis and snug closure to cover the prosthesis with living tissue are essential in groin incisions. Avoid dead space.

It is unnecessary to resuture Poupart's ligament because herniation does not occur along a prosthesis, and it is better if flexion of the thigh cannot compress the graft.

Copious irrigation of the incision with bacitracin solutions and antibiotics given preoperatively and intraoperatively as well as postoperatively are all helpful in preventing infection, but careful closure is essential. We prefer interrupted silk in the deeper layers.

Postoperative care

Beware of postoperative phlebitis. Some of these aneurysms can cause venous compression, edema, and possibly undetected phlebitis before the operation.

164

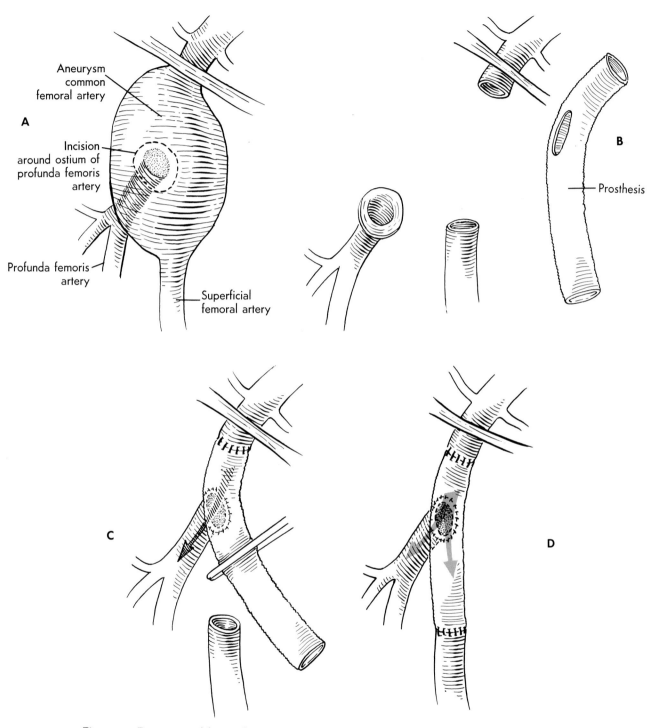

Fig. 6-10. Resection of femoral aneurysm and three-way anastomosis. **A,** Aneurysm. Dotted line shows incision to save cuff at orifice of profunda femoris artery. **B,** Incision in graft for anastomosis to profunda femoris artery. **C,** Proximal anastomosis completed and flow restored into profunda femoris artery. **D,** Three-way anastomosis completed.

165

Extensive dissections in the groin inevitably interrupt lymphatic vessels, but bed rest for seven days keeps lymph flow at a minimum and helps the wound layers to heal and seal.

ANASTOMOTIC FALSE ANEURYSMS

The wall of the usual or true aneurysm is the stretched and dilated wall of the artery. False aneurysms result from a leak in the artery wall through which a pulsating hematoma develops whose wall is connective tissue pushed aside and also formed in reaction around the hematoma. The development of false aneurysms after arterial trauma are discussed in Chapter 10.

The anastomotic aneurysm due to a tiny disruption of a suture line is more common in the femoral area than elsewhere, and there are special considerations in the repair at this site. It is now a rare complication when proper precautions are observed. In almost all reported cases, silk sutures were used to suture the prostheses to the artery. Experimental studies have shown that silk loses its tensile strength during implantation, and although arterial silk is satisfactory for joining two living blood vessels, it will weaken and may permit disruption between a prosthesis and an artery. In the first edition of this atlas, we suggested and we now require the use of Dacron or other synthetic suture material that is not biologically degradable and that is of suitable strength for all anastomoses of prostheses.

The use of woven prostheses is followed by a higher incidence of false aneurysms than the use of the more flexible knitted fabrics. Knitted prostheses are therefore preferred.

False aneurysms appear more commonly in the groin than elsewhere; but they are frequently multiple, so that when one is found, arteriograms should be performed to visualize the other anastomoses.

False aneurysms may occur with all types of anastomosis, end-to-end or end-to-side, but are rare unless a prosthesis is used. The prosthesis never knits or joins end to end with the artery, and its integrity requires sturdy suture material and sturdy arterial wall. The reinforcement of anastomoses by external grafting as described in Chapter 4 may be helpful. Reinforcement, however, is only an adjunct, and the surgeon must rely mainly on a wide cuff of sturdy arterial wall. In aortic aneurysms, 5 mm. cuff is customarily used and is easily made with the larger vascular needle. In end-to-side anastomoses or patch angioplasties, a 2 to 3 mm. edge of the artery is incorporated into the suture line without narrowing the lumen.

Infection at the suture line may lead to disruption and false aneurysms and hemorrhage, but infection is usually evident before the aneurysm or hemorrhage occurs. Treatment of infected prostheses is discussed in a separate section; however, any suspicious collection of fluid near a false aneurysm or disruption should be smeared and cultured for microorganisms.

Operations for anastomotic aneurysms at the groin

The most frequent cause of anastomotic aneurysm at the groin is disruption of the suture line between the end of a prosthesis and the common femoral artery. The principles are applicable to the same problem at other sites. Most of these grafts have been passed under the inguinal ligament (Fig. 6-11).

The operation must correct the cause or presumed causes of the suture line failure, meanwhile maintaining or restoring flow to the leg. The best operation includes

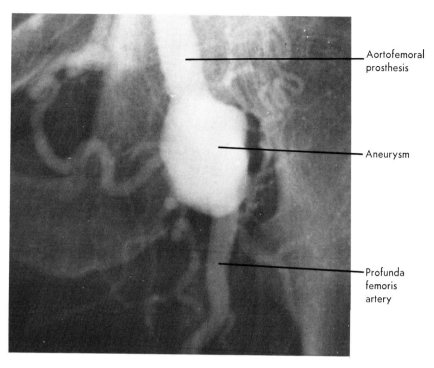

Aortofemoral
prosthesis

Aneurysm

Profunda
femoris
artery

Fig. 6-11. Arteriogram showing anastomotic aneurysm in left groin. Superficial femoral artery is occluded. Profunda femoris artery fills faintly.

(1) making a new anastomosis with Dacron suture instead of silk, (2) making the anastomosis into relatively normal or sturdy artery, (3) avoiding tension by splicing a new piece to lengthen the graft, and (4) replacing woven tubes with more flexible knitted Dacron in the segment near the anastomosis.

For procedures to follow when the disruption results from infection, see Chapters 1 and 5. Infection will be limited to the groin if sufficient time elapsed before infection occurred to permit the normal fibrous layer to form a tight sheath and to grow into the pores of the graft. If infection is recent, it will probably extend along the whole length of the graft. However, the principles of treatment are the same: (1) establish a new bypass through an uninfected route, and (2) remove the infected prosthesis. For the discussion of alternate routes for bypass, see Chapter 5 and the section on the bypass operation to the profunda femoris artery in the midthigh earlier in this chapter.

The technical problems in the resection and repair of anastomotic aneurysms in the groin are mainly (1) obtaining control proximally and distally without tedious and hazardous dissection in the fibrous tissue at the previous operative site around the prosthesis and around the sac; (2) reinforcing the suture line, since sturdy artery may not be accessible without extensive dissection and large risks; (3) problems arising from poor outflow.

Procedure

Incision and exposure

See the procedures for surgical treatment of femoral aneurysm described earlier in this chapter. The incision may extend above the inguinal ligament as described.

The prosthesis proximal to the aneurysm will be pulsating and readily palpated beneath the skin. Incision over it with careful strokes of the sharp knife will reveal the sturdy Dacron prosthesis. The surrounding fibrous tissue is densely adherent but can be peeled away from a short segment of the prosthesis so that a clamp can be applied vertically to occlude the prosthesis. It is difficult and unnecessary to dissect behind the prosthesis. It is probably lying on the artery or vein.

Proximal and distal control

With large aneurysms, obtaining control distally may be feasible only by boldly opening the sac and putting balloon catheters into the orifices of the profunda femoris, common femoral, and superficial femoral arteries as described earlier (Figs. 4-10, C, and 5-5, B). After preclotting a piece of tube prosthesis and patch material, inject 3,000 units of heparin and clamp the prosthesis. The pulsation in the aneurysm should dampen considerably.

Opening the sac may reveal only a small disruption and may not permit you to enter the artery to occlude the back-bleeding orifices. Usually, however, pressure and suction controls the bleeding, and you can quickly tease the edge of the prosthesis away from the artery. If it can not be teased easily, snip close to the prosthesis and trim the edge later. When you can see the orifices, insert and inflate the balloon catheters. Detach the whole suture line.

COMMENT: *The balloon catheters devised by Noon are short and have different sizes of balloons adequate for most orifices. Inflate the balloons slowly and only enough to control the ooze and back bleeding.*

Reconstruction—grafting

Since the weakness is at the suture line, the remainder of the artery is probably sturdy, and the outflow probably is and will remain satisfactory. Trim the edge of the arteriotomy so that new sutures are made in healthy tissue. Splice a new piece or segment of prosthesis into place if tension seems excessive. Use 4-0 Dacron sutures, and pass the needle 3 mm. from the edge of the arteriotomy. Follow the usual flushing maneuvers, check back bleeding, and restore flow.

Reinforcement of suture lines—external grafting

For external grafting at a bifurcation such as in the common femoral artery, the same principles are followed as described earlier. It requires circumferential dissection of the common femoral and superficial femoral arteries; this may be difficult because of scarring from the previous surgery. However, external grafting is the only feasible way to reinforce such a suture line. The profunda femoris artery does not need to be dissected so that is free but may be dissected only close to the orifice.

Fig. 6-12 shows a method of external grafting for reinforcement. A knitted Dacron bifurcation graft is needed that is large enough to wrap around the widest part. The hole for the profunda femoris artery must be accurately placed. This hole and the crotch are the two fixed and accurately located features. The slit and hole for the profunda femoris artery are made only after the crotch is sutured so that it is snug anteriorly. Then cut the slit and hole for the artery in the correct location. Last of all, wrap the external graft around the posterior wall of the common femoral artery, and trim the excess and suture the graft so that it is snug, to complete the reinforcement.

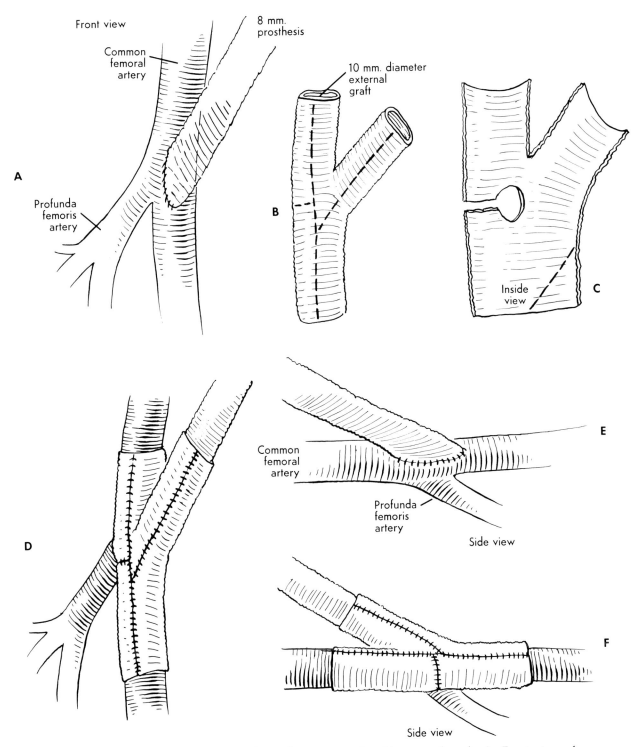

Fig. 6-12. Reinforcement of end-to-side anastomosis with external graft. **A,** Front view of aortofemoral anastomosis redone after anastomotic aneurysm. **B,** Bifurcation prosthesis for external graft. Dotted lines show incisions. **C,** Open inside view of **B. D,** Front view of external graft in place. **E,** Side view of aortofemoral anastomosis before application of external graft reinforcement. **F,** Side view after external graft is in place.

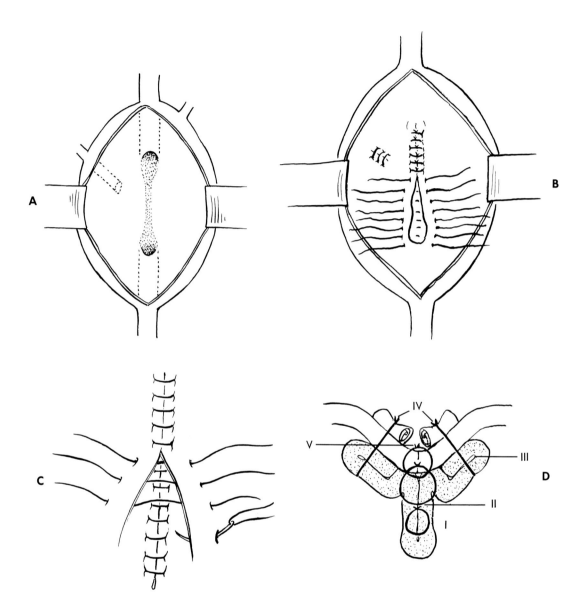

Fig. 6-13. For legend see opposite page.

Fig. 6-13. Matas' obliterative endoaneurysmorrhaphy.

A, "Interior of large aneurismal sac of the fusiform type exposed by retraction. The two openings lead respectively to the parent trunk on the proximal (cardiac) and peripheral sides, and the groove between them represents the continuity of the arterial walls blending with the aneurismal sac. This was the type of sac observed in cases 1, 2, and 4, reported in the text. The orifice of one collateral or branch originating in the sac is shown, and a large collateral opening into the main trunk near the orifice of communication, on the cardiac side, is indicated by the dotted line."

B, "Shows the orifices in the aneurismal sac in process of obliteration by suture. The first plane of sutures may be made with fine silk, but chromicized catgut is preferred. The sutures are applied very much like Lambert's sutures in intestinal work; the first plane of sutures should be sufficient to secure complete hemostasis.

"The orifice of the collateral vessel on the left upper side of the sac is shown closed by three continuous sutures."

C, "This shows a second row of sutures, a technical detail of the operation which is advantageous, but not necessary in every case.

"The first row of sutures has been completed and the arterial orifices have been obliterated. As the walls of the sac are usually relaxed, it is easy to insert a second series of sutures which add security to the first row, and, in addition, reduce the size of the cavity which is to be obliterated by inversion of the skin and surplus sac walls at a later stage in the operation. This second row of sutures is applied as in the first series, by either the continuous or interrupted method, with a curved needle, and Nos. 1, 2, or 3 chromic catgut. A large surface of the sac is thus brought in apposition, and the best opportunity given for adhesion by plastic or exudative endo-arteritis. If the floor of the sac is rigid or too adherent to the underlying parts, this second row may be omitted, and the operation can be advanced to the last step— i.e., obliteration of the sac after suture of the orifices."

D, "Sectional diagram showing method of obliterating the aneurismal sac in the *fusiform* type of aneurism with two openings. In this class of cases [**A, B,** and **C**] the tunics of the parent artery blend with the sac, and the arterial channel cannot usually be restored.

"The diagram shows the first row of sutures (I), which obliterates the orifice of the artery at the bottom of the sac. The second row of sutures is shown higher up (II), and also the effect of this row in reducing the capacity of the sac. The obliteration of the remaining part of the cavity by the folding in or inversion of the sac walls, with the attached overlying skin, is shown in III.

"The function of the deep sutures (IV) tied over gauze pads, and of the more superficial skin sutures (V) in obtaining firm contact of the opposed surfaces, is also shown. This drawing is purely schematic; it gives an exaggerated idea of the size of the sac walls, and is chiefly intended to give an idea of the position of the sutures and other parts."

(From Matas, R. J.: An operation for the radical cure of aneurism, based upon arteriorrhaphy, Ann. Surg. 37:161-196, 1903.)

False aneurysm sac—obliterative aneurysmorrhaphy

If the false aneurysm sac is large or densely adherent to adjacent veins and nerves, perform the Matas' endoaneurysmorrhaphy, suturing and obliterating the sac from the inside, folding it over the prosthesis with multiple rows of continuous Dacron sutures. It is dangerous and unnecessary to resect the adherent sac.

Fig. 6-13 is a copy of Matas' highly schematic drawing showing the technique for obliteration of the sac of a popliteal aneurysm with multiple interrupted silk sutures. We use continuous Dacron sutures. There is no back bleeding from false aneurysm sacs because there are no branches. The sac may be very large and irregular in shape. The drawings from Matas' original articles in 1903 and 1920 are highly schematic. Few popliteal aneurysms will be so symmetrical, and false aneurysms will all be in odd shapes; therefore, Matas' precise rows of sutures need not be attained.

Closure of incision and postoperative care

The closure of the incision and postoperative care are the same as those described on p. 142.

F.B.H.

References

Matas, R. J.: An operation for the radical cure of aneurism, based upon arteriorrhaphy, Ann. Surg. **37**:161-196, 1903.
Matas, R. J.: Ann. Surg. **71**:403-427, 1920.

7

Occlusive disease in the lower extremity

INTRODUCTION

Arteriosclerotic occlusive disease below the common femoral artery is still one of the most challenging problems in vascular reconstructive surgery. Legs in danger because of occlusive disease below the inguinal ligament can frequently be saved or salvaged by the procedures described in this chapter. The patterns of atherosclerotic occlusive disease in the abdominal aorta and iliac vessels are described in previous chapters. Atherosclerotic narrowing of the profunda femoris artery at the groin is likewise emphasized and illustrated in Chapter 6. A leg may be endangered by atherosclerotic occlusions of the superficial femoral and popliteal arteries, but in order to plan operations well the surgeon must have a map of the entire arterial system from the abdominal aorta to the ankles furnished by arteriograms. The technique of aortoiliofemoral arteriography via the needle at the groin will supply this information. Films of the ankle and foot are obtained with delayed exposures as described in the subsequent section on distal tibial bypasses. Vein grafts to the distal ends of tibial arteries or even the dorsalis pedis artery on the foot have salvaged many legs that were previously inoperable. The vein grafts remain open even with low flow, as demonstrated by these procedures and by the coronary artery bypass operations.

Atherosclerosis in the thigh and leg causes symptoms only when it is widespread; therefore, localized operations are of no value. Localized operations in which the profunda femoris artery is reopened are the sole exception to this rule. Plaques and occlusions occur most frequently in the zone of the superficial femoral artery at the adductor canal, but when a patient has severe intermittent claudication or if the leg is in peril, there will be widespread narrowing or multiple areas of occlusion elsewhere. Plaques and occlusions occur most frequently at bifurcations, namely, at the origin of the superficial femoral artery and at the origins of the large branches below the knee, namely, the anterior and posterior tibial and the peroneal arteries.

Long-term follow-up of results has clarified the policy and assisted in the choice of operations. Thromboendarterectomy in the superficial femoral and popliteal arteries is commonly followed by narrowing and occlusion of the endarterectomized segment and is seldom performed if veins are available for the bypass operation. Bypasses with living veins are clearly superior to disobliteration of long segments by thromboendarterectomy. Furthermore, vein grafts can now be extended from the groin all the way to the foot to restore flow and save legs in suitable cases, as described later.

173

The improved prostheses, including the so-called velour Dacron prosthesis, offer some advantages over the previous fabric prostheses and may be used provided that they do not cross the knee joint. Few patients who need surgery will have such localized disease. The bovine heterograft will be useful in a rare case in which veins are not available. Thromboendarterectomy is still performed as a last resort.

The outlook for patients with intermittent claudication is excellent, although they are, of course, more prone to complications of atherosclerosis elsewhere than is the general population, and their life expectancy is shorter than that of the general population. An operation of any sort is rarely indicated solely for intermittent claudication. A rare patient will need restoration of flow so that he can continue his work. Older and retired people are seldom obliged to earn their living with their legs and need an operation only when the leg is in peril.

The first section in this chapter deals with the surgical exposure of the various parts of the popliteal artery. Further details regarding the choice and extent of operation are explained in the appropriate sections.

In operations on the lower extremity, the importance of the deep femoral artery cannot be overemphasized. At any time that the common femoral artery is exposed and opened, the orifice of the profunda femoris artery should be inspected and be cleared of any constricting arteriosclerotic plaque. In many patients the profunda femoris artery has proved to be capable of nourishing the entire lower extremity.

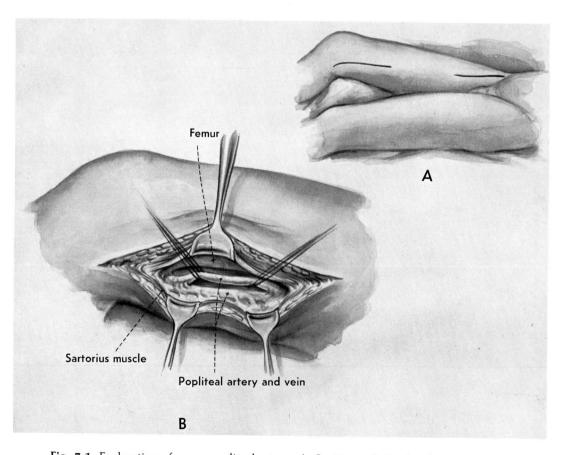

Femur

Sartorius muscle

Popliteal artery and vein

A

B

Fig. 7-1. Exploration of upper popliteal artery. A, Incisions. B, Popliteal exposure.

In these as well as in other patients with borderline arterial circulation, lumbar sympathectomy should be employed frequently.

EXPLORATION OF POPLITEAL ARTERY

The common diseases involving the popliteal artery are atherosclerotic occlusive disease, popliteal aneurysm, and embolism. The medial approach as illustrated in this discussion is most advantageous for surgical treatment of occlusive disease, embolism, and injuries. The midline posterior approach is rarely useful. Important advantages of the medial approach are as follows:

1. Incisions can easily be extended upward and downward as the operative findings may dictate.
2. The popliteal artery is more accessible by the medial approach, particularly in its proximal and distal portions.
3. The artery is easily drawn forward toward the skin when the knee is flexed.
4. The tibial nerve and the popliteal veins are more easily avoided.
5. The patient is in the supine position, so that the surgeon may work simultaneously in the groin and in the abdomen without repositioning.

The popliteal artery may be considered in three divisions. The proximal or upper portion begins at the adductor hiatus, the midportion lies between the heads of the gastrocnemius muscle at about the level of the knee joint, and the distal portion lies behind the upper parts of the tibia and fibula. The upper part of the popliteal artery is commonly affected by occlusive disease extending distally from the adductor canal (Hunter's canal). Plaques are commonly seen at the branching of the distal portion of the popliteal artery.

Procedure

Exploration of proximal portion of popliteal artery

1. Place the patient in the supine position with the thigh slightly abducted and externally rotated and the knee flexed and supported. The surgeon stands at the opposite side of the table.

2. Begin the incision medial and anterior to the saphenous vein in the lower part of the thigh and extend it downward to the lower border of the patella (Fig. 7-1, *A*). The saphenous nerve may cross the incision and can be divided or retracted gently. The saphenous vein should be preserved in case manipulation of the popliteal vein predisposes to thrombosis or in case it is needed as a vein graft.

3. Open the deep fascia anterior to the sartorius muscle and retract the muscle posteriorly.

4. Identify the posterior edge of the vastus medialis muscle with blunt dissection and retract it anteriorly. Divide the adductor tendon to mobilize the artery (Fig. 7-1, *B*).

5. Identify the popliteal artery, which is the most superficial cordlike structure palpable through the exposure. Divide the overlying fascia and the sheath of the artery.

6. Mobilize a considerable length of the artery so that it can be easily drawn up into the incision with an umbilical tape.

COMMENT: *The tibial nerve and the popliteal vein lie posteriorly and well away from the proximal portion of the artery. The nerve need not be dissected out or otherwise disturbed. The vein is not usually troublesome posteriorly and laterally; but frequently*

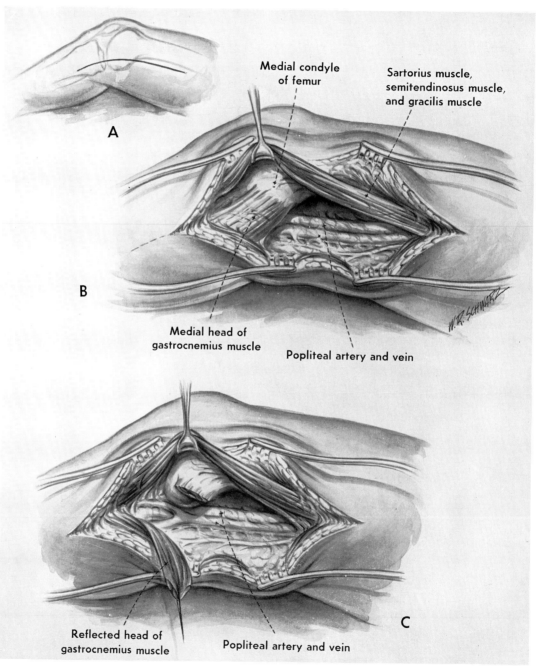

Fig. 7-2. Exploration of midportion of popliteal artery. **A,** Incision. **B,** Retraction of hamstring muscles to expose upper popliteal artery and origin of gastrocnemius muscle. **C,** Division of medial head of gastrocnemius muscle to reveal midportion of popliteal artery.

the popliteal or superficial femoral vein is double, and one of the channels may lie anterior and medial to the artery.

Exploration of midportion of popliteal artery

The medial approach is useful if occlusive disease involves the upper portion of the popliteal artery. Arteriotomy of the midportion of the popliteal artery is also preferred for embolectomy by the retrograde flush method.

The midportion of the popliteal artery is approached by mobilizing the hamstring muscles and tendons and retracting them posteriorly. The exposure is extended by dividing the medial head of the gastrocnemius muscle where it attaches to the medial condyle of the femur (Fig. 7-2, *B* and *C*).

1. Extend the skin incision employed for the proximal end of the popliteal artery distally, anterior to the saphenous vein and nerve, and as far distal as the medial tibial condyle (Fig. 7-2, *A*).

2. Incise the deep fasica along the anterior edge of the sartorius and the hamstring muscles. Occasionally it is preferable to incise along the posterior edge of these muscles and to retract them anteriorly (Fig. 7-2, *B*).

3. Identify the medial head of the gastrocnemius muscle and divide it close to its ligamentous origin. Leave 1 or 2 cm. of the tendinous attachment to facilitate suture later and to avoid opening the knee joint (Fig. 7-2, *C*).

4. Turn the distal divided end of the gastrocnemius downward and medially. Note and spare the motor nerve and the arterial branches that enter the muscle at a somewhat lower level.

5. Incise the sheath of the popliteal artery. It may be necessary to divide venous tributaries that cross the artery. The popliteal vein is not troublesome, except distally. The tibial nerve is posterior and well out of the way.

6. Flexion of the knee relaxes the artery so that it is readily drawn close to the skin level.

Exploration of distal portion of popliteal artery

Distal exposure is suitable for surgical treatment of occlusive disease proximal to this level or arterial injuries, arteriotomy for popliteal embolectomy, and the like. Arteriotomies in the distal portion of the popliteal artery should be closed with vein patch to avoid narrowing. The technique of patch angioplasty is described on p. 158 and illustrated in Figs. 6-4, 6-5, 6-6, and 13-5, *D* to *G*.

1. Place the patient in the supine position with the leg externally rotated, the thigh abducted, and the knee moderately flexed.

2. Make an incision 8 to 10 cm. long along the posteromedial border of the tibia, below the medial condyle, and extending upward to the knee joint (Fig. 7-3, *A*).

3. Incise the deep fasica overlying the gastrocnemius muscle along the posterior edge of the tibia (Fig. 7-3, *B*).

4. Retract the medial head of the gastrocnemius muscle posteriorly away from the tibia, and expose the origin of the soleus muscle from the posterior aspect of the tibia. Elevate the thigh on a folded sheet or towel in order to flex the knee slightly and allow the calf muscles to drop downward.

5. Divide the tendons of insertion of the sartorius and other medial hamstring muscles that are attached to the medial condyle of the tibia.

6. Identify the popliteal vein along the medial edge of the soleus muscle. Dissect

177

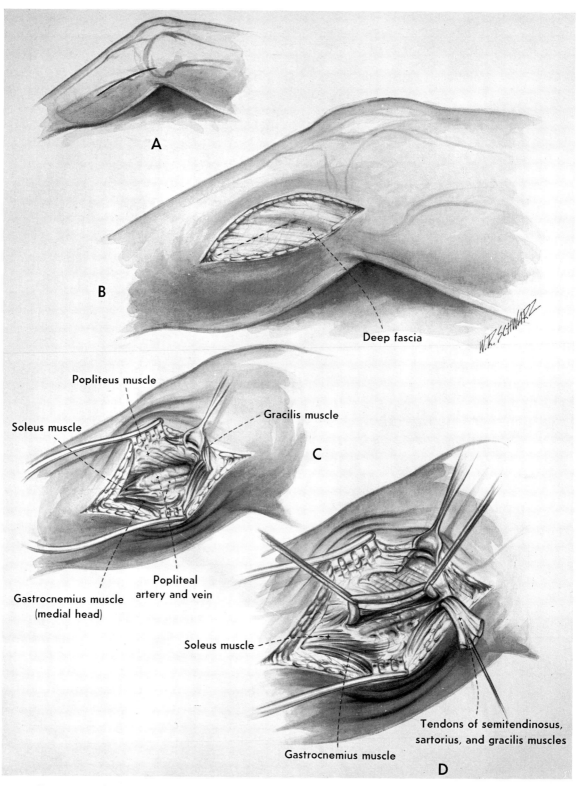

Fig. 7-3. Exploration of distal portion of popliteal artery. **A,** Incision. **B,** Incision in deep fascia at posterior border of tibia. **C,** Distal portion of a popliteal artery uncovered by retraction of muscles. **D,** Distal portion of popliteal artery dissected free and drawn up toward skin. The knee is bent.

this and retract it anteriorly with a small vein retractor to uncover the popliteal artery (Fig. 7-3, C).

7. Identify the origin of the anterior tibial artery on the opposite side of the popliteal artery. The point of origin is almost perpendicular to the popliteal artery. After a very short course, the anterior tibial artery penetrates a hiatus in the interosseous membrane between the tibia and fibula.

COMMENT: *In an occasional patient the anterior tibial artery originates at a higher level. Another variation is the trifurcation, that is, simultaneous origin of the three outflow branches at one point. Normally, however, the popliteal artery continues another few centimeters before it terminates by division into the posterior tibial and the peroneal arteries.*

8. Expose the distal portion of the popliteal artery by dividing the attachments of the soleus muscle to the tibia for 2 to 5 cm.

9. Separate the popliteal veins from the artery at the site of the proposed arteriotomy. The popliteal vein at this low level is frequently double. Arteriotomy at the origin of the anterior tibial artery permits local endarterectomy of stenosing plaques at that level, and attachment of the graft at this site assures perfusion of the anterior tibial artery by the flow from the graft.

10. With the knee flexed and the medial tendons divided, the artery is readily drawn forward into the incision (Fig. 7-3, D).

11. A tunnel can be made ready for the bypass, or an endarterectomy stripper can be readily passed upward.

FEMOROPOPLITEAL BYPASS WITH VEIN GRAFTS
Introduction

Femoral bypass is a useful procedure to restore normal pulsatile flow and to heal ischemic lesions in the foot or leg that are caused by atherosclerotic occlusions in the superficial femoral artery. Intermittent claudication alone is not a sufficient indication for operation unless it is disabling.

Operability may be determined by preoperative angiography, which should show uninterrupted blood flow from a patent popliteal artery into at least two of the major branches. When in doubt, the surgeon should obtain a new arteriogram with slower injection of larger volumes of dye and multiple delayed exposures that gives a map of the arteries all the way to the foot.

Candidates for bypass of the femoral artery should be chosen carefully. Patients with late changes (that is, muscle wasting in the calf, loss of hair, nail changes, and absent distal pulses) have obliterative disease that is too extensive for vascular reconstructive surgery. Some patients with extensive atherosclerosis of the femoral and popliteal arteries are good candidates for long bypass with vein grafts to the distal end of the tibial arteries.

If stenoses are present proximally, they must be relieved by an appropriate earlier or simultaneous operation such as aortoiliac bypass or endarterectomy.

Bypass with a long saphenous vein graft is less likely to be complicated by postoperative thrombosis than bypass with a Dacron prosthesis. Vein grafts are preferable for patients with borderline outflow. Prosthetic materials may be employed when bypassing to the proximal portion of the popliteal artery. When the saphenous vein is missing, diseased, or too small, the cephalic vein from the arm can be used and spliced to the short saphenous vein. The Sparks mandril as discussed later will form a living graft in situ, but a period of six weeks is required before the graft can be connected and conduct blood.

Preoperative care

Preoperative care should be thorough. Arteriograms must demonstrate patency of the major vessels proximal and distal to the proposed bypass. The risk to life in operations on the leg alone is small, but evaluation of cardiopulmonary and renal function is essential.

The skin should be prepared with antiseptic soap (pHisoHex or Septisol) for several days preoperatively.

Procedure

Place the patient in the supine position with the thigh slightly abducted and externally rotated and the knee flexed and supported laterally. Prepare and drape the entire groin, thigh, leg, and foot.

Two surgeons work simultaneously at the upper thigh and at the knee to remove the vein for grafting. Then one surgeon exposes the common femoral artery while his teammate prepares the vein. When the graft is ready, the proximal anastomosis is performed by the first surgeon while the teammate exposes the popliteal artery.

COMMENT: *With detailed arteriograms, there is seldom any doubt about operability; however, the vein prepared should always be longer than what you expect to need.*

Procurement of vein graft

A suitable vein is essential, and sufficient length of veins of adequate caliber can almost always be obtained. Rarely this will require the splicing of segments of vein from the opposite leg or arm. And it may be necessary to splice segments after excising narrowed or doubled parts of the vein.

1. Incise the skin over the full length of the saphenous vein at least 4 inches down the calf from the site of the intended anastomosis (Fig. 7-4, *A*). After reversal and anastomosis are completed, the vein will be replaced in its subcutaneous bed in the thigh. The tunnel or course of the vein distally depends on the site of implantation.

COMMENT: *Two surgeons work simultaneously, beginning at the groin and the lower leg. When we procured grafts through three separate incisions, we sometimes damaged them in dissecting them from under the intervening skin.*

2. Trace the vein superiorly and inferiorly, dissecting close to the vein so that it is thin, shiny, and blue.

COMMENT: *It saves time to dissect off most excess adventitia while the vein is in situ. Leave blood running through the vein until the vein is ready to be removed.*

3. Ligate the large tributaries in situ. Some small ones may be overlooked until the vein is distended later with saline solution.

4. Uncover only the main saphenous vein, and do not undermine the skin edges.

COMMENT: *Occasionally near the knee it is difficult to decide which large tributary is the main channel, and it may be necessary to trace both (Fig. 7-6, A).*

5. Excise the doubled segments of veins. Occasionally the saphenous vein is doubled, dividing into two parallel large tributaries that rejoin. It is usually better to excise and discard such doubled segments and splice two large ends together so that no part of the graft will be less than 5 mm. in diameter. We remove the saphenous

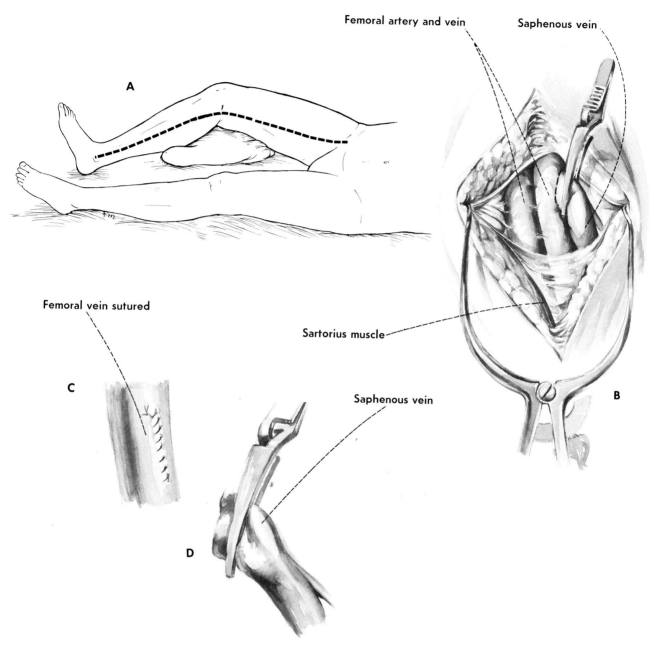

Fig. 7-4. Femoropopliteal artery bypass—vein graft procurement. A, Incision. B, Exposure of upper end of saphenous vein. Dotted line shows incision for detachment of saphenous vein. C, Closure of common femoral vein by suture after detachment of saphenous vein. D, Upper end of saphenous vein.

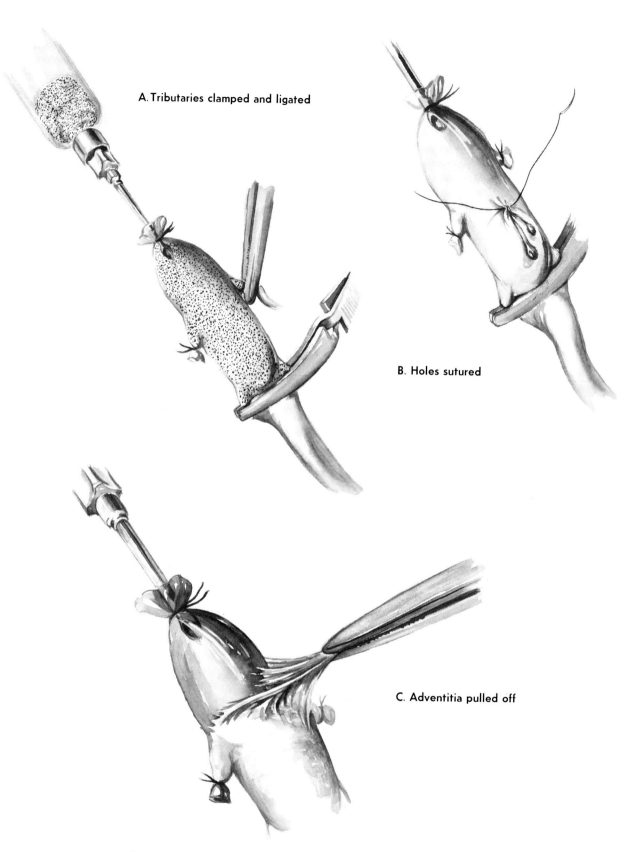

A. Tributaries clamped and ligated

B. Holes sutured

C. Adventitia pulled off

Fig. 7-5. Femoropopliteal artery bypass. Preparation of vein graft.

vein all the way from the groin to the ankle for the distal bypasses described later. The saphenous vein in the lower leg and down to the ankle is large and of uniform caliber.

6. Excise thin, undermined skin edges or they will slough.

7. Ligate the saphenous vein flush with the common femoral vein to conserve length. No cuff is needed on the common femoral vein if a continuous vascular suture is used (Fig. 7-4, *C*).

Preparation of vein graft

While one surgeon exposes the common femoral artery, the other prepares the vein graft at the separate sterile table. Bowls of sterile saline solution with 5,000 units of heparin per 500 ml., 5-0 monofilament vascular sutures, and fine vascular instruments are needed. This is a good time in which to practice with the loupe, and the magnification is helpful in revealing imperfections in the vein graft.

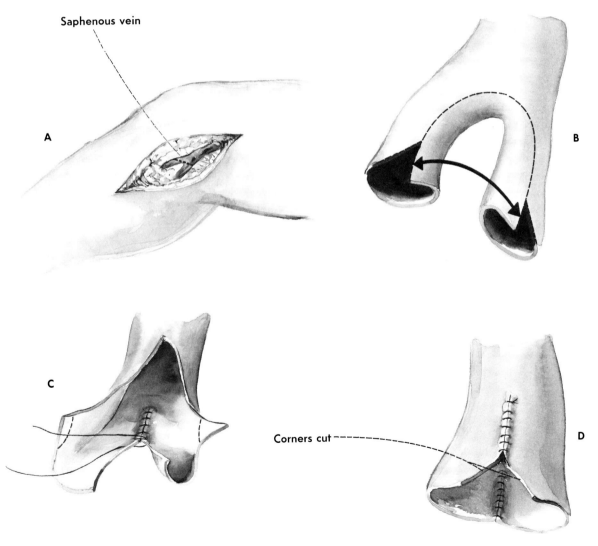

Saphenous vein

Corners cut

Continued.

Fig. 7-6. Preparation of vein graft. **A** to **D**, Maneuvers to utilize short vein.

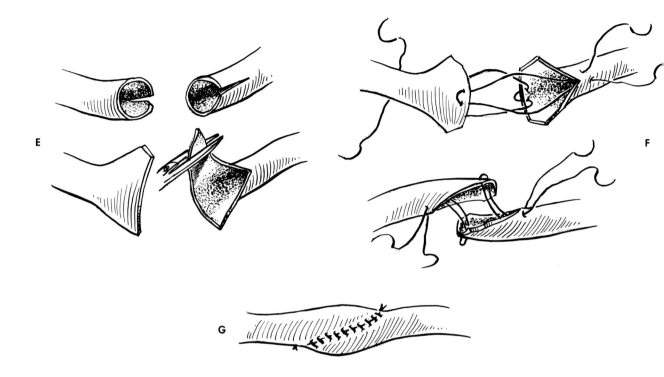

Fig. 7-6, cont'd. Preparation of vein graft. E to G, End-to-end splicing of vein graft. E, Ends trimmed. F, First sutures. G, Completed anastomosis. (E to G adapted from Linton, R. R.: Some practical considerations in surgery of blood vessel grafts, Surgery 38:817-834, 1955.)

1. Remove the vein to a separate small table. Rinse it with heparin in saline solution. Tie the distal end of the vein over a beaded cannula, clamp the opposite end, and distend the vein with heparin in saline solution (Fig. 7-5, A). This reveals small tributaries and leaks and enlarges the lumen of the vein somewhat. Ligate or suture branches and tributaries (Fig. 7-5, B).

2. Remove the adventitia of the vein so that it will dilate further. Pull off the adventitia with fine thumb forceps (Fig. 7-5, C), or rub it off with moist gauze while the vein is distended with heparin in saline solution under pressure.

COMMENT: *Several maneuvers previously described to lengthen short grafts are occasionally useful but seldom needed. Uncover at least 2 to 4 inches more vein than you expect to need. You will find that the troublesome part is usually near the knee and that it is simpler to excise a segment and reanastomose two ends (Fig. 7-6, E to G) than to perform the maneuvers in Fig. 7-6, B to D.*

Exposure of common femoral artery

1. Extend the skin incision superiorly over the femoral pulsation to about 2 cm. above the inguinal ligament, and open the superficial fascia (Fig. 7-7).

2. Open the femoral arterial sheath directly over the artery and dissect upward and downward. Identify the profunda femoris and the superficial femoral branches of the common femoral artery.

3. Palpate the artery carefully. Plaques at the bifurcation of the common femoral

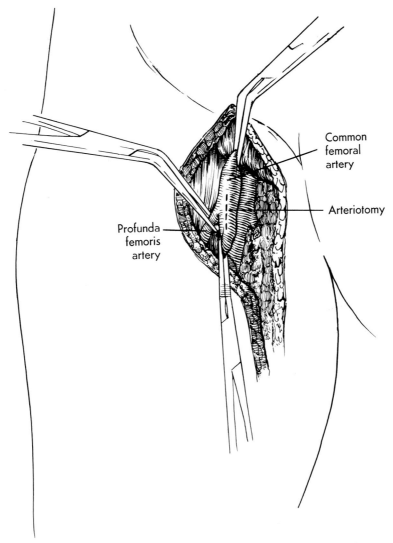

Common
femoral
artery

Arteriotomy

Profunda
femoris
artery

Fig. 7-7. Femoropopliteal bypass vein graft. Exposure for common femoral arteriotomy and proximal anastomosis.

artery are usually not demonstrated by the arteriograms of the anteroposterior view. Therefore, the arteriorotomy will be made over the bifurcation. Tapes are necessary about the common femoral, superficial femoral, and profunda femoris arteries. Arteriotomy over the bifurcation will permit inspection of the interior of the artery and examination of the orifice of the profunda femoris artery. Plaques are frequently localized at the exit of the profunda femoris artery and may be removed by local endarterectomy prior to anastomosis. (See Chapter 6.)

COMMENT: *Attachment of bypass grafts to the proximal end of the superficial femoral artery is never advisable in operations for atherosclerosis, no matter how normal the artery seems. Atherosclerotic plaques frequently form in the proximal end of the superficial femoral artery at the bifurcation of the common femoral artery and obstruct the inflow, so that such grafts quickly fail.*

Femoral arteriotomy

1. Inject 3,000 units of heparin in 30 ml. of saline solution into the common femoral artery.

2. Immediately apply occluding clamps. DeBakey angled clamps are convenient for controlling the common, superficial, and deep femoral vessels (Fig. 7-7).

3. Make a short longitudinal arteriotomy at about the junction of the profunda femoris and superficial femoral arteries. Begin the arteriotomy with a knife, and complete it with the Potts angled scissors. The arteriotomy is one and one-half to two times the diameter of the artery. If the ostium of the profunda femoris artery is narrowed, a local endarectomy is performed at this time.

Proximal end-to-side anastomosis of vein graft and artery

While one surgeon performs the proximal anastomosis, the other exposes the popliteal artery. The technique of end-to-side anastomosis is illustrated in Fig. 7-8. The vein is living and must be kept moist at all times. The proximal anastomosis is done first so that clamps can be released and the vein can be distended under pressure, dilated, and stretched during the remainder of the operation.

1. Reverse the vein so that the distal end is anastomosed at the common femoral artery. Trim the end as diagrammed in Fig. 7-8, *A*.

2. Use double-armed monofilament 5-0 or 6-0 polyethylene or polypropylene suture, and start the anastomosis with a vertical suture (Fig. 7-8, *B*).

COMMENT: *Avoid the error illustrated in Fig. 7-8, C. The tributary is useful when available as illustrated in Fig. 7-8, D and E. The vein must always be left loose at the acute angle and not stretched except at the very tip of the anastomosis. This permits the takeoff portion to "hump up" and not be stretched tight or be flattened.*

3. Continue the suture from vein to artery, inserting the needle close to the edge of the vein at the acute angle, but elsewhere, 2 mm. from the edge of the vein and 1.5 mm. from the edge of the artery (or only 1 mm. if the artery is thick).

4. Suture a portion of the lateral edge of the vein graft to the artery with a continuous over-and-over stitch, using one of the ends of the double-armed suture.

5. Suture the medial edge of the vein and artery with the other end of the suture.

6. Stretch the tip of the graft, lengthening the arteriotomy if necessary to fit the stretched tip, ensuring that the graft will take off obliquely from the artery.

7. Continue one of the sutures around the upper end of the arteriotomy to meet the other suture. End the suture line by tying the two ends securely (Fig. 7-8, *G*). Open the proximal clamp momentarily to flush the graft (Fig. 7-8, *G*).

8. Clamp the tip of the graft so that it throbs and dilates. Cover the graft and keep it moist.

Exploration of popliteal artery

Because femoral bypass is rarely performed for intermittent claudication, the atherosclerosis is extensive and involves the proximal end of the popliteal artery. When performed for more advanced arterial insufficiency, the bypass is almost always attached to the distal end of the popliteal artery and occasionally to the tibial arteries in the lower calf (Figs. 7-10 and 7-12).

The skin incision for removal of the saphenous vein is satisfactory for the popliteal exposure.

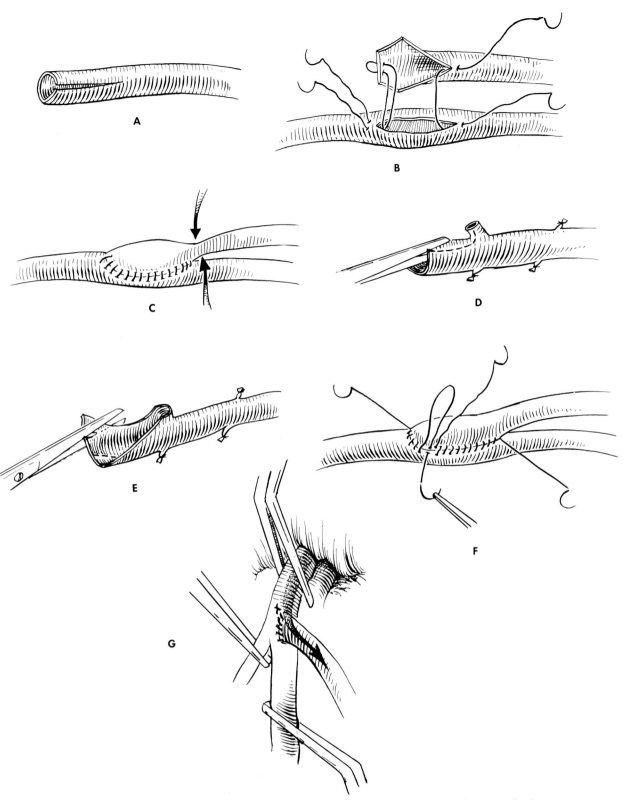

Fig. 7-8. Vein graft—proximal end-to-side anastomosis. **A** and **B,** Cut and trim end of vein graft. **B,** Start anastomosis at acute angle. **C,** Common error. **D** and **E,** One way to avoid error in **C.** When this is not feasible, stenosis as in **C** is avoided by leaving a long tip on graft and letting it "hump up" without tension. **F,** Completion of anastomosis at side. **G,** Flush out graft to remove any clots from graft and any sludge or clots accumulated above the clamp.

187

1. Flex the knee. Then incise the deep fascia 1 cm. posterior to the posterior border of the tibia and dissect as described on p. 177 and illustrated in Fig. 7-3.

COMMENT: *Good modern arteriograms are usually a good guide, but occasionally a wide popliteal artery seen on the arteriogram is found to have a narrow cross section like a ribbon when it is palpated.*

2. Divide the medial head of the gastrocnemius muscle near its attachment to the femur. Even though exposure may be satisfactory without this maneuver, the gastrocnemius muscle in its normal position would displace and possibly compress the vein graft. Later the muscle may be reattached to the deep fascia along the posterior border of the tibia.

3. Divide the tendons inserted medially on the upper portion of the tibia if they limit the exposure.

4. See the detailed description on p. 177 and drawings in Figs. 7-2 and 7-3 of the anatomy and technique. The popliteal artery is tethered by the origin of the anterior tibial artery, which penetrates the interosseus membrane between the tibia and fibula. Proximal to this, the popliteal artery can be mobilized and drawn up so that it is easily accessible.

5. The popliteal vein lies medial to and covers the artery. Dissect the vein so that it is free and retract it anteriorly so that the graft will not cross it after anastomosis. Sometimes the vein is doubled. The entrance of the anterior tibial vein should be noted and not torn.

6. Palpate the popliteal artery and select the site for anastomosis where the artery is not unduly thickened and where no obvious stenoses are palpable distally and where "adequate" outflow is seen on the arteriograms.

COMMENT: *Outflow is clearly adequate if two of the three major branches are not narrowed. Sometimes only one open vessel has adequate outflow to maintain patency for considerable periods of time; however, the rate of progression of arteriosclerosis at the branching origins of these outflow arteries is variable. We suspect that arteriosclerosis will progress more rapidly and obstruct such major branches more quickly than it progresses in the muscular portions of the tibial arteries farther down the leg. Time may prove that distal tibial bypass (Figs. 7-10 and 7-12) may last longer than femoropopliteal anastomosis with only one outflow vessel or very narrow outflow vessels.*

7. Make the arteriotomy 1.5 cm. long in the medial side of the popliteal artery after occluding the vessel proximally and distally. The fine-toothed arterial clamps can be placed so that they hold the artery forward for arteriotomy and anastomosis. The previous heparin injection in the common femoral artery is sufficient. Irrigate with heparin in saline solution.

Fig. 7-9. Distal tibial or popliteal anastomosis of vein graft. **A,** First suture at proximal, that is, acute, angle. **B,** First suture tied. **C,** Continuous suture of inferior edge. **D,** Continuous suture of superior edge. **E,** New suture at tip of graft and distal end of arteriotomy. **F,** Suture tied and then continued proximally. **G,** Completed anastomosis; sutures meet and are tied at side. (From Auer, A. I., and Hershey, F. B.: Bypass vein grafts to distal tibial or dorsalis pedis arteries, Mo. Med. **70:**93-100, 1973.)

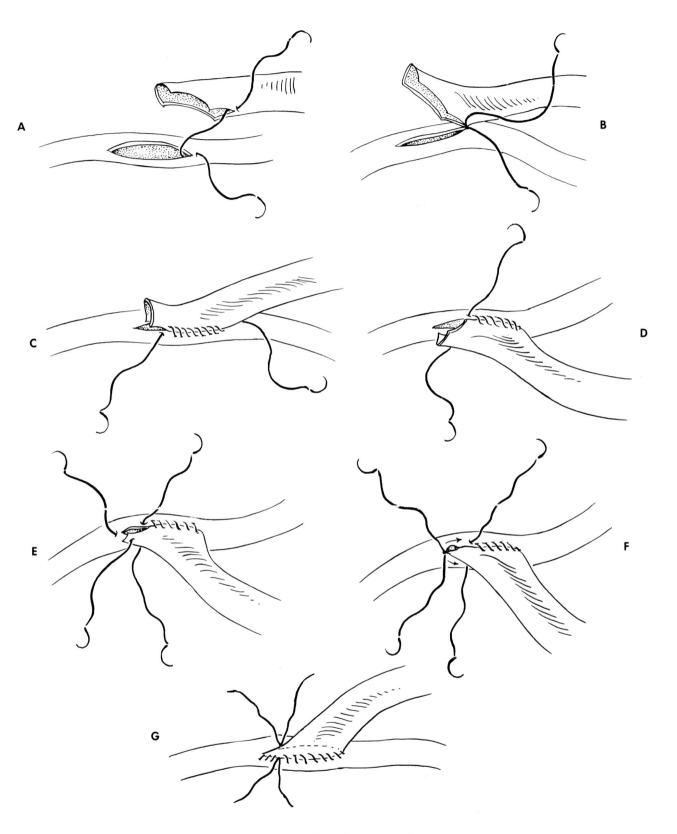

Fig. 7-9. For legend see opposite page.

Drawing vein graft down and making the tunnel

No tunnel is needed in the thigh when the graft has been removed with the long continuous incision. The graft may be placed in the subcutaneous bed from which it was removed. In a very thin thigh, a tunnel may be made beneath the sartorius muscle as described in the Sparks mandril technique. The graft must not be twisted in the tunnel.

1. Straighten the leg, draw the vein graft down, and estimate the length needed to reach the arteriotomy without excessive tension.

COMMENT: *The graft has been covered and kept moist and throbbing with blood, stretching and lengthening, after the proximal anastomosis and during the exposure of the popliteal artery. The graft must be a little taut, since it will stretch a little more during and after the anastomosis; but the graft should be cut so that excess is left at the tip to be trimmed later.*

2. Flex the knee. Cut the graft as shown in Figs. 7-8, *A* and *B*, and 7-9, *A*, but leave more at the tip than is illustrated. Then the forceps will pinch only part of the tip that is later trimmed.

3. Flush the graft. The jet should shoot past the foot of the table. Then reapply the clamp to the graft close to the tip.

Popliteal anastomosis

Use 4-0 or 5-0 monofilament polyethylene or polypropylene suture with two small needles and a fine needle holder.

1. Start the suture at the proximal end of the arteriotomy as diagrammed in Fig. 7-9, *A* and *B*. The needle passes 1 mm. from the edge.

2. Continue along one side, progressing distally with over-and-over continuous sutures passing from vein graft to the artery (Fig. 7-9, *C*). Go half way along the arteriotomy. Hold only the tip of the vein graft in the forceps and trim this tip later.

3. Do the same on the other side (Fig. 7-9, *D*).

4. Trim the tip of the vein graft (not illustrated); then place another double-needle polypropylene suture at the tip of the vein graft (Fig. 7-9, *E*), and tie it down.

5. Finish the anastomosis with these sutures by sewing proximally in the direction of the arrows (Fig. 7-9, *F*) to join and tie the suture to the one that was started at the other end of the arteriotomy.

6. Remove clamps from the popliteal artery to flush it and to check back bleeding; then reapply them.

7. Flush the vein graft, and reapply the clamp on it. Then tie the sutures. Remove the clamps on the popliteal artery, and then slowly remove the clamp on the vein graft.

COMMENT: *The sutures should be pulled snug, but if there is a little bleeding from the suture line, gentle pressure with Gelfoam is sufficient to stop it. Do not pinch or occlude the artery or the graft.*

8. Check pulsations in the popliteal artery proximally and distally, and check pulsations in the foot.

COMMENT: *If the result is in doubt, an intraoperative arteriogram is easily performed by inserting an 18-gauge needle in the vein graft and injecting 20 ml. of Conray (60%). The x-ray film in a sterile pillowcase or sterile Mayo table cover is placed under the leg. No Bucky tray is needed. One film suffices. The needle hole is closed with one vascular suture. Fogarty catheters are readily passed through small incisions in the vein graft whenever this maneuver is indicated. Any imperfection in the anastomosis or any intimal flap must be corrected.*

9. Irrigate the incisions with bacitracin solution and close the wounds. Use multiple layers of fine silk in the groin. In the popliteal incision, do not resuture tendons that might displace or compress the graft. It is unnecessary to suture the medial head of the gastrocnemius muscle; however, it can be sutured to the anterior edge of the deep fascia at the posteromedial border of the tibia. We close the popliteal fascia with continuous suture with 2-0 chromic catgut. Subcutaneous fascia in the thigh is closed with fine plain catgut, and the skin everywhere is closed with fine nylon continuous sutures. Excise any undermined or thin skin. Avoid dead space in which lymph or serum might accumulate. No drains are needed; avoid constricting bandages.

Postoperative care

The pressure of a tight bandage behind the knee is avoided. Keep the limb slightly elevated, and check the pedal pulses regularly. The pedal pulses may not be palpable immediately. If they are palpable but later disappear, reoperation is necessary at once.

Bed rest for seven to ten days is necessary until the incision has healed. After that time, gradual flexion of the knee may be allowed. However, the knee must not be flexed past 90 degrees. Crossing of the legs and all pressure behind the knee should be avoided. Patients may stand and take a few steps a week after surgery, using a cane.

If there is any tendency toward development of edema, elastic bandages are worn for several months.

Complications of bypass vein grafts in leg

Early thrombosis is almost always due to some technical error and is correctable. Prompt reoperation usually permits correction of an intimal flap, a narrowed suture line, and so forth without placement of a whole new vein graft. If the occlusion goes unrecognized overnight, restoration of flow is followed by swelling that requires fasciotomy of the calf (Chapter 10).

Hemorrhage postoperatively should be a rare occurrence. When it occurs in the first twelve to twenty-four hours, it is due to some correctable imperfection of the anastomosis or of the graft. Delayed hemorrhage results from infection. Infection is present even when there is no pus and none of the other signs of infection are evident. Attempts at repair of late hemorrhage will *always* fail, and the best treatment is ligation of the involved vessels and grafting via a new route in clean tissue.

Thrombophlebitis is difficult to recognize after extensive arterial operations. Patients who have had previous episodes of phlebitis should receive small prophylactic doses of heparin, but ordinarily it is unnecessary to use anticoagulants postoperatively. If the presence of thrombophlebitis is suspected, an ascending phlebogram is helpful in making the diagnosis before the risks of therapeutic doses of heparin are assumed.

Some edema of the foot is common and appears to be due to disruption or ligation of lymphatic vessels in the groin. With elastic support, the edema is controlled and usually disappears after a few months and lymphangiograms show that collateral channels have developed.

Hypesthesia or anesthesia due to trauma to the medial femoral cutaneous nerve overlying the common femoral artery or to the saphenous nerve in the medial thigh is temporary and seldom troublesome. Ischemic neuritis that has been prolonged is healed slowly and may be troublesome for some months.

Late occlusion can usually be avoided by careful follow-up to note recurrence of symptoms, that is, intermittent claudication, development of murmurs or bruits in the graft, changes in the pulses or Doppler sounds (Chapter 10). Arteriograms should be obtained for any of the above indications, since correction before thrombosis occurs may be easy. The arteriograms may also demonstrate clamp injury in the artery, anastomotic aneurysms, stenoses in the graft, or diaphragms or septa formed by thickened valve cusps. The angiographic changes may appear minor but should be corrected promptly. As more vein grafts are recovered at autopsy at various intervals after coronary bypass, atherosclerosis and various other pathological changes may be revealed and elucidated. About two thirds of vein grafts in the legs will be patent for five years, and vigilant follow-up might salvage some of the legs in which grafts fail.

BYPASS VEIN GRAFTS TO DISTAL PARTS OF TIBIAL ARTERIES

Amputations can sometimes be prevented by long bypass vein grafts anastomosed to arteries in the lower leg or foot. Abundant flow is sometimes achieved, since the peripheral resistance is low. Flow rates through vein grafts anastomosed to the distal parts of tibial arteries with bidirectional outflow may equal the flow rates measured after popliteal anastomoses with good outflow. The small size of the arteries at the site of anastomosis requires meticulous technique, and the loupe has been useful.

Detailed arteriograms are needed. Multiple films taken after long delay frequently reveal distal parts of vessels satisfactory for anastomosis.

This bypass graft may be useful in cases of arteriosclerosis obliterans, thrombosis of popliteal aneurysms, femoropopliteal vein grafts, or trauma obliterating the distal end of the popliteal artery and the proximal end of the tibial arteries.

We have not performed this operation for intermittent claudication but have performed it only when the leg was in danger. The risk is small. The only contraindications are recent myocardial infarction, renal failure, or gangrene proximal to the foot. Diabetes is no contraindication.

Arteriography

Satisfactory arteriograms reveal the distal end of the abdominal aorta and its branches, the arteries in both thighs, and the arteries in the affected leg and foot in detail.

1. Introduce the No. 160 Seldinger needle into the common femoral artery.

2. Demonstrate the aorta and arteries in the thighs with several films taken after injection of 50 ml. of Conray (60%) at a pressure of 225 pounds per square inch or sufficient pressure to empty the syringe in three to four seconds.

3. Demonstrate the arteries of the lower leg and foot by slow injection (of ten seconds duration) of 30 to 50 ml. of Conray (60%). A series of films should be taken ending twenty to thirty seconds after injection.

COMMENT: *The injected dye perfuses collateral vessels to reach the foot in twenty to thirty seconds. Nonvisualization of an artery does not mean that there is occlusion unless two films three to five seconds apart show dye in other vessels at that level. Refilling of the anterior tibial artery may be very slow when the other two main arteries are occluded.*

4. Repeat the injection with different timing if necessary in order to obtain lateral views of the foot and see the dorsalis pedis artery or large lateral tarsal collateral arteries.

COMMENT: *A total dose of 150 ml. of Conray (60%) is well tolerated because only a small amount reaches the renal arteries before recirculation. Good arteriograms make it unnecessary to explore doubtful arteries and are a good guide.*

Procedure for bypass vein graft to distal parts of tibial arteries

The upper end of the vein graft is attached at the common femoral artery because the atherosclerosis progresses upward in the superficial femoral artery and occludes its origin. Indeed, it is already totally occluded in most cases. Furthermore, arteriotomy at that site permits dilation of the orifice of the profunda femoris artery or local endarterectomy, which is frequently necessary.

Occasionally in a case of trauma or thrombosed popliteal aneurysm, there may be a suitable superficial femoral or popliteal artery for the proximal anastomosis.

See the discussion on p. 185 and illustrations in Figs. 7-7 and 7-8 of techniques of proximal anastomosis.

Profundaplasty has been performed in one third of our cases together with local thromboendarterectomy of the common femoral artery in order to assure adequate inflow for the graft and to restore flow via the profunda femoris artery. These plaques on the posterior wall were not visible in the routine anteroposterior views of arteriograms. In all these cases there was widespread atherosclerosis elsewhere, and in several cases femorofemoral bypass was needed to bring the inflow for the graft and the profunda femoris artery across from the other common femoral artery (Fig. 5-1).

Make the distal anastomosis at the midportion of the most normal part of the longest open segment. In many cases, only one satisfactory vessel is needed to perfuse and save the leg. Discontinuity at the ankle is no contraindication, but of course, it is encouraging when one or more main arteries continue into the foot. Satisfactory vessels have been at least 2 mm. in diameter at the site of anastomosis.

Procurement and preparation of vein graft

Two surgeons can operate simultaneously and shorten the procedure, which is otherwise very tedious. The two surgeons procure the vein graft, one starting at the groin and the other at the ankle. Then while one prepares the vein, the other exposes the common femoral artery. While one surgeon completes the proximal anastomosis, the second surgeon exposes the site for distal anastomosis. While one surgeon completes the distal anastomosis, the first surgeon closes the proximal incisions.

Sufficient length of veins of adequate caliber (5 mm. at the minimum) can always be obtained. The length of the vein graft must not dictate the site of implantation.

Remove the long saphenous vein from the medial malleolus at the ankle all the way to the groin. One long continuous incision uncovers the vein without risking injury to the vein and without undermining the skin edge. After reversal and anastomosis are completed, the vein will be replaced in its subcutaneous bed in the thigh. The course of the vein below the knee depends, of course, on the site of distal implantation. Narrowed, doubled, or otherwise unsuitable parts of the vein may occur in the midportion. These should be excised and discarded and the vein spliced by oblique anastomosis (Fig. 7-6, *D* to *F*).

Details of the procurement and preparation are given earlier in this chapter (see Figs. 7-4 and 7-5). The only difference in this procedure is the length required.

Exposure of posterior tibial artery

The posterior tibial artery is most easily accessible and is preferred when it is suitable. Good arteriograms avoid needless dissection. At the ankle the artery is superficial, but in the calf the collateral circulation through the numerous muscular branches is abundant; only time will tell which area is preferable. In the calf, the artery is accompanied by the pair of veins that have many cross connections and muscular tributaries.

Fig. 7-10, *A* shows the surgical anatomy of the middle and distal portions of the posterior tibial artery. The proximal part can be uncovered by dividing the remaining medial attachments of the soleus muscle. A long skin incision is made to procure the vein graft, but the fascial incision 1 cm. posterior to the tibia is made only long enough to uncover the site for anastomosis and is seldom more than 4 inches long.

In the midcalf, after the deep fascia is incised, the attachments of the soleus muscle to the posterior border of the tibia must be reflected so that the gastrocnemius and soleus muscles are retracted posteriorly. The flexor digitorum longus muscle on the posterior surface of the tibia is retracted anteriorly and separated from the soleus muscle. The posterior tibial artery, the paired veins, and the nerve lie in this groove.

At the ankle, a new skin incision is needed posterior to the incision for removal of the vein (Fig. 10, *B*). The overlying skin is already open proximally. The fascial incision is only long enough to uncover the site for anastomosis. The exposure is shown in Fig. 7-10, *C*.

Exposure of peroneal artery

The peroneal artery will be the only suitable or the most suitable outflow vessel in some cases. It is close to the posterior tibial artery, only 2 cm. lateral to it. We approach the peroneal artery from the medial side of the leg. The vein graft lies medially, and sometimes we divide the tendons attached to the upper medial part of the tibia so that the vein graft can lie without angulation or compression. Fig. 7-11 is a cross section of the midportion of the leg showing the medial approach.

Fig. 7-10. Posterior tibial artery. **A,** Anatomical relationships; view after separation of attachments of soleus muscle to tibia. For superior extension and more proximal exposure, continue to detach soleus muscle. For exposure of proximal end of posterior tibial artery, cut arch of soleus muscle where popliteal artery goes beneath it, and trace it inferiorly (see Fig. 7-3). **B,** Incision for exposure of distal end of posterior tibial artery. **C,** Surgical exposure of distal end of posterior tibial artery. (From Auer, A. I., and Hershey, F. B.: Bypass vein grafts to distal tibial or dorsalis pedis arteries, Mo. Med. **70:**93-100, 1973.)

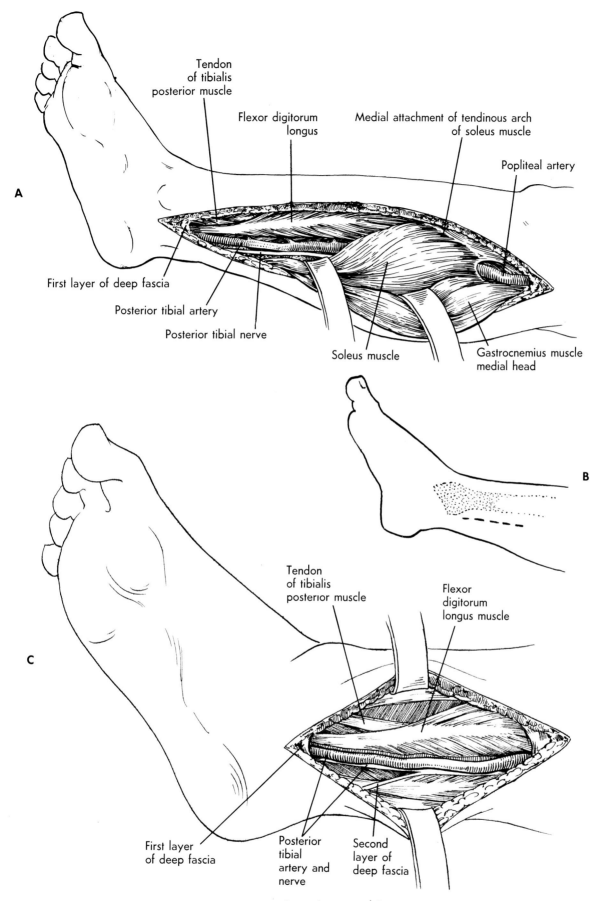

A

Tendon of tibialis posterior muscle

Flexor digitorum longus

Medial attachment of tendinous arch of soleus muscle

Popliteal artery

First layer of deep fascia

Posterior tibial artery

Posterior tibial nerve

Soleus muscle

Gastrocnemius muscle medial head

B

C

Tendon of tibialis posterior muscle

Flexor digitorum longus muscle

First layer of deep fascia

Posterior tibial artery and nerve

Second layer of deep fascia

Fig. 7-10. For legend see opposite page.

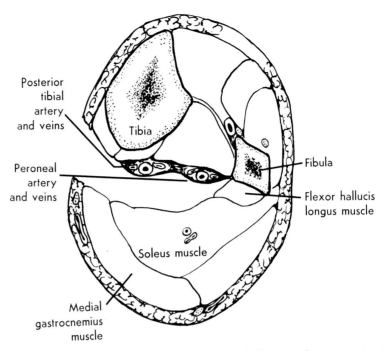

Posterior
tibial
artery
and veins

Peroneal
artery
and veins

Tibia

Fibula

Flexor hallucis
longus muscle

Soleus muscle

Medial
gastrocnemius
muscle

Fig. 7-11. Cross section of midportion of leg showing medial approach to posterior tibial artery and adjacent peroneal artery. (From Auer, A. I., and Hershey, F. B.: Bypass vein grafts to distal tibial or dorsalis pedis arteries, Mo. Med. **70**:93-100, 1973.)

The incision is similar to the approach to the posterior tibial artery, which is encountered first.

Retract the posterior tibial neurovascular bundle anteriorly. In the lower part of the leg deep to this is the tibialis anterior muscle (not shown in Fig. 7-11), which is also retracted anteriorly. The peroneal artery is only 1.5 to 2 cm. away. If the peroneal vessels are not encountered nearby, you have probably followed the septum between the soleus and the flexor hallucis longus muscles and gone too far posteriorly.

The vein graft will lie medially. Some tibial attachments of the gastrocnemius muscle may have to be incised to prevent too much deviation or compression of the graft.

Exposure of anterior tibial artery

Fig. 7-12 illustrates the surgical approach to the upper or midportion of the anterior tibial artery, via an anterolateral incision in the leg. Separate the muscles as diagrammed. Divide the cross connections between the paired veins that accompany the artery. Make the tunnel through the popliteal space and through the interosseous space well below the normal fascial hiatus. This avoids the veins that pass through the interosseous membrane at the hiatus and would be easily torn. The approach to the midportion permits bidirectional outflow, that is, proximal as well as distal. The proximal part of the anterior tibial artery is the portion least accessible and most often occluded.

The incision in skin and fascia lies a finger breadth lateral to the crest of the tibia in the lower third of the leg. The fascial incision is lateral to the prominent

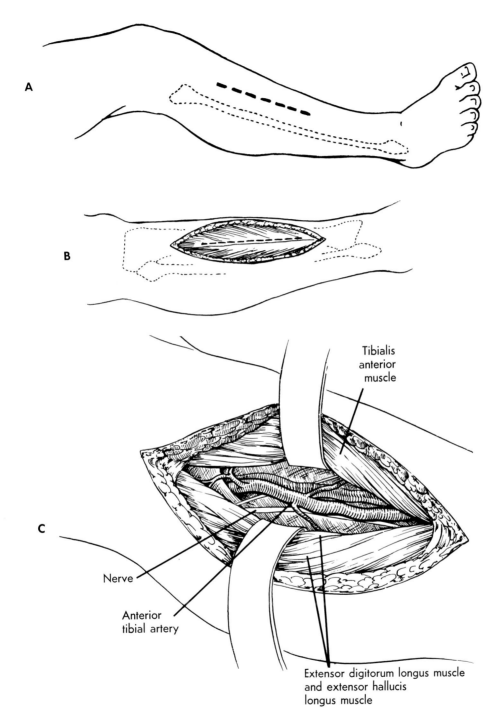

A

B

C

Tibialis
anterior
muscle

Nerve

Anterior
tibial artery

Extensor digitorum longus muscle
and extensor hallucis
longus muscle

Fig. 7-12. Surgical exposure of anterior tibial artery. **A,** Incision. **B,** Incise fascia at dotted line. **C,** Reflect fibers of tibialis anterior muscle from its origin on intermuscular septum and retract it anteriorly. (From Auer, A. I., and Hershey, F. B.: Bypass vein grafts to distal tibial or dorsalis pedis arteries, Mo. Med. **70:**93-100, 1973.)

anterior tibial tendon, which lies close to the tibia. In the midportion of the leg, go between the anterior tibial and the extensor digitorum longus muscles. Slightly deeper in the midportion, the extensor hallucis longus muscle screens or overlies the anterior neurovascular bundle. This must also be retracted laterally. The nerve that has curved around the head of the fibula lies lateral to the anterior tibial artery.

Exposure of dorsalis pedis artery

The dorsalis pedis artery is very superficial and accessible between the tendons on the dorsum of the foot as shown in Fig. 7-13. Lateral arteriograms of the foot show more detail without the interfering opacity of the bones of the foot.

Distal anastomosis

Measure the length of the graft with the leg straightened and the vein lying in its bed or tunnel without rotation and without tension. Cut the end so that there is a little excess at the tip. This is useful for handling the vein and can be trimmed later.

Anastomosis of the vein graft to these arteries only 2 to 3 mm. in diameter requires gentle precise technique. The technique of suture is illustrated in Fig. 7-9, A to G, and described on p. 190. The magnification obtained with a 2.5× binocular loupe is of considerable help, and this loupe has a convenient focal length and adequate depth of field. The artery and branches are occluded with neurosurgical aneurysm clips (Schwartz or Mayfield) instead of toothed clamps. Ophthalmic scissors and forceps have fine tips. Handle the vein with the forceps applied only to the adventitia or to the tip of the graft, which can be trimmed later. The arteries are thin and fragile, so that no tension is permitted on these grafts. The 5-0 or 6-0 monofilament polypropylene sutures glide through the artery and vein easily. Pull them through and set them carefully without buttonholing or tearing the edge of the artery. Restore flow after the usual flushing maneuvers as described on p. 190.

Intraoperative arteriograms

Intraoperative arteriograms show rapid and complete filling of the vessels of the calf proximally and distally and onto the foot. They will detect any imperfections of the anastomosis, thrombi or emboli, and the like. Follow the technique described earlier. The No. 2 Fogarty catheter is the largest permissible in these arteries.

Closure

Examine the position of the vein graft with the knee flexed and with the knee straight. The graft must be in a roomy plane or tunnel and must not be compressed or deviated. Divide any tendons medially that appear to cause angulation of the graft.

Fig. 7-13. A, Dorsalis pedis artery. Dotted line shows incision between first and second metatarsal bones. **B,** Arteriogram showing vein graft to dorsalis pedis artery. **C,** Arteriogram showing vein graft to posterior tibial artery. (From Auer, A. I., and Hershey, F. B.: Bypass vein grafts to distal tibial or dorsalis pedis arteries, Mo. Med. **70:**93-100, 1973.)

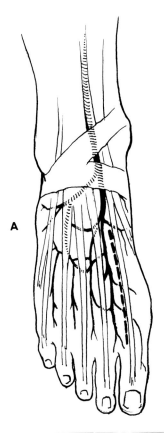

A

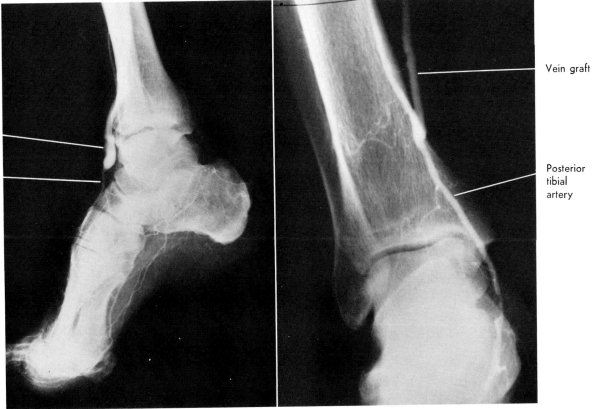

Graft

Dorsalis
pedis
artery

B

Vein graft

Posterior
tibial
artery

Fig. 7-13. For legend see opposite page.

199

Close the superficial fascia in the thigh over the graft, and in the lower leg likewise close the deep fascia with continuous sutures of fine catgut. Close the skin loosely with continuous sutures of fine nylon. Excise thin or undermined devitalized skin edges.

Debridement or toe amputation may be performed at the conclusion of the operation whenever it is indicated.

Postoperative care and complications

See pp. 191-192.

SILICONE MANDRIL METHOD FOR FEMOROPOPLITEAL ARTERY BYPASS

Introduction

The Sparks mandril is a device that is used to grow a reinforced autogenous artery graft in situ for use as a femoropopliteal bypass. A period of six weeks is required for the graft to form. Sparks has used the device since the middle of 1967. Our own experience with this is limited to a few cases, but it appears to be promising for nonurgent cases and therefore is included in this atlas.

The mandril is that part of a mold that shapes the inner surface. It is implanted at the site at which the graft is needed; after the graft has formed, the mold is withdrawn, and the living hollow tube is connected to the arteries above and below, to bypass the obstructed femoral and/or popliteal arteries (Sparks, 1972 and in press).

The mandril is a flexible silicone rubber rod that is covered with a special Dacron mesh that serves as reinforcement of the tube. The Dacron fabric is designed to permit rapid ingrowth of a smooth living lining. This fabric differs therefore from the present Dacron grafts whose lining is mostly Dacron thread between small pores that fill with fibrin and some pores that later fill with tufts of collagenous tissue. Unlike previous Dacron grafts, these autogenous grafts have a smooth living lining, and Sparks states that they can be implanted across the knee joint with a high rate of success.

Indications

Sparks prefers the mandril technique for femoropopliteal bypass in any case in which the patient's condition permits a delay of six weeks between implantation and anastomosis of the graft. He states that this requires less surgery than the vein graft bypass and that this procedure guarantees a suitable uniform graft. Furthermore, it conserves the saphenous vein in case it is needed for coronary bypass. Sparks implants the mandril when he obtains the arteriogram if it indicates the potential need. Thus far we have implanted the mandril in patients in whom the saphenous veins are not available or are not suitable for use because of varicosities, previous phlebitis, or previous operations on these veins. We implant mandrils in legs at the time of arteriography, sympathectomy, abdominal vascular surgery, or operations on the opposite leg.

Sparks has used the mandril method of arterial grafting for other operations also, namely, femorotibial bypass, iliofemoral bypass, axillofemoral bypass, iliac artery replacement, and as arteriovenous shunts in the upper extremity for renal dialysis. The mandril can also be implanted on the abdominal or chest wall to form a graft for later transplantation elsewhere—for example, as a renal artery bypass.

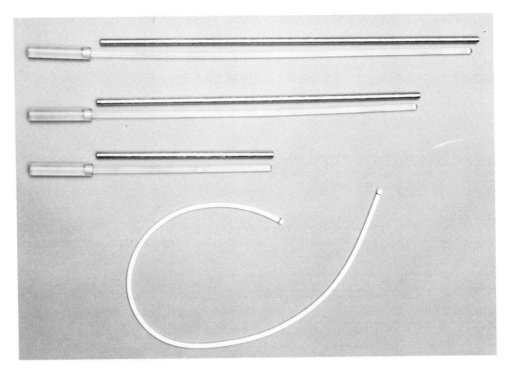

Fig. 7-14. Sparks mandril and tunnelers for its insertion. The tunnelers are hollow steel tubes with plastic obturators. There are three lengths.

Mandril design features

The mandril assembly consists of a flexible silicone rubber rod (mandril) and two siliconized coarse knitted Dacron tubes that have been specially prepared for the purpose. Each tube is knitted with 70-denier, hard-twist, 2-ply Dacron thread. The inner tube contains larger interstices than the outer one. They provide a finished graft of great strength and of ideal thickness and flexibility. The mandril assembly and instruments are shown in Fig. 7-14.

The tunneling tools are hollow stainless steel tubes and a solid bullet-nosed handle-obturator. There are three lengths of tubes. The mandril can be inserted from midcalf to the groin through two small incisions.

The silicone mandril with its knitted Dacron coverings is implanted for a period of six weeks. At the end of this time, a strong, tough tube of connective tissue, with the knitted Dacron tubes contained within its walls, surrounds the mandril. The flexibility of the mandril is about the same as that of an artery of the same diameter distended with arterial pressure. The mandrils available in diameters of 6 and 7 mm. are optimal for replacing arteries from 3 to 9 mm. in diameter.

Grafts grown by the mandril method have a wall thickness of 25/1,000 to 30/1,000 inch. The smooth living lining is collagenous connective tissue. Encapsulated within this wall are the two layers of siliconized knitted Dacron tube that act as a superstructure to impart great strength to the graft. The primary purpose of the outer knitted tube is to provide strength and resistance of intraluminal pressure. The inner knitted tube guarantees the growth of a cushion of tissue inside the outer tube and consequently guarantees the graft against rupture through interstices. In addition, the inner tube adds its own strength to the wall. The growth of the graft is complete six weeks after implantation of the mandril. Grafts harvested at six weeks have been found to be indistinguishable from grafts harvested at three years. Presumably a mandril can be left in place indefinitely and the graft harvested at any time after six weeks.

The mandrils are received in a sterile package ready for implantation. If the mandrils are contaminated, they can be removed from the package and wrapped and autoclaved with gas or steam by usual techniques.

The following is Sparks' detailed description and illustrations of the procedure for femoropopliteal artery bypass. There are two stages: first the implantation of the mandril assembly and then, six weeks later, the removal of the silicone core and anastomosis of the graft.

First stage—implantation of mandril
Indications

The mandril is implanted where it is needed in patients who may need bypass grafting in the near future. The sterile mandril assembly is implanted *beneath the deep fascia* of the thigh, parallel to the femoropopliteal artery. This is conveniently done at the time of arteriography while the patient is anesthetized.

Preparations

The entire abdomen, the pubic region, and the lower extremity are meticulously prepared and scrubbed in the evening and again in the morning before surgery. Prophylactic doses of antibiotics are given intramuscularly in the evening and again in the morning prior to surgery.

With the patient in the supine position under either general or spinal anesthesia, the abdomen and extremity down to the ankle are again prepared and are draped so that the leg and thigh can be flexed during the operation.

Procedure
Distal incision for implantation

Make an incision 4 to 5 cm. in length along the anterior border of the sartorius muscle just above the knee joint, and open the deep fascia to enter Hunter's canal. Pass the index finger through this incision inferiorly into the popliteal space and then withdraw it.

COMMENT: *It is important to thoroughly dissect the tunnel inferiorly with the finger at the level of the incision and superiorly so that the mandril will lie deep under the*

Fig. 7-15. Silicone mandril method for femoropopliteal artery bypass. First stage—implantation of Sparks silicone mandril. **A,** Incision made through deep fascia anterior to sartorius muscle. Hollow tunneler in place beneath deep fascia. Mandril assembly introduced distally. **B,** Tunneler introduced proximally beneath deep fascia. Mandril assembly in place distally. **C,** Tunneler emerging at groin incision and withdrawn through distal incision. Mandril inserted proximally into hollow tunneler.

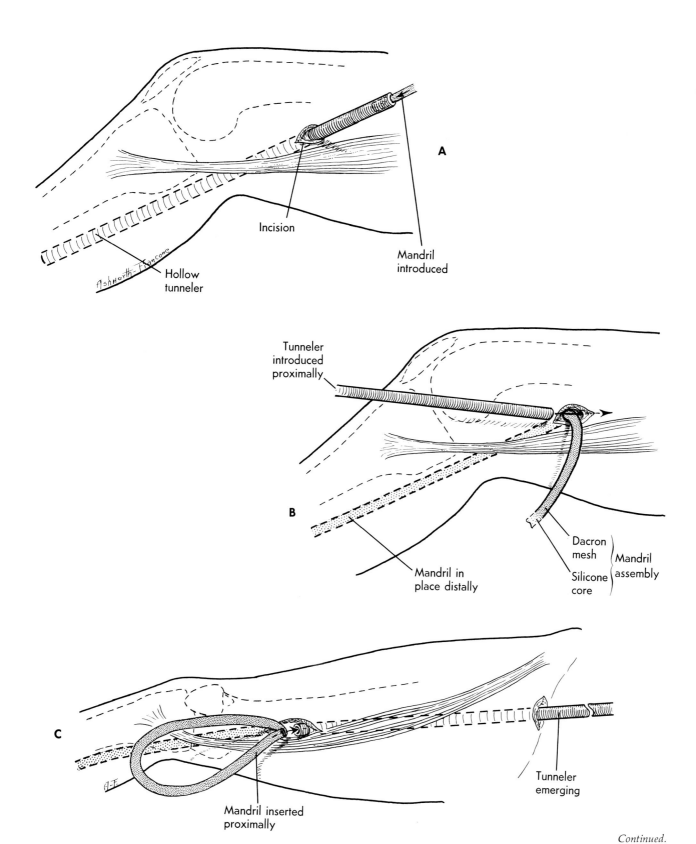

A

Incision

Mandril
introduced

Hollow
tunneler

Tunneler
introduced
proximally

B

Mandril in
place distally

Dacron
mesh

Silicone
core

Mandril
assembly

C

Mandril inserted
proximally

Tunneler
emerging

Fig. 7-15. For legend see opposite page.

Continued.

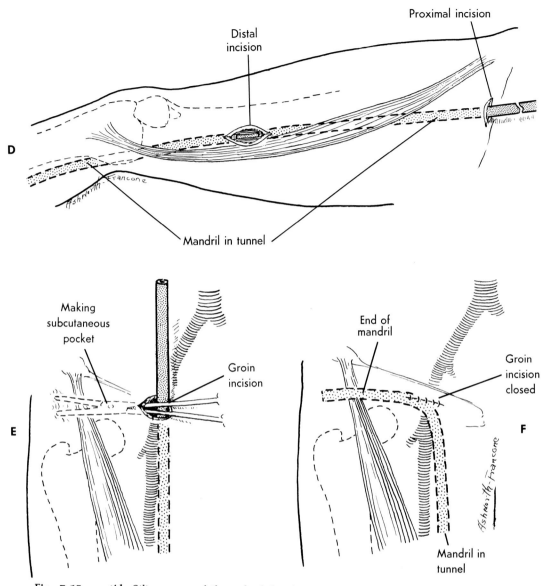

Fig. 7-15, cont'd. Silicone mandril method for femoropopliteal artery bypass. First stage—implantation of Sparks silicone mandril. **D,** Mandril in tunnel. Distal incision ready for closure. **E,** Blunt dissection laterally making a subcutaneous pocket for proximal end of mandril. **F,** Implantation of mandril completed and proximal incision closed.

deep fascia when implanted and will not angle superficially. A properly dissected tunnel is of great importance to the proper function of the subsequent graft.

Introduce the short tunneler into the incision and inferiorly through the popliteal space for a distance of 4 inches or more below the knee (Fig. 7-15, *A*). To do this, flex the knee and angle the tunneler so that it can be palpated. It should pass immediately under the deep fascia and under the tendon of the sartorius muscle and other tendons that attach to the posteromedial border of the tibia and should lie approximately 1 cm. posterior to the posteromedial border of the tibia. Withdraw the obturator, and fill the tunneler partially with a solution of 1 million units of penicillin and 1 Gm. of streptomycin in 100 ml. of distilled water. Pass one end of the mandril throughout the length of the tunneler; leave it loose in the tunneler while you withdraw the tunneler, leaving the mandril in place.

COMMENT: *Flexion of the knee causes longitudinal motion of the mandril if the mandril is stuffed into the tunnel and compressed or coiled. This gliding motion prevents ingrowth of the fibrous tissue into the mesh. Do not stretch the mandril, since this may disturb the predetermined relationship between the mandril and the knitted Dacron tubes. This relationship is carefully determined during the manufacturing process.*

Proximal incision and implantation

Make an incision 3 cm. in length over the common femoral artery, and incise the deep fascia. With a sterile marking pen, draw a line on the skin between the two incisions. Pass the tip of the index finger distally beneath the deep fascia and beneath the sartorius muscle. From the thigh incision, pass the fingertip up beneath the deep fascia and beneath the sartorius muscle.

COMMENT: *Do not tunnel through the muscle. One graft that lay in a bed of muscle had insufficient fibrous tissue growth into the pores of the mesh.*

Introduce the medium-length tunneler under the deep fascia and under the satorius muscle, and push it proximally to the groin incision as shown in Fig. 7-15, B, following the line on the skin. Pass the tunneler out through the groin incision, and withdraw it until the lower end of the tunneler barely is in view in the lower incision. Pass the entire exposed portion of the mandril up the tunneler to the groin (Fig. 7-15, C), and withdraw the tunneler through the groin incision. This leaves the mandril in place, with some excess emerging at the groin (Fig. 7-15, D). Estimate the length needed and divide the mandril midway between two ligatures (not shown), which are tied tightly approximately 1 cm. apart at a distance of approximately 5 cm. from the groin incision. The ligatures are essential to prevent slippage or migration of the Dacron tube that covers the silicone mandril. A subcutaneous tunnel is fashioned laterally (Fig. 7-15, E), and the free end of the mandril is passed into the lateral tunnel (Fig. 7-15, F) and sutured to the inguinal ligament.

COMMENT: *The bend in the mandril is essential to prevent motion or migration of the mandril; motion or migration prevents ingrowth of sturdy tissue into the mesh.*

Closure

Instill the solution of penicillin and streptomycin into the tunnels from the groin wound. Close the incisions carefully with interrupted nonabsorbable sutures in the subcutaneous fascia as the first layer and in the skin as a second layer.

Postoperative care

The patient is given 600,000 units of aqueous penicillin G and 0.5 Gm. of streptomycin at 6- and 12-hour intervals, respectively. The patient is discharged from the hospital on the first postoperative day with a prescription for ampicillin to be taken in the dosage of 0.5 Gm. every six hours for five days. Previous activity is resumed after hospital discharge. The sutures are removed five days later in the physician's office. The patient may return to the hospital for the grafting operation after six weeks.

Second stage—femoropopliteal artery bypass

After six or more weeks, the surgeon operates on the patient again to remove the mandril core and anastomose the hollow living graft. When the patient is readmitted to the hospital, the same meticulous preparations are made as were used prior to implantation of the mandril, including prophylactic therapy with antibiotics.

The patient is placed in the supine position, and the abdomen and involved lower extremity are prepared with Betadine and draped so that the extremity is free to be moved in the field. The foot is wrapped separately.

Our indications for femoropopliteal artery bypass are chiefly ischemic lesions and pain at rest, as described on p. 179. If further experience confirms the safety and effectiveness of the mandril method, possibly intermittent claudication will be sufficient indication for completing the bypass.

Procedure

Incision

Make an incision 10 to 12 cm. in length slightly posterior to the upper posteromedial border of the tibia, and curve it gently over the popliteal space (Fig. 7-16, *A*). Incise the deep fascia along the posteromedial border of the tibia, exposing the new graft and mandril and the medial head of the gastrocnemius muscle (Fig. 7-16, *B*). Mobilize the mandril and the new graft.

COMMENT: *Do not dissect too close to the graft and mandril. There is no harm in leaving a small amount of fat on the graft when it is adherent. Normally there is a fine areolar plane of cleavage around the graft. You may see the Dacron mesh faintly, but do not dissect so close that the mesh is plainly revealed.*

Exposure of distal end of popliteal artery

Flex the knee. Then mobilize the medial head of the gastrocnemius muscle and divide it with cautery superiorly near its tendinous attachment. Later, during the wound closure, this muscle is sutured to the deep fascia along the posteromedial border of the tibia, thus allowing the graft to lie freely in the popliteal space. The medial head of the gastrocnemius muscle in its normal position would lie in the path of the graft. Mobilize the distal 5 cm. of the popliteal artery and vein by blunt and sharp dissection. At this level, the artery lies lateral to the vein. The vein should be slightly retracted anteriorly and the artery mobilized so that it is posterior to the vein. The graft when attached will lie posteriorly and not obstruct the vein. Palpate the popliteal artery to select the most suitable site for grafting (Fig. 7-16, *C*). Cut off the end of the mandril and graft proximal to the ligature around them; this frees the mandril at this end of the graft.

Exposure of common femoral artery and proximal end of graft

Make an oblique incision over the common femoral artery close to the inguinal ligament. Mobilize the new graft and mandril and reflect them out of the way. Dissect and identify the common femoral artery and the origins of the superficial femoral and profunda femoris arteries (Fig. 7-16, *D*).

COMMENT: *We prefer vertical incisions because they are more easily extended to correct any narrowing of the profunda femoris artery that might be encountered.*

Cut off the end of the mandril and graft just proximal to the ligature so that they lie free within the new graft.

Withdraw the mandril slightly. Grasp the upper end of the mandril with an Allis clamp and withdraw it from the graft until the popliteal end is a short distance above the anticipated site of the distal anastomosis.

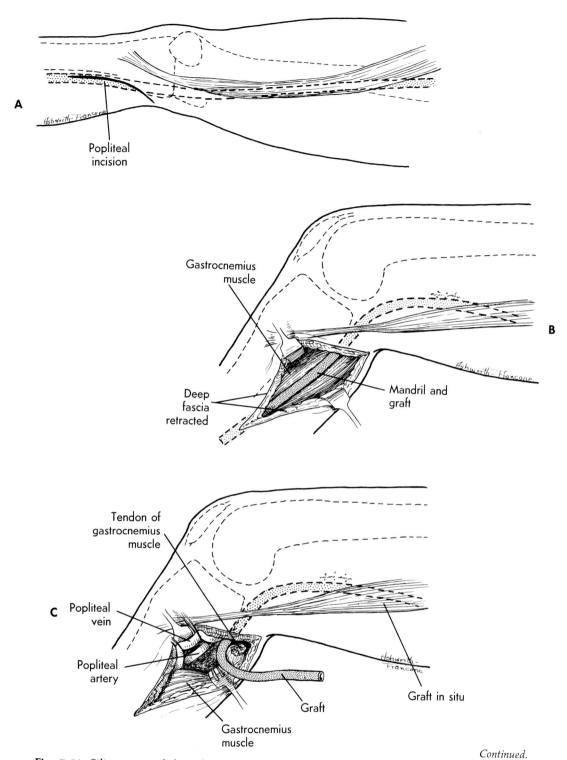

Popliteal
incision

Gastrocnemius
muscle

Deep
fascia
retracted

Mandril and
graft

B

Tendon of
gastrocnemius
muscle

C Popliteal
vein

Popliteal
artery

Graft

Graft in situ

Gastrocnemius
muscle

Continued.

Fig. 7-16. Silicone mandril method for femoropopliteal artery bypass. Second stage—bypass with autogenous graft formed in situ by Sparks silicone mandril. **A,** Popliteal incision. **B,** Deep fascia incised and retracted. Mandril and graft uncovered. **C,** Tendon of gastrocnemius muscle divided and muscle retracted. Popliteal artery and vein uncovered at site of anastomosis. End of graft mobilized.

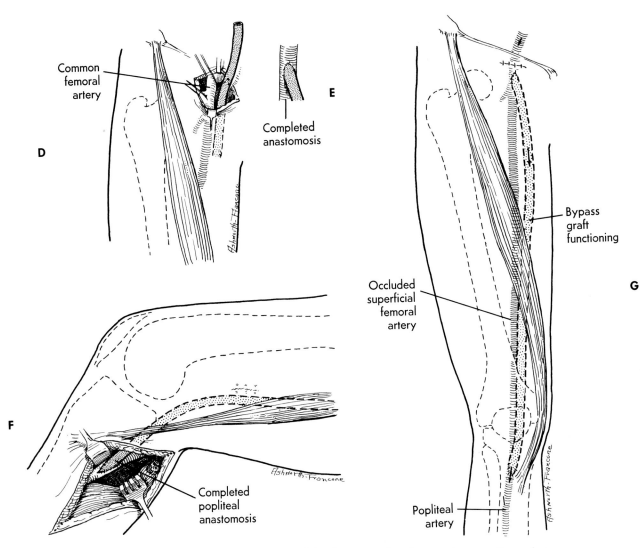

Fig. 7-16, cont'd. Silicone mandril method for femoropopliteal artery bypass. Second stage—bypass with autogenous graft formed in situ by Sparks silicone mandril. **D,** Common femoral artery exposed at site of anastomosis. **E,** Proximal anastomosis completed. **F,** Popliteal anastomosis completed. **G,** Bypass graft functioning.

COMMENT: *Leave the mandril in place while the popliteal anastomosis is being made. This avoids possible rotation of the graft.*

Popliteal arteriotomy

Inject 6,000 units of heparin intravenously. Apply umbilical tape tourniquets to the popliteal artery proximal and distal to the intended site of arteriotomy. Tighten the upper tourniquet, and inject heparin into the distal runoff vessel. We use a syringe with 22-gauge needle and inject 25 ml. of a solution of 1,000 units of heparin in 100 ml. of normal saline solution. Then tighten the distal tourniquet immediately.

Make an incision 1.5 cm. in length in the medial side of the popliteal artery, and irrigate the occluded segment with normal saline solution. Straighten the leg. Cut the graft on a 45-degree angle at the level of intended anastomosis. The oblique cut leaves an oval aperture for anastomosis. The length of this oval may be increased by incising the graft wall proximally from the upper angle of the oblique end. The final length of this oval should be approximately the same as the length of the incision in the popliteal artery. Trim any corners or sharp angles in this oval produced as a result of the longitudinal incision.

COMMENT: *These grafts are short and flexible but not elastic and are fixed in situ in their midportion. Judge the length carefully. We leave a little excess at the tip to be trimmed later.*

Popliteal anastomosis

Anastomose the graft to the popliteal artery, using a continuous stitch of 5-0 Tevdek suture. Start at the acute angle of the proximal end, and suture halfway along each side. Leave the distal half of this anastomosis for completion just before the graft is ready to function.

COMMENT: *The sutures must include more of the edge of these grafts than is customarily included when suturing vein grafts, in order to include 2 to 3 mm. of the embedded fabric. The needle can be passed through the graft 2 to 3 mm. from the edge without narrowing the sides of the anastomosis. The critical parts are the two ends of the arteriotomy. Interrupted sutures are tedious, and furthermore, continuous sutures prevent ravelling or running of the loose Dacron mesh at the cut edge.*

The detailed drawings in Fig. 7-9 show our method of popliteal anastomosis. Fig. 7-16, *F*, shows the completed anastomosis done by Sparks.

Femoral anastomosis

Occlude the upper end of the common femoral artery with a delicate artery clamp. Occlude the origins of the superficial femoral and profunda femoris arteries with bulldog clamps. Make an incision 1.5 cm. in length anteriorly in the common femoral artery. The lower end of this arteriotomy may extend to within 0.5 cm. of the distal end of the common femoral artery but no closer. (The reason for this is that the femoral artery is usually more diseased and thicker walled at the distal end than it is a short distance above.)

COMMENT: *We disagree with Sparks and prefer arteriotomies close to the origin of the profunda femoris artery so that any narrowing can be corrected at this time. The attachment of the graft will widen the arteriotomy.*

Irrigate the lumen with normal saline solution. Withdraw the mandril completely, cut off the end of the graft at a 45-degree angle, and prepare the end in the same manner as described for the lower end. Anastomose the graft to the common femoral artery with a continuous 5-0 Tevdek suture. Sparks starts with double-armed mattress suture at each end and sutures each side from both ends, making the knot midway between the two ends. This graft, which is 6 mm. in diameter, is wider and just as sturdy as a vein graft. However, the sutures must include 2 to 3 mm. of the edge of the graft in order to have a secure hold in the embedded Dacron reinforcement.

Flushing and restoration of flow to popliteal artery

Remove the distal tourniquet from the popliteal artery and note the back bleeding. If the back bleeding is poor, pass a Fogarty balloon catheter or a Fogarty irrigating catheter or both distally at this time.

COMMENT: *One case of multiple aneurysms occurred after Fogarty catheter thrombectomy; therefore, if it is ever necessary to pass Fogarty catheters in a mandril-grown graft, do not stretch or dilate the graft more than you would a normal artery.*

If the back bleeding is satisfactory, reapply the distal tourniquet. Then loosen the proximal tourniquet on the popliteal artery to allow forward bleeding and then reapply it, and irrigate the isolated segment of popliteal artery with normal saline solution. Complete the popliteal anastomosis.

Remove the clamps or occluding tourniquets in sequence as follows: First remove the proximal tourniquet on the popliteal artery. Next remove the clamps on the superficial femoral and profunda femoris arteries. When the graft fills with blood, remove the proximal clamp on the common femoral artery slowly. Apply gentle pressure to the anastomoses with gauze sponges if there is slight leakage. Two minutes after removal of the clamp on the upper end of the femoral artery, remove the distal tourniquet on the popliteal artery, reestablishing circulation to the lower leg (Fig. 7-16, *G*).

Note pulsations in the graft and the popliteal artery distal to the anastomosis. Remove the covering from the foot and palpate for pulses.

Intraoperative arteriogram and closure

Insert an 18-gauge needle into the common femoral artery or the upper end of the graft. Inject 20 ml. of Conray (60%) to make an arteriogram of the lower end of the graft and the runoff vessels. (See p. 190.)

Irrigate the incisions with the antibiotic solution, and close the wounds in layers, using fine silk. In closing the popliteal incision, suture the medial head of the gastrocnemis muscle to the deep fascia at the posteromedial border of the tibia throughout the length of the incision so that the muscle will not press on or deviate the graft. Apply sterile dressings to the incisions, and wrap the leg with elastic bandages from the toes to the upper thigh.

Postoperative care

Postoperatively the patient is given aqueous penicillin G, 600,000 units every six hours, and streptomycin, 0.5 Gm. every twelve hours for six days. Throughout the postoperative hospital stay, the head of the patient's bed is kept flat and the foot is kept elevated 30 degrees. Ambulation is started on the morning after surgery. The patient must neither stand still nor sit with his feet down. The leg is rewrapped twice daily for the first six postoperative days, and then the wrapping is changed to a good-quality knee-length elastic stocking. The sutures are removed on about the seventh postoperative day, and ordinarily the patient is discharged between the seventh and tenth postoperative days with instructions to neither stand still nor sit with his feet down and to continue to wear the elastic stocking when he is not in bed as long as there is any tendency toward swelling in the extremity.

COMMENT: *We agree with Sparks that postoperative phlebitis or lymphedema is more easily prevented than treated. Other complications of femoropopliteal bypass operations have been discussed previously.*

FEMORAL ENDARTERECTOMY
Introduction

If there is an available vein for bypass, we do not employ closed-loop endarterectomy of the superficial femoral artery. As in bypass grafting, an adequate outflow tract is necessary, and diffuse atherosclerotic disease involving the popliteal artery and its branches is a contraindication. Vein bypass is superior to extensive endarterectomy; however, sometimes veins may not be available. Open endarterectomy of long segments of the femoral artery, closed by angioplasty with a long strip of vein, is a poor operation and leads to mural thrombi and early occlusion. Bypass prostheses should be available whenever endarterectomy is begun in case the femoral bypass procedure should become desirable.

Procedure
With endarterectomy loops

1. Prepare the skin for several days in advance. Place the patient in the supine position, with the thigh abducted and externally rotated and the knee flexed and supported. All levels of the popliteal artery are readily approached by the medial route (pp. 174-179).

2. Expose the common femoral artery in the goin. The proximal incision should expose the common femoral artery and permit endarterectomy at the branching of the profunda femoris and superficial femoral arteries. Identify the common femoral artery and its branches and isolate them with umbilical tapes.

3. Expose the popliteal artery as described on pp. 174-179.

4. Inject 20 mg. of heparin into the popliteal artery distally, and apply an angled arterial clamp. Give an additional 50 mg. of heparin intravenously.

5. Make a transverse arteriotomy at the distal end of the occlusion, extending to the occluded area proximally and into relatively normal artery distally (Fig. 7-17, A).

COMMENT: *Transverse arteriotomies are now preferred instead of longitudinal incisions as illustrated in Fig. 7-17.*

6. Separate the diseased intima and the thrombotic core from the media for a distance of several centimeters. The Freer elevator or a suitably shaped scissors is used for transecting the intima where it is suitably thin. The correct plane of clevage is marked by the circular muscular fibers of the tunica media.

7. Distally, bevel the intima and suture it to the arterial wall with a double-armed mattress suture of 5-0 arterial suture. Pass the suture from within outward, tying it outside the artery.

8. Place the open loop of the stripping instrument over the end of the core, hold the end of the core for countertraction, and gently advance the stripper upward (Fig. 7-17, B).

COMMENT: *Distal introduction of the stripper ensures that it will not be too large for the artery as it is passed upward in the direction of increasing arterial diameter. Various types of closed-loop strippers are available. Loops may also be improvised from stiffer steel wire if no instruments specifically designed for endarterectomy are available.*

9. Inject 20 mg. of heparin into the common femoral artery, and place arterial clamps on the common femoral artery above the disease process and on the profunda femoris artery. Make a longitudinal arteriotomy at the bifurcation of the common

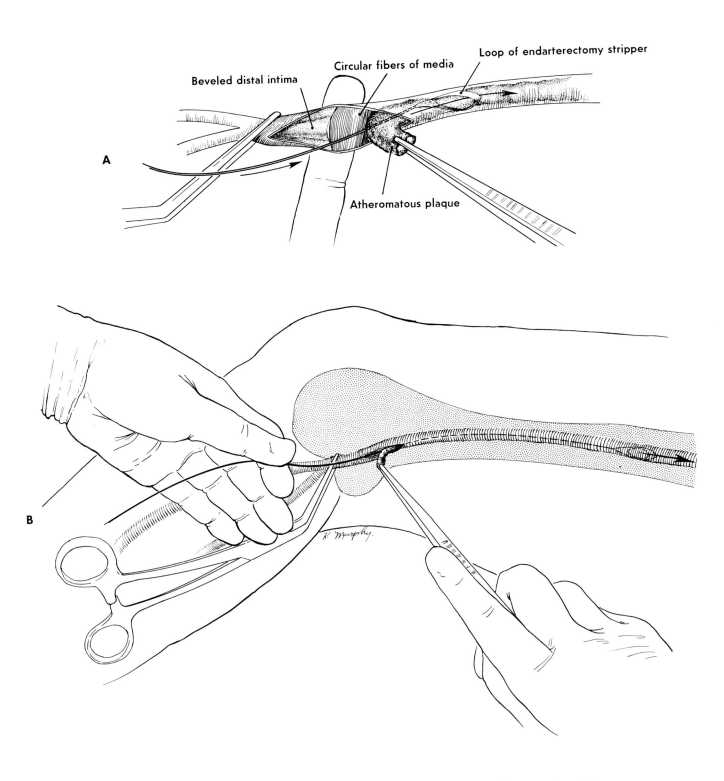

Fig. 7-17. Femoral endarterectomy. **A,** Begin endarterectomy by introducing stripper into popliteal artery. **B,** Pass stripper proximally.

femoral artery to allow visualization of disease at the ostium of the profunda femoris branch.

10. Pass the stripper from below as far as the profunda femoris artery. Separate diseased intima from the media in the region of the bifurcation, and tease any plaque from the ostium of the profunda femoris artery. Divide the intima above any thick plaques.

COMMENT: *Do not attempt blind endarterectomy at major arterial bifurcations. If the stripper becomes arrested, another skin incision and arteriotomy will be necessary, or endarterectomy can be abandoned and a bypass prosthesis can be anastomosed to the upper and lower arteriotomies.*

11. Withdraw the stripper through the popliteal incision and the core from above. Introduce a polyvinyl catheter the same size as the stripped segment of artery for its full length and irrigate with heparin in saline solution (0.1%). Back bleeding from collateral branches usually causes oozing.

COMMENT: *Remnants of attached intima are the cause of many failures. Those surgeons who advocate endarterectomy use many supplementary maneuvers. LaVeen passes size 01 tube gauze through the artery. A spring-handled nasal speculum prevents the gauze from dragging at the edge of the arteriotomy.*

12. Perform an intraoperative arteriogram. Even small irregularities shown on the films are cause for concern, and such defects should be corrected by flushing, by drawing tube gauze through the artery, or by transverse arteriotomy at the site. The arteriography is most readily performed through a whistle-tipped cardiovascular catheter held in the endarterectomized artery with a Javid clamp or umbilical tape.

The portable x-ray machine and the 14-by-17-inch grid-front cassette are the only pieces of radiographic equipment needed. The cassette is dropped into a sterile pillowcase. The entire leg has been prepared and draped as usual. The leg is lifted so that the film can be positioned accurately beneath it.

Irrigate the artery with heparin in saline solution to estimate the volume of contrast medium needed to fill the artery.

Inject a slightly larger volume of Conray 400, expose the film, release the distal clamp, irrigate again, and begin closure while the films are being developed.

Closure of distal and proximal arteriotomies

1. Close the distal arteriotomy first, using a continuous 5-0 Dacron, Tevdek, polyethylene, or polypropylene arterial suture. The catheter stent is in place to prevent narrowing during the closure.

COMMENT: *If the popliteal artery is small, a patch of vein or prosthesis is sutured between the edges of any longitudinal arteriotomy to prevent narrowing. (See patch angioplasty, Fig. 6-7 and pp. 157 and 158.)*

2. Partially close the proximal arteriotomy.

3. Withdraw the catheter stent that was used for irrigation, leaving the artery full of heparin in saline solution.

4. Cross-clamp the superficial femoral artery, and momentarily release the clamp on the common femoral artery to flush out clots. Next release the clamp on the profunda femoris artery to check back bleeding.

5. Finish closure of the proximal arteriotomy, releasing the clamps on the popliteal, superficial femoral, and profunda femoris arteries before tying the suture. Last, slowly release the clamp on the common femoral artery.

Closure of popliteal and groin incisions

Close the popliteal incision, suturing all except the adductor tendon. Since anticoagulants will be used, a drain should be inserted; but this should not lie close to an arteriotomy. Close the fascia and skin. In closing the groin incision, be careful to eliminate all dead space.

Postoperative care

1. Avoid circumferential dressings.

2. Heparin, 30 mg. to 60 mg., should be given intravenously every four hours to prolong the clotting time. These frequent intravenous injections are made painlessly via a Teflon cannula inserted in a forearm vein for several days. The needle is inserted into a rubber cap over the hub. Frequent intravenous injections of small doses of heparin maintain a more constant heparin effect.

3. Bed rest is advisable for a period of seven to ten days.

4. If the leg becomes ischemic, reoperate at once. Be prepared for intraoperative angiography, retrograde flushing, bypass grafting, or patch angioplasty.

F.B.H.

References

Sparks, C. H.: Silicone mandril method of femoropopliteal artery bypass, Am. J. Surg. **124**:244-249, 1972.

Sparks, C. H.: Silicone mandril method for growth of reinforced autogenous femoropopliteal artery grafts in situ, Ann. Surg. **177**:273, 1973.

8

Aneurysms of the popliteal artery

Aneurysms of the popliteal artery are dangerous. Complications are very common because these aneurysms are compressed with flexion of the knee. Even small aneurysms are hazardous. Embolism from contents of the sac, acute thrombosis, and rupture may occur. Popliteal aneurysms are frequently bilateral.

The diagnosis is usually made by palpation of the lesion. Arteriograms are needed to demonstrate outflow distal to the popliteal artery, size of the proximal and distal portions of the popliteal artery, and presence of collateral circulation. Lateral views show the artery and aneurysm best. Arteriograms will not always reveal the aneurysm. They may show only the channel through the laminated clot lining the sac. Arteriograms showing occlusion of the distal popliteal artery should not discourage the surgeon unduly. Many times the obstruction is due to embolism from debris that is readily removed.

Operation for aneurysm of the popliteal artery is advisable even though the popliteal outflow is absent or poor. The purpose of the operation is to remove the aneurysm and to restore normal blood flow to the leg. Any sizable or symptomatic aneurysm should be removed if the patient is a reasonable surgical risk and if there is no established distal gangrene.

Distal occlusion by propagation of thrombosis or by the distal embolization of atheromatous debris often precipitates acute vascular insufficiency in unrecognized or neglected popliteal aneurysms. Reconstruction and limb salvage are difficult after these complications.

CHOICE OF OPERATION

The type of operation performed is adapted to the needs of the patient. There are two phases to the operation: first the treatment of the aneurysm and then the restoration of flow to the lower leg. Fig. 8-1 shows various types of operations.

Arteriography is helpful in planning the operation. It maps the outflow and serves as a guide, and it may indicate the need to bypass stenoses proximal or distal to the aneurysm.

Aneurysms need not be removed. A large one causing compression in the popliteal space can be evacuated of its contents, but the sac that is adherent to veins and nerve need not be removed. Sacs can be obliterated by the Matas' endoaneurysmorrhaphy. Embolism from small aneurysms can be prevented by ligating and dividing the popliteal artery distal to the aneurysm if it is small and there is no compression of adjoining structures. Flow through genicular arteries originating from the aneurysm can be maintained by permitting the normal inflow into the aneurysm. Some long

215

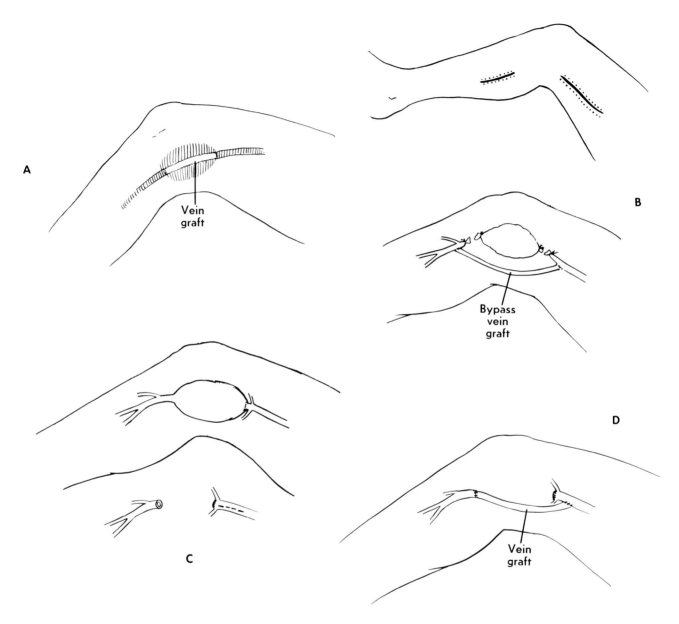

Fig. 8-1. Various operations for popliteal aneurysm. **A,** Intrasaccular resection and end-to-end anastomosis with vein graft. **B,** Ligation and exclusion and bypass vein graft. **C,** Resection and proximal closure by suture instead of ligation. **D,** Vein graft with proximal bypass.

E

F

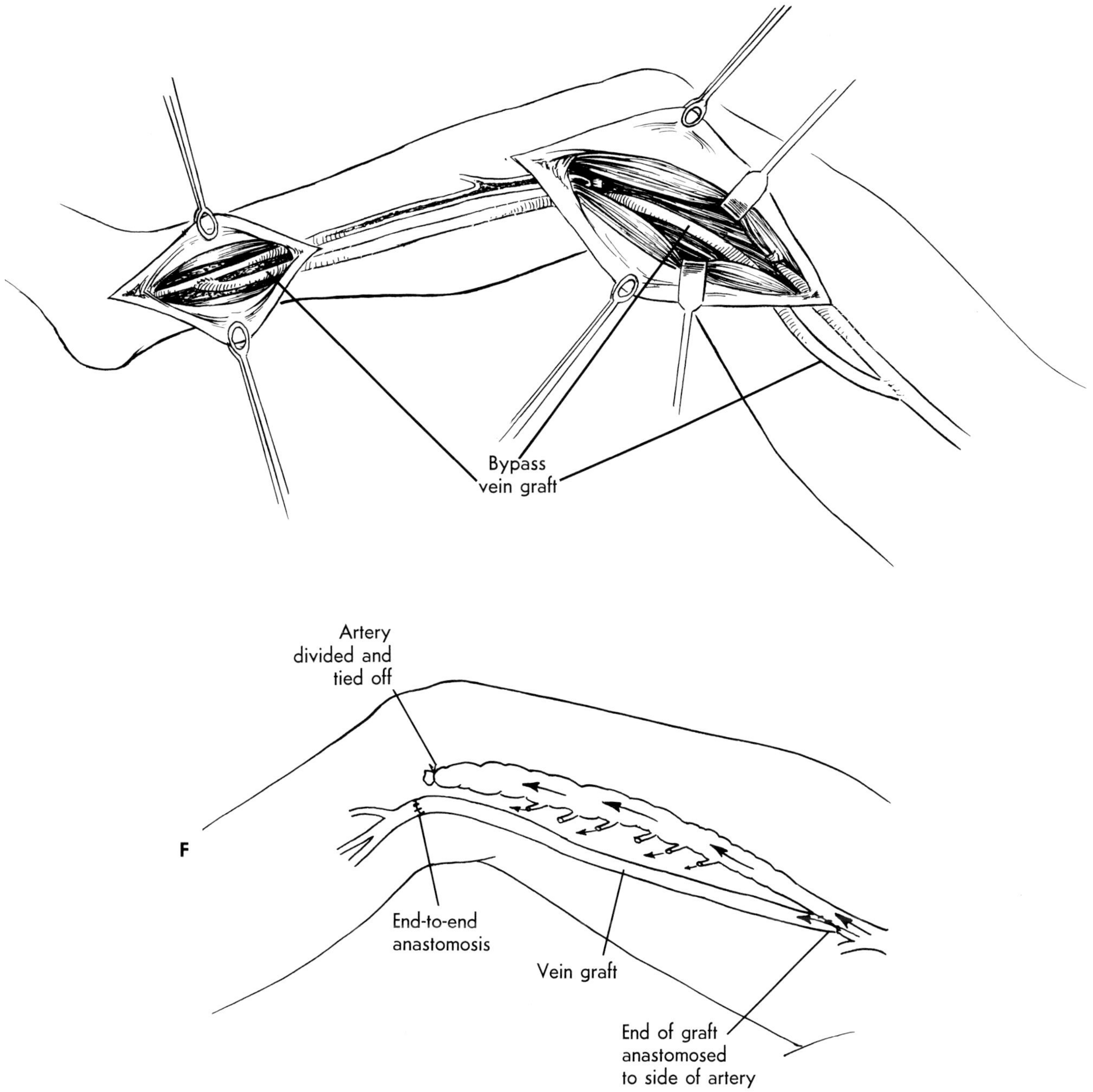

Bypass
vein graft
Artery
divided and
tied off
End-to-end
anastomosis
Vein graft
End of graft
anastomosed
to side of artery

Fig. 8-1, cont'd. Various operations for popliteal aneurysm. **E,** Bypass vein graft to distal end of posterior tibial artery. **F,** Bypass vein graft excluding popliteal aneurysm and ectasia of femoral artery, which was source of emboli. (**E** adapted from Evans, W. E., Conley, J. E., and Bernhard, V.: Popliteal aneurysms, Surgery **70:**762-767, 1971.)

popliteal aneurysms are not large in diameter and are accompanied by lesser sacculations and bulges along the superficial femoral artery. The distal division and ligation prevents embolism, and the vein graft can originate from the side of the normal proximal part of the femoral artery. Continuity need not always be restored when the outflow is very poor and the collateral circulation is sufficient. In rare cases, the aneurysm may be excised or disconnected and the sac obliterated without restoring continuity. Collateral branches close to the aneurysm should be preserved. Oversewing the proximal part of the popliteal artery permits excision close to the collateral vessels (Fig. 8-1, C). Excision without restoration of continuity relieves local pain or pressure and prevents embolism, but it is rarely indicated and rarely performed. Lumbar sympathectomy is a helpful adjunct for such cases.

Restoration of continuity is almost always essential. The end-to-end anastomosis with a vein graft is the usual method of restoring continuity. The bypass technique may also be helpful in some cases (Fig. 8-1, B and D).

Aneurysms are frequently accompanied by occlusion and stenosis of the distal end of the popliteal artery and the proximal ends of the tibial and peroneal arteries. When the outflow is poor, the distal end of the vein graft may be implanted further down the leg as a bypass into the distal end of one of the tibial arteries (Fig. 8-1, E).

A saphenous vein graft is usually used for restoring continuity. Vein grafts are ordinarily preferable across the knee joint because prostheses become encased in fibrous tissue, become stiff, and kink when flexed; but short segments of prosthesis 8 to 10 mm. in diameter have served very well in several cases for many years. The use of prostheses is justified only to restore continuity when the arteries are large, the gap is short, and prolonging of the surgery to procure a living graft seems to be unwise.

Autologous living artery, larger than a vein graft, is probably the ideal graft; it is seldom used but should not be forgotten. The patient's external iliac artery may be resected and replaced by a prosthesis, and the patient's external iliac artery may be transplanted to replace his popliteal aneurysm. This is the preferred graft if infection is present.

Thrombosis in aneurysms may extend proximally and distally and the use of Fogarty balloon catheters or retrograde flush techniques discribed in Chapter 9 may be useful. When the major branches cannot be cleared of thrombi, the vein graft is attached distally to one of the tibial arteries (Fig. 8-1, E). Tendons need not be divided when bypass grafts can be inserted into accessible arteries proximally and distally.

SURGICAL APPROACH TO POPLITEAL ANEURYSMS

The medial approach is very satisfactory for the surgical treatment of all aneurysms. The medial incision allows better access to the proximal and distal parts of the artery and can be extended easily into the thigh or lower leg whenever necessary for large aneurysms or for bypass grafts.

The posterior approach was occasionally used for aneurysms of the popliteal artery because the popliteal vein and the nerve trunks traversing the fossa are more accessible by this approach. They are frequently found to be adherent to a large sac. The proximal and distal portions of the popliteal artery, however, are deep, and the posterior incision is not easily extended.

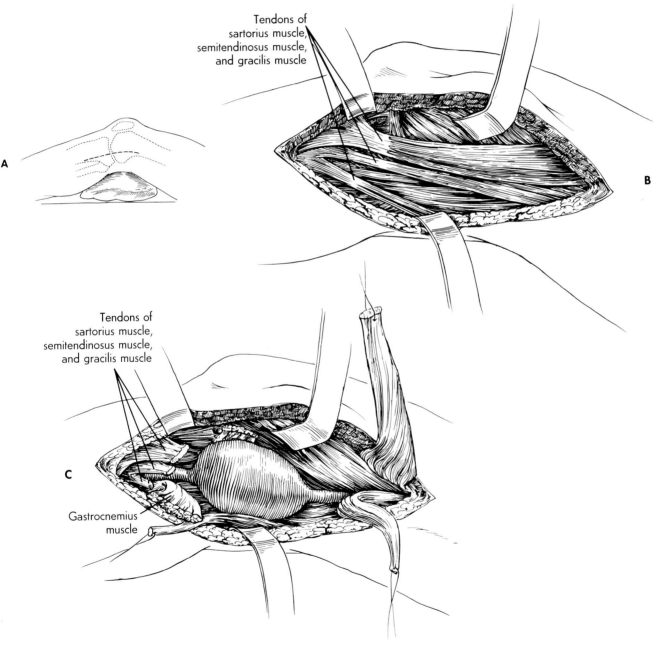

Tendons of
sartorius muscle,
semitendinosus muscle,
and gracilis muscle

A

B

Tendons of
sartorius muscle,
semitendinosus muscle,
and gracilis muscle

C

Gastrocnemius
muscle

Fig. 8-2. Medial exposure of popliteal aneurysm. **A,** Incision. **B,** Exposure. **C,** Popliteal aneurysm after division of tendons.

Medial approach to popliteal aneurysms

The anatomy of the popliteal artery and the technique used to expose it are discussed in Chapter 7 and illustrated in Figs. 7-1 to 7-3. Fig. 8-2, *A,* shows the medial incision, and Fig. 8-2, *B,* shows the muscles after the deep fascia is opened medially. More flexion of the knee will permit retraction of the muscles, and for small aneurysms, it is ordinarily sufficient to divide the medial head of the gastrocnemius muscle close to its insertion.

COMMENT: *Tendons need not be divided for small aneurysms or for other aneurysms that can be ligated proximally and distally and left in situ (Fig. 8-1, B). Not all aneurysms need be resected, and tendons need not be divided when bypass grafts can be inserted into accessible arteries proximally and distally.*

Procedure

1. With the patient lying in the supine position, prepare and drape the affected leg from the groin to the ankle, and prepare and drape the opposite thigh for procurement of the saphenous vein graft.

2. Incise the skin from the posterior border of the tibia to the posterior aspect of the femur (Fig. 8-2, *A*).

COMMENT: *Work in the anterior area and avoid the saphenous vein. It is a useful collateral vein about the knee if popliteal vein thrombosis occurs.*

3. Open the popliteal fascia. Retract the muscles and tendons that insert on the medial condyle of the tibia. One or more of the tendons may be divided if necessary (Fig. 8-2, *C*).

4. The aneurysm is then encountered; if it is large, divide the medial head of the gastrocnemius muscle near its attachment to the condyle of the femur (Fig. 8-2, *C*).

5. Mobilize the popliteal artery proximal and distal to the aneurysm for proximal and distal control.

Intrasaccular resection of popliteal aneurysms

It is unnecessary to dissect the aneurysm so that it is free of the veins and nerve; in very large aneurysms, this is not only unnecessary but also tedious and hazardous because they may be densely adherent.

1. Inject 3,000 units of heparin into the artery, and apply the DeBakey angled clamps proximally and distally as illustrated in Fig. 8-3, *A.*

2. Divide the artery above and below the aneurysm. Check the back bleeding, and if the outflow distally is in doubt, perform an intraoperative arteriogram and continue the operation while films are developed.

3. Open the sac longitudinally, remove the contents of the sac, and close the orifices of any bleeding vessels with figure-of-eight sutures (Fig. 8-3, *B* and *C*).

Fig. 8-3. Popliteal aneurysm—intrasaccular resection and end-to-end anastomosis with vein graft. **A,** Sac opened after proximal and distal control obtained. **B,** Sac contents evacuated, and orifices of bleeding vessels ligated. **C,** Figure-of-eight stitch ligature about bleeding orifice. **D,** V incision to enlarge end of vein graft. **E,** Oblique incision to enlarge end of vein graft. **F,** Vein graft sutured for end-to-end anastomosis.

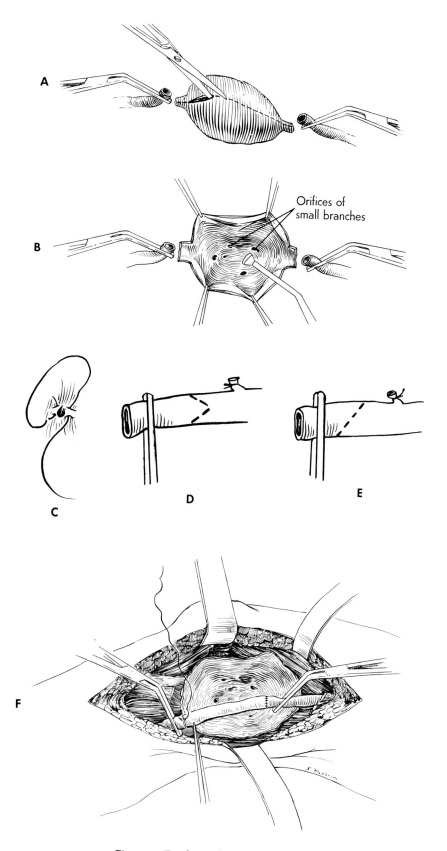

A

B

Orifices of
small branches

C

D

E

F

Fig. 8-3. For legend see opposite page.

221

COMMENT: *The sac can be opened along a line that does not cross the popliteal vein. The nerve is safe on the lateral side.*

4. Small bleeding vessels in the edge of the sac or in the lining can be touched lightly with cautery.

Procurement and preparation of vein graft

A generous length of the saphenous vein is removed from the opposite thigh. There should be an inch or more of excess length. The sites of proximal and distal anastomosis must be decided before this is done to ensure removal of sufficient length of vein. The preparation of the vein, that is, ligation of its tributaries and stripping away of excess adventitia to permit its dilation, is described in Chapter 7 and illustrated in Figs. 7-4 and 7-5 in full detail. The vein is always smaller than the atherosclerotic artery, and several maneuvers are useful with small veins: (1) meticulous stripping away of adventitia while the vein is distended with pressure of saline solution or stretched with hemostats; (2) trimming of the end obliquely or in a V shape (Fig. 8-3, *D* and *E*); (3) for the proximal anastomosis of a small and a large artery, suturing of the end of the vein to the side of the dilated artery; and (4) for easy anastomosis, sometimes trimming of the end of the vein graft as in Fig. 7-6.

Restoration of continuity—vein graft

End-to-end anastomosis with the reversed vein graft is illustrated in Fig. 8-4. The triangulation of the vein makes it easier to handle, avoids folding and wrinkling, and permits precise anastomosis.

1. Reverse the vein, and perform the proximal anastomosis first.

2. Insert three double-armed mattress sutures of 4-0 monofilament polypropylene into the end of the vein at equidistant points. Hold two of the sutures as guide sutures while placing the other through the artery. Pass the suture at least 1 mm. from the edge of a thin vein (Fig. 8-4, *A*).

3. Pass these triangulating sutures through the edge of the artery and tie them (Fig. 8-4, *B*). Use these sutures to hold the ends so that they are steady.

4. Sew a continuous suture between each mattress stitch. Sew from the vein to the artery (Fig. 8-4, *C*).

5. End the continuous suture by tying it to the next mattress suture (Fig. 8-4, *D*).

6. Repeat this between the other mattress sutures in the same fashion (Fig. 8-4, *E*).

7. Release the proximal arterial clamp to flush the artery, and apply a bulldog clamp to the end of the graft so that it distends under arterial pressure and dilates and lengthens.

8. Straighten the leg to judge the length of graft needed, reapply the proximal arterial clamp, and cut the graft so that it will reach with modest tension. It may be cut obliquely or in a slight V as shown in Fig. 8-3, *D* and *E*.

9. Reapply the bulldog clamp close to the end of the graft, and allow the graft to distend with arterial pulsation.

10. Place the triangulating mattress sutures and perform the distal anastomosis in the same fashion after checking the back bleeding.

COMMENT: *The triangulation technique is very helpful with end-to-end anastomoses with vein grafts. Interrupted sutures may be used instead of continuous sutures between the guy sutures.*

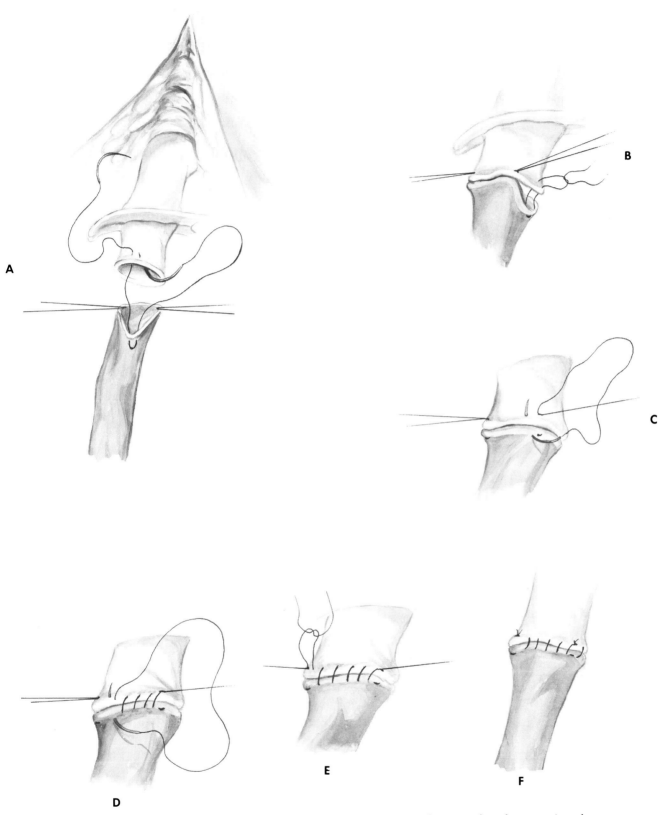

Fig. 8-4. Triangulation technique for end-to-end anastomosis of vein graft and artery. A and B, Triangulating sutures passed through artery and tied. C to E, Continuous suture of everted edges. F, Completed proximal anastomosis.

223

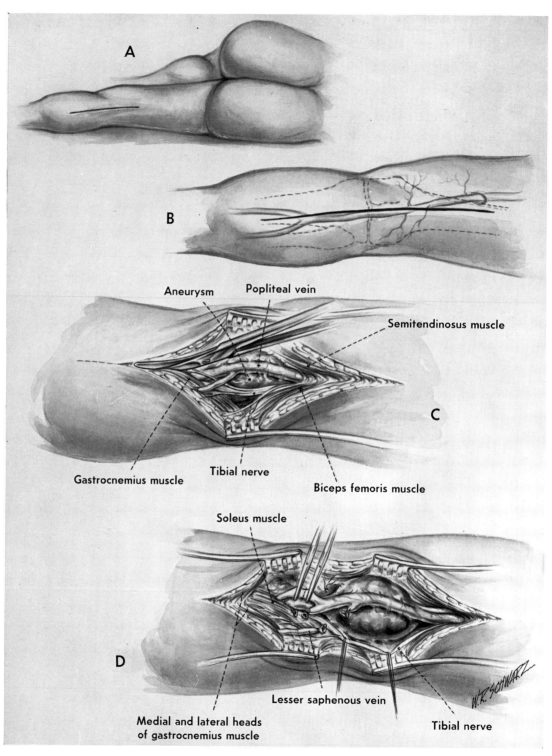

Fig. 8-5. Midline posterior approach to popliteal aneurysm. **A,** Position. **B,** Incision. **C,** Exposure of aneurysm by retraction of muscles. **D,** Dissection of vein and nerves from aneurysm.

11. Release the distal clamp first to note any leaks and to express any air. Release the proximal clamp and check pulses distally.

Closure

1. Leave the sac in place and do not resect it.
2. Resuture any divided tendons with 0-0 Mersilene.
3. Close the popliteal fascia with continuous sutures of 2-0 chromic catgut and the subcutaneous tissue with fine catgut.
4. No drains are needed.
5. Close the skin with continuous sutures of fine nylon.

Midline posterior approach to popliteal aneurysms

The midline posterior approach is the classical approach and is suitable for small aneurysms. It is difficult to extend the incision proximally or distally as the artery goes deeper, and of course, it is difficult to obtain the saphenous vein from the thigh without turning the patient.

Procedure

1. Place the patient in the lateral position, with the affected leg down and the opposite leg flexed (Fig. 8-5, *A*). Prepare and drape the entire thigh, leg, and foot.
2. Make a long midline posterior or S-shaped incision, placing the superior limb of the incision more medially (Fig. 8-5, *B*).
3. Open the popliteal fascia, avoiding the medial popliteal (tibial) nerve, which crosses from medial to slightly lateral superficial to the popliteal artery, giving off several branches on the way.

Proximal control

1. Retract the biceps femoris muscle laterally and the hamstring muscles medially (Fig. 8-5, *C*).
2. Identify the popliteal artery deep in the incision and slightly medial as it emerges from the adductor canal. The artery will usually be tortuous and dilated. Spare the superior genicular artery and other collateral vessels.
3. Retract and spare the overlying popliteal vein when possible. The vein may be densely adherent to the aneurysmal sac. The medial popliteal and the lateral popliteal (peroneal) nerves lie close together superiorly.
4. Pass umbilical tape around the artery preparatory to clamping.

Distal control

1. Retract the heads of the gastrocnemius muscle.
2. Free the popliteal vein from the artery distally. There may be two veins distally.
3. If necessary because of dense adhesions to the aneurysm, divide tributaries of the popliteal vein (Fig. 8-5, *D*).
4. Pass umbilical tape about the artery preparatory to clamping.

Intrasaccular resection of aneurysm

Follow the technique described in detail earlier (see Fig. 8-3).

Reconstruction by end-to-end anastomosis of vein graft

Follow the technique described in detail earlier (see Fig. 8-4).

F.B.H.

9
Acute arterial occlusion—emboli

INTRODUCTION

The possibility of physically removing emboli from major arteries has been appreciated for a number of years, and attempts go back to 1895. The first completely successful embolectomy was done in 1911. In spite of this early start, Haimovici in 1950 reported 330 unselected cases of embolism in 228 patients, only a few of whom were treated surgically. Complete recovery was noted in only 29.5% of cases, early death in 11.3%, and development of gangrene in 28%. What did emerge from studies such as this, which is only representative of a number of others, is that careful follow-up and autopsy information showed the source of arterial emboli to be the left side of the heart in 96% of the cases. Consequently, myocardial infarction or even silent infarction or arrythmias must always be sought as the source of embolism.

In the last twenty years awareness of this condition and the decline in incidence of rheumatic heart disease have probably decreased the overall incidence of embolic disease. The more widespread routine use of anticoagulants has certainly been part of the picture of decrease, as has been the correction of cardiac arrhythmias by cardioversion.

Analysis of the tabulated cases of embolism show a peak in the fourth, fifth, and sixth decades of life. Multiple emboli occur frequently. There is no marked sex difference. The incidence of embolism in various arteries show a peak of about 33% to 35% in the common femoral, with the leg accounting for over 50% of diagnosed distal emboli. Only about 10% of emboli lodge at the aortic bifurcation, and the axillary, brachial, radial, and ulnar arteries in the hand are affected in perhaps only 15% of the total cases.

All emboli in major arteries should be removed, even if the limb is viable and the collateral circulation seems to be adequate. Embolectomy prevents proximal and distal propagation of the clot and prevents irreversible ischemic changes in the limb. No arbitary time limit should be set, since limbs may be salvaged hours or even days after embolism by retrograde flushing or extraction of remote clots with balloon catheters. Major exceptions to this policy should be made with moribund patients or patients with established gangrene. Surgery is performed with the use of local or spinal anesthesia at low risk. When emboli arise in seriously diseased hearts, the mortality of both nonoperative and operative treatment is high.

Several new concepts need emphasis:

1. Maximum collateral circulation develops within a few hours, and further im-

provement with vasodilators, sympathetic nerve blocks, and the like cannot save legs with major ischemia. Only operation restores normal blood flow.

2. Frequently legs remain viable and can be saved even after much delay. The clot propagates distally. However, distant clots can be extracted readily with balloon catheters. As long as the distal arterioles are still open and there is no extensive propagating thrombophlebitis, the limb is probably still viable and is worth the risk of operation.

3. Multiple emboli, distal thrombosis or "tail thrombi," and fragmented or migratory emboli are more common than we realized and are the most frequent cause of postembolectomy "spasm." Intra-operative arteriograms used routinely reveal the presence of these clots, and balloon catheters extract them.

Diagnosis of embolism is usually not difficult. The classic clincial picture of arterial embolism is that of a patient with some thrombogenic cardiopathy leading to formation of an embolus and sudden arterial occlusion. The pulses disappear distal to the site of occlusion, and the coincident onset of acute arterial insufficiency is manifested by ischemic pain, coldness, pallor, loss of sensation, and finally, loss of motor function and obvious gangrene. As a rule, emboli lodge at the sites of major arterial bifurcations. These areas are also the most common places for atherosclerotic narrowing of the blood vessels, and embolism or acute thrombosis may be superimposed on this narrowing.

The classic picture just described is present perhaps 80% of the time, with sudden onset being the most reliable diagnostic clue. Slow progression and even silent symptoms may be noted in 10% to 15% of cases of distal emboli. Presumably these are small and fragmented and announce themselves only by propagation of the clot proximally. Showers of small emboli from aneurysms or from ulcerated arteriosclerotic plaques may propagate distally into the feet, producing small infarcts of the toes that have a rather typical appearance. The same condition may be seen less rarely in the hand, and of course, it manifests itself in the brain by a polymorphic picture of neurological symptoms. Embolic occlusion of the middle cerebral artery may now be amenable to surgical treatment using microvascular techniques and using the external temporal artery to shunt blood to the devascularized middle cerebral area.

Special problems

Diagnostic problems arise when there are multiple emboli in the same extremity, when embolic occlusion is superimposed on arteriosclerosis, when embolic occlusion is incomplete, or when an embolic occlusion is present without an apparent source for the emboli. Late and repeated embolism, embolism of the visceral branches of the aorta, and embolism associated with long-term anticoagulation treatment pose special therapeutic problems. Some of these diagnostic and therapeutic problems and their solutions may be summarized as follows:

1. Embolism or acute thrombosis superimposed on arteriosclerotic narrowing may require either bypass or endarterectomy in association with thrombectomy.

2. Embolism originating in an aneurysm or thombosis of an aneurysm should be treated by excision of the aneurysm.

3. Clot propagated distally should be removed by retrograde flushing or balloon catheters.

4. Restoration of circulation after prolonged ischemia may be followed by massive edema of the limb and this, in turn, requires fasciotomy.
5. Multiple emboli in the same extemity are frequently unrecognized. Intraoperative arteriography or second incisions may be required to remove a more distal embolus in the same extemity if the balloon catheter cannot be passed.
6. Repeated embolism may require reoperation, sometimes on the same extremity.
7. Embolism secondary to intracardiac surgery continues to be a problem. We do not, however, see this any longer as a result of mitral valvulotomy, as we did in the past. It is desirable to have a preoperative record of pulses prior to any open-heart surgery and to observe the limbs for emboli frequently thereafter.

Balloon catheters (Fogarty)

The balloon catheter devised by Fogarty is a significant advance in vascular surgery and an indispensable instrument in embolectomy. Proximal emboli (that is, at the aortic or iliac bifuraction) and peripheral emboli at or below the knee can be extracted through a single arteriotomy in the femoral artery. Routine passage of the balloon catheter distally before an arteriotomy is closed frequently extracts distal fragments of clot and improves the results of the operation. The adequacy of back bleeding is difficult to judge, and profuse back bleeding may occur from proximal collateral channels even while the distal end of the popiteal artery is still occluded.

The balloon catheter has other uses such as (1) extraction of clot from the iliac veins and vena cava (see femoral vein thrombectomy, Fig. 17-4) and (2) passage down the leg prior to the last iliac anastomosis after resection of the abdominal aorta.

The balloon catheters are 80 cm. long, are available in sizes 4 Fr. to 7 Fr., and have delicate inflatable balloons at the tip. The catheter passes through the clot readily without dislodging it (Fig. 9-1, A). After the catheter is passed, the balloon is inflated (Fig. 9-1, B) with the correct volume of saline solution. The catheter is withdrawn, extracting the clot ahead of it (Fig. 9-1, C). The balloon is fragile and ruptures if it is overdistended. It glides by narrow places (Fig. 9-1, D) because when resistance is encountered, the fluid is displaced into the proximal part of the balloon.

The embolectomy catheter is not an unmixed blessing. It must be used carefully and atraumatically. Rough usage can result in the balloon's breaking or in the spiral wire-wound tip's catching in the arterial wall. The latter condition is manifested by inability to move the catheter without force even though the balloon is deflated. The embolectomy catheter must be used with care when it is passed below the popliteal artery in the lower extremity.

Preoperative and postoperative medical and surgical teamwork

The site of the embolus must be localized by palpation, oscillometry, or arteriography. When pulses are absent in the opposite extremity, associated arteriosclerotic disease should be strongly suspected. A grid cassette and x-ray machine should be in the operating room for intraoperative arteriography. Skin preparation and draping should include the whole extremity, so that retrograde flushing may be performed without interruption of the operative procedure to prepare and drape the extended surgical field. Bleeding, clotting, and prothrombin times should be obtained preoperatively, since anticoagulant therapy may be necessary in the postoperative period.

228

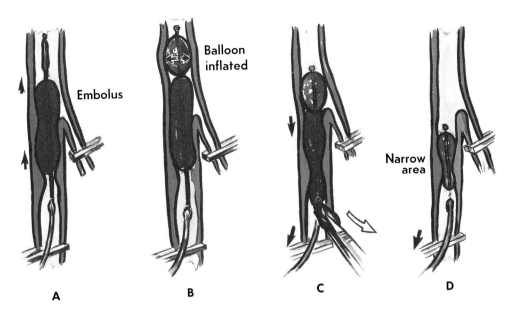

Fig. 9-1. Balloon catheters (Fogarty) for embolectomy. **A,** Catheter passes through clot. **B,** Balloon is inflated. **C,** Catheter is withdrawn, extruding clot. **D,** Delicate balloon deforms to pass narrow area.

Failure to restore circulation may be caused by unrecognized distal embolism, and arteriograms or distal exploration may be needed if the limb is still in peril. The use of anticoagulants is indicated for prevention of recurrent mural thrombi or when the surgical procedure has included endarterectomy. Anticoagulants seldom lead to serious complications in groin incisions that are carefully closed—popliteal incisions should be drained and abdominal incisions should be avoided if immediate anticoagulant therapy is intended.

Medical-surgical teamwork is essential, since all the patients have serious associated medical problems. Although small emboli in the distal end of the popliteal or brachial artery do not imperil the limb, there is no medical method to restore sufficient flow after major arterial occlusions. The medical treatment is concerned with the following problems:

1. Treatment of the heart disease. The internist will avoid excessive use of digitalis or diuresis, which may predispose to further thrombosis. A special problem is the occasional case of left ventricular failure precipitated by embolic obstruction of the abdominal aorta. Embolectomy may relieve the heart strain and may usually be accomplished with the use of local anesthesia by introducing balloon catheters via the femoral arteries (Fig. 9-2).

2. Management of the ischemic limb. Extremities may survive without operation when small emboli plug only the distal end of the brachial or popliteal artery. In bedridden or poor-risk patients, these emboli need not be removed. The ischemic limb should be protected from injury or pressure and kept at room temperature in a slightly dependent position. Active cooling causes vasoconstriction of the skin and active warming increases blood requirements, and both are harmful. In a slightly dependent position, the limb is usually more comfortable, the veins are full, and the color improves.

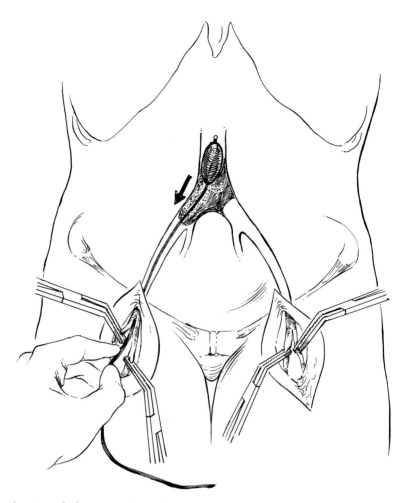

Fig. 9-2. Aortic embolectomy with balloon catheter introduced via femoral arteries. Details of groin incisions shown in Fig. 9-3.

3. Vasodilation of the collateral arteries is desirable, but vasodilation elsewhere is useless or possibly even harmful to an ischemic limb. Vasodilator drugs or physiological stimuli to vasodilation such as warming the patient's body are not used. Sympathetic nerve block causes vasodilation in the affected extremity but will not save a limb when major ischemia is present. Sympathetic nerve block may be helpful in patients with minor ischemia unless contraindicated by anticoagulant treatment.

4. Anticoagulants, beginning with heparin, should be used to prevent formation of more clots in the heart. Despite their use in high dosage, however, multiple or recurrent embolism occurs very frequently.

AORTIC BIFURCATION EMBOLECTOMY
Choice of procedure

The abdominal approach is seldom necessary now, but preparations must be made for both the abdominal and the femoral approach, since either route alone may not be satisfactory. The patient is placed in the supine position, and the entire abdomen, the groin areas, and the thighs are prepared to a point slightly below the knees. In most patients, balloon catheters can be passed up normal common femoral and iliac arteries, and the embolus lodged at the bifurcation of the aorta can be removed by withdrawal of the catheter. This is the preferred approach because general anesthesia is unnecessary and heparin may be given postoperatively more safely. Laparotomy and arteriotomy at the bifurcation are described later.

Femoral approach—aortic embolectomy by retrograde catheterization of femoral arteries

Indications and preparation

Aortic or iliac bifurcation embolectomy via the femoral arteries may be done with the use of local infiltration anesthesia and is preferable. In some patients laparotomy may become necessary. Therefore, the entire abdomen should be prepared and draped, and atropine should be included in the preanesthetic medication. Heparin may be given preoperatively, since the bleeding produced in the small incisions is not particularly troublesome. The balloon catheters (Fogarty) are preferred, although the open-ended polyvinyl cardiovascular catheters and suction are also described and are still useful.

Procedure
Retrograde aortic embolectomy with balloon catheters

1. Make a vertical incision over both common femoral arteries extending from Poupart's ligament superiorly downward for a distance of 6 to 7 cm. (Fig. 9-3, *A*). Open the fascia over the arteries. If there is no clot at the bifurcation of the femoral artery, distal control of the vessels may be obtained proximal to the profunda femoris (deep femoral) artery.

2. Dissect around the common femoral arteries, and pass umbilical tape around the artery above and below the proposed arteriotomies.

3. Slowly inject 20 mg. of heparin in 20 ml. of saline solution into the femoral artery. Lift the distal umbilical tapes and apply arterial clamps to both femoral arteries. In this location soft-jawed clamps* or delicate pediatric clamps with 1 mm. line jaw† are ideal and least traumatic.

4. Make a 1 cm. vertical incision between the umbilical tapes on one femoral artery.

5. Pass the large (6 Fr.) balloon catheter proximally in the femoral artery until the tip is well above the navel.

6. Inflate the balloon with the *correct* amount of sterile saline solution, and withdraw the catheter and the embolus. This is followed by forceful arterial bleeding.

7. Apply an arterial clamp above the femoral arteriotomy.

8. Release the distal clamp on the femoral artery. Back bleeding may be brisk from proximal collateral vessels, but we always pass the appropriate-sized balloon catheter distally in the femoral artey to remove fragments of clot distal in the popliteal artery.

9. Pass the 4 Fr. size balloon catheter distally as far as it will go gently, inflate

---

*Supplied by Edwards Laboratories, Santa Ana, Calif.
†Available from Pilling Co., Ft. Washington, Pa.

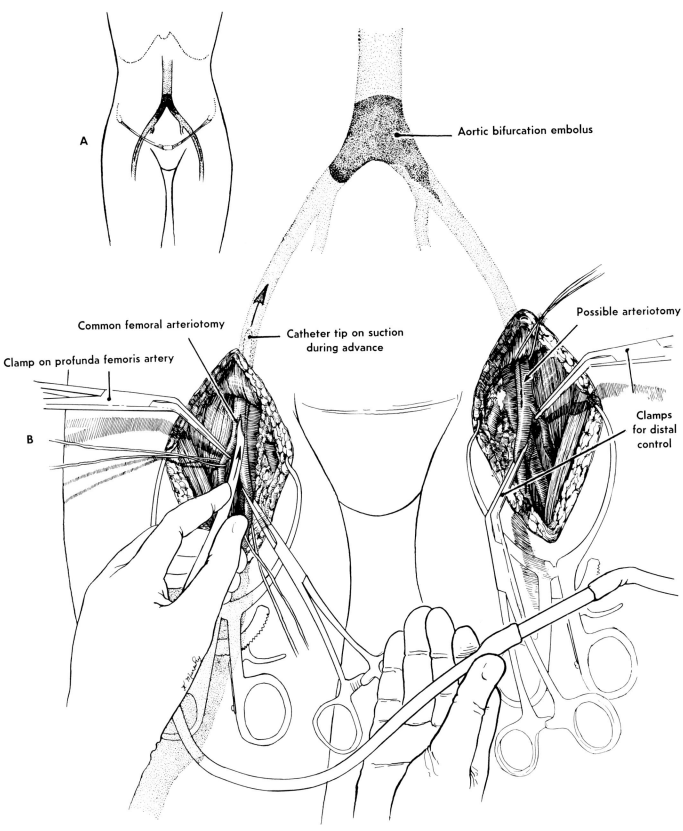

Fig. 9-3. Aortic embolectomy by retrograde method. **A,** Incisions. **B,** Simultaneous control of both femoral arteries and retrograde catheterization.

Aortic bifurcation embolus

Common femoral arteriotomy

Clamp on profunda femoris artery

Catheter tip on suction during advance

Possible arteriotomy

Clamps for distal control

B

A

232

the balloon with the correct amount of sterile saline solution, and withdraw the balloon. Unexpected distal small emboli are frequently removed.

COMMENT: *The surgeon holds the inflating syringe in one hand while withdrawing the inflated catheter with the other hand. If resistance is encountered at narrow areas, the balloon is deflated slightly.*

10. Pass the balloon catheter into the profunda femoris artery also, inflate the balloon, and withdraw the catheter.

11. Close the arteriotomy with 5-0 arterial suture.

12. Make an arteriotomy of the opposite femoral artery, where fragments of embolus from the aortic bifurcation usually have been swept down to be arrested by the occluding clamp that was placed prior to the proximal passage of the balloon catheter into the aorta.

13. The passage proximally and distally of appropriate-sized balloon catheters guarantees that the iliac, femoral, popliteal, and profunda femoris arteries are all open. Repeat the procedure described for the opposite side.

Retrograde aortic embolectomy with suction catheters

1-4. The incision, exposure, femoral arteriotomy, and other procedures are the same as those described in the first four steps for retrograde aortic embolectomy with balloon catheters.

5. Choose a catheter that fits rather snugly into the arterial lumen and has an oblique opening at the tip. A glass connector is used to connect the suction catheter to the remainder of the suction apparatus. Cut a hole in the side of the suction tubing close to the glass connector to control suction (Fig. 9-3, *B*). Pass the catheter upward toward the heart, and observe for bleeding through the glass connector. A glass T tube or Y tube may also be used as a connector and makes the hole in the tubing unnecessary.

6. Bleeding through the glass connecting tubing ceases when the catheter tip passes the hypogastric artery and touches the embolus. Advance the catheter until bleeding stops. At this point, turn on the suction line and apply suction to the catheter by closing the hole or the side arm with the thumb. Withdraw the catheter slowly as suction holds the clot against its tip. As the clot is extracted, clamp the femoral artery proximal to the arteriotomy. It may be necessary to pass the catheter several times.

7. Repeat the procedure on the other side. At this point, pieces of embolus may have been pushed over to the side that was originally cleared, and a second aspiration may be necessary to obtain an abundant, forceful, and pulsatile flow of blood from both sides.

COMMENT: *The combined abdominal and femoral approach may be necessary if catheters cannot be passed readily or if they do not clear the obstruction (Fig. 9-3, B).*

8. Check back bleeding from both the deep femoral and the superficial femoral arteries by removing the distal occluding clamps. Rinse the blood clot away. Reapply the clamps, and suture the arteriotomy with 4-0 arterial suture as a continuous over-and-over suture. Close the femoral sheath and fascial layers carefully, avoiding dead space where oozing blood could accumulate during anticoagulant therapy.

Postoperative care

Anticoagulants may be used more safely with the femoral approach, since an occasional hematoma in the groin incision is easily noted and managed. Vigorous heparinization is advisable at the time of surgery and for a short period thereafter. The more extensive the embolus or its propagating thrombus is, the more urgent is the need for anticoagulants. Some patients' blood is hypercoagulable, and they will require more-than-average doses of anticoagulant. Postoperative care includes medical management of associated heart disease.

Abdominal approach

Because the abdominal approach is used only after the femoral approach with retrograde catheters has failed and because retrograde catheters fail mainly because of atherosclerotic narrowing, the embolectomy may have to be supplemented with endarterectomy. However, the classic abdominal aortic embolectomy is described.

Procedure

1. Make a long paramedian incision from the pubis to well above the umbilicus (Fig. 9-4, *A*). Expose the aortic bifurcation by packing off the sigmoid colon to the left and the small bowel to the right. For further details, see Chapter 3. Incise the peritoneum over the bifurcation, and observe the location of the embolus.

COMMENT: *The retroperitoneal approach to the bifurcation is also simple, but mobilization of the peritoneum over a large area results in more oozing in the heparinized patient.*

2. Incise the peritoneum over both iliac arteries distal to any apparent clot, and pass umbilical tapes about the arteries. Slowly inject 20 mg. of heparin into each iliac artery, and apply the arterial clamps. (See Fig. 9-4, *B*.)

3. Application of clamps to the iliac vessels ensures prevention of distal propagation of the embolus. Dissect around the aorta carefully above the embolus. It may not be necessary to elevate the aorta, since it may be clamped vertically as well as cross-clamped. Enough of the aorta should be exposed that a vertical clamp can be applied without damaging the vena cava. Most careful dissection, therefore, must be done on the right side. When the aorta is fairly well exposed, a vertical clamp can be applied as a test. Do not close the clamp immediately. (See Fig. 9-4, *B*.)

4. Open the proximal portion of the iliac artery on the side where the embolus is largest. As the blood pressure extrudes the embolus, close the aortic clamp. (See Fig. 9-4, *C*.)

5. Open the iliac clamps one at a time to check for complete removal of the embolus (Fig. 9-4, *C*). A brisk gush of blood should result. If back bleeding is not abundant, pass a catheter attached to suction distally to remove any remaining thrombus (Fig. 9-4, *D*). Pass balloon catheters down one or both iliac arteries to make certain that they are clear and to extract any distal thrombus. This may avoid arteriotomy at the groin level.

6. Close the arteriotomy with a continuous over-and-over suture of 3-0 or 4-0 arterial suture. Before the last few stitches are taken, release both the iliac clamps to fill the arteries with blood and to extrude any air within the artery. Finish the arteriotomy closure and tie the stitches.

7. Release the aortic clamp slowly and check pulses in the iliac vessels, the groins, and the politeal fossae. If pulses are not present in the groin, the femoral arteries must be explored before the abdomen is closed. Secondary emboli must be removed at this time, and any arteriosclerotic occlusions present must be treated. Blood clot in or distal to the iliac arteries may be removed by femoral arteriotomy

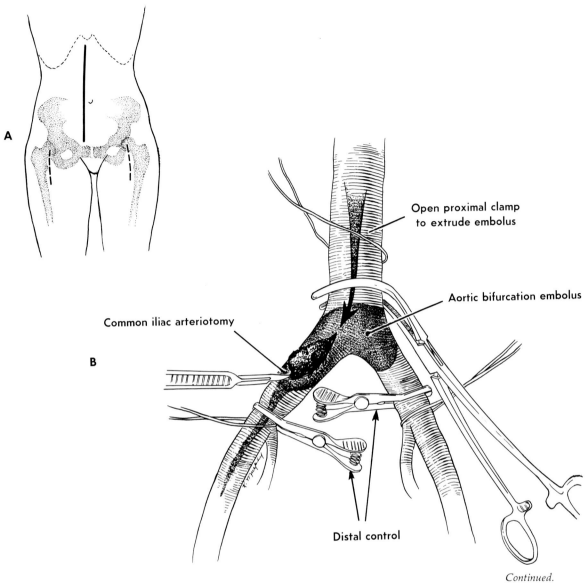

Fig. 9-4. Transabdominal aortic bifurcation embolectomy. A, Incisions. B, Extrusion of embolus.

Continued.

and retrograde extraction with catheters as described earlier in this chapter. Popliteal or pedal pulses may be slow to return, particularly in patients with cardiac disease, prolonged occlusion, and spasm.

FEMORAL EMBOLECTOMY

Indications

The femoral artery must be explored for embolus when there is acute arterial insufficiency of the leg and pulses are absent below the bifurcation of the common femoral artery. Since the procedure may be done with the use of local infiltration anesthesia, there are no contraindications except established gangrene.

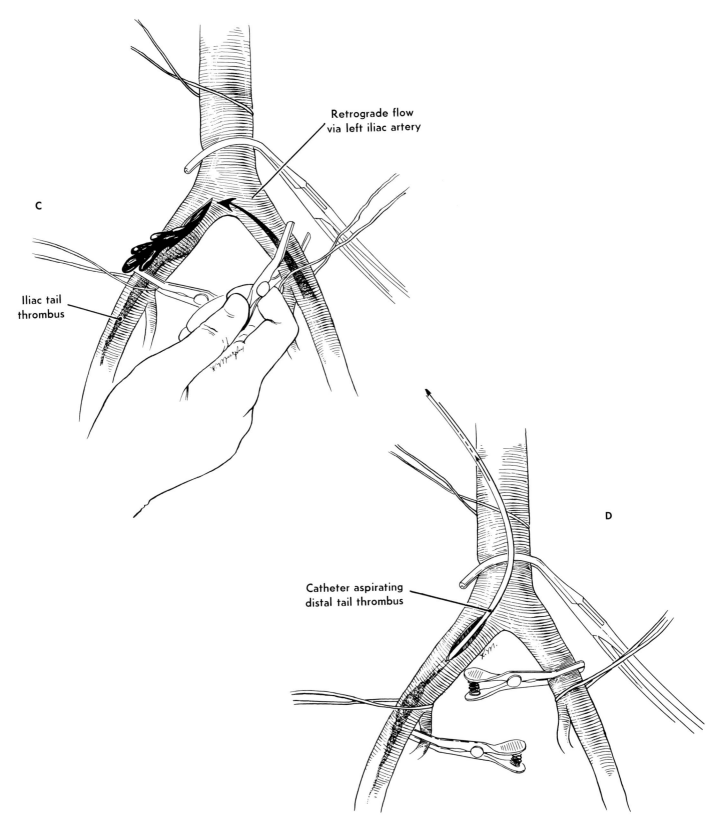

C

Retrograde flow
via left iliac artery

Iliac tail
thrombus

D

Catheter aspirating
distal tail thrombus

Fig. 9-4, cont'd. Transabdominal aortic bifurcation embolectomy. **C,** Check back bleeding from other iliac artery. **D,** Remove tail thrombus if present.

Note that the bifurcation of the common femoral artery is the most common location (in about 33% of cases) of clinically troublesome and diagnosed peripheral emboli. Clot may propagate both proximally and distally, but it is not unusual to find several inches of organized thrombus located proximally.

Preparation

Preoperatively the entire leg and foot should be prepared and draped so that the popliteal and posterior tibial arteries are accessible for retrograde flushing and to facilitate intraoperative arteriography if it is needed.

Procedure

1. Make a longitudinal incision over the course of the femoral artery (Fig. 9-5, A). Superiorly the incision extends to the inguinal ligament, and inferiorly it should be distal to the bifurcation of the common femoral artery. Diagnosis is confirmed by a visible embolus and by the absence of pulsation at the femoral bifurcation.

2. Dissect around the superficial femoral artery, and apply an arterial clamp distal to the embolus to prevent displacement and distal migration of the thrombus.

3. Dissect and pass an umbilical tape around the common femoral and profunda femoris arteries. Because of the very brief operation time, it is usually unnecessary to inject heparin.

4. Cross-clamp the common femoral artery. Make a short vertical arteriotomy in the common femoral artery.

5. Release the distal clamp on the superficial femoral artery. Carefully pull the embolus out, being careful to withdraw it slowly in order not to lose any propagating tail thrombus in the superficial femoral or the profunda femoris artery.

6. Pass the Fogarty balloon catheter (4 Fr.) distally as far as possible without force. Inflate the balloon gently, and withdraw the catheter to extract any distal fragments. Pass the Fogarty irrigating catheter and instill 30 ml. of dilute heparin solution as it is withdrawn. Clamp the superficial femoral artery. These balloon catheters are described in further detail on pp. 228 and 229.

7. Pass a small Fogarty balloon catheter into the profunda femoris artery and repeat the procedure just described.

COMMENT: *Poor back bleeding may signify the need for endarterectomy of the orifice of the profunda femoris or dilation of the orifice. Good back bleeding may be present even when distal fragments of clot are present, and the balloon catheters should be used in all cases to extract these distal fragments.*

8. Open the clamp on the common femoral artery. Proximal clot may be extruded spontaneously. If there is no spontaneous vigorous bleeding, most of the clot may still be present above the bifurcation of the common femoral artery. It is then necessary to pass a balloon catheter or suction tip proximally. Reapply the clamp after forceful pulsatile flow is observed (Fig. 9-5, E).

9. Rinse away blood clots, and close the arteriotomy with an over-and-over stitch of 4-0 or 5-0 arterial suture (Fig. 9-5, F). Release the distal clamp momentarily before the last stitch is placed to allow back bleeding to extrude any air in the lumen.

10. Close the femoral sheath and subcutaneous fascia carefully to prevent collections of serum, blood, or lymph.

COMMENT: *Calcification of the media of the femoral artery may render it fragile and interfere with closure. A secure closure can be obtained by suturing adventitia only,*

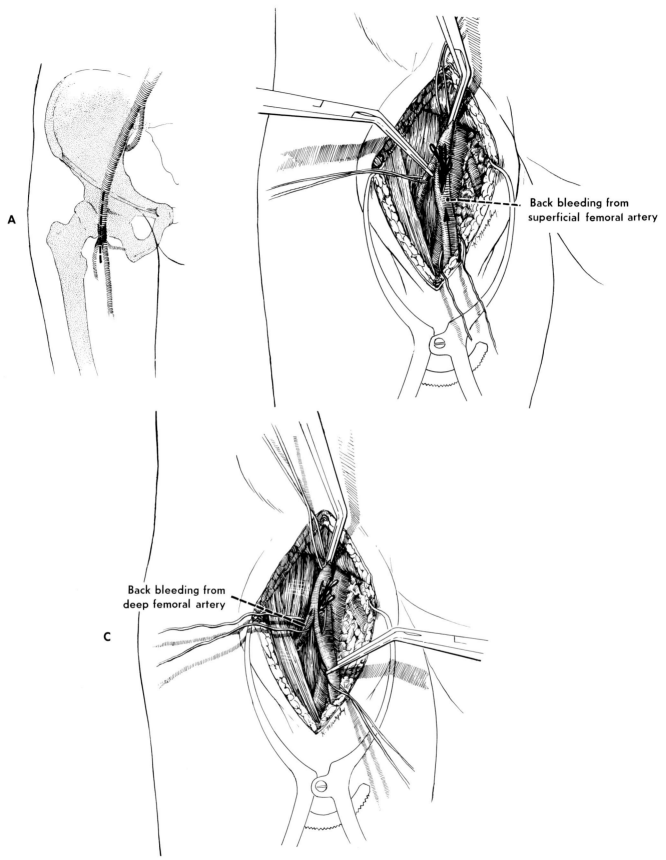

Fig. 9-5. Femoral embolectomy. A, Incision. B, Check back bleeding from superficial femoral artery. C, Check back bleeding from deep femoral artery (profunda femoris).

238

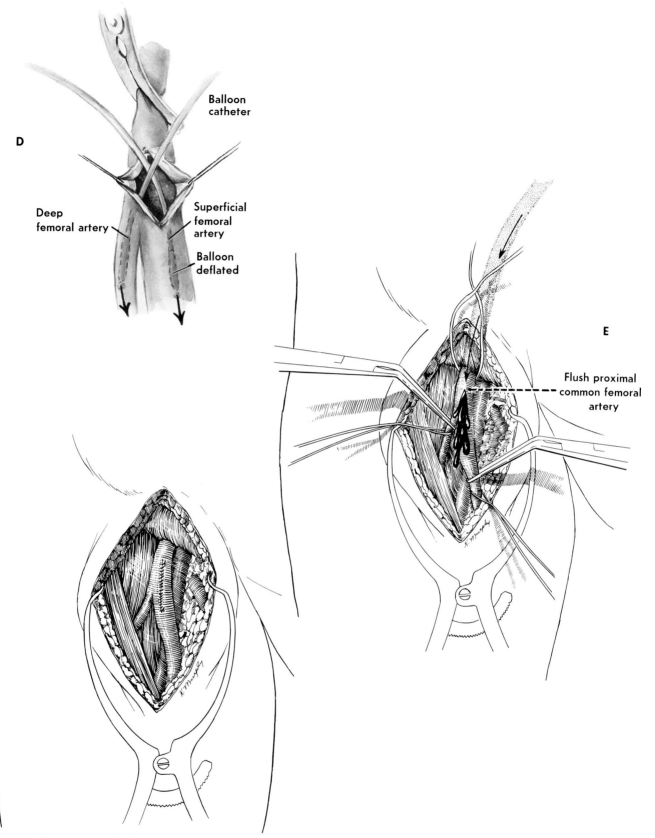

Fig. 9-5, cont'd. Femoral embolectomy. **D,** Pass balloon catheters into superficial and deep femoral arteries. **E,** Flush proximal artery. **F,** Closure of arteriotomy.

Within the illustration:
Balloon catheter
Deep femoral artery
Superficial femoral artery
Balloon deflated
D
E
Flush proximal common femoral artery
F

as after endarterectomy. If necessary, the suture line may be reinforced with a sleeve of prosthesis (Fig. 3-10, C), or the diseased part of the arterial wall may be trimmed away and the defect closed with a patch of prosthesis or vein.

Postoperative care

Anticoagulants may be used to prevent further thrombus formation in the heart. Careful closure of the incision obliterates dead space and helps to prevent hematoma when it is necessary to use anticoagulants.

DELAYED EMBOLECTOMY—FASCIOTOMY
Indications

Operation is sometimes delayed because of poor facilities or the desperate condition of the patient, and delay may cause new complications. However, we have restored circulation and saved limbs even after a delay of many hours or days, and embolectomy or arterial repair must not be denied because of any arbitrary time limit. The distal thrombosis does not become inaccessible in the tiny arterioles until irreversible muscle damage has occurred. This is signified by the development of rigor of the muscle. This rigor resembles thrombophlebitis, and there is probably an element of such phlebitis present. It is a doughy edematous hardness, somewhat less tender than acute thrombophlebitis, with variable amounts of clinically observed pain.

Heparin injections may be useful to prevent or limit distal propagation of the clot. However, these tail thrombi or other distal thrombi that are not continuous with the original embolus may form. Balloon catheters have made it possible to remove these remote thrombi from the main channels without separate incisions.

When severe ischemia has persisted six to twelve hours, restoration of flow is followed by severe swelling that may imperil the extremity. Edema is confined by closed fascial compartments and compresses the capillaries, resulting in muscle necrosis and gangrene. After delayed embolectomy, this dangerous edema is manifested by tightness and/or firmness of the calf of the leg without visible subcutaneous swelling or pedal edema.

Fasciotomy is frequently necessary if embolectomy has been delayed longer than six to twelve hours, particularly if the collateral circulation has been poor. However, prophylactic fasciotomy cannot be prescribed after any arbitrary time limit. The indications for fasciotomy are disappearance of pedal pulses that had been restored by embolectomy, recurrent pain, numbness or pallor of the limb, and stiffness or tightness of the calf muscles.

Procedure—fasciotomy of leg

1. Make a long incision in the skin and fascia in the posteromedial aspect of the calf. The skin incision need not be as long as the incision in the fascia, which can be slit with the scissors proximal and distal to the skin incision.
2. Cut the fascia proximally and distally until pale muscle no longer bulges through the incision. Observe the return of color to the bulging muscle and to the foot. Note and mark the pedal pulses.
3. Incise the skin and fascia over the anterior tibial muscle compartment also.

COMMENT: *Whenever fasciotomy of the leg is indicated, both fascial compartments must be opened. Rarely, fasciotomy of the anterior compartment only is needed for the "anterior tibial syndrome."*

4. Close the skin partially at the ends of the incision unless closure causes tension.

5. Apply dressings, leaving the foot exposed for inspection and for palpation of the pulses. The edema rapidly subsides, so that the dressings become soaked and must be changed daily. Secondary closure of the skin in five days is usually feasible.

COMMENT: *The Pilling Company makes an instrument for accomplishing fasciotomy subcutaneously. On a busy vascular service this is a convenience but not a necessity. The important matter is to recognize the necessity for relief of pressure in the tight fascial compartments of the leg or arm.*

RETROGRADE ARTERIAL FLUSH

Retrograde flush procedures are seldom needed since the advent of the balloon catheters to remove other clots in the extremity. Balloon catheters, however, may be difficult to pass below the bifurcation of the popliteal artery. Retrograde arterial flush beginning at the ankle becomes necessary when the balloon catheter does not remove a thrombus that has extended distally from the popliteal artery and there is poor back bleeding after popliteal embolectomy. Persistent arterial insufficiency after embolectomy may also be due to multiple distal emboli.

If flushing of the posterior tibial artery is not successful, flush may be attempted via the dorsalis pedis artery.

Occasionally, squeezing the calf or wrapping it with a sterile snug Esmarch bandage from the toes proximally has extruded clots or assisted the flushing procedure. We have never regretted using these procedures. Flushing the posterior tibial artery will occasionally yield a branched clot. If perchance no clot is found, no harm has been done.

Procedure
Flush of posterior tibial artery

1. Make a vertical incision posterior to the medial tibial malleolus (Fig. 9-6, *A*).
2. Divide the thickened fascia of the laciniate ligament (flexor retinaculum). Identify the posterior tibial nerve or the medial and lateral plantar nerves, the posterior tibial artery, and the posterior tibial vein between the tendons of the flexor digitorum longus and the flexor hallucis longus muscles.
3. Isolate the posterior tibial artery, and occlude it distally with a rubber-shod bulldog clamp. Incise the artery longitudinally proximal to the clamp (a very small incision will do), and insert a No. 13 to No. 15 thin-walled beaded cannula in the proximal direction. Secure the cannula with a temporary ligature. (See Fig. 9-6, *B*.)
4. Attach a 50 ml. large-bore syringe filled with warm heparin in saline solution. Empty the syringe rapidly and forcefully. Sometimes more than one irrigation may be necessary. Remaining clot will be extruded from the popliteal arteriotomy and should be followed by a profuse flow of clear saline solution.
5. Close the popliteal arteriotomy with a simple over-and-over suture of continuous 5-0 suture. If it appears that such a closure will constrict a small popliteal artery, use a small patch of vein or prosthesis so that constriction is avoided.
6. Remove the proximal popliteal clamp, and observe the pulsatile flow into the syringe at the ankle.
7. Remove the temporary ligature about the cannula at the ankle, remove the cannula, and close the arteriotomy in the posterior tibial artery with a few fine inter-

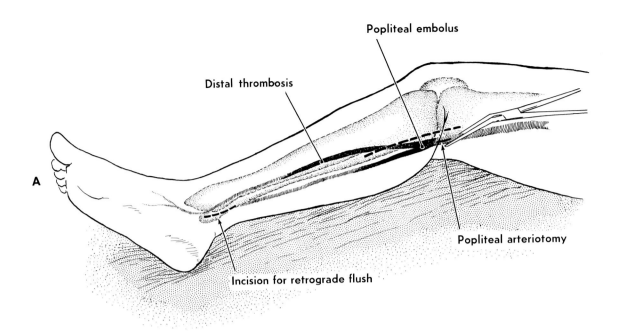

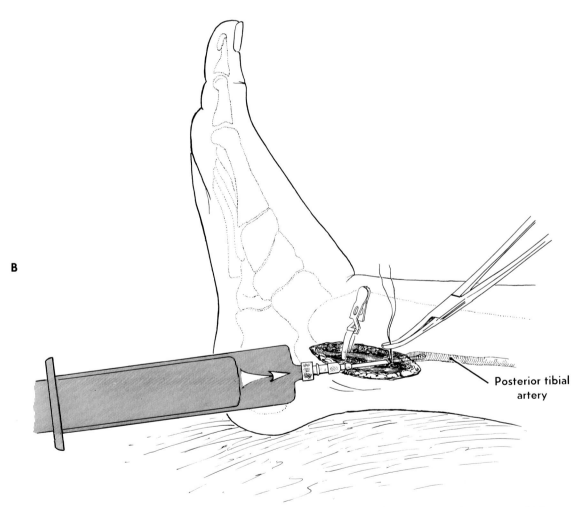

Fig. 9-6. Retrograde arterial flush at ankle. A, Incisions. B, Cannulation of posterior tibial artery at ankle.

rupted sutures of 6-0 or 7-0 silk placed in the adventitia only. Apply Gelfoam or oxidized cellulose and gentle pressure over the arteriotomy until leakage ceases. Close the incision.

Retrograde flush of dorsalis pedis artery

1. Expose the dorsalis pedis artery by a transverse incision on the dorsum of the foot, about 1 inch below the malleoli.

2. Divide the deep fascia (inferior extensor retinaculum or ligamentum cruciatum cruris).

3. Locate the artery between the tendons of the extensor hallucis longus and the extensor digitorum longus muscles.

4. Isolate the artery, occlude it distally, and flush by the technique discribed for the posterior tibial artery.

COMMENT: *We have never regretted the incision at the ankle, even when retrograde flushing of one of the vessels was unsuccessful. Opening only one of the main arteries at the foot and calf may save the leg.*

CRITIQUE OF RESULTS OF EMBOLECTOMY

Extensive review of comparative results for embolectomy dating from 1948 to the present may be found in the papers of the Committee on Vascular Surgery (1972) and of Thompson (1970). Both of these tabulations, which include series of operative cases ranging in numbers from 25 to 156 and totaling 951 cases, reflect a high mortality of patients afflicted with emboli. It must be remembered that in almost all cases, underlying cardiac disease is the source of the embolus. Consequently, reported mortality ranges from 12% to 81%, with an average of about 30%. Limb salvage is accomplished in about 80% of cases.

In our experience few of the deaths are related to the surgical procedure, but most result from the patient's underlying cardiac disease. Some deaths may be related to shock in the immediate postoperative period, and this in turn may be due either to pulmonary embolization or to something similar to "crush syndrome," which arises when blood flow is restored to an ischemic limb. In the groin the femoral vein may be inspected and even opened in a search for possible thrombophlebitis in this location. Embolectomy patients should be treated postoperatively in the intensive care unit or cardiac care unit because of the anticipated mortality.

Our own experience is not greatly different from the averages noted above. Almost all cases involving the aortic bifurcation or lower extremity are treated regardless of condition unless the presence of gangrene is established or the patient is moribund. We do not think that such aggressive criteria essentially changed the overall mortality rate, but for those who recover, the amputation rate is markedly decreased.

C.H.C.

References

Baird, R. J., et al.: Emboli to the arm, Ann. Surg. 160:905-909, 1964.

Committee on Vascular Surgery (DeWeese, J. A., Chairman): Optimal resources for vascular surgery, Circulation 46:A-305–A-324, 1972.

Haimovici, H.: Peripheral arterial embolism; a study of 330 unselected cases of embolism of the extremities, Angiology 1:20-45, 1950.

Key, E.: Embolectomy in circulatory disturbances in extremities, Surg. Gynecol. Obstet. **36**:309-316, 1923.

Thompson, J. E., et al.: Arterial embolectomy: a 20 year experience with 163 cases, Surgery **67**:212-220, 1970.

10

Vascular injuries

INTRODUCTION

Interruption of the major artery to an extremity causes gangrene in a high percentage of instances. The general subject of injuries has been under intense investigation since World War I. Some of this history is documented in Chapter 1. From World War I there were only a few reports of attempts to repair injuries on the Allied side, those by Bernheim, Goodman, and Makins (see Chapter 1 references). German surgeons later reported similar but somewhat more extensive experiences. Excellent material following this period may be obtained from the extensive study of DeBakey and Simeone (1946) who summarized the extensive experiences of World War II. In this collection of 2,471 acute arterial injuries, the overall amputation rate was 49% after arterial ligation, and there were few attempts at direct repair and only three end-to-end anastomoses. In the recent Viet Nam experiences, which are not completely collected, Rich (1972) cited the amputation rate in 950 major arterial injuries as 13.5. Among these injuries, the popliteal artery stands out as it almost always does in large reviews as being the site of injury where the largest number of amputations are necessary, the current low rate being 29.5%, or approximately the same as the rate in civilian experiences.

All surgeons must be acquainted with the principles and techniques of treating arterial injuries because prompt reconstruction and restoration of arterial blood flow is essential. Complications in untreated patients are as follows: (1) secondary hemorrhage, (2) false aneurysm, (3) peripheral propagation of thrombosis, (4) distal embolism, and (5) irreversible ischemic change in muscle and nerve.

Even if a limb remains viable, usefulness is impaired because of arterial insufficiency. Fibrosis, contractures, claudication, or other signs of interference with blood flow and nutrition may appear.

Although there is great variation in the nature of each particular traumatic injury to a great artery or a great vein, it is both possible and convenient to break these down by anatomical location for the purposes of analysis and discussion.

Penetrating trauma

Arterial injury should be suspected of being present when there is any penetrating trauma near a large artery, particularly in the neck, groin, axilla, or popliteal areas. Further indications of arterial injury are (1) pulsatile bleeding; (2) active bleeding; (3) distal arterial insufficiency; and (4) pulsating, extensive, or enlarging hematoma.

If a patient has a penetrating abdominal wound, major vascular injury should be suspected of being present if shock does not respond to rapid transfusion of 1,500 ml. of blood. For wounds of extremities, pressure dressings will stop the bleeding temporarily. Thoracic and abdominal hemorrhages usually require operation to arrest bleeding before the shock can be treated.

Venous injury may be as damaging and difficult to treat as arterial injury, although it may be initially less spectacular.

Nonpenetrating trauma

Arterial insufficiency can follow nonpenetrating trauma from dislocations and fractures about the knee or elbow or from compression of arteries in the tight fascial compartments of crushed extremities. Compression-occlusion may also result from massive venous occlusion or from the interstitial edema that follows restoration of arterial circulation after prolonged ischemia from other causes. After nonpenetrating injury, loss of pulses, coldness, pallor, progressive hypesthesia, anesthesia, and paralysis are danger signs and indicate the urgent need for accurate diagnosis and surgical exploration or other treatment.

Traumatic vasospasm may occur in patients with nonpenetrating arterial injury. If the arterial insufficiency is severe and is not relieved immediately and dramatically by sympathetic nerve block, the artery in which the injury is suspected of being present should be explored immediately. Return of pulses after sympathetic nerve block is reassuring, but increase in skin temperature and color alone merely signifies improvement in collateral flow and does not exclude arterial injury. The diagnosis of traumatic vasospasm must be verified and treated by operation. The condition is myogenic in origin and is independent of nervous control but responds to topical application of papaverine. Spasm, when present, is often accompanied by contusion and thrombosis, and resection of a section of damaged artery will be necessary.

No such problem of spasm or contraction is present in venous injuries, at times making them just as treacherous and dangerous to the patient as an arterial injury although less spectacular at the moment. In the limbs, of course, venous hemorrhage is much more easily controlled by pressure. This is not true internally. It should always be remembered that venous injury in the neck can become a source of air embolism, and such wounds should be covered at once. If embolism is suspected of having occurred, the immediate treatment is to place the patient with the right side up in the Trendelenburg position, which will allow air bubbles to localize in the right atrium and the inferior vena cava.

Methods of repair

The method of repair varies with the type, severity, and location of the injury. Lateral repair of tangential injuries is seldom advisable. If debridement is unnecessary or very limited, closure of the laceration with a patch of vein or prosthetic material prevents narrowing at the closure. End-to-end anastomosis is performed when the ends can be approximated. If adequate debridement of the artery prevents anastomosis without extensive mobilization of the artery, the use of a vein graft or prosthetic tube is preferable. Extensive mobilization tends to sacrifice collateral vessels and may put the anastomosis under undue tension.

Various arterial substitutes have been used, and arterial homografts enjoyed extensive use during the Korean War. However, the thrombosis rate in homografts is high. The patient's own living vein is preferable. The saphenous vein is sturdy and needs no external support. Vein grafts are always preferable in small arteries.

Of the various prosthetic materials available, knitted Dacron of moderate pore size is highly satisfactory. Prostheses of this and other material are available in a wide range of sizes. However, prostheses less than 8 mm. in diameter should not be used. Prostheses are necessary in large arteries such as the iliac artery because vein grafts dilate and form aneurysms in these locations and all forms of external support have failed. Prostheses or vein grafts must be covered with living tissue.

Preoperative and postoperative care

Preoperative care should include antibiotic therapy, tetanus and gas-gangrene prophylaxis, blood replacement, and immobilization of the injured extremity. Successful anastomosis results in prompt postoperative improvement. For reasons that are not clear, pedal pulses may not return for a period of six or eight hours. Theoretical reasons for this delay are (1) vasoconstriction persisting because of inadequate blood replacement, (2) reflex vasoconstriction from excessive tension on the anastomosis, (3) air embolism from residual air in the arteries, and (4) distal thrombosis or embolism. Sympathectomy or sympathetic nerve blocks are not necessary postoperatively when arterial continuity has been restored and are useless when it has not been restored. The only treatment indicated if arterial insufficiency recurs is reoperation. Vasoconstricting drugs, local heat, and excessive elevation of the extremity should be avoided. The limb should be immobilized for a period of ten to fourteen days.

Principles of surgical treatment

The essentials of surgical treatment in arterial injury may be briefly summarized as follows:

1. Early exploration and definitive treatment, preferably anatomical restoration. Early operation is desirable not only to prevent gangrene in some cases but also to prevent thrombosis of outflow tracts that might prevent a later successful repair.
2. Adequate surgical exposure secured by a longitudinal incision along the course of the artery.
3. Proximal and distal control of the artery and vein before incision into a hematoma or false aneurysm.
4. Removal of distal clot by balloon catheters (pp. 228 and 229) or by the retrograde flush technique (pp. 241-243) if there is inadequate back bleeding from the distal arterial segment.
5. Restoration of continuity of all major or critical arteries.
6. Correct care of remainder of wound, including drainage when indicated, coverage of arterial anastomoses, and fixation of fractures.
7. Early recognition of and fasciotomy for closed-space injuries or edema.

REGIONAL CONSIDERATIONS
Neck, supraclavicular region, and upper thorax

Injuries in the neck, supraclavicular region, and upper thorax have a high mortality, and many patients with such injuries do not survive long enough to reach a hospital. Rapid control of hemorrhage is essential. Exposure of the subclavian artery requires resection of the clavicle. However, proximal control at the origin of the artery

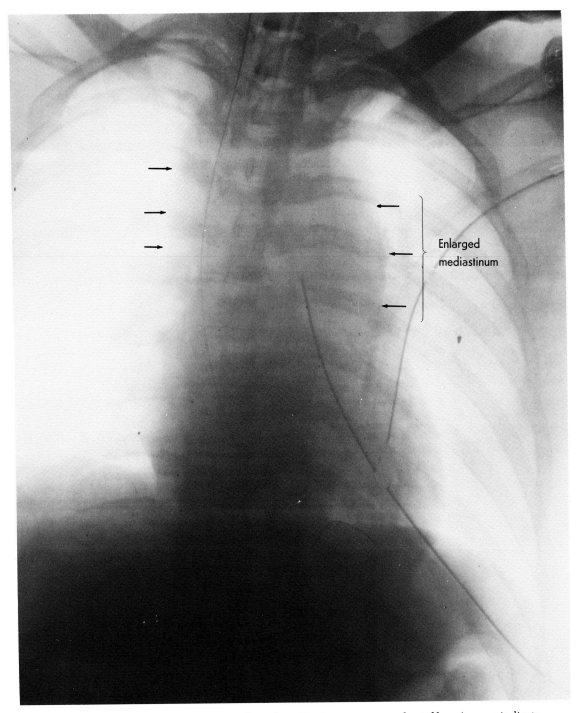

Fig. 10-1. Ruptured thoracic aorta. Enlarged mediastinum seen on chest film. Arrows indicate the outline of the mediastinal hematoma.

may become necessary. The origin of the subclavian artery and other great vessels is approached by splitting the upper part of the sternum. Details of these exposures are found in the discussion of the upper extremity in Chapter 16.

Associated injury of the great veins may require ligation or repair of the subclavian or internal jugular veins. The superior vena cava should not be ligated. The innominate, subclavian, or jugular veins may be either repaired or ligated. Ligation of the great arteries in the superior mediastinum and neck should be avoided. Injuries of these vessels that do not kill instantly can usually be repaired. Gangrene of the arm may follow ligation of the second and third portions of the subclavian artery. Massive cerebral necrosis and death follow ligation of the innominate artery in 9% of patients. Morbidity after ligation of the common carotid artery is even higher, reaching 20% to 30%.

Aneurysm in the upper thorax and first portion of the subclavian artery can be approached safely only after adequate exposure to permit proximal control of the great vessels.

Thorax and abdomen

Many injuries of the heart and aorta are incompatible with survival. Whereas military injuries are somewhat unpredictable, civilian injuries show a fairly high number of ruptured thoracic aortas due to automobile accidents. Not many persons with such injuries survive to reach the hospital; but with better transportation, evacuation, and emergency room care, it is anticipated that perhaps more of these unfortunate individuals will reach the operating room.

Diagnosis must be made rapidly. A plain film of the chest shows a widened mediastinum if the aorta has ruptured in the thoracic area. This condition is illustrated in Fig. 10-1. The changes in the abdomen are more subtle: one must look for obliteration of the psoas muscle shadow on the left, or perhaps in an older person with an aneurysm, the eggshell-thin calcification at its borders may be seen.

There is little time for special studies and arteriography. The patient must be taken to the operating room and exploratory surgery done. In cases of both thoracic and abdominal injuries, there may be some few persons whose cases are not so urgent. In the abdomen the retained blood may tend to act as a tampon to stop the hemorrhage, so that one can delay opening the abdomen until blood is ready. In the chest, the injury occasionally spares the adventitia; and although it can dissect upward and downward, causing enlargement of the mediastinum with the other symptoms of cough, dysphagia, pain, shortness of breath, and perhaps some neck vein distension or differential blood pressure in the upper extremities, the mainstream of blood may be contained for an indefinite period of time. Nevertheless, delay is not advisable because of the poor prognosis without immediate surgery.

To stop hemorrhage from the aorta, the surgeon must immediately cross-clamp the aorta, running the risk of causing hemiplegia. In spite of the increased theoretical risk, there is not statistical evidence that it is actually greatly increased. In the abdomen a Foley catheter passed upward from the injury may be expanded within the lumen of the aorta and used to stop the acute blood loss.

Intrathoracic traumatic rupture of the aorta affects chiefly the young, with the peak age distribution lying in the decade from age 15 to age 25 years.

Other sources of intra-abdominal and retroperitoneal injuries are hemorrhage from mesenteric vessels after blunt trauma to the upper abdomen, injury to the retroperitoneal duodenum, and injury to the kidney. Most retroperitoneal hemorrhages can be treated conservatively. Occasionally there is massive loss of blood from a torn renal pedicle or similar injury just as there is massive blood loss from rupture of the spleen or rupture of the liver. All such injuries require prompt attention to the hemorrhage as a lifesaving measure.

Abdominal viscera

In the case of renal hemorrhage when the kidney is not totally destroyed or torn away from its pedicle, the surgeon must begin treatment by uncovering the site of bleeding. If the artery is intact, only venous bleeding need be contended with, and pressure can be maintained to control bleeding as the site is found. The left renal vein can be ligated without sacrificing the kidney as long as it has some distal tributaries that provide collateral circulation. The right renal vein is short and wide and must be repaired if possible.

COMMENT: *Even small holes of the vena cava will bleed massively, and when they are finally uncovered, local pressure over a small laceration will suffice until the edges of the tear can be brought together. See detailed description later.*

A massive hemorrhage can result from even slight laceration of the spleen. This condition is well known and is, of course, quite well managed by immediate splenectomy.

Massive injuries to the liver are much more difficult to deal with. The principles of hemostasis and mattress suturing and drainage are well known for laceration of the peripheral portion of the liver. If hematoma appears near the hepatic hilum and all else appears well, it is probably best to leave this condition alone, particularly if the anatomy is obscure at the time.

Subhepatic and intrahepatic injuries to the vena cava, however, are catastrophic and are seldom managed successfully. The suggestions that follow, which are those of Blaisdell and others, may be helpful. There is always a major liver injury, and conversely, the presence of caval injury or hepatic artery injury must be suspected when the liver fractures or perforations are central and approach the hilum. The first step in management is to expose the subhepatic portion of the vena cava by reflecting the entire right retroperitoneal part of the colon. This requires a long abdominal midline incision.

1. Mobilize the right colon by dividing the lateral peritoneal reflections, beginning with the cecum and the terminal portion of the ileum. At the hepatic flexure, the peritoneum and subadjacent fat may bleed, and hemostasis may be necessary. The mesentery of the right colon and ileum is easily separated from the perinephric fat and drawn medially to uncover the duodenum.

COMMENT: *This approach uncovers the entire infrahepatic portion of the inferior vena cava and right retroperitoneal area so that associated urologic, pancreatic, and duodenal injuries may be visualized and treated.*

2. Mobilize the duodenum with a Kocher maneuver. This maneuver is extended until the subhepatic part of the vena cava and the renal veins are exposed, and the portal vein is rolled anteriorly and can be inspected along with the head of the pancreas.

3. The renal arteries are now accessible for temporary occlusion.

4. A long 38 Fr. to 36 Fr. plastic chest drainage tube or cuffed endotracheal tube must now be inserted (Fig. 10-2, *A* and *B*). This can be done from below

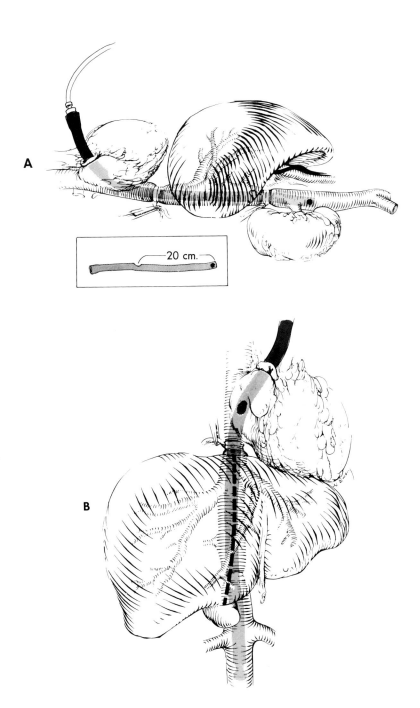

Fig. 10-2. A, Lateral view of internal shunt in inferior vena cava. A 34 Fr. catheter is inserted through right atrial appendage into inferior vena cava. Tip is just below renal veins. Side hole lies in atrium. Proximal end of catheter may be used for transfusion or may be clamped. **B,** Anterior view of internal shunt in inferior vena cava. Tapes encircle vena cava above and below liver, isolating laceration of vena cava in hilum of liver. Internal shunt is a No. 34 plastic chest drainage tube that conducts blood to the heart from kidneys and lower half of body. (Reproduced with permission from Schrock, T., Blaisdell, F. W., and Mathewson, C.: Management of blunt trauma to the liver and hepatic veins, Arch. Surg. **96:**698-704, 1968.)

or through an extension of the abdominal incision through the sternum or through a right fifth interspace extension of the abdominal incision. In order to achieve a complete bypass, it is necessary to secure the catheter above. If an endotracheal tube or Foley catheter is used, inflation of the bag alone may be successful. If it cannot be placed initially from below or if a catheter is not secure, take the following steps:

a. Open the pericardium in the midline or close to the right atrial appendage.
b. Grasp the right atrial appendage with an auricular clamp or Satinsky clamp, and place a purse-string suture of 2-0 silk.
c. Insert the catheter through the tip of the auricle, tightening the purse-string suture around it as it is advanced into the inferior vena cava below the renal vein.

COMMENT: *In either case, side holes are cut in the catheter just below the auricle. This allows a better upward drainage. Umbilical tapes are placed around the inferior vena cava inside the pericardium and as close below the liver as possible compatible with the injuries noted. The intrahepatic portion of the vena cava is now isolated, but blood may return from the lower half of the body via the shunt. Placement of a vascular clamp across the portal triad and across the portal vein completes isolation and devascularization of the injured site. Hepatic artery ligation if necessary should be done as far proximally as possible; while a serious step, this is not inevitably fatal.*

Cardiac injury

It may be impossible to distinguish injury to the great vessels at the root of the heart from injury to the heart itself, but frequently differential diagnosis can be made on the basis of immediate x-ray findings and on the basis of the fact that pericardial tamponade may cause some hypotension with poor peripheral pulses out of proportion to any obvious blood loss.

Those patients who are salvageable are found to have relatively small wounds in the ventricles. The quickest approach to these is through anterior left thoracotomy. After the distended pericardium is opened, a suture is placed through the apex of the heart, which is now elevated, as a search for the injury is made. Whereas a stab wound may cause only a single injury, a small-caliber bullet may leave two wounds in the heart, one anterior and one posterior; the latter is sought for by elevating the heart with the traction suture.

Iliac artery

In regard to the leg, the prognosis is about the same as for the common femoral artery in that gangrene will result in about 80% of patients if the circulation is interrupted. Note that this is not true in cases in which arteriosclerosis has slowly occluded the iliac artery. Indeed, in such occlusions, the incidence of distal gangrene is lower than if the occlusion involves the popliteal, superficial femoral, or more distal vessels.

Management is often complicated by associated abdominal injuries. The distal portion of the iliac artery may be exposed in conjunction with the femoral artery by dividing the inguinal ligament. This should be done without hesitation to obtain proximal control and to stop hemorrhage. Ligation of the external iliac or common femoral vein may lead to massive edema. Therefore, these veins should also be repaired when possible. Restoration of continuity of the iliac artery is absolutely essential. When primary suture is not possible, a prosthetic tube must be inserted. Vein grafts are neither large enough nor strong enough to replace the iliac and larger arteries. If the procedure is to be long, the use of a plastic or Silastic shunt is advisable to preserve distal blood flow and prevent the formation of small clots. The same is true in procedures in other peripheral areas described subsequently.

Femoral artery

Interruption of the common femoral artery results in gangrene in about 80% of patients. Associated atherosclerosis may be troublesome in older persons and may require more extensive exploration and replacement than indicated by the injury alone. The great saphenous vein from the opposite leg can be used as a replacement, but prosthetic materials are satisfactory for replacement of the common femoral artery.

Injury to the superficial femoral artery produces gangrene in 45% to 55% of patients. The accompanying vein may be ligated with little risk of subsequent edema of the leg. The saphenous vein is the best replacement for the superficial femoral and popliteal arteries.

Brachial and axillary arteries

Gangrene is much less likely to occur after interruption of arteries in the upper extremities than in the lower extremities. Interruption of the brachial artery above the profunda brachii artery, however, results in gangrene in about 56% of patients, whereas gangrene results in only 25% when ligation is below the profunda brachii artery. The brachial artery is easily exposed by a longitudinal incision along the medial side of the biceps muscle. Continuity should be restored whenever possible to avoid disability as well as the risk of gangrene.

Details of exposure of the brachial artery in the antecubital fossa and the upper arm are described in the discussion of the upper extremity. If the injury is above the midarm, adequate exposure will usually require division of the tendon of the pectoralis major muscle. The veins may be divided and ligated. Injured brachial arteries can usually be reanastomosed. When reconstruction requires a graft, one of the arm veins or the saphenous vein is the best replacement.

Noncritical arteries in lower leg and forearm

Penetrating injury or nonpenetrating injury may impair circulation in the lower leg or forearm. Arteries may be injured with or without associated fractures. Swelling within the tight fascial sheaths can cause arterial insufficiency by compression. The volar aspect of the forearm is the best location for fasciotomy in this location through a longitudinal incision. Below the knee, anterolateral and posteromedial incisions release pressure in the anterior and posterior compartments. Fasciotomy interrupts the vicious cycle in which impairment of capillary circulation leads to further edema. The objection that incision can interrupt collateral circulation through the skin is a theoretical one, and the skin and fascia, which tolerate ischemia better than muscle or nerve tissue, will survive and heal if deep circulation is restored. Without restoration of circulation to the muscle, fibrosis and contracture will ensue.

Occasionally, injury to a "noncritical" artery will result in arterial insufficiency because collateral circulation has been compromised, so that primary repair is indicated. The technique of anastomosing small arteries is given on pp. 266-268. This requires special instruments and sutures and meticulous technique for best results.

Popliteal artery

The popliteal artery is frequently injured by penetrating missiles or after distal femoral fractures. Posterior displacement of the distal fragment of a broken femur may compress or occlude the artery and injure the veins. Interruption of both the saphenous and popliteal veins can lead to massive edema that will require fasciotomy. This edema may not appear until arterial continuity has been restored.

Fractures of the upper portion of the tibia may result in avulsion of the anterior tibial artery from the distal end of the popliteal artery where the anterior tibial artery passes through a strong fascial sheet into the anterior compartment of the leg. This injury usually cannot be repaired; however, the continuity of the popliteal artery itself must be evaluated by arteriograms.

Continuity can be restored by anastomosing the distal end of the popliteal artery to the posterior tibial artery. Surgical approaches to the popliteal artery are shown in Chapter 7. The artery is small; therefore, end-to-end anastomosis must be precise. When debridement makes the use of a graft necessary, a saphenous vein graft is preferred. The incidence of failure and gangrene after repair of the popliteal artery is higher than that for any other major vessel, being about 25% to 35% (Korean War statistics). Without primary repair, however, the leg amputation rate after popliteal artery injury is 78% (World War I and World War II statistics). At the present time popliteal injuries are still resulting in gangrene at a rate of 29% to 33% (Viet Nam statistics).

Associated venous injury

The accompanying veins are almost always injured in penetrating arterial wounds. Formerly it was believed that ligation of the veins would improve the circulation of the injured extremity and would reduce the incidence of gangrene when the artery was ligated. Ligation of veins may be necessary in debridement of gunshot wounds, but an occasional knife wound can be successfully repaired. No immediate harm will result from ligation of veins, but edema and stasis ulceration almost invariably follow interruption of the common femoral or external iliac veins. When all the veins of an extremity are thrombosed, massive edema may interrupt the arterial circulation by compression within the tight fascial compartments in the forearm or in the lower leg. If this happens, fasciotomy is necessary and repair of the veins and/or thrombectomy should be considered.

Vascular injury during elective surgical procedures
Inferior vena cava

The inferior vena cava may be injured during a number of procedures (for example, right nephrectomy, right lumbar sympathectomy, or right retroperitoneal lymph node dissection). Usually the source of bleeding is a small tear that results from traction on a small tributary. Bleeding is profuse but usually can be easily controlled by the local pressure of a small sponge on the fingertip—large bulky packs may prove to be ineffective and always prevent visualization of the injury. Repair is simple after application of an Allis forceps or a sidewise partially occluding clamp such as the Satinsky clamp and can be accomplished without further mobilization and without obtaining proximal and distal control of the vein.

It is important to remember that blood loss from either surgical or traumatic injury to the vena cava can be massive. Although only slight pressure is required for

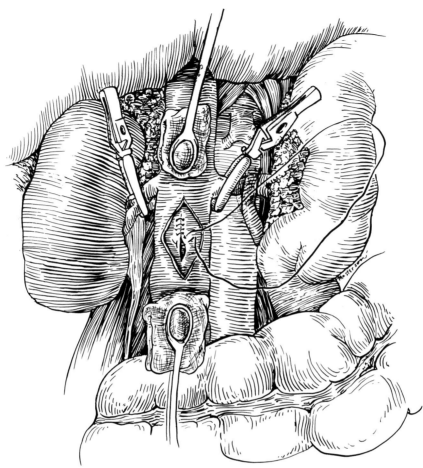

Fig. 10-3. Exploration of inferior vena cava. Transvenous suture repair of injury to posterior wall of vena cava.

local control, other matters may not be pursued until such injuries are either controlled or repaired.

When searching for an injury, start from below and occlude the upward flow of blood in the vena cava with a sponge stick (see Fig. 10-3). Coming upward, gently roll or retract or withdraw the gauze pack until the edge of the leak is encountered. Digital pressure may be necessary to prevent inflow from lumbar veins.

Of course, if the vena cava is badly damaged, the surgeon may resort to ligation. The indications for inferior caval ligation are as follows: (1) severe and complicated injuries; (2) multiple injuries; (3) poor condition of the patient, persisting hypotension, or lack of blood for replacement; and (4) electively when the risk of postoperative embolism seems to be high, such as with associated fractures of the legs or pelvis. Postoperative management of a ligated vena cava is discussed in Chapter 18.

If not ligated, the inferior vena cava, the right renal vein, and other major abdominal veins should be repaired.

One maneuver that is most useful with the vena cava is that illustrated in Fig. 10-3, in which the anterior wall of the vena cava is opened in order to suture conveniently a relatively inaccessible tear in the posterior wall. Posterior and anterior lacerations in this case are closed with continuous over-and-over sutures with vascular suture material.

Portal vein

The portal vein may be injured in pancreatoduodenal resections (Whipple operation). The vein may be invaded by cancer or may be adherent because of accompanying pancreatitis. Injury usually occurs as the operator uses his finger to dissect bluntly through the venous tunnel under the pancreas. To avoid injury to the vein, uncover it by dividing the pancrease to the left of the midline, and lift the proximal end of the divided pancreas anteriorly and to the right, approaching the portal vein and the superior mesenteric artery from the left side. Small branches may then be visualized and ligated as the vein is uncovered.

Left iliac vein and artery

The left iliac vein and artery may be injured during removal of a fifth lumbar herniated nucleus pulposus. If the anterior part of the annulus fibrosus is ruptured, the underlying vein may be torn. Hemorrhage is profuse and occurs immediately. Laparotomy is necessary if packing of the intervertebral space does not arrest the hemorrhage. If both artery and vein are injured, arteriovenous fistula may result. When shock follows an operation or occurs during an operation for herniated disk in the low lumbar region, this injury must immediately be suspected of being present and must be sought.

Left hepatic vein

The left hepatic vein may be injured during mobilization of the left lobe of the liver for abdominal vagectomy. This vein is more superficial than expected but is covered with a dense fibrous sheath that is readily distinguished from the areolar tissue between the left lobe and the diaphragm.

Hepatic artery

The hepatic artery may be resected with gastric cancer or during gastrectomy for duodenal ulcer. The right hepatic artery is occasionally ligated during cholecystectomy. In such instances, when the injury is recognized, the blood flow must be restored to the liver, and the end of the splenic artery may be implanted into the side or anastomosed to the distal end of the hepatic artery. End-to-end anastomosis may be feasible.

Puncture wounds of arteries

Arterial puncture is usually innocuous. However, we have observed false aneurysms and arteriovenous fistulas following venipuncture near the femoral and brachial arteries and in the popliteal and brachial arteries secondary to puncture by Kirschner wires or Steinmann pins or arterial puncture for retrograde catheterization.

More recently the widespread use of arterial catheterization has resulted in tears, small aneurysms, and other seemingly minor injuries to the femoral and brachial arteries. Patients subjected to these procedures should be examined prior to the procedure for distal pulses and should be watched closely afterward and not discharged from the hospital. Frequently the procedure is done by a radiologist, who resorts to compression rather than one or two fine sutures for repair. If no cutdown has been done, as is usual in the femoral artery, a small aneurysm may not be noted for several weeks until local hemorrhage has subsided. This condition is more usual when patients are catheterized to evaluate them for hypertension.

Although many small aneurysms are of the traumatic type and will disappear in a few weeks, elevation of the intima and accidental occlusion are more serious and should be attended to at once.

FALSE ANEURYSM AND ARTERIOVENOUS FISTULA

False aneurysms and arteriovenous fistulas are usually the result of penetrating injuries to blood vessels. When an artery is completely severed, the ends retract and contract and often the hemorrhage stops spontaneously. If, however, a vessel is partially severed, only the cut portion of the vessel is able to retract. The wound is held open, allowing rather profuse hemorrhage. If the soft tissue wound associated with the vascular wound is large, the hemorrhage is visible externally. When associated soft tissue wounds are small and there is no opportunity for external blood loss, blood may be trapped in muscle and fascial planes, with formation of a pulsating hematoma. The blood clot and the hematoma acquire a laminated organized exterior. The blood in the center of the hematoma remains fluid and is free to flow in and out of the tear in the arterial wall.

Organization of the wall of the hematoma produces a fibrous tissue sac lined with a glistening intima-like layer. Such false aneurysms assume shapes according to the contour of the surrounding anatomical structures. Accompanying veins and nerves are commonly incorporated into the walls of this false aneurysmal sac.

When the associated veins are injured in addition to the artery, blood escaping under high pressure from the site of the arterial injury may follow the path of least resistance, enter into the vein, and form a fistulous tract. Such fistulas are prone to develop where the artery and vein are enclosed in a common sheath. Commonly, the false aneurysmal sac makes up a portion of the fistulous lesion. If two veins accompany the artery, all three vessels can become involved. The feeding artery proximal to the fistula usually becomes larger than normal, and the associated veins become enlarged and thickened.

Differential diagnosis

The following points help to differentiate false aneurysms from arteriovenous fistulas:

1. Arteriovenous fistula is usually accompanied by continuous rough vibratory thrill that is easily palpated. Auscultation reveals a rough, machinery-like murmur. False aneurysms have a murmur only during systole or perhaps not at all.
2. Large arteriovenous fistulas are accompanied by a rapid pulse rate that slows when the fistulous tract is manually occluded (Branham's sign).
3. Dilatation of superficial veins is usual with arteriovenous fistula.

There are no systemic manifestations of a false aneurysm, but large arteriovenous fistulas cause cardiovascular manifestations. Branham's sign, a decrease in pulse rate with compression of the fistula, has already been mentioned. Early in the formation of arteriovenous fistulas there may be a decrease in both systolic and diastolic blood pressure, but after a time the systolic pressure tends to recover. With the increase

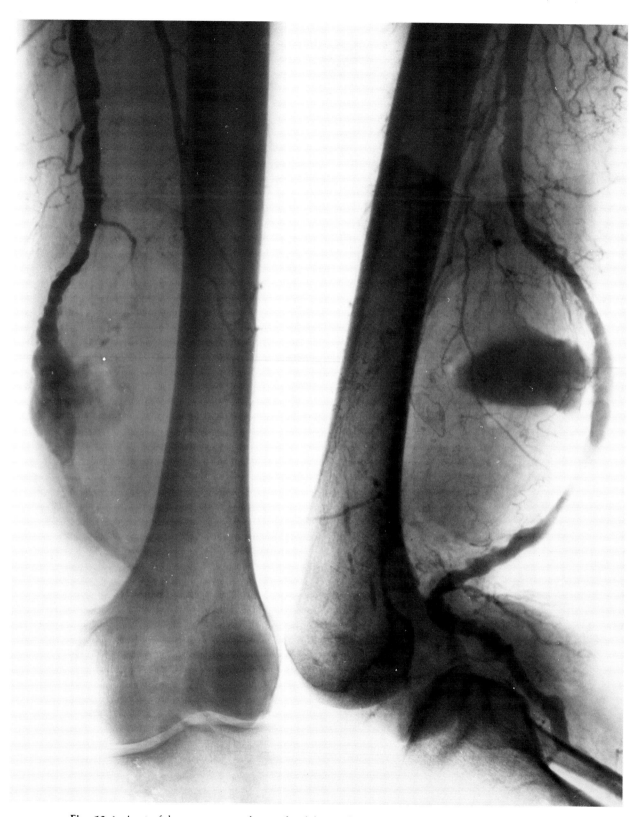

Fig. 10-4. Acute false aneurysm of superficial femoral artery due to arteriosclerosis and trauma.

in blood volume and the increased work load on the heart, there may be gradual dilatation of the heart and later hypertrophy and cardiac failure.

Certain local changes may accompany arteriovenous fistulas. These are cool skin, trophic changes in the skin and appendages, edema, ulceration, cyanosis, pallor, and perhaps gangrene distal to the site of the fistula. The area near the fistula itself is usually warmer to the touch, and oscillometric readings are increased locally.

Although not always necessary, arteriography may be employed in differential diagnosis.

Surgical treatment

The goal of treatment is to eliminate the fistula and to restore normal arterial flow. Repair may be undertaken as soon as the patient's general condition permits and the associated soft tissue injuries are healed. Delay permits further dilatation of the aneurysmal sac and of associated veins and other complications and disability. The expanding sac may erode bone and damage adjacent nerve trunks. In long-standing fistulas, troublesome scarring, ectopic bone formation, and dilatation of all regional veins and their collateral vessels may develop.

Years ago quadruple ligation was the best treatment, and delay in operation was advised in order to allow development of collateral circulation. Quadruple ligation eliminated the fistula but was frequently followed by crippling arterial insufficiency. Therefore, this procedure is now used only for small, noncritical arteries.

Small fistulas in large vessels may occasionally be exposed and closed by transvenous repair. This method is subject to the limitations of primary lateral arteriorrhaphy already mentioned. Sometimes a false aneurysm may be closed laterally, or the fibrous wall may be used for the support of a vein graft. The operation of endoaneurysmorrhaphy (intrasaccular suture and repair) was first described by Matas in 1888. The procedure was invented because proximal and distal ligation in a case of aneurysm of the brachial artery had failed. Most such operations have become unnecessary and undesirable since the technique of arterial replacement has been developed. Therefore, if at all possible, a Dacron arterial prothesis or vein graft should be employed and should be sutured to normal artery proximal and distal to the excised aneurysm.

EXPLORATION OF GUNSHOT WOUND OF FEMORAL ARTERY AND VEIN

Stab wounds cause little surrounding damage. Low-speed bullets tend to push surrounding tissues aside. High-speed missiles enter the tissue, often leaving an unimpressive wound of entrance and/or exit. As the momentum of the missile is expended in the tissues, however, the phenomenon of cavitation takes place, and the underlying damage may be great. In the example of exploration that follows, typical widespread damage of a high-speed missile in the surrounding tissues is assumed and illustrated.

Restoration of arterial continuity is essential for all wounds of major arteries. However, the most meticulous arterial suture may fail unless infection is forestalled by debridement and unless there is correct treatment of associated injuries such as fractures. These important matters have been discussed in various books and articles and are not discussed here.

Adequate exposure requires long incisions over the course of the artery. Details of the surgical approach to various parts of the femoral and popliteal arteries are described and illustrated in Chapters 3 to 8. In the drawings included in those chapters as well as in the illustrations in this chapter, the drapes and skin towels are omitted in order to show clearly the anatomical landmarks.

In the appraisal of the amount of resection or type of treatment, it is usual to underestimate the extent of injury. One must look for minimal clues that may indicate damage. Concussion or spasm of injured arteries that does not respond to local applications of 2% papaverine solution requires resection of the portion of the artery. Such specimens usually show subintimal damage and thrombosis. Tangential repair of arteries or veins should be reserved for knife wounds. The partial or tangential lacerations that are the result of gunshot wounds require resection. In gunshot wounds the accompanying vein is usually injured. Its repair is seldom successful. Because of the high velocity of the bullet, arterial injury is usually more extensive than anticipated, and the usual error is to resect insufficient artery. If two of the three major veins of the thigh are injured or occluded, massive and dangerous edema may result in gangrene. Prophylactic fasciotomy of the calf is mandatory for such patients, and restoration of venous continuity with a graft from the opposite leg should be considered. If the accompanying vein has been injured, it should be preserved. There is no evidence that ligation of the accompanying vein improves blood flow to the injured extremity.

The method used to restore arterial continuity depends in part on the length of the defect after the resection and on the location of the injury. Primary end-to-end anastomosis is seldom practicable for defects longer than 2 cm. without extensive dissection for mobilization of the artery proximally and distally and without sacrifice of collateral vessels. Saphenous vein grafts or prostheses are preferable for longer defects. Autogenous vein grafts are preferable in the superficial femoral or popliteal artery. Experience has shown that they do not need support by surrounding muscle or fascia. The saphenous vein is sturdy, will not dilate, and is suitable for replacement of the femoral or brachial arteries. The cephalic and brachial veins are thin walled. The saphenous vein graft is procured from the normal leg when the accompanying superficial femoral or popliteal vein is injured. Knitted prostheses of Dacron are available in various diameters and lengths and should be used in large arteries such as the common femoral artery because vein grafts in these locations will dilate despite external support with fascia, pericardium, and the like. The techiques for use of such prostheses are described in the discussion of occlusive disease in the lower extremity.

It must be remembered that veins are not elastic and therefore the vein graft must not be too short. The veins are so thin walled that the edges at the cut end, fold, wrinkle, and collapse unless held by mattress sutures. Triangulating mattress sutures are essential. In this fashion the ends can be held open, manipulation with forceps can be avoided, and accurate placement of sutures is assured.

The most meticulous arterial suture may fail because of infection, improper fixation of associated fractures, or postischemic swelling in closed fascial compartments. Infection is usually the result of contamination and inadequate debridement. Adequate debridement of wounds from high-velocity missiles may result in sizable defects of soft tissue. Arterial anastomoses should be covered by living tissue, and muscle or skin flaps must be mobilized for this purpose. Dead space collects serum that can become infected, and this must not be permitted. Radical debridement of soft tissue is unnecessary for most civilian gunshot wounds. Drains may be placed in soft tissue and led out through a small separate and dependent drainage incision. They are not placed in contact with vascular anastomoses and are removed early.

Fasciotomy of the calf or forearm may be necessary to prevent compression of arteries and arterioles by edema within the tight fascial envelope. Fasciotomy is mandatory after popliteal artery injuries because of the associated venous outflow injury and obstruction. Fasciotomy should be done prophylactically in other instances when venous outflow is seriously impaired or when ischemia of the muscles of the calf has persisted over twelve hours. In such cases the muscle swells markedly when arterial continuity is restored. Swelling of muscle inside tight fascial compartments is evident only by firmness of the calf. Any evidence of arterial insufficiency of the foot in the presence of a firm calf is sufficient indication for fasciotomy. The surgeon will observe the edematous muscle bulge through the incision and be gratified at the return of distal pulses.

Procedure

Debridement of femoral artery and vein

1. Make a long incision over the course of the femoral artery (Fig. 10-5, A). Do not hesitate to divide the inguinal ligament if this is necessary to obtain proximal control of the bleeding.

2. Identify the femoral artery and the femoral vein, and obtain proximal control using serrefine arterial clamps before approaching the actual area of injury (Fig. 10-5, B). For occlusion of the veins, rubber-shod bulldog clamps are satisfactory and somewhat less traumatic. The superficial femoral vein usually has sizable posterior branches that also must be controlled. Approach the injury site by dissecting progressively from normal tissues toward the area of hematoma. In the drawing the superficial femoral artery is almost completely divided and the vein has a through-and-through perforation.

3. Debride from 1 to 2 cm. of artery at each end of the wound (Fig. 10-5, C). Closely inspect the adventitia for tiny hematomas at the origins of small branches. The intima of the artery should be normal at the site of transection. Temporarily remove the distal clamp to observe back bleeding and to aspirate distal clots that may have formed during the period of occlusion. After the injured segment of artery has been resected, the remainder of the vessel retracts rather markedly.

4. Prepare the ends of the artery for anastomosis by trimming off any adventia that might protrude into the edges of the anastomosis (Fig. 10-5, D). In some instances, arterial continuity may be restored by end-to-end anastomosis. In most gunshot wounds, however, adequate debridement leaves a considerable gap. Divided arteries retract, so that a gap of 6 to 7 cm. may result from resection of half that amount of artery. In this instance, a 6 cm. vein graft was necessary. Measure the length of graft required without traction on the arterial clamps and make the vein graft a few centimeters longer than necessary.

5. Ligate the accompanying superficial femoral vein if repair is not feasible (Fig. 10-5, E).

Procurement of saphenous vein graft

1. Expose the saphenous vein in the upper thigh through a longitudinal incision (Fig. 10-5, F).

2. Uncover a sufficient length of vein. Ligate small tributaries prior to division

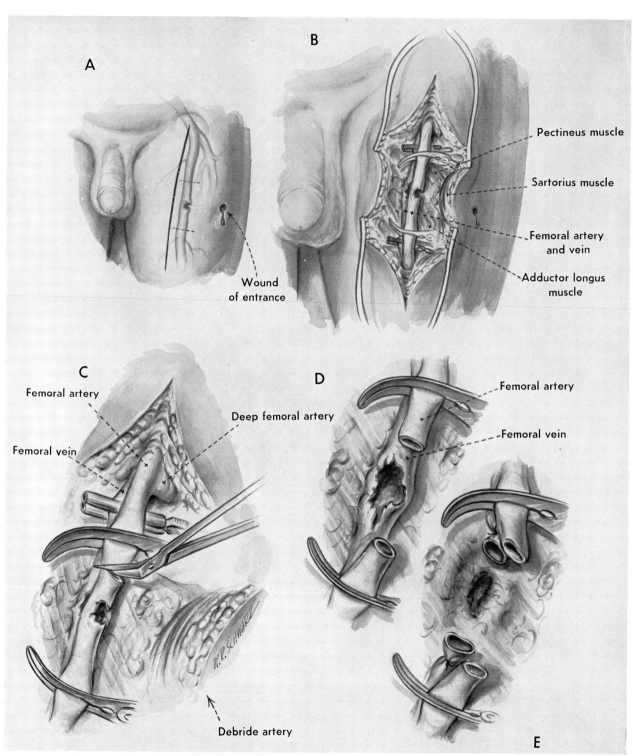

Fig. 10-5. Vein graft for gunshot wound of femoral artery. **A** and **B**, Exploration of wound of femoral artery and vein. **C** and **D**, Debridement of femoral artery and vein. **E**, Vein ligated.

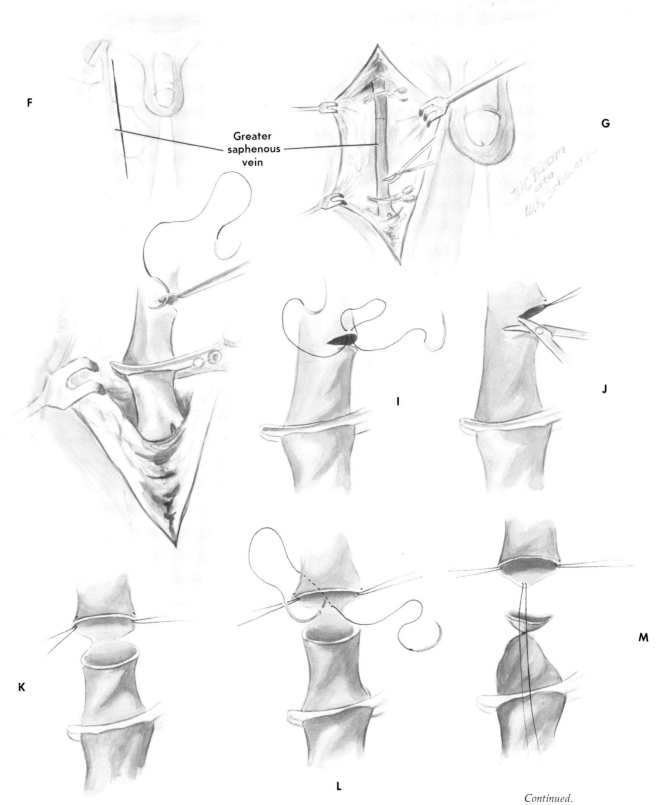

Greater saphenous vein

F

G

J

I

K

L

M

Continued.

Fig. 10-5, cont'd. Vein graft for gunshot wound of femoral artery. **F** to **M,** Procurement of saphenous vein graft. **F,** Incision. **G,** Partial division of vein. **H** and **I,** First triangulation suture. **J,** Further division of vein graft. **K,** Second triangulation suture. **L** and **M,** Third triangulation suture.

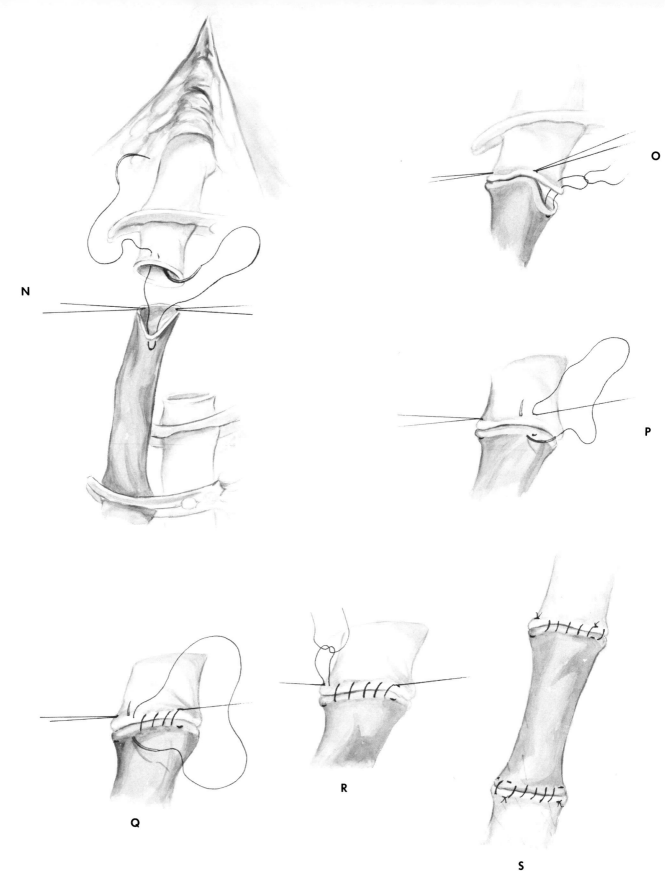

Fig. 10-5, cont'd. Vein graft for gunshot wound of femoral artery and vein. **N** to **S**, End-to-end anastomosis of vein graft and femoral artery. **N** and **O**, Triangulation sutures passed through artery and tied. **P** to **R**, Continuous suture of everted edges. **S**, Completed vein graft.

of the vein. Employ sharp Potts arterial scissors to partially divide the vein distally (Fig. 10-5, *G*). Then place the first guide suture. Fig. 10-5, *I* to *M*, shows placement of other guide sutures before complete division of the vein.

3. Pass a double-armed 5-0 arterial suture through the vein distally, 0.5 mm. from the edge, for use as a horizontal everting mattress suture (Fig. 10-5, *H* and *I*). Hold both ends in a rubber-shod bulldog clamp. Continue division of the vein (Fig. 10-5, *J*).

4. Place the second suture one third of the distance around the circumference of the vein (Fig. 10-5, *K*).

5. Place a third horizontal everting mattress suture in the vein so that the three stitches form an equilateral triangle (Fig. 10-5, *L*).

6. Apply a toothed bulldog clamp proximally. Complete the division of the vein so that it is several centimeters longer than necessary (Fig. 10-5, *G*). *The vein must be reversed when it is inserted.*

COMMENT: *Divide the vein so that is is 1 to 2 cm. longer than necessary and place the triangulation sutures at the other end after completion of the first anastomosis. The judgment of the correct length for the vein graft is easier after the first anastomosis is completed, particularly if the graft is close to a joint.*

End-to-end anastomosis of vein graft and femoral artery

1. Insert, in the fashion illustrated, the previously placed guide sutures at the end of the vein into the prepared end of the artery as shown in Fig. 10-5, *N*. *Reverse the direction of the vein.*

2. Tie the mattress sutures without traction on the arterial clamps (Fig. 10-5, *O*). When the sutures are tied, the resulting eversion of the edges facilitates the remaining maneuvers.

3. Hold the suture line taut by placing traction laterally and medially on one of the limbs of the previously placed mattress suture. Sew the vein to the artery with small stitches about 0.5 mm. from the edge of the vessels, using an over-and-over continuous suture (Fig. 10-5, *P*).

4. Continue until the next mattress suture is reached (Fig. 10-5, *Q*).

5. End the continous suture by tying it to one limb of adjacent mattress suture (Fig. 10-5, *R*). Release the proximal clamps to flush the proximal artery of the graft.

6. Reapply the bulldog clamp to the distal end of the vein graft to allow it to distend and lengthen under arterial pressure after release of the proximal arterial clamp.

7. Determine the correct length of the vein graft with the graft distended. If the graft is near a joint, judge the length with the joint extended and flexed.

8. Reapply the proximal arterial clamp, divide the vein graft partially, and place the first mattress suture for triangulation. Divide the graft more, and place the second and third triangulation sutures as shown in Fig. 10-5, *H* to *M*.

9. Perform the distal anastomosis as described previously in steps 1 to 5 and illustrated in Fig. 10-5, *N* to *R*.

10. Before closing the last sutures, flush by the graft by momentarily releasing the proximal and distal clamps. Then tie the last suture. Remove the distal clamp until the graft fills with blood, and then slowly and intermittently release the proximal clamp. Bleeding from the needle holes or from the suture line will stop after five minutes. That the saphenous vein is slightly narrower than the artery should not

be a cause of concern. Arteriograms in six or eight weeks will show that the vein has accommodated itself and is the same size as the artery.

11. Reconstruct the femoral sheath and soft tissues about the vein. Debridement of soft tissues need not be radical for wounds caused by low-velocity missiles. Associated injuries should be treated. The fascia of the thigh is closed loosely.

ANASTOMOSIS OF SMALL ARTERIES
Introduction

Restoration of continuity by direct vessel anastomosis should be performed in all traumatic interruptions of major arteries. When collateral circulation has been compromised, this principle must be extended to smaller vessels below the elbow and below the knee. Newer indications for this procedure are experimental organ transplantation, reimplantation of a severed limb, and microneurosurgery in which blood is shunted from the superficial temporal artery into the middle cerebral artery when it is occluded. Such vessels can be anastomosed with a fair rate of success by use of meticulous surgical technique. In emergency treatment of injuries of such vessels, use of hemostats to clamp severed vessels should be avoided. Wide operative exposure of the vessel at the site of injury is essential. If the injury is relatively old (that is, over twenty-four hours), extraction of the thrombus distal to the site of injury may prove to be difficult. However, this should be attempted, both by direct methods and by retrograde flushing.

The technique of anastomosis to be described employs fine 7-0 silk or monofilament suture on small atraumatic needles. The surgeon should make use of every aid to render his work precise, including adequate lighting and a binocular loupe. He should sit and arrange the field so that his elbows or forearms are supported. Microsurgery on very fine blood vessels using the binocular microscope has been described by Jacobson. This facilitates anastomosis of these small vessels. The Nakayama stapler has been useful in our laboratory.

Instrumentation, magnification, and general principles

Fine instruments may be obtained from companies specializing either in eye instruments or in the microvascular instruments devised by Jacobson.* For very fine vessels, a vise or rack is available on which the bulldog clamps illustrated in Fig. 10-6 can be supported.

For magnification, binocular loupes are almost universally available; however, they have the defect of limited magnification, on the order of 2× to 2.5×. Beyond this magnification, the special optics of a surgical microscope are necessary in order to provide more magnification. A number of these instruments are marketed in an almost constantly changing variety. The Xonix stereoscope† is unique in that it is mounted on the operator's head and has a self-contained light source that provides maximum flexibility.

When an ultrasmall or microscopic anastomosis is to be attempted, it is also necessary that the assistant be provided with some magnification and that both surgeon and assistant have provision made to rest their forearms on a solid object. This requires ingenious arrangement of tables, sandbags, and other equipment. It is impos-

---

*Manufactured by V. Mueller, Division American Hospital Supply Corp., Chicago, Ill.
†Manufactured by Xonix, Inc., Walthon, Mass.

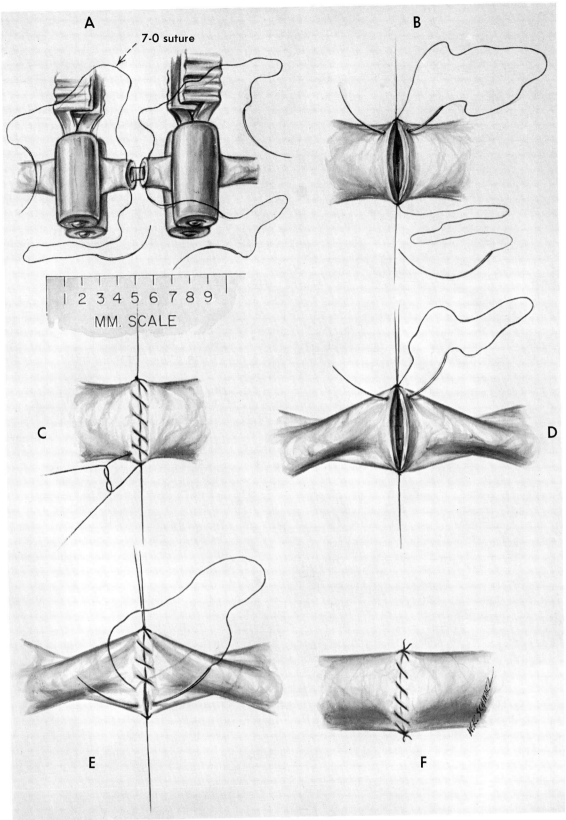

Inside the figure, the following labels appear:

A

7-0 suture

B

1 2 3 4 5 6 7 8 9
MM. SCALE

C

D

E

F

Fig. 10-6. Anastomosis of small arteries. **A,** First sutures. **B** and **C,** Continuous suture of anterior row without excision or narrowing of lumen. **D** and **E,** Posterior row of continuous sutures. **F,** Completed anastomosis.

sible to do this fine work using the entire arm, that is, with no forearm rest and with the elbow and shoulder joints moving about.

It is axiomatic that man can do only what the eye can see. In this respect, the operator's hand is usually a more precise instrument than the eye, and perhaps at the present time, about 6× to 10× magnification is the practical limit of the surgeon's hand, his instruments, and his suture materials.

Procedure

1. Debride the injured vessel. Occlude the vessel proximally and distally with rubber-shod bulldog clamps. Wash blood clot from the ends of the vessels with warm saline solution or warm 0.1% heparin in saline solution. Two stay or guide sutures are now inserted with double-armed fine silk sutures at opposite ends of the vessel (Fig. 10-6, *A*).

COMMENT: *After injury, small arteries may be highly spastic. Smooth muscle spasm may be overcome by topical applications of pledgets soaked with 2% papaverine solution. If this is ineffective or unavailable, the ends of the vessels must be mechanically dilated by very gently spreading the tips of a fine hemostat within the lumen of the vessel. At this stage and before the anastomosis has begun, the distal portion of the vessel must be cleared of thrombus by using a wire loop or a small balloon catheter or by retrograde flushing.*

2. Have the assistant place traction on the tied guide sutures. Begin the anastomosis of the vessel with a simple over-and-over stitich, sewing toward yourself (Fig. 10-6, *B*).

3. When the end of the row is reached, tie the suture (Fig. 10-6, *C*).

4. Pass the three pieces of thread at one end to the assistant, and rotate the vessel 180 degrees (Fig. 10-6, *D*). Complete the remainder of the suture line with a simple over-and-over stitch (Fig. 10-6, *E*).

5. The suture line is completed in a manner similar to that used for the first row (Fig. 10-6, *F*).

COMMENT: *The operator should feel a pulsatile flow of blood when the anastomosis is complete and the bulldog clamps are released. If the vessel remains spastic, a sponge soaked in warm (not hot) saline solution may be employed in an attempt to relax muscle spasm and increase blood flow locally. It may be necessary to perform intraoperative angiography in order to assure patency of the anastomosis and the distal vessels.*

In this and other chapters, we have illustrated the use of double-armed sutures. It is obvious that the same procedures may be carried out with single-armed sutures. The double-armed suture allows the surgeon to sew in either direction from either end of the anastomosis. In addition, if one of the threads should break—and this is not

Fig. 10-7. Nakayama stapler for anastomosis of a small vessel. **A,** Nakayama clamps. **B,** Stapling rings. **C,** Stapling ring recessed in clamp. **D,** End of vessel drawn through ring and everted over prongs. **E,** Approximate two clamps to join two ends of vessel. **F,** Open clamp to free ring anastomosis.

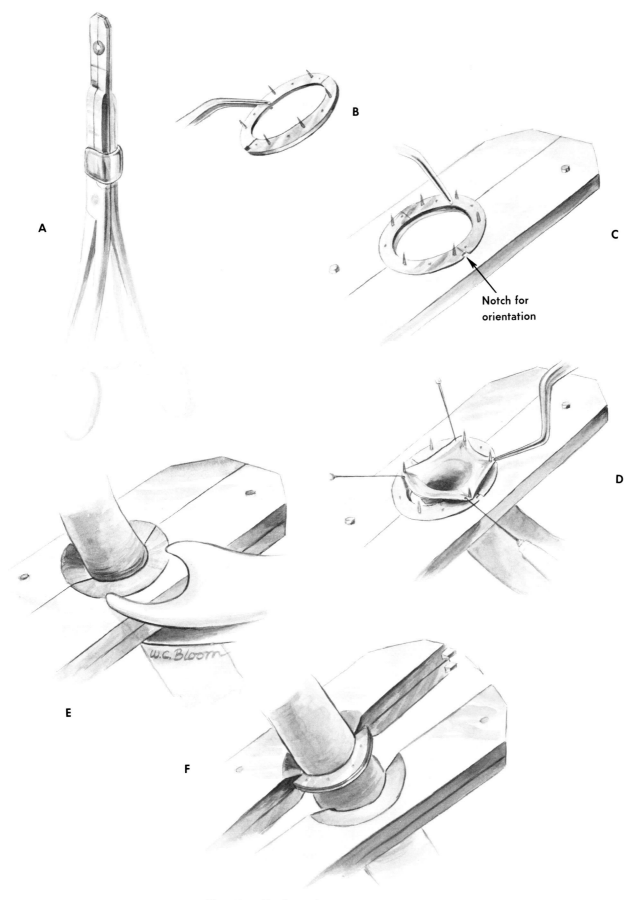

Fig. 10-7. For legend see opposite page.

Notch for orientation

269

unusual when very fine material is used—the spare suture and needle are available and the anastomosis can proceed without delay.

To avoid damage, vascular sutures should never be grasped or tagged with a hemostat unless it is rubber shod. Preferably, traction on these fine sutures should be exerted directly through the gloved hand of the operator or his assistant without the intervention of an instrument.

ANASTOMOSIS OF SMALL VESSELS WITH NAKAYAMA STAPLER

We have used the Nakayama vascular stapler* for rapid and accurate anastomosis of normal arteries or veins 2 to 4 mm. in diameter. The vessels are anastomosed with two thin metal rings with prongs and holes that act as staples. Each of the two flat rings of stainless steel or tantalum has six tiny prongs and six holes (Fig. 10-7, B). One ring is placed in the opening of the jaw of the clamp (Fig. 10-7, C) and is held in place by closing the clamp. The prongs project upward and will pass into the holes of the opposite ring at the time of the anastomosis. To orient the prongs of one clamp with the holes of the other ring, the rings are rotated until a notch on the ring lies opposite a scored mark on the jaw of its holding clamp. With a small hook provided for this purpose, the cleaned end of the vessel is drawn through the ring and everted over the prongs (Fig. 10-7, D). This most difficult step of the procedure requires practice in the laboratory. It is facilitated by gently dilating the end of the vessel with a small hemostat. The edges of the vessel must be forced down over each prong of the ring individually with the use of the fine tissue forceps. The vessel may be more firmly fixed on the prongs by a stylet of appropriate size. The other end of the anastomosis is similarly fixed to the ring in the other holding clamp.

The ends of the vessel are joined when the jaws of the two clamps are approximated (Fig. 10-7, E). The projections on the face of one clamp fit into indentations in the other clamp. A small clip holds the two clamps together. A special pliers is applied to the ends of the clamps so that its notched jaws surround the projecting vessels. This pliers is closed very firmly to drive the prongs of each ring through the opposite vessel into the holes of the other ring. The prongs are bent as they are pressed against the plate of the holding clamp. The pliers and clip are removed and the clamps opened to free the rings (Fig. 10-7, F). The anastomosis may be made more watertight by further compression of the rings with a strong hemostat throughout their circumference.

An end-to-side or side-to-side anastomosis may be constructed by drawing the edges of an opening in the side of a vessel through the hole of the ring and everting over the prongs in the same manner.

With practice, the anastomosis can be accomplished in about half the time required to suture vessels of the same size. The intimal surface is uniformly smooth and free of foreign material since the rings and traumatized vessel edges lie outside the lumen. The union is strong and seldom leaks. Reloading is simple and rapid.

---

*Devised by Prof. Komei Nakayama, Chiba University Medical School in Japan. The instrument and staples are available in the United States from V. Mueller, Division American Hospital Supply Corp., Chicago, Ill. The Nakayama stapler has been used extensively with great success on more than fifty canine renal transplants by Dr. Thomas Sheridan in our laboratory.

Other rings may be sterilized separately and inserted into the clamps at the operating table.

There are three important limitations of the stapler:

1. The eversion over the prongs requires that the vessel edges be pliable.
2. The anastomosis is permanently surrounded by a rigid ring that prevents expansion and growth. Dr. Nakayama reports observing aneurysmal dilatation of the vessel distal to the ring in some dogs. The staple rings are scored for the purpose of being fractured by bending after completion of the anastomosis to make expansion possible. However, this often results in unacceptable leaking.
3. In our experience, the apparatus is not useful for ureteral or bile duct anastomosis because of stricture formation. The lumen of the thick-walled tube (such as a dog ureter) is narrowed where the entire circumference must pass through the circle. This is less significant for thin-walled tubes.

The apparatus has been very useful in renal artery anastomosis in dog kidney transplants and clinically for anastomosis of the radial and ulnar arteries.

LIMB REIMPLANTATION

Only a few operations of limb reimplantation have been done, and we have had no personal experience with any of them. When the occasion arises, however, an emergency exists. The severed limb must be immediately preserved in iced saline solution and washed through with cold heparin in saline solution and/or with low–molecular weight dextran. While one surgical team is doing this and attending to any necessary debridement, another team prepares the site of severance or avulsion of the limb for reimplantation.

No general rule for reimplantation can be given. If there is much soft tissue loss, this must be made up for by removal of some bone. The severed long bones are stabilized by internal fixation, following which the blood vessels are anastomosed. Because of the edema after this type of surgery, anastomosis of the vein is usually carried out first, although some surgeons advocate the opposite sequence. When circulation to the limb has been restored, there is ample time for the remainder of the surgical procedure.

C.H.C.

References

Amato, J. J., and Rich, N. M.: Temporary cavity effects in blood vessel injury by high velocity missiles, J. Cardiovasc. Surg. 13:147-155, 1972.

Amato, J. J., et al.: High-veolocity arterial injury: a study of the mechanism of injury, J. Trauma 11:412-416, 1971.

Clegg, J., and Charlesworth, D.: Traumatic rupture of the thoracic aorta, J. Cardiovasc. Surg. 13:206-208, 1972.

DeBakey, M. E., and Simeone, F. A.: Battle injuries of arteries in World War II; an analysis of 2,471 cases, Ann. Surg. 123:534-579, 1946.

Drapanas, T., and Hewitt, R. L., et. al.: Civilian vascular injuries: a critical appraisal of three decades of management, Ann. Surg. 172:351-360, 1970.

Hershey, F. B.: Secondary repair of arterial injuries, Am. Surg. 27:33-41, 1961.

Jacobson, J. H.: The development of microsurgical technique. In Donaghy, R. M. P., and Yaşargil, M. G.: Micro-vascular surgery, St. Louis, 1967, The C. V. Mosby Co.

Jacobson, J. H.: Microsurgery. In Current problems in surgery, Chicago, 1971, Year Book Medical Publishers, Inc.

Meyer, J. A., et al.: Traumatic rupture of the aorta in a child, J.A.M.A. **208**:527-529, 1969.

Pate, J. W., et al.: Traumatic rupture of the thoracic aorta, J.A.M.A. **203**:1022-1024, 1968.

Patman, R. D., et al.: The management of civilian arterial injuries, Surg. Gynecol. Obstet. **118**:725-737, 1964.

Rich, N. M.: Vascular injuries, Bull. Am. Coll. Surg. **57**:35-40, 1972.

Rich, N. M., and Hughes, C. V.: Vietnam vascular registry: a preliminary report, Surgery **65**:218-226, 1969.

Richards, A. J., Jr., et al.: Laceration of abdominal aorta and study of intact abdominal wall as tamponade: report of survival and literature review, Ann. Surg. **164**:321-324, 1966.

Smith, R. F., et al.: Fracture of long bones with arterial injury due to blunt trauma, Arch. Surg. **99**:315-324, 1969.

11

Operations on the abdominal visceral arteries

SUPERIOR MESENTERIC ARTERY
Sudden occlusion

Sudden occlusion of the superior mesenteric artery has received the major attention of vascular surgeons because of the dramatic nature of the disease, the almost always fatal outcome, and the possiblity of reversal by early surgery. Although the condition has been known for some time, particularly in conjunction with embolic disease, in 1957 Shaw and Rutledge were the first to report a successful embolectomy with reversal of ischemia and survival.

Some patients may survive because of excellent collateral circulation, but as a rule, sudden occlusion of the superior mesenteric artery will produce gangrene of the major portion of the intestine. In this instance, the superior mesenteric artery and its branches act much in the manner of an end-artery even though this is not in fact the case anatomically.

A few patients may survive such a disaster after massive resection of the infarcted intestine. However, it is obviously preferable to salvage the ischemic tissues by early diagnosis, early operation, and treatment to restore the arterial flow. Unfortunately, early diagnosis is difficult.

Sudden occlusion is usually embolic or thrombotic in origin. Chronic occlusion (discussed later) is more likely to present problems in diagnosis and treatment. Both embolectomy and aortic–superior mesenteric artery bypass are performed in the accessible portion of the superior mesenteric artery after it emerges beneath the pancreas.

Symptoms

The patient initially complains of sudden severe upper abdominal pain. It is not cramping; it is agonizing. It is not associated with anterior abdominal symptoms such as guard or rebound initially. In these respects, it somewhat resembles pancreatitis, although vomiting is not as inevitable. Temperature and initial blood cell counts and x-ray films of the abdomen are unremarkable. At this stage, a diagnosis is made by an alert medical or surgical team, with the knowledge of the existence of a source of embolus. After a quiescent period, the signs and symptoms of peritonitis usually appear, but at this time gangrene of the intestine is well established.

Diagnosis

The diagnosis is perhaps most easily made when fibrillation or a recent myocardial infarct alerts the physician to the possibility of embolism. Results of early laboratory work can be equivocal, although a markedly elevated white blood cell count is not infrequent. We have demonstrated an early and marked elevation of the level of serum lactic dehydrogenase in most of the patients. At times, infarction of the intestine is observed without organic occlusion, usually in conjunction with shock, the administration of known vasoconstrictors, or some other form of cardiovascular failure, and in particular, in conjunction with aortic insufficiency. In this respect, the splanchnic bed exhibits the same reactivity and necrotic responses that are seen precipitating renal failure and histological renal damage in shock. Mesenteric vascular occlusion may occur in children. This may be primarily arterial, primarily venous, or combined. In most of the patients no specific etiological factor could be identified.

As always, intestinal infarction can be polymorphic and due to causes other than superior mesenteric artery occlusion. Small emboli may reach distal branches of the main artery, and small segments of the intestine may be selectively affected by infarction. These cases, however, are usually diagnosed and treated with a great deal more success than those cases of massive small-bowel necrosis resulting in almost complete small-bowel resection.

Treatment

In acute occlusion of the superior mesenteric artery, early correct diagnosis and abdominal exploration will make possible the restoration of pulsatile blood flow by embolectomy or endarterectomy. The point of narrowing is usually 0.25 to 1 cm. distal to the aortic orifice of the superior mesenteric artery. About one half of the fresh occlusions are confined to the superior mesenteric artery with normal distal branches and are therefore correctable by operation. If operation is done very early, the bowel may appear to be normal but without pulsation of the superior mesenteric artery. If the bowel is dark and discolored, viability may still be retained. In such cases, if blood flow can be successfully restored, careful postoperative observation and reexploration in twenty-four to forty-eight hours is advisable to detect and resect any segment of intestine that has not recovered.

Mesenteric angina

In addition to the acute occlusions of the superior mesenteric artery, partial obstruction may result in cramping pain, particularly after meals. Such pain is analogous to the ischemic work pain of intermittent claudication in skeletal muscle. Usually both the celiac axis and the superior mesenteric artery must be affected by occlusive disease to produce symptoms. The collateral circulation is so abundant that surgical treatment may be limited to revascularization of the superior mesenteric artery by aortic–superior mesenteric artery bypass with a Dacron prosthesis or with an autogenous vein graft.

As always there are exceptions to the rule above. Matz and Kahn in 1968 reported complete asymptomatic occlusion of the celiac, superior mesenteric, and inferior mesenteric arteries in a 74-year-old man, with all occlusions demonstrated angiographically. Their review of the literature revealed the first such complete obliteration, with the visceral blood supply coming through extraperitoneal collateral vessels, described by Chiene in 1869.

At this point (1973) we do not know precisely what conditions are necessary for slowly occurring arterial stenosis in the arteries that supply the intestines to become clinically manifest. Lumbar aortograms sometimes show an asymptomatic superior mesenteric artery stenosis. In an attempt to define the problem, Koikkalainen and Köhler (1971) performed angiography of the abdominal aorta in 153 patients, many of whom had disease elsewhere, particularly in the lower limbs. They found stenosis or occlusion in some of the abdominal visceral arteries in 53.6% of the cases, with the greatest number of changes being in the celiac artery (36%). As might be expected, complete occlusion was frequently found in the inferior mesenteric artery; this condition is known to be marginally asymptomatic. Abdominal angina, however, could be verified in only 5 (3.3%) of these patients.

As a result of these studies and our own experience, it is possible to state only that the clinical diagnosis may be confirmed by angiography but cannot be made by angiography alone. The same uncertainty with regard to selective angiography therefore also exists with attempts to make a quick diagnosis of sudden occlusion of the superior mesenteric artery.

Symptoms

Symptoms of mesenteric angina include abdominal pain after meals, constipation, and weight loss. The pain is cramping in nature, develops shortly after ingestion of food, and lasts one or two hours. The patients have malabsorption and exhibit a high fat content in the feces and occult blood in the stools. Physiologically, the deficiency in blood flow to the small intestine may be confirmed by the decreased absorption of D-xylose. The cause is usually atherosclerotic occlusion or narrowing of the superior mesenteric and celiac arteries.

Many of these patients have been extensively examined and x-ray studies of them done before the diagnosis of mesenteric artery insufficiency is suspected. This circumstance combined with the fact that the patient is elderly should raise the index of suspicion to the point that the surgeon resorts to absorption tests and arteriograms.

Diagnosis

The diagnosis is made either by translumbar or by retrograde percutaneous aortography. It may be helpful and necessary to take films in the lateral decubitus position to better visualize the celiac axis and its branches. To do this by the translumbar route, it is safer to introduce a flexible Teflon catheter than to use a rigid needle. A confirmatory sign of superior mesenteric occlusion is the finding of an enlarged meandering inferior mesenteric and/or left colic artery bringing collateral circulation to the ischemic superior portion of the intestine.

In a few cases we have seen diffuse arteriosclerosis of the splanchnic arteries combined with severe signs and symptoms but with much less peripheral arteriosclerosis than one would anticipate.

In differential diagnosis one must consider nonsclerotic stenosis of the celiac axis. Although the symptoms are quite similar, celiac axis compression is usually a disease of younger persons, differentiated usually at the time of arteriography (Fig. 11-4) and remedied by releasing the artery from the surrounding fascial bands of the crus or right crural ligament of the diaphragm.

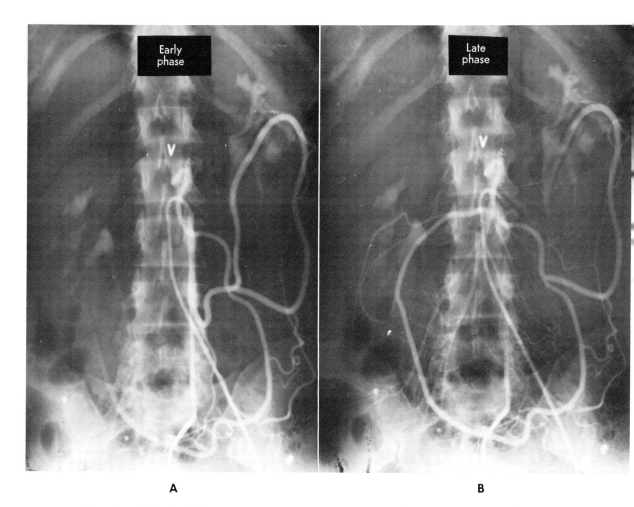

Early phase

Late phase

A   B

Fig. 11-1. Selective inferior mesenteric arteriogram in case of mesenteric angina due to occlusion of superior mesenteric artery with stenosis of celiac axis. **A,** Film soon after injection shows meandering mesenteric artery. **B,** Later film shows occluded superior mesenteric artery filled by collateral flow.

Treatment

In chronic cases of intestinal angina, bypass of the superior mesenteric artery obstruction with a vascular prosthesis is employed to revascularize the intestine. The celiac axis need not be revascularized. The superior mesenteric artery is best vascularized by a direct bypass from the aorta. Endarterectomy is more difficult and unnecessary.

Surgical exposure
Anesthesia

General anesthesia or high continuous spinal anesthesia maintained by giving small intermittent doses of the anesthetic agent is satisfactory. For this surgery high in the abdomen, adequate relaxation is essential. Usually fluids must be given vigorously, since a large amount of interstitial fluid has already been lost into the wall of the intestine. If the condition has progressed, the patient is a candidate for septice-

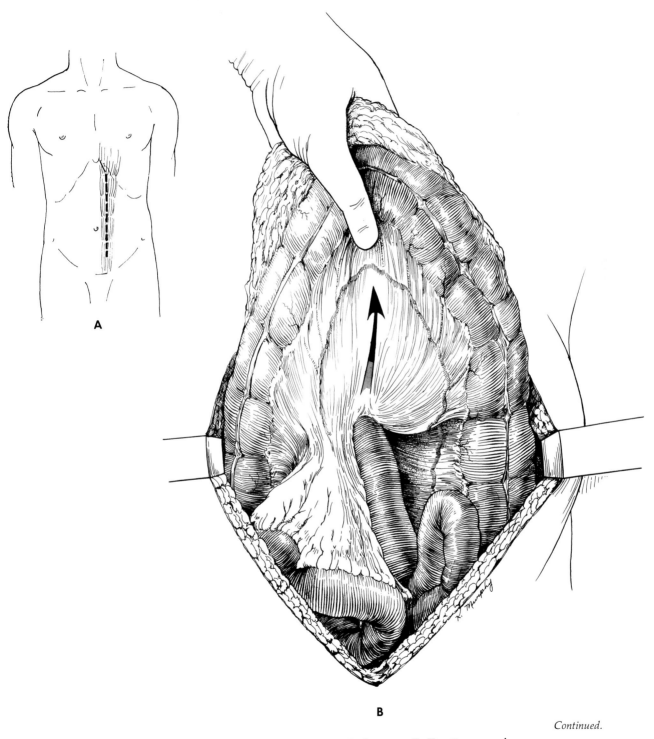

A

B

Continued.

Fig. 11-2. Exposure of superior mesenteric artery. **A,** Incision. **B,** Traction on colon, mesocolon, and middle colic artery.

277

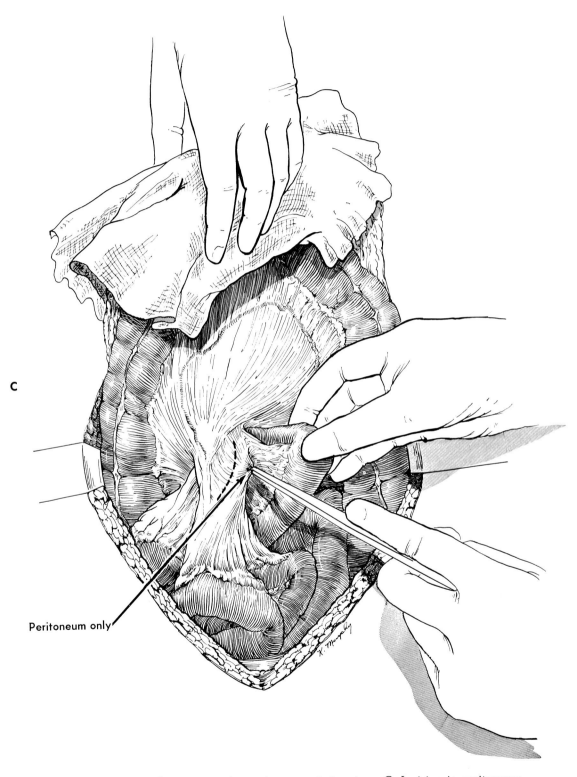

C

Peritoneum only

Fig. 11-2, cont'd. Exposure of superior mesenteric artery. **C,** Incision in peritoneum.

278

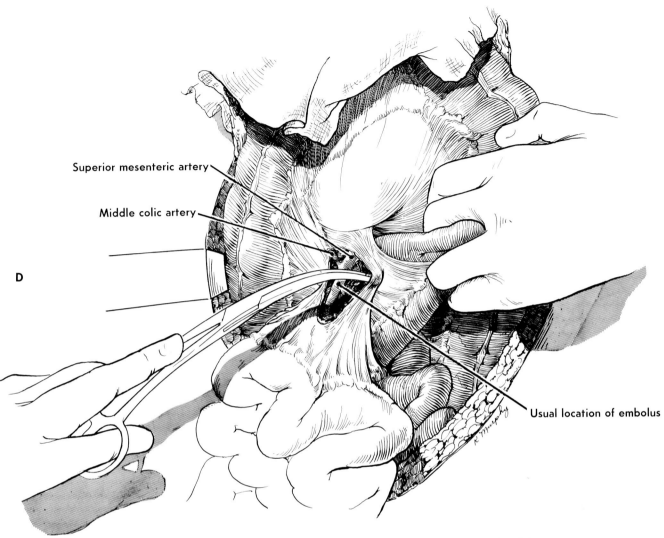

Superior mesenteric artery

Middle colic artery

D

Usual location of embolus

Fig. 11-2, cont'd. Exposure of superior mesenteric artery. **D,** Artery has been freed from surrounding tissues.

mia from gram-negative organisms and shock; both the surgery and anesthesia teams should be prepared for this event.

Procedure

Exposure of superior mesenteric artery for embolectomy or bypass

The following procedure exposes enough of the superior mesenteric artery for performing an adequate embolectomy. The usual site for lodgment of an embolus is at the origin of the middle colic artery. The superior mesenteric artery narrows considerably at this branch. When further exposure of the superior mesenteric artery is necessary, the extended exposure procedure may be used, or the balloon catheter may be passed into the proximal portion of the superior mesenteric artery to extract proximal emboli.

279

1. Open the abdomen through a long left paramedian or a midline incision (Fig. 11-2, *A*).

2. Retract the transverse colon upward and retract the most proximal portion of the jejunum to the left. When retracting, make certain that tension has been placed on the middle colic artery. This maneuver both elevates and fixes the superior mesenteric artery and facilitates the subsequent dissection. (See Fig. 11-2, *B*.)

3. Pick up the parietal peritoneum just to the right of the duodenojejunal flexure with a fine thumb forceps. Make a longitudinal incision in the peritoneum approximately 4 cm. long. The superior mesenteric artery will appear in the fatty tissue immediately beneath the incision and can be kept relatively superficial by continued traction on the colon and the jejunum (Fig. 11-2, *C* and *D*). Isolate the artery by blunt dissection with small rolls of umbilical tape. When the artery has been visualized, dissection can be carried out along its anterior aspect, exposing 3 or 4 cm. of the vessel.

Exposure of retropancreatic portion of superior mesenteric artery

1. Expose the distal portion of the superior mesenteric artery as detailed in the preceding procedure.

2. Beginning at the top of the peritoneal incision, extend the incision in the parietal peritoneum to the left along the lower border of the pancreas for 6 to 8 cm.

3. Gently and carefully divide the peritoneal attachment of the duodenojejunal flexure and the ligament of Treitz so that the duodenojejunal flexure can be retracted inferiorly. Retraction should be gentle to protect the first jejunal branches that enter the bowel from the superior mesenteric artery at this point.

4. Clamp, ligate, and divide the *inferior* mesenteric vein.

5. Dissect along the anterior surface of the mesenteric artery carefully, tunneling under the pancreas. The inferior pancreatic artery may be divided. As the dissection proceeds, place a narrow Deaver retractor under the inferior edge of the pancreas, rolling the pancreas anteriorly and exposing the origin of the superior mesenteric artery from the front of the aorta.

Restoration of blood flow

The principles and techniques of embolectomy, including the use of balloon catheters, patch angioplasty, localized endarterectomy, and bypass grafting, are described elsewhere in this book. The bypass prosthesis must be at least 8 mm. in diameter and connect the side of the superior mesenteric artery to the side of the aorta or to the side of another prosthesis. Saphenous vein grafts deserve a trial in this site as bypass tubes or for patch angioplasty.

Aortic–superior mesenteric artery bypass
Procedure

1. Prepare and expose the superior mesenteric artery as for thrombectomy or embolectomy (Fig. 11-2, *A* to *D*).

2. Expose the anterior surface of the aorta by enlarging the incision in the mesentery of the small intestine or by reflecting the mesentery to the right and incising the posterior peritoneal reflection over the aorta.

3. Select a site on the anterior wall of the aorta that is relatively free of atherosclerosis and calcification. This may be quite high. Prepare about 4 to 6 cm. of the

anterior aortic wall for anastomosis by stripping it of perivascular lymphatic vessels and other material. Circumferential exposure is not necessary.

4. Place a curved partially occluding clamp on the anterior aortic wall. Make a small anterior incision, rinse it with heparin in saline solution, and attach a vein graft or Dacron prosthesis by the usual end-to-side suture technique using 4-0 arterial polyethylene or Tevdek.

COMMENT: *Monofilament sutures glide easily through the thin-walled superior mesenteric or renal arteries.*

5. Adjust the length of the graft or prosthesis. If the aorta was exposed to the left of the root of the mesentery, a tunnel must be made through the mesentery to the superior mesenteric artery.

6. Temporarily occlude the superior mesenteric artery with tapes or vascular clamps. Make a short longitudinal incision on the posterior or lateral wall of the artery, rinse it with heparin in saline solution, and again proceed with end-to-side anastomosis. Before completing the last few stitches, check back bleeding from the mesenteric side and then flush the graft from the aortic side. Complete the anastomosis (Fig. 11-3). Before closing, check the arterial supply of the small intestine for pulsation.

COMMENT: *If the operation is performed for acute mesenteric artery occlusion in which the viability of bowel is still in doubt, take a "second look" twenty-four hours after revascularization is done. The delay permits further recovery of viable bowel and the demarcation of the bowel whose recovery is doubtful. At reoperation, bowel resection will be safe and less extensive.*

MESENTERIC AND INTESTINAL VEINS
Mesenteric and intestinal infarct

Infarction and edema of the small intestine can also originate from the venous side. It is almost impossible to make a reliable preoperative diagnosis, since the onset is slow and insidious. There is a tendency toward initial localization of pain or tenderness in the right lower quadrant, but epigastric pain and vomiting may also be an initial complaint.

The condition should be suspected of being present in those patients who have other conditions that would lead to thromboembolic disease, such as carcinoma of the lung or the pancreas, and in patients who have known thromboembolic disease, such as thrombophlebitis of the limb or pulmonary embolism.

The condition evolves from rather vague complaints of abdominal pain and tenderness to the signs and symptoms of peritonitis requiring surgical intervention. If the diagnosis is made early, anticoagulation may be helpful, particularly if the process has originated peripherally. Naitove and Weismann (1965) collected thirty-four cases plus their own and noted that nonoperative treatment produced a mortality of 100%, versus 21% for surgical treatment. Surgical mortality was zero among patients receiving anticoagulants versus 50% among patients receiving no anticoagulants, with the number of patients in each group being approximately equal.

The usual treatment is localized resection of the affected intestine. Fontaine and associates in 1969 reported emergency thrombectomy in four patients, with one recovery without intestinal resection and three recoveries that involved additional intestinal resection.

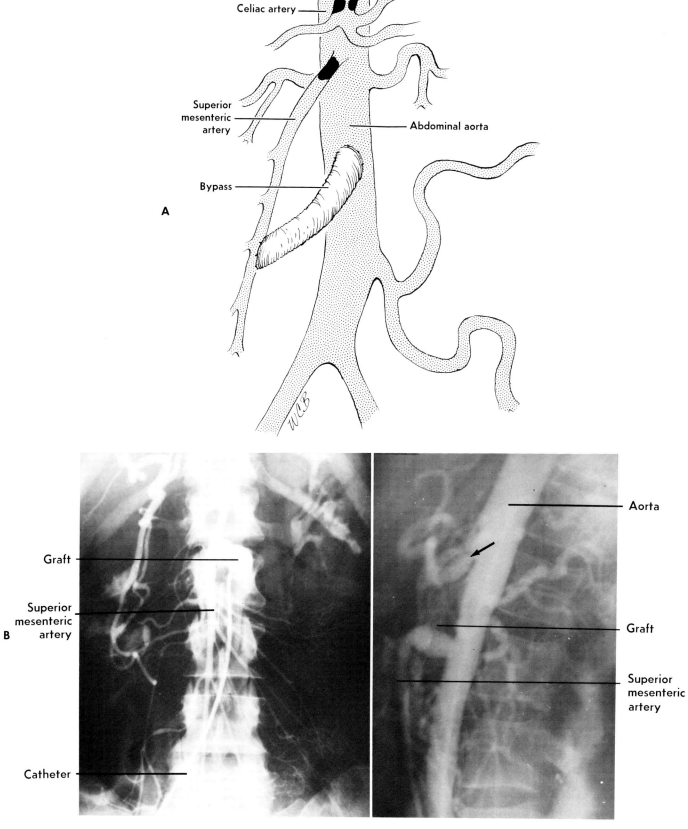

Fig. 11-3. For legend see opposite page.

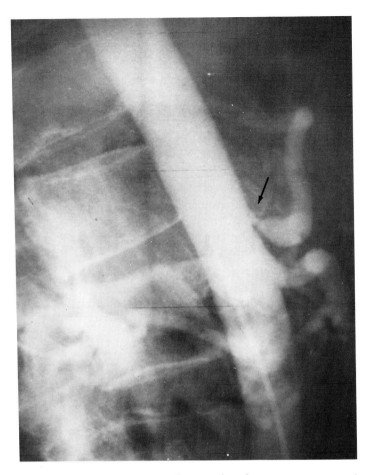

Fig. 11-4. Celiac artery compression. Lateral view of midstream aortogram. Arrow points to narrowing at origin of celiac artery. The patient was a 42-year-old man with pain after eating and 20-pound weight loss. All other x-ray films and studies were normal. He was relieved of all symptoms after patch angioplasty and regained normal weight. The postoperative angiogram was normal. In addition to compression by extrinsic bands, there was a coarctation or stricture of the artery wall that was widened with a patch angioplasty.

Fig. 11-3. A, Aortic–superior mesenteric artery bypass for occlusion of superior mesenteric artery with narrowing of celiac artery. **B,** Aortic–superior mesenteric bypass prosthesis. Anteroposterior view of selective arteriogram. Catheter introduced into aorta by transfemoral route. **C,** Aortic–superior mesenteric bypass graft. Lateral view of arteriogram. Note that graft is only 2 to 3 cm. long connecting abdominal aorta and superior mesenteric artery. Proximal portion of superior mesenteric artery is occluded. Arrow denotes stenosis of proximal portion of celiac artery.

CELIAC ARTERY
Aneurysm

Celiac artery aneurysm is a relatively rare condition but should demand the surgeon's attention because of the high death rate associated with rupture of the aneurysm. Among 44 cases collected and reported by Miller and Royster in 1971, there were thirty-two deaths from rupture of the aneurysm.

The diagnosis is made by noting a nontender pulsatile abdominal mass, and by using selective angiography.

Surgically, exposure may be gained through the gastrohepatic omentum or through a thoracoabdominal incision on the left. Only a few surgically treated cases have been reported, with the surgical procedure ranging from excision of the aneurysm and reimplantation of the celiac axis, to ligation of the left gastric, common hepatic, and the splenic arteries as they arise from the aneurysm, with or without splenectomy. The procedure of ligation of the celiac axis and removal of the aneurysm is both possible and successful. The hepatic artery in such cases must be ligated as far proximally as possible. The superior mesenteric artery may aberrantly arise from a common trunk with the celiac artery and should be preserved, bypassed, or reimplanted.

Compression syndrome

The syndrome of celiac artery compression is seldom diagnosed clinically until arteriograms are made (see Fig. 11-4). Typically patients with this syndrome are young and complain of rather relentless upper abdominal pain. Usually other conditions are sought for first, with negative results, and perhaps the gallbladder is removed. There is no weight loss or vomiting, and pain may be intermittent or follow fluid ingestion. Arteriosclerosis is not a major factor. An epigastric bruit makes one strongly suspect the presence of the syndrome, but it must be confirmed by selective retrograde angiography. Compression is best appreciated in lateral views of films of the area.

Surgical treatment is simple, mechanical, and effective. The celiac axis is freed from surrounding fibrous tissue; usually there is an abnormally low attachment of the right crural ligament of the diaphragm.

COMMENT: *The celiac artery at this level is overlain and surrounded by the large celiac ganglion of the sympathetic nervous system. Since ganglionectomy here may result in severe and intractable diarrhea, we recommend that it not be removed.*

SPLENIC ARTERY
Aneurysm

Aneurysm of the splenic artery has been recognized since 1770. Clinically the highest incidence is in the older decades of life, but there is a large enough and significant enough incidence in young women to cause the female-to-male ratio to be about 2 to 1. The condition is probably recognized more often in women because of the number of patients in whom the condition becomes symptomatic during the last trimester of pregnancy, when the aneurysm tends to rupture. The exact reason for the association of this condition with pregnancy is not understood. Other etiological factors, which are not much different from those in arterial aneurysm elsewhere, include congenital aneurysm, atherosclerosis, mycotic aneurysm, and aneurysm associated with systemic hypertension. Whether or not portal hypertension has any etiological relationship is uncertain.

Diagnosis may be made by ordinary abdominal x-ray films; these sometimes will show concentric or eggshell calcification either isolated or multiple in the left upper quadrant to the left of the first lumbar vertebra. The best confirmation of the diagnosis is obtained, of course, by selective angiography or translumbar aortography.

Elective surgery is advisable if the aneurysm is large, if the patient has hypertension, or if there is risk of rupture during pregnancy. These aneurysms do not seem to have the deadly potential of similar pathological conditions in the celiac artery.

HEPATIC ARTERY
Aneurysm

Aneurysms of the hepatic artery are relatively rare, as are those of the arteries discussed previously in this chapter. Abraham and associates in 1971 cited a previous collection of 175 cases and included one of their own, bringing the current total to 176.

The diagnosis is usually a surprise; 80% of the patients are first seen with a ruptured aneurysm, usually associated with pain, blood loss, jaundice, and bleeding into the biliary tract. As in aneurysms of the splenic artery, round calcification in the right upper quadrant may be a suggestive sign on plain x-ray films of the abdomen. Also when aneurysms have not ruptured, such upper gastrointestinal studies as gallbladder visualization or upper gastrointestinal series may show the indentation of an aneurysm on adjacent organs.

Treatment is difficult. The right hepatic artery is a common location for the condition, and ligation at this level carries with it a high mortality. When the aneurysm is located within the liver, resection of the involved lobe must be considered. Perhaps the best reconstructive maneuver after excision is to use the splenic artery as a conduit for blood to the liver. Another helpful maneuver is to preserve the gastroduodenal artery if the aneurysm is proximal to it.

The morbidity and mortality usually connected with ligating the hepatic artery or the right hepatic artery are, we believe, real considerations that cannot lightly be set aside. Therefore, every attempt should be made to secure normal blood flow to the liver.

INFERIOR MESENTERIC ARTERY

Occlusion of the inferior mesenteric artery is more common and a good deal more innocuous than similar occlusion of the superior mesenteric artery. This artery is frequently interrupted in excising abdominal aortic aneurysms, without any consequences. Ligation should always be done close to the aorta to preserve collateral vessels. In spite of this usually favorable experience, infarct of the descending colon due to occlusion of the inferior mesenteric artery has been reported. The condition can mimic diverticulitis in elderly persons. Sigmoidoscopic examination of the colon, if done early, will usually reveal color changes in the mucosa both in patients who have frank infarctions and in those who have only recently suffered occlusion of the inferior mesenteric artery and are complaining of the bloating cramps and ileus that accompany an ischemic condition that does not progress to complete infarction. The clinical picture can also resemble that of diverticulitis, and the x-ray picture may suggest obstruction. If the surgeon does not resort to laparotomy, he can make the diagnosis by sigmoidoscopy or colonoscopy or by suggestive x-ray film changes.

It is probable that in those cases in which the descending colon suffers complete infarction, the collateral circulation, particularly that from below, was incomplete or insufficient. In such cases the infarcted bowel must be resected.

C.H.C.

References

Abraham, R. A., et al.: Hepatic artery aneurysm, Angiology **22**:134-140, 1971.

Bull, S. M., et al.: Mesenteric venous thrombosis following splenectomy: report of two cases, Ann. Surg. **162**:938-940, 1965.

Cornell, S. H.: Severe stenosis of the celiac artery. Analysis of patients with and without symptoms, Radiology **99**:311-316, 1971.

Fontaine, R., et al.: Intestinal mesenteric infarct of venous origin in 2 previously unreported patients: place of thrombectomy in treatment, J. Chir. **97**:145-160, 1969.

Jackson, B. B.: Occlusion of the superior mesenteric artery, Springfield, Ill., 1963, Charles C Thomas, Publisher.

Koikkalainen, K., and Köhler, R.: Stenosis and occlusion in the coeliac and mesenteric arteries. A comparative angiographic and clinical study, Ann. Chir. Gynaecol. Fenn. **60**:9-24, 1971.

McCort, J. J.: Infarction of the descending colon due to vascular occlusion: report of three cases, N. Engl. J. Med. **262**: 168-172, 1960.

Martinez, N. S., and Khan, A. H.: The relentless symptom complex of undiagnosed celiac artery compression, Angiology **23**:198-204, 1972.

Matz, E. M., and Kahn, P. C.: Occlusion of the celiac, superior mesenteric and inferior mesenteric arteries. Angiographic demonstration in an asymptomatic patient, Vasc. Dis. **5**:130-136, 1968.

Miller, D. W., Jr., and Royster, T. S.: Celiac artery aneurysm: rationale for celiac axis ligation with excisional treatment, Vasc. Surg. **5**:42-47, 1971.

Naitove, A. and Weismann, R. E.: Primary mesenteric venous thrombosis, Ann. Surg. **161**:516-523, 1965.

Shaw, R. S., and Rutledge, R. H.: Superior-mesenteric artery embolectomy in the treatment of massive mesenteric infarction, N. Engl. J. Med. **257**:595, 1957.

12

Renovascular hypertension

RENAL HYPERTENSION

Reconstructive vascular procedures can restore blood flow and can usually correct hypertension caused by renal artery obstruction. This type of hypertension is the clinical counterpart of the renal hypertension first demonstrated by Goldblatt, who induced hypertension experimentally by restricting renal blood flow. Humoral substances (the renin-angiotensin system) are released by the ischemic kidney under certain circumstances. Renin levels are affected by many mechanisms and physiological changes, so that measurement of renin is not yet conclusive for the diagnosis of renovascular hypertension. When there is bilateral stenosis, comparison of renin levels between the two kidneys is useless. Specimens obtained from the renal veins after stimulation by hydralazine may be more reliable than basal levels of renin. Renal ischemia is probably a relatively uncommon cause of elevated blood pressure. However, as many as 25% of hypertensive patients are said to have varying degrees of renal arterial abnormalities.

In screening hypertensive patients for conditions that are correctable surgically, the surgeon should suspect that renal ischemic lesions are present in association with the following circumstances:

1. When long-standing hypertension suddenly becomes severe
2. When malignant hypertension arises suddenly, particularly in a middle-aged or older patient
3. When signs or symptoms of renal infarct precede the development of hypertension (a history or findings of unilateral renal pain and hematuria are suggestive)
4. When a hypertensive patient is unusually young and does not have a family history of hypertension

When hypertension of renal origin is suspected of being present, excretory urography with early films is the most readily available test of renal function. Films taken one to three minutes after injection may show a delay in excretion by the involved kidney. In some instances, an increase in the filtration factor on the affected side has resulted in the appearance of the contrast medium in greater density in the affected kidney fifteen to thirty minutes after injection. If this is not kept in mind, the diagnosis may be missed. The affected kidney may be somewhat smaller than the normal one.

Separated renal function tests are helpful when carefully performed and evaluated. When blood flow to the kidney is impaired, the glomerular filtration rate and the effective renal plasma flow are correspondingly reduced. On the constricted side, the output of sodium and of water will be reduced. In unilateral pyelonephritis or partial infarction of the kidney, the urinary sodium levels usually remain the same. It should not be forgotten that arterial stenosis can protect the parenchyma of the kidney distal to the stenosis, so that even though this organ shows decreased function compared to its mate, it may actually be more normal and, as a consequence, superior in function once the arterial obstruction is corrected.

Renal arteriography is the most important study for accurate location and confirmation of the diagnosis. The method of percutaneous retrograde catheterization described in Chapter 2 is usually applicable, although for patients with associated occlusive lesions of the aorta or iliac arteries, we prefer translumbar aortography. A sequence of films of the kidneys obtained with the changer is useful but not essential. Films of the oblique view are needed to see the proximal portions of those renal arteries that arise from the posterior wall of the aorta.

Renal ischemia and constriction may result from atherosclerotic plaques, thrombosis, embolism, congenital or acquired stenosis, thromboangiitis, external pressure by aneurysm, fibrous bands, tumors, or trauma. Of those named, atherosclerosis is the most common cause in older adults, and fibromuscular hyperplasia of the renal artery is the lesion most commonly encountered in young patients.

Indications for operation

Arterial reconstructions of the renal arteries are among the more difficult, since the renal arteries are small, short, and not easy to expose. For success, restoration of normal pulsatile pressure is required, not just improved flow. Therefore, correct choice of operation and precise technique are required.

Operation is not ordinarily indicated in persons over 65 years of age. The person must be a good risk for major vascular surgery. Also, clearly, no operation is justified as long as the hypertension can be controlled by medical management.

Surgical procedures

The purpose of surgical reconstruction is to restore normal pulsatile blood flow to the affected kidney. The ideal surgical candidate is a relatively young patient who has recently become hypertensive who has no atherosclerotic disease in the coronary or cerebral arteries. When reconstruction of the artery is not feasible, nephrectomy is performed. Nephrectomy is elected when the renal artery is completely occluded or the kidney is very atrophic. Various procedures to restore flow may be used according to the situation encountered (Fig. 12-1).

The procedures for atherosclerotic stenosis are frequently different from the operations for fibromuscular dysplasia because the latter is usually more diffuse and distal. Intraluminal dilation of the septa is frequently the preferred operation for fibromuscular dysplasia (see Chapter 13). Thromboendarterectomy, excision of the fibrous constriction with end-to-end anastomosis, bypass prosthesis or vein graft, splenorenal anastomosis on the left side, or implantation of the renal artery into a new site on the aorta may each be appropriate for stenosis. In doubtful cases, the pressure in the renal artery distal to the stenosis should be measured at exploration. If significant pressure difference cannot be demonstrated across the suspicious area, the correction of stenosis is only prophylactic.

Of all the surgical procedures mentioned, direct aortorenal bypass grafting is probably the most useful and the most widely applicable. In elderly patients with

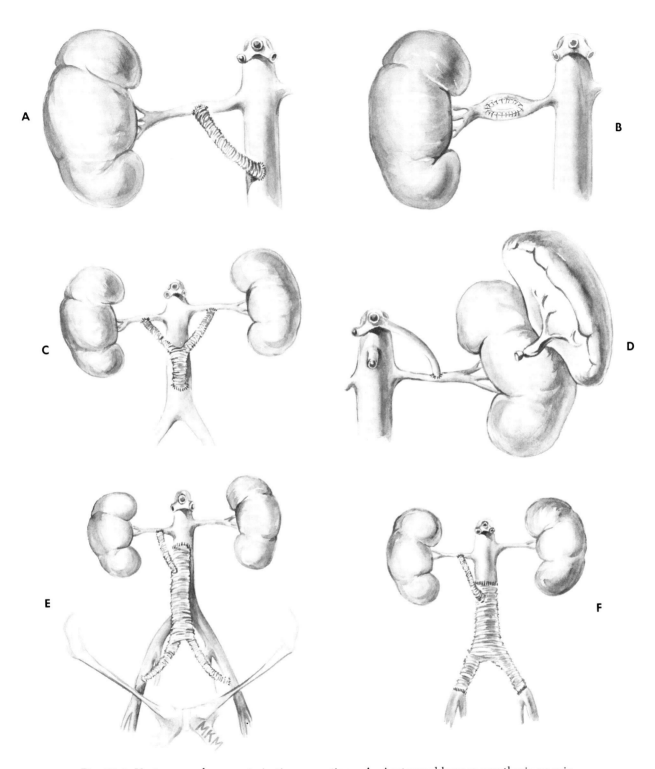

Fig. 12-1. Various renal revascularization operations. **A,** Aortorenal bypass prosthesis or vein graft. **B,** Patch angioplasty. **C,** Bilateral aortorenal bypass prosthesis. **D,** Splenorenal arterial anastomosis. **E,** Renal artery bypass from aortoiliac bypass prosthesis. **F,** Renal artery bypass from prosthesis for aortic resection.

atherosclerotic disease, this procedure may be done bilaterally or may be combined with prosthetic replacement of the aorta or with aortofemoral bypass procedures.

Anterior approach to kidney

For patients with atherosclerotic occlusions, the anterior approach must be employed, since it allows inspection of both kidneys, better exposure of the proximal ends of the renal vessels, and access to the aorta. The most useful exposure is through a long midline or paramedian incision.

Exposure of both kidneys is facilitated by several adjuncts: (1) a small sandbag beneath the eleventh and twelfth ribs and the flank to push the kidney forward, (2) an additional assistant to retract the costal margin, (3) elevation of the renal arteries by the special renal artery clamps, and (4) special deep retractors with blades 2 inches wide.

Anterior approach to proximal portions of renal arteries

Atherosclerotic lesions involve the proximal part of the artery. The exposure is an upward continuation of the exposure of the lower abdominal aorta (Fig. 3-2).

1. Make a long midline incision (Fig. 12-2, *A*). Mobilize the small bowel to the right, divide the ligament of Treitz, and reflect the duodenum to the right (Fig. 12-2, *C*).

2. Divide the inferior mesenteric vein where it crosses the aorta at the inferior border of the pancreas.

3. Isolate and lift the left renal vein with umbilical tape, and ligate and divide the adrenal and ovarian or spermatic veins (Fig. 12-2, *D* and *E*).

COMMENT: *In cases in which the aorta will be divided for concurrent aortic grafting, the maneuver illustrated in Fig. 12-3, A, displaces the renal vein posteriorly and out of the way.*

4. Retract the mesocolon upward and laterally.

5. Divide the inferior mesenteric artery if it is necessary to retract the left mesocolon laterally.

6. For access to the proximal part of the right renal artery, between the inferior vena cava and the aorta, dissect the inferior vena cava so that it is free and so that the medial edge can be rolled laterally and held laterally with a narrow deep Deaver retractor (Fig. 12-2, *E*).

7. Mobilize the proximal portions of the renal arteries and uncover the front and sides of the nearby aorta preparatory to clamping it. The origin of the superior mesenteric artery will be visualized just above the renal arteries, emerging from beneath the pancreas.

8. Palpation of the renal arteries, possibly measurement of the arterial pressure in the aorta and renal arteries, and review of the arteriograms are helpful in choosing the correct operation.

9. After choice of the operation is made, whether endarterectomy or bypass grafting, arterial clamps of appropriate size and shape are chosen so that when they are applied, they lift the renal artery anteriorly and hold the inferior vena cava and left renal vein aside (Fig. 12-2, *F*).

COMMENT: *When a concurrent operation on the abdominal aorta involves division of the aorta, the renal arteries and aorta are more accessible after the divided aorta is transposed to the front of the left renal vein (Fig. 12-3, A).*

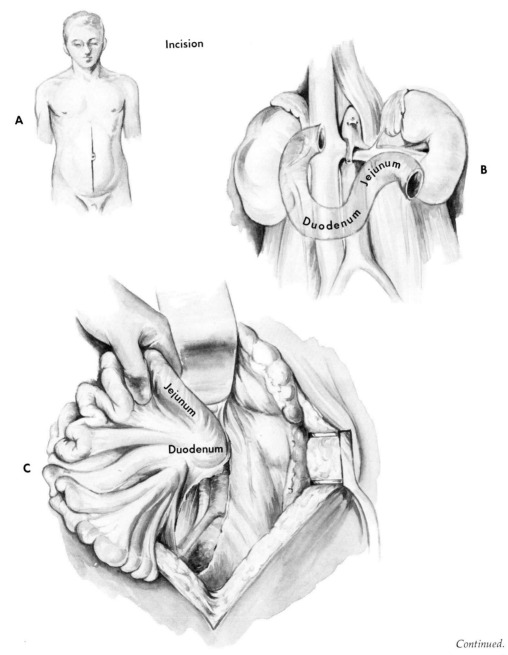

Incision

A

B

Jejunum

Duodenum

C

Jejunum

Duodenum

Continued.

Fig. 12-2. Exposure of renal arteries—midline anterior approach. **A,** Incision. **B,** Anatomical relationships of structures overlying renal arteries. **C,** Peritoneal incision and division of ligament of Treitz.

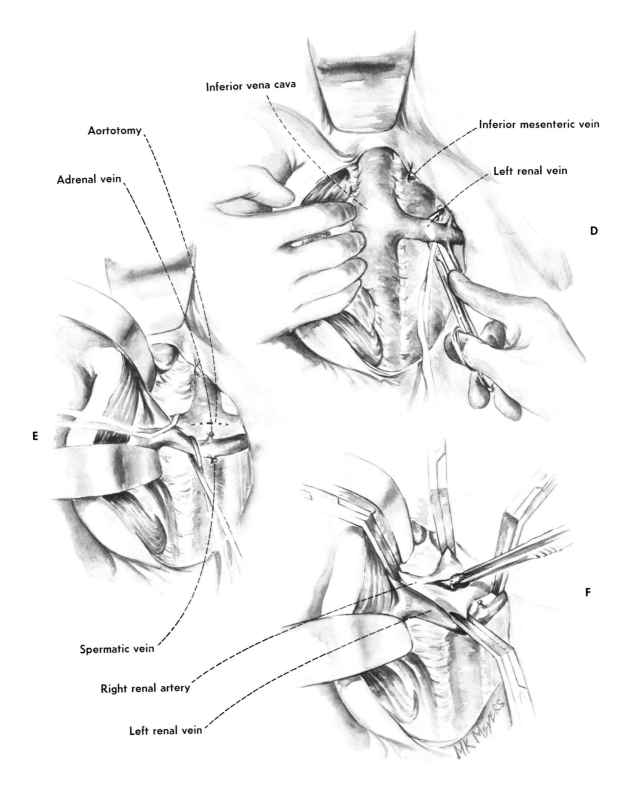

Inferior vena cava

Aortotomy

Adrenal vein

Inferior mesenteric vein

Left renal vein

D

E

Spermatic vein

Right renal artery

Left renal vein

F

Fig. 12-2, cont'd. Exposure of renal arteries—midline anterior approach. **D,** Mobilization of left renal vein. **E,** Aortotomy at origin of both renal arteries. **F,** Endarterectomy of orifices of both renal arteries through incision in aorta.

292

Bilateral renal endarterectomy

Bilateral renal endarterectomy is employed when the obstructing plaques are only in the proximal parts of the renal arteries. The endarterectomy may include adjacent plaques in the aorta. It is seldom, if ever, necessary to suture distal intima after removal of short plaques, since the distal intima will be normal. If the plaques extend farther than 1 cm. into the renal artery, bypass is preferred so that the renal arteriotomy can be short.

The choices of incisions for the endarterectomy are illustrated. If an incision extends onto the origin of the renal artery, close it with a patch angioplasty.

The surgical exposure is made via the anterior midline approach previously described and illustrated in Fig. 12-2.

1. Clamp the aorta below the superior mesenteric artery with a coarctation or angle clamp applied vertically and below the renal arteries likewise. This inferior clamp will hold the left renal vein out of the way (Fig. 12-2, *F*).

2. Inject heparin above and below this clamp (a total of 50 mg.).

3. Clamp the aorta above the renal arteries in the same fashion.

4. Temporary occlusion of the lumbar arteries posteriorly is obtained by the proper application of coarctation or angle clamps with the tips close together posteriorly or by the use of the S-shaped Craaford clamp inferiorly applied as illustrated in Fig. 4-4.

5. Transverse aortotomy is begun with the No. 15 blade, and the incision is lengthened with the Potts vascular scissors after it has been ascertained that control has been obtained by the aortic clamps (Fig. 12-2, *E*).

6. Apply the spring-handled renal artery clamp distally on the renal artery with the tip of the clamp 1 to 2 cm. deeper than the artery, which is thereby held forward and is more accessible. The clamp also holds the inferior vena cava or renal vein aside (Fig. 12-2, *F*).

7. Endarterectomy is performed by finding the plane of cleavage at the edge of the arteriotomy or aortotomy and developing this plane around the orifice of and into the proximal end of the renal artery. Tease the plaque out. Inspect the tip of the plaque that is removed. If it is thin, the distal intima is most likely normal. However, if you are in doubt, you should extend the incision onto the renal artery to permit inspection of the distal intima, which must be sutured if it is loose.

8. Irrigate the arteriotomy with dilute heparin solution to flush out detritus and to reveal loose tags of intima. The beaded cannula and syringe are useful for instilling heparin into the renal arteries.

9. Ascertain the diameter of the renal artery with Bakes dilators if you are in doubt about the caliber.

10. Release the proximal and distal aortic clamps momentarily to flush out any small clots and other material.

11. Suture the aortotomy with 4-0 or 5-0 arterial suture. If the incision extended onto the renal artery, close it with a patch angioplasty to avoid narrowing of the renal artery. Uncrimped plastic prosthesis is sewn easily and is preferred.

12. Cover the arteriotomy with Gelfoam and apply gentle pressure while you release first the distal aortic clamp, then the proximal aortic clamps, and finally the renal artery clamps.

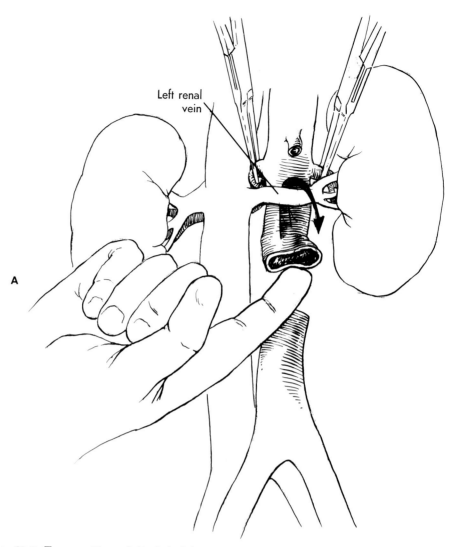

Fig. 12-3. Transposition of divided abdominal aorta for improved access to renal arteries. **A,** Divided aorta brought anterior to left renal vein.

Renal endarterectomy during operations on abdominal aorta

Occlusive disease or aneurysm of the abdominal aorta is sometimes associated with renovascular hypertension and renal artery stenosis. The renal arteries are more accessible after the divided aorta is transposed to the front of the left renal vein (Fig. 12-3).

1. Inject heparin and apply clamps as shown.

2. Divide the aorta low enough to permit a long arteriotomy close to the renal arteries after the transposition.

COMMENT: *The aortic clamp can be placed proximally above the superior mesenteric artery when endarterectomy is needed more proximally, and it may be preferable to place the clamp vertically.*

3. Mobilize sections several centimeters in length of the renal arteries; then apply

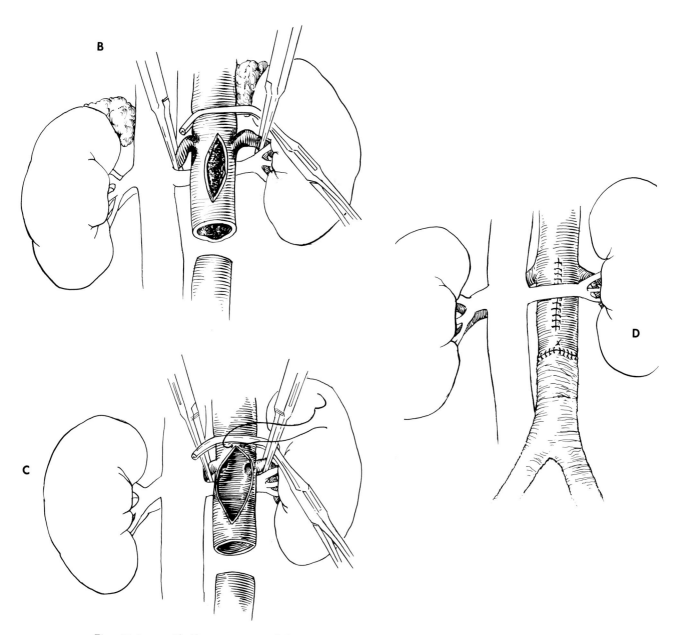

Fig. 12-3, cont'd. Transposition of divided abdominal aorta for improved access to renal arteries. **B,** Renal artery clamps placed distally so that proximal portions of renal arteries are accessible. **C,** Endarterectomy completed. **D,** Aortic bypass graft sutured with end-to-end anastomosis.

the special renal artery clamps so that a 2 cm. section of the proximal end of the renal artery humps up between the clamp and the aorta (Fig. 12-3, *B*).

4. A long arteriotomy on the aorta gives access to the orifices of the renal arteries and permits careful endarterectomy (Fig. 12-3, *B*). Develop the plane of cleavage between aortic plaque and adventitia first so that the aortic plaque is a handle while you dissect around the plaque in the renal orifices. The clamp on the renal artery should cause the proximal end of the artery to prolapse toward the aorta.

5. Gently tease out the plaque in the renal arteries by dissecting around it while maintaining gentle traction. Plaques are usually localized to the proximal 1 cm. portion of the renal artery and can be teased out with a thin tip.

COMMENT: *Loose intimal flap in the renal artery is a constant worry. When it is suspected of being present, it will usually be easier to place a bypass prosthesis distal to the flap than to try to correct the flap intraluminally.*

6. Close the arteriotomy with running sutures (Fig. 12-3, *C*). Then flush the proximal portion of the aorta and each renal artery.

7. Replace the aortic clamp below the renal arteries and restore flow to the renal arteries before completing the closure of the aortotomy.

8. Proceed with the aortic operation. Fig. 12-3, *D*, shows the aortic bypass graft placed with end-to-end anastomosis below the endarterectomy incision.

COMMENT: *In cases of aortic and renal artery stenosis, there usually is fairly generalized atherosclerosis of the iliac arteries and bypass grafts are needed (see Chapter 4).*

Bypass operations for renal artery stenosis

Bypass procedures are preferred when atherosclerotic plaques occupy more than the proximal 1 cm. portion of the renal artery. During a bypass procedure, the renal artery need be occluded only briefly, since the renal arteriotomy for bypass procedures never exceeds 8 mm. If local endarterectomy and patch angioplasty are done in such cases, longer arteriotomies are required.

The varieties of bypass procedures are illustrated in Fig. 12-1. The renal anastomosis is always distal to the arteriosclerotic plaque and the aortic anastomosis is inferior to it. Turbulence does not appear to be a problem, no doubt because the grafts are short. The aortic anastomosis may be to the side of the aorta or to the side of an aortic prosthesis if such is needed to replace the abdominal aorta.

Operations for congenital anomalies and fibromuscular dysplasia require special techniques because of their unique location and the longer life expectancy of the patients. These are discussed later.

Right renal artery bypass

The midline anterior approach was previously described and illustrated (Fig. 12-2). Good exposure of the proximal 2 to 3 cm. portion of the right renal artery is obtained by retracting the inferior vena cava to the right and the left renal vein inferiorly. Deep and narrow Deaver and Harrington retractors are essential.

1. Palpate the artery, and review the arteriograms to determine whether bypass or endarterectomy is necessary. Use a bypass if an endarterectomy would require arteriotomy longer than 10 mm.

2. Cut the end of an 8 mm. fine-knitted DeBakey or Weaveknit prosthesis obliquely, and preclot it by filling it with blood.

COMMENT: *Vein grafts in this location have a high flow and are prone to form an-*

eurysms and therefore should be used only for children or for persons with long life expectancy.

3. Prepare the site for the aortic anastomosis of the bypass graft. Although sidewise clamping of the aorta is theoretically advantageous, it is usually easier and preferable to cross-clamp the aorta for the fifteen to twenty minutes needed to anastomose the graft to the aorta.

4. Cross-clamp the aorta with vertical clamps.

5. Inject 20 mg. of heparin proximally and distally.

6. Incise the anterolateral aspect of the aorta or aortic prosthesis vertically for a distance of 10 mm.

7. Empty the preclotted graft and suture it to the aortotomy, using a double-armed 4-0 monofilament arterial suture.

8. Flush out the distal part of the aorta by releasing the distal clamp and reapplying it momentarily. Release the proximal clamp to flush out the proximal part of the aorta via the bypass tube.

9. Restore flow through the aorta after the graft is clamped close to the anastomosis. When the aortic clamps are released, any slight bleeding from the suture line is controlled by Gelfoam and gentle pressure.

10. Cut the distal end of the graft transversely at a length that reaches the renal artery without tension.

11. Lift the right renal artery with the tape around it preparatory to heparin injection and clamping. Have renal artery clamps ready.

COMMENT: *It is surprising that a 2 to 3 cm. section of the artery is accessible between the vena cava and the aorta. However, dissection is required to free the artery. Then apply the special spring-handled long-bladed clamp distally on the renal artery so that the proximal portion bows anteriorly (Fig. 12-3, B).*

12. Inject 10 mg. of heparin into the right renal artery.

13. Quickly apply the clamp distally with the artery held up and the inferior vena cava retracted far to the right. Apply the clamp at 30 degrees to the perpendicular so that it can be rotated superiorly for better access to the posterior row of sutures.

14. Apply the renal artery clamp proximally in the same fashion.

15. Make the arteriotomy 8 mm. long distal to the obstruction and on the anteroinferior aspect of the renal artery. Place small retracting stitches in the renal artery first. Hold these up while incising the renal artery with a No. 11 blade. Complete the arteriotomy with the angled Potts scissors.

16. Begin with the posterior row of sutures to anastomose the end of the bypass graft to the side of the right renal artery. Sew this back row of continuous sutures from inside the lumen. Use 5-0 arterial or polyethylene monofilament sutures, which glide easily through the thin-walled renal artery. Turn the handles of the renal artery clamps superiorly to rotate the posterior edge of the renal arteriotomy so that it is more anterior and more accessible.

17. Start the double-armed arterial suture at one end of the arteriotomy, and pass the needle through the artery and graft separately. Then pull the stitch into place, approximating the edges, using your forceps to guide the suture and edges and to avoid tearing the renal artery. A blunt nerve hook is useful.

18. Complete the posterior row, and continue the same suture anteriorly. Flush and fill the prosthesis before tying the last suture. Flush and fill the prosthesis by releasing the proximal renal artery clamp. Then tie the last suture.

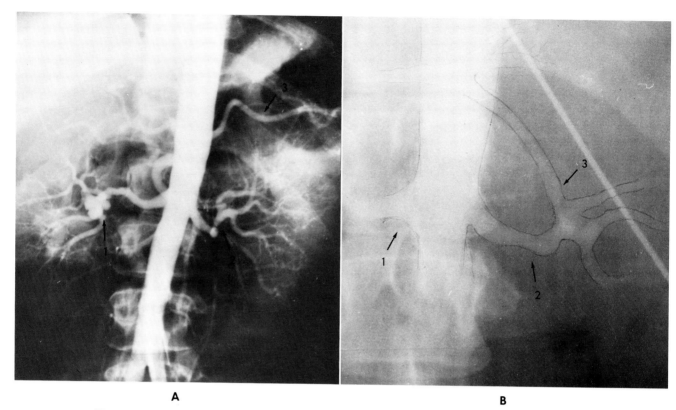

A   B

Fig. 12-4. Renal arteriograms in fibromuscular dysplasia. **A,** Preoperative film: **1,** multiple aneurysms in right renal artery; **2,** stenosis in left renal artery; **3,** splenic artery. **B,** Postoperative splenorenal arterial anastomosis: **1,** right renal artery; **2,** left renal artery; **3,** splenorenal anastomosis.

19. Release the distal renal artery clamp. Control of minor bleeding at the suture line with gentle pressure and Gelfoam must not obstruct the renal artery. Slowly release the clamp at the aortic end of the graft to restore full flow to the kidney. Then remove the proximal clamp on the renal artery.

20. Cover the prosthesis with soft tissue of the mesentery of the colon so that the duodenum is not in contact with the graft. This procedure prevents graft-enteric fistulas.

RENOVASCULAR HYPERTENSION DUE TO FIBROMUSCULAR DYSPLASIA

Fibromuscular dysplasia of the renal arteries is a rare cause of renovascular hypertension, but it is particularly troublesome because the disease usually involves most of the renal artery, may extend distally into the branches of the renal artery, and is frequently bilateral.

The disease has been recognized in various essential peripheral arteries such as the renal, coronary, internal carotid, cerebral, and popliteal. It doubtlessly occurs elsewhere but is asymptomatic in areas in which the collateral circulation is adequate.

The renal arteriograms (Fig. 12-4) show multiple short areas of stenosis with intervening dilation, giving a beaded appearance. The stenotic areas may not be obvious at operation, but the beaded areas are small aneurysms whose walls may be so thin that the blood may be seen swirling inside. In the thin bulging areas, the

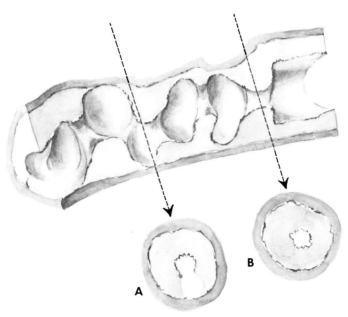

Fig. 12-5. Fibromuscular stenosis of renal artery with multiple microaneurysms (cross section **A**) and intervening fibromuscular thickenings with narrowings of lumen (cross section **B**). (Redrawn from Bernatz, P. E.: Arch. Surg. 85:608-616, 1962.)

media and internal elastic lamina are degenerated or absent. In the stenotic areas, the media is thickened by loose myxomatous tissue, or the stenosis may be due mainly to intimal thickening (Fig. 12-5). Periarterial fibrosis is seldom troublesome.

The arteriographic appearance is characteristic. There is no evidence of atherosclerosis elsewhere. The patients are young (with an average age of 35 years) and frequently have an audible murmur over the upper abdomen and flank.

Surgical procedures

Many operations have been utilized because of the extent and variety of pathological condition encountered. The difficulties for the surgeon arise because the disease usually extends to the bifurcation of the renal artery. The maneuvers to expose the distal renal artery at the hilum of the kidney are illustrated in Fig. 12-6. Access to the distal portion of the left renal artery seldom requires reflection of the colon, since the inferior mesenteric vein can always be divided and the mesocolon can be divided a considerable distance without encountering the arterial supply to the colon (Fig. 12-6, *B*). For access to the distal portion of the right renal artery, frequently rotation of the kidney anteriorly is required, since the right renal vein is short and sturdy and difficult or impossible to retract.

Dilation as first proposed for carotid fibromuscular dysplasia is usually the best operation. When grafting is necessary and feasible, autogenous vein or artery is the preferred graft material. Vein bypass from the aorta to the renal artery resembles the technique described earlier for prosthesis except that the anastomosis may be at the hilum of the kidney and may be end-to-end anastomosis of the vein graft and the distal portion of the renal artery or even a branch of it.

The splenic artery can be readily divided distally and anastomosed to the left

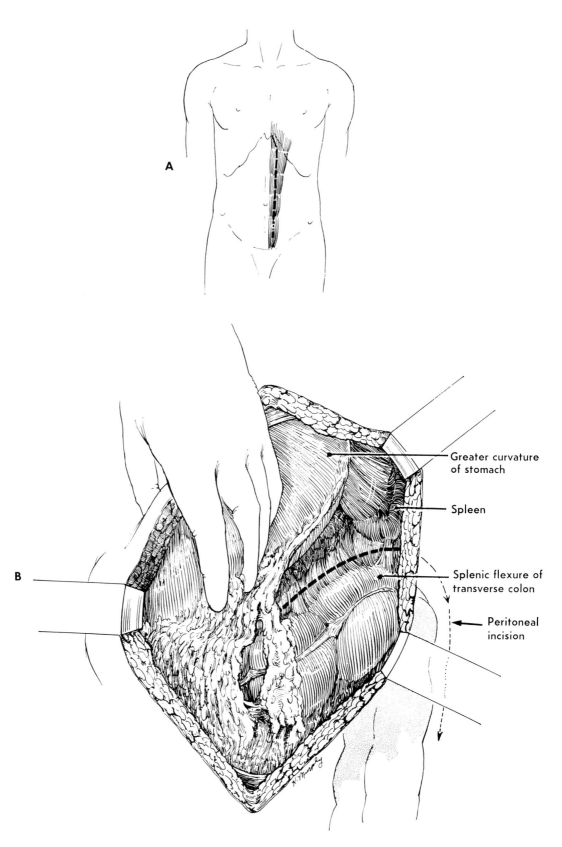

Fig. 12-6. Extended exposure of left renal artery. **A,** Incision. **B,** Peritoneal incision to uncover left kidney.

Greater curvature
of stomach

Spleen

Splenic flexure of
transverse colon

Peritoneal
incision

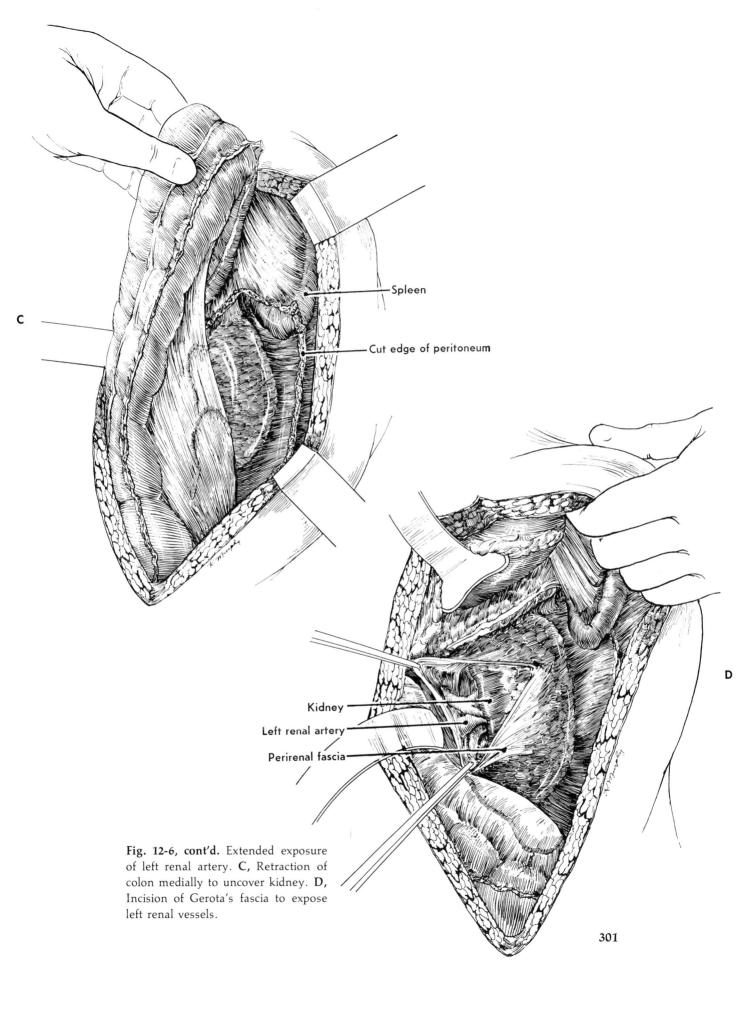

C

Spleen

Cut edge of peritoneum

Kidney

Left renal artery

Perirenal fascia

D

Fig. 12-6, cont'd. Extended exposure of left renal artery. **C,** Retraction of colon medially to uncover kidney. **D,** Incision of Gerota's fascia to expose left renal vessels.

301

renal artery without sacrifice of the spleen (Fig. 12-4, B). The body and tail of the pancreas are elevated anteriorly to gain access to the splenic artery without mobilizing the spleen or sacrificing it.

When accessory renal arteries are involved, partial nephrectomy or, in other inoperable situations, total nephrectomy is regrettable but necessary. In occasional patients, suspension of the kidney (nephropexy) to straighten the course of the renal artery is said to relieve the pressure gradient. In one patient, we widened the lumen of two stenotic primary branches of the renal artery with a vein patch in the shape of a Y whose base extended onto the main renal artery.

Intraluminal dilation for renal fibromuscular dysplasia

Intraluminal dilation was first proposed for treatment of fibromuscular dysplasia portions of the internal carotid artery but appears to be promising for treatment of renal fibromuscular dysplasia also. The thin septa are easily stretched or ruptured, but the artery is also thin and the dilators must be passed under direct vision. One can see blood swirling in the thin-walled portions of the artery. The dilator must not be passed blindly, and an attempt must be made to steady and support the artery with a finger behind the hilum while the dilator is passed. The dilator will encounter resistance at the septa, and a distinct give is felt as the dilator passes through these septa or diaphragms. The arteriotomy must be made in a normal sturdy part of the proximal part of the renal artery or aorta. Bakes common duct dilators have a malleable handle that can be bent to any desirable shape and that is stiff enough that the tip of the dilator can be accurately and safely directed. The smallest Bakes dilator must be ground so that it is smaller, that is, 1.5 to 2 mm. in diameter.

Extended approach to distal portions of renal arteries by anterior approach

The anterior midline transperitoneal approach is preferred over the flank approach. The anterior approach gives access to the aorta for bypass grafting or to the other renal artery for bilateral lesions.

Reflection of the colon is illustrated but is seldom needed to expose the full length of the left renal artery. The proximal parts of the left renal artery and vein are uncovered alongside the aorta as described on p. 290 and illustrated in Fig. 12-2. The inferior mesenteric vein is divided with impunity, and the medial part of the mesentery of the splenic flexure covers the hilum of the kidney. The mesentery is avascular between the left colic and middle colic arteries for at least several inches. The incision in the mesentery can be extended along the inferior border of the pancreas.

Reflection of the splenic flexure and descending colon gives access to the kidney for inspection and biopsy, as well as full exposure of the distal renal vessels. It also facilitates splenorenal arterial anastomosis.

1. The long midline incision has been made, and usually the proximal part of the renal artery and abdominal aorta are exposed as illustrated in Fig. 12-2.

2. Incise the posterior parietal peritoneum in the left gutter. It may be necessary to continue this up and medially to reflect the splenic flexure.

3. Uncover the kidney by retracting the splenic flexure and descending colon anteriorly and to the right (Fig. 12-6, B). Identify the ureter and renal pelvis.

4. Incise Gerota's fascia to expose the kidney and its hilum (Fig. 12-6, C and D).

5. If the aorta has not already been uncovered by the midline approach, it is

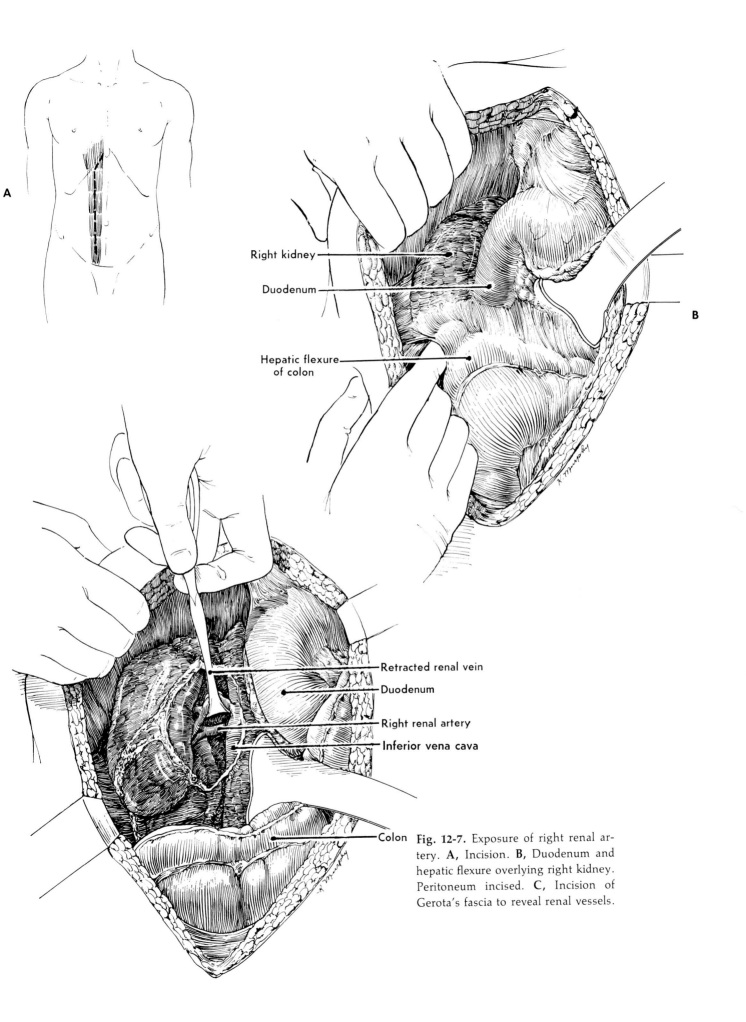

A

B

Right kidney

Duodenum

Hepatic flexure
of colon

Retracted renal vein

Duodenum

Right renal artery

Inferior vena cava

Colon

Fig. 12-7. Exposure of right renal artery. **A,** Incision. **B,** Duodenum and hepatic flexure overlying right kidney. Peritoneum incised. **C,** Incision of Gerota's fascia to reveal renal vessels.

easily accessible by further mobilization of the mesocolon. The inferior mesenteric vein may be divided if it is in the way, or the surgeon may lift it anteriorly and tunnel beneath it to the origin of the renal artery from the aorta.

Extended anterior approach to distal part of right renal artery and kidney

1. Make a long right paramedian or midline incision (Fig. 12-7, *A*).

2. Divide the avascular attachment of the hepatic flexure of the colon (Fig. 12-7, *B*) and retract it downward.

3. Mobilize the duodenum and head of the pancreas medially after incising the peritoneum to the right of the second portion of the duodenum (Kocher maneuver).

4. Dissect the lateral (right) border of the inferior vena cava and the right renal vein so that they are free. The right renal vein lies over the renal artery and is shown retracted in Fig. 12-7, *C*. Sometimes the right renal vein is so short, broad, and sturdy that it cannot be retracted enough. In such a case, mobilize the kidney and rotate it anteriorly to reveal the renal artery. When distal fibromuscular dysplasia occurs only in the right kidney, the best approach is the posterior approach through the flank incision. The proximal part of the right renal artery is accessible between the inferior vena cava and the aorta.

5. Access to the distal part of the aorta for a bypass may be obtained by tunneling under the mesentery of the small bowel and uncovering the distal portion of the aorta as illustrated in Fig. 3-2.

F.B.H.

13
Cerebral arterial insufficiency

INTRODUCTION

Localized extracranial occlusive lesions of the innominate, common carotid, internal carotid, subclavian, or vertebral arteries can usually be corrected. Most often the underlying disease is atherosclerosis, either at the origins of the great vessels from the aortic arch or distally in the neck. The more common sites of atherosclerotic disease are illustrated in Fig. 13-1. The best surgical results are obtained in patients with intermittent symptoms, partial occlusions, and no persistent neurological defect.

Postoperative arteriograms show that endarterectomized carotid arteries, once opened, remain patent and smooth for many years.

Medical success in treating hypertension has brought about a marked decrease in hemorrhagic stroke and a corresponding increase in the number of "strokes" that are due to occlusive vascular disease and/or thrombosis. Currently, the condition of the stroke victim usually must be regarded as nonhemorrhagic.

Signs and symptoms

Signs and symptoms are variable, and the correlation of symptoms and specific arteriographic findings has proved to be most difficult.

The circle of Willis is perfused by both carotid and vertebral arteries and is a splendid arrangement that can maintain and distribute blood flow despite narrowing or occlusion of one or more of the inflow arteries. If the circle is intact and occlusion develops gradually, collateral circulation develops and there may be few symptoms. However, most patients cannot tolerate acute occlusions without suffering significant neurological damage.

It is difficult sometimes to associate specific sites of extracranial arterial narrowing with specific symptoms because the collateral circulation is variable and because variable sites of intracranial atherosclerosis may accompany the correctable extracranial stenoses.

With internal carotid artery occlusion, the classic picture of homolateral visual disturbance and contralateral sensory and motor disturbance is rather rare. When atherosclerosis affects the origins of the vertebral arteries, the "basilar artery syndrome" may be produced—cortical visual loss, cerebellar and cranial nerve symptoms, and bilateral motor and sensory symptoms. As a rule, interference with the circulation from both vertebral arteries is necessary to produce this picture, provided that there is no disease in the intracranial portion of the vertebral arteries or the basilar artery itself. If arteriography shows one vertebral artery to be normal, visualization of the opposite vessel is not necessary.

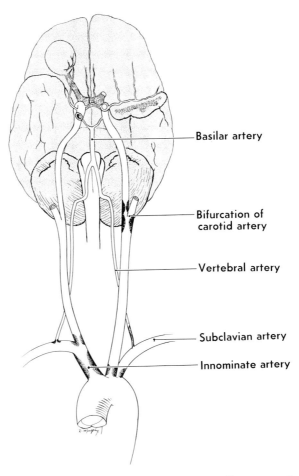

Basilar artery

Bifurcation of carotid artery

Vertebral artery

Subclavian artery

Innominate artery

Fig. 13-1. Usual sites of extracranial occlusive disease affecting cerebral circulation.

Arterial insufficiency involving the aortic arch or the carotid vessels produces recurrent hemiplegia, aphasia, paresthesias, syncope, and visual disturbances that may be unilateral or bilateral. When the aortic arch is involved, decreased pulses and decreased blood pressures in the arms may be noted. Claudication in the arm is rare. Systolic murmurs referable to the areas of narrowing may be audible. Palpation of the internal carotid pulse in the tonsillar fossa is unreliable.

Arteriograms are essential to demonstrate extracranial occlusions, and they offer the best estimate of the degree of obstruction. A 20 mm. Hg pressure gradient across the stenotic area is clincially significant, and such a significant fall in the pressure gradient may be predicted if there is a 50% reduction in the arterial lumen as seen on the preoperative arteriogram. Ulcerated plaques cause transient attacks by embolism from particles and small fibrin thrombi and should be removed even though they do not cause significant obstruction in the neck. Regrettably, there are no reliable arteriographic signs of ulceration (Fig. 13-2). The method of arteriographic survey by right transbrachial-cerebral combined with left carotid arteriography is described in detail in Chapter 2. This method shows both carotid arteries and the right vertebral artery and is sufficient for almost all cases.

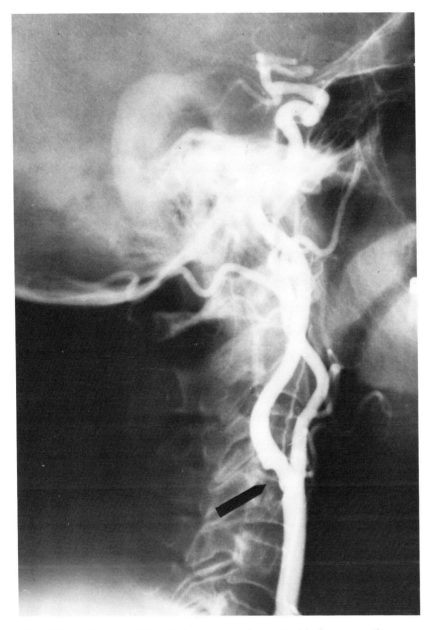

Fig. 13-2. Carotid arteriogram. Ulcerated plaque is shown by black arrow. There are no reliable arteriographic signs of ulceration of these plaques.

The pathological causes of extracranial occlusions or narrowing are usually atheromatous plaques at the major bifurcations. Tortuosity of the internal carotid artery may cause symptoms by kinking. Vertebral artery occlusions may result from external pressure by osteophytic spurs, constricting bands, and the like. Compression of the opposite carotid artery usually causes prompt slowing of the waves on the electroencephalogram. Compression can be released before untoward symptoms or alarming attacks develop. These tests and complete neurological work-up are essential. A coincidental brain tumor was found in several of our patients with extracranial arterial occlusion.

Reconstructive procedures and choice of operation

The surgical objective is to restore normal flow and pressure to the circle of Willis and to relieve symptoms due to small emboli from the surface of the ulcerated plaques. Operations relieve ischemic and embolic attacks and restore cerebral blood flow. Operations prevent strokes, but like other procedures on patients with atherosclerosis, they may not prolong life. The life expectancy of these patients is short because complications of atherosclerosis may occur in the heart or kidneys or elsewhere.

The best results from arterial vascular reconstruction of the extracranial portions of the cerebral circulation are obtained in patients with intermittent neurological signs and symptoms and no residual neurological damage. Surgical results are poor in patients with recent or progressive strokes. The results of a current cooperative clinical study clarify indications and contraindications for carotid endarterectomy. The risks are higher when both internal carotid arteries are narrowed.

The surgical procedures currently in use are endarterectomy, patch angioplasty, and bypass grafting. The bypass method is most applicable when obstruction involves the origins of the great vessels at the aortic arch, whereas endarterectomy is more applicable to the common and internal carotid arteries. The preferred procedure for localized plaque at the origin of the internal carotid artery is localized endarterectomy with patch angioplasty.

Narrowing at the origins of the vertebral arteries may be treated by endarterectomy of the subclavian artery and patch angioplasty at the origin of the vertebral arteries.

Fig. 13-3. Varieties of internal shunts for carotid artery. **A,** Javid shunt. **B,** Javid shunt inserted in common and internal carotid arteries. **C,** Polyvinyl flexible tubes with diameters 12, 14, and 16 Fr. Ligature at upper end permits withdrawal via small aperture without bending of tube. **D,** Shunt being withdrawn from internal carotid artery just prior to completion of patch angioplasty. **E,** Tapered vinyl tubing with outside diameter 5 to 14 Fr. To assure maximum flow, estimate size of internal carotid artery and cut off excess taper to within 2 cm. of desired diameter. Long pieces can be used like the Javid shunt, or shorter pieces can be cut and used as in **F.** (**A** and **B,** Javid shunt No. CB 7954 1852 supplied by U. S. Catheter and Instrument Corp., Glen Falls, N. Y. **C** and **D,** Polyvinyl tubes No. 1885 supplied by U. S. Catheter and Instrument Corp., Glen Falls, N. Y. **E,** Tapered tube 5M0287 [old code U510] supplied by Travenol Laboratories, Inc., Morton Grove, Ill.)

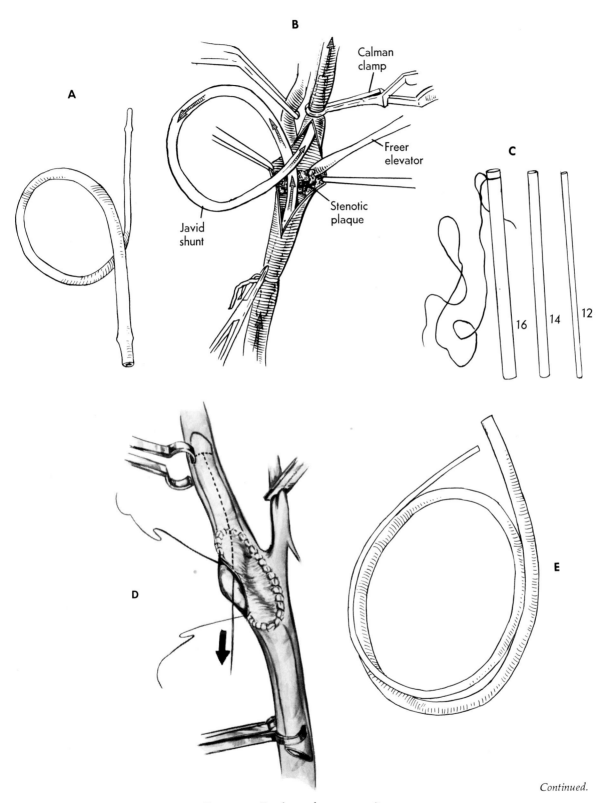

A

B

Calman clamp

Freer elevator

Stenotic plaque

Javid shunt

C

16   14   12

D

E

Fig. 13-3. For legend see opposite page.

Continued.

309

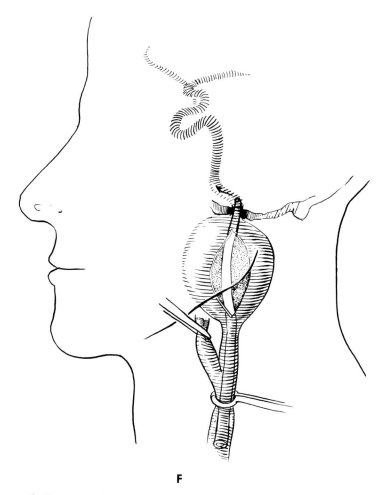

F

Fig. 13-3, cont'd. Varieties of internal shunts for carotid artery. **F,** Tapered shunt wedged into internal carotid canal during operation for aneurysm extending up to base of skull. (Tapered tube 5M0287 supplied by Travenol Laboratories, Inc., Morton Grove, Ill.)

Operations for tortuosity, external compression, and the like are improvised according to the situation encountered. Symptoms referable to tortuosity may be relieved by nothing more than surgical mobilization. In some patients, the internal carotid artery may be detached and reimplanted at a lower level.

It has been widely held that a completely occluded internal carotid artery is inoperable. This is usually true. However, we believe that recent occlusions with definite contralateral symptoms should be explored. Operability can be determined at low risk by opening the internal carotid artery above the bifurcation and not clamping the common or external carotid arteries. Particularly when embolism may be the cause of the occlusion, we have employed the Fogarty balloon catheter, passing it distally as far as the carotid siphon. By this method, otherwise inaccessible clots can be extracted. In a few cases excellent back bleeding from the distal part of the internal carotid artery has been obtained and flow restored.

Special measures to support the cerebral circulation are helpful. The anesthesiologist should maintain blood pressure and ensure adequate oxygenation. An internal shunt allows longer periods of occlusion with safety, and clamps and plastic tubing suitable for shunting are always included in the surgical setup (Fig. 13-3).

Internal shunts

The internal shunts are simple, they conduct a large flow, and no additional needle punctures and the like are required. The internal shunt permits ample operating time for a long arteriotomy, complete endarterectomy, careful reattachment of the intima, and secure closure. It also permits safe operation with the use of general anesthesia on patients with stenosis or occlusion in the opposite carotid artery. We have never regretted using them.

We have used the three varieties illustrated in Fig. 13-3. For most purposes the long Javid shunt is preferred. The short vinyl tubes are also effective. They are removed by traction on a tie at the upper end as illustrated in Fig. 13-3, *B* to *D*. The tapered catheter (Fig. 13-3, *E*) can be wedged into the orifice of the internal carotid artery at the base of the skull; therefore, no clamp around the upper portion of the internal carotid artery and shunt is needed. This is essential for operation on high aneurysms of the extracranial portion of the internal carotid artery (Fig. 13-3, *F*).

CAROTID ENDARTERECTOMY
Indications, signs, and symptoms

Carotid endarterectomy is the removal of atherosclerotic plaques at the carotid bifurcation; it is done to restore normal pulsatile blood flow in the internal carotid artery, relieve cerebral arterial insufficiency, and prevent internal carotid artery thrombosis. The usual indication is localized stenosis at the carotid bifurcation, producing a narrowing of 50% or more in one arteriographic view. Plaques that are ulcerated cause transient attacks by recurrent embolism from tiny emboli and should be removed even though there is no mechanical obstruction or significant stenosis. Basilar artery insufficiency can usually be relieved by correction of internal carotid artery stenosis, which increases pressure and flow in the circle of Willis.

The signs and symptoms are discussed at greater length on p. 305 and in general are intermittent motor weakness, paresthesia, aphasia, and visual disturbances.

Arteriographic visualization of the cerebral circulation is best accomplished by right transbrachial-cerebral arteriography combined with arteriography of the left common carotid artery. It must be demonstrated that the partial stenosis is symptomatic and the atherosclerotic block is extracranial. Neurological consultation is helpful and has revealed coincidental tumors. Carotid artery compression during electroencephalography is a safe and significant test of flow through the opposite carotid artery and cross cerebral collateral circulation. When compression of a carotid artery causes slowing of the alpha waves in the electroencephalogram, there is significant obstruction of the cerebral flow from the opposite side.

Occasionally, a complete unilateral carotid occlusion will be found without significant neurological defect. Operation is not advisable if there is generalized cerebral arteriosclerosis, if complete occlusion of the internal carotid artery has been present for more than one week, or if there is an acute or progressing stroke.

Anticoagulant treatment has been used by some physicians in preference to surgery. However, anticoagulants do not remove the obstruction and frequently fail to relieve the symptoms. Patients with intracerebral occlusions or thromboses may benefit from anticoagulant therapy, and anticoagulants appear to be helpful in some

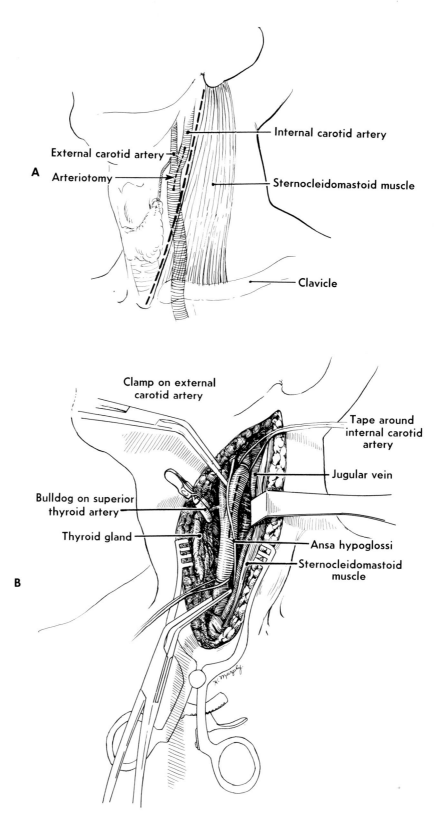

Fig. 13-4. Carotid endarterectomy with patch angioplasty. **A,** Incision. **B,** Exposure of carotid bifurcation.

cases in which there are vertebrobasilar symptoms. Agents to decrease platelet adhesion and prevent platelet thrombi are being tested.

Anesthesia

Carefully administered light general anesthesia is preferred in order to maintain blood pressure and consequent cerebral blood flow across areas of critical stenosis. The suggestion has been offered that the addition of carbon dioxide to the anesthetic mixture will result in additional cerebral vasodilation and total blood flow. At this time, we prefer routine internal shunting. This step takes only a few minutes and allows unhurried meticulous surgery, long arteriotomy, and patch angioplastic closure. Improved catheters, techniques, and special clamps have simplified the shunt procedure (Fig. 13-3).

Procedure

Place the patient in the supine position, turning his head slightly away from the side to be operated on. Avoid hyperextension of the head and neck if there is associated basilar artery insufficiency.

Exposure

1. Incise the skin along the anterior border of the sternocleidomastoid muscle (Fig. 13-4, *A*). In short necks, carry the incision to the mastoid process.

2. Retract the sternocleidomastoid muscle and the internal jugular vein laterally. Divide the anterior facial vein, the cervical fascia, and the omohyoid muscle.

3. Open the sheath of the common carotid artery near the bulb. Infiltrate the tissue near the bifurcation with local anesthetic.

4. Expose the front of the common carotid artery for about 2 cm. above and below the bifurcation. Avoid embolism from the surface of the plaque. Uncover the vessels, but do not lift or disturb the bifurcation until the internal carotid artery is clamped. Employ careful perivascular dissection and separate the artery from the internal jugular vein. Divide or retract the ansa hypoglossi.

5. Expose the internal carotid artery up to the parotid gland. Dissect along the posterior border of the internal carotid artery first, in order to avoid the hypoglossal nerve, which crosses it. Expose a section several centimeters in length of the external carotid artery as well. Occlude the superior thyroid artery with a temporary ligature or a Schwartz clip. Identify the hypoglossal nerve. Rarely, the plaque is long or the neck is short, and the hypoglossal nerve must be retracted upward.

COMMENT: *The amount of exposure necessary varies according to the length of the atherosclerotic plaque. It is not necessary to free the entire artery except where clamps will be applied. Umbilical tapes are used around the internal shunt but are unnecessary when Javid or Calman clamps are available to hold the shunt in place (Fig. 13-5, B).*

Preparation of Dacron prosthesis patch

1. Cut a strip of thin Dacron intracardiac patch material about 5 to 10 mm. in width and several centimeters longer than the intended arteriotomy. The thin intra-auricular cardiac patch material is best.

2. Tag the lower end with a 2-0 black silk suture, and round the corners of the opposite (upper) end.

3. Place a double-needle 5-0 arterial suture through the upper tip of the patch.

313

4. Preclot the patch with a small amount of blood from the incision or from the jugular vein.

Arteriotomy and insertion of internal shunt

1. Inject 3,000 units of heparin. Clamp the internal and then the common and external carotid arteries (Fig. 13-4, *B*).

COMMENT: *The DeBakey angled clamps are ideal for this purpose, since the handles lie flat and out of the way of the operator.*

2. Incise the anterolateral aspect of the internal carotid and the common carotid arteries for the full length of the plaque to be removed and an additional 5 mm. The incision divides the plaque close to its edge. Check for back bleeding from the internal carotid artery.

3. Insert the internal shunt as diagrammed in Fig. 13-5, *A*, and secure it in place with Calman or Javid clamps. If these special clamps are not available, loops of umbilical tape secured by a hemostat may be improvised.

COMMENT: *The best shunt is the Javid tube illustrated in Fig. 13-3. It is easily turned from side to side or retracted as you dissect inside the artery. Other soft, thin-walled polyvinyl tubing 10 to 14 Fr. in diameter can also be used. Prior to insertion of these short shunts, tie a stout suture at the upper end of the internal shunt for traction during its removal later.*

4. Restore flow to the internal carotid artery via the shunt by removing the occluding clamps on the carotid arteries.

Endarterectomy

1. Develop a plane of cleavage between the plaque and the media of the artery (Fig. 13-5, *A*). Tease the plaque away from the arterial wall, and dissect it with a Freer elevator. The circular muscular fibers of the arterial media appear beneath the plaque as it is removed. Sometimes the media is adherent to the plaque, and the only remaining layer of the arterial wall is the adventitia. This is thin but sturdy.

2. Free the plaque until it is attached superiorly by thin, normal intima. Lengthen the arteriotomy if necessary. With blood flowing through the internal shunt, there is no hurry, and thickened intima superiorly almost always can be removed. It is almost never necessary to leave loose thick intima, which formerly needed to be reattached and held in place with sutures.

3. Free the plaque inferiorly down into the carotid bulb, and tease it out of the orifice of the external carotid artery. One can readily work around the internal shunt. Fig. 13-5, *C*, shows how the shunt can be rotated to the left.

COMMENT: *It is permissible to perform blind endarterectomy only in the external carotid artery, that is, the technique of loosening plaque and pulling it out of the artery until it is teased out. The external carotid artery should be freed up so that it can prolapse toward the orifice and the plaque inside can be loosened and extruded. The plaque comes off under direct vision if it is short, and in such a case, the endarterectomy is not truly blind even though the incision does not extend onto the external carotid artery.*

4. The plaque in the common carotid artery below the stenosis is usually 1 mm. thick. This continues proximally and does not need to be removed. Use the deeply curved endarterectomy scissors to cut away the stenotic portion. Trim any loose edge inferiorly with the scissors.

COMMENT: *The arteriotomy can be lengthened superiorly, but it is never necessary*

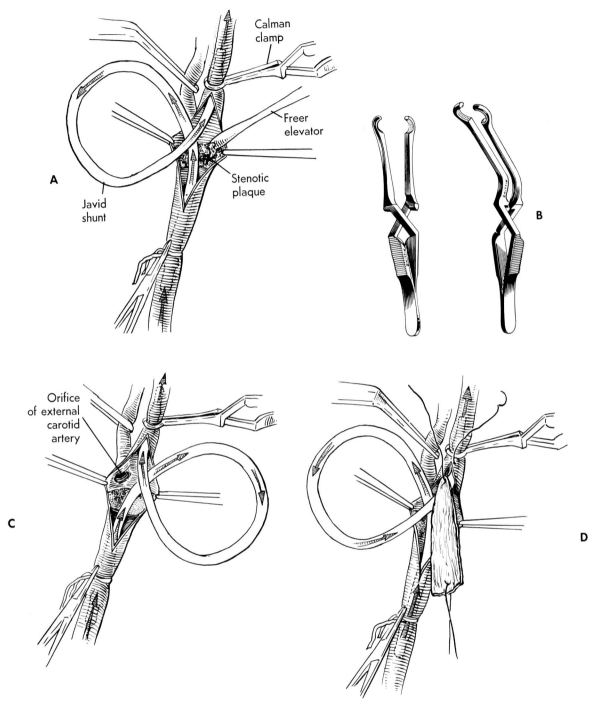

Calman
clamp

Freer
elevator

Stenotic
plaque

A

Javid
shunt

B

Orifice
of external
carotid
artery

C

D

Continued.

Fig. 13-5. Carotid endarterectomy with internal shunt and patch angioplasty. **A,** Javid shunt in place. Stenotic plaque peeled away. **B,** Calman clamps to hold internal shunts in place. **C,** Shunt rotated for completion of endarterectomy. **D,** Patch angioplasty begun.

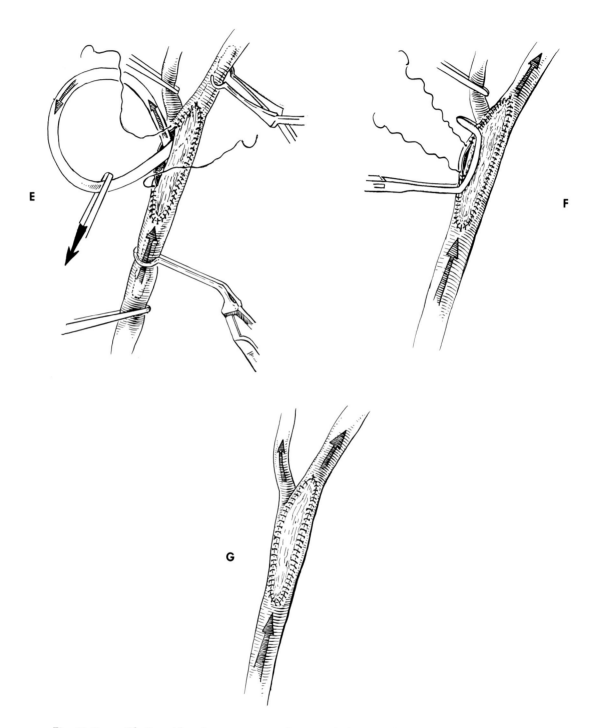

Fig. 13-5, cont'd. Carotid endarterectomy with internal shunt and patch angioplasty. **E,** Shunt being withdrawn from internal carotid artery. **F,** Flow restored to internal carotid artery during completion of patch angioplasty. **G,** Patch angioplasty completed.

to extend it more than 1 to 2 cm. inferiorly. A small strip of thickened intima is safely left proximally in the common carotid artery.

5. Irrigate the lining of the artery with heparin in saline solution, and inspect it carefully to wash out debris or tease out fragments still attached. Any loose shreds of media should be teased away to leave a smooth lining.

Closure of arteriotomy by patch angioplasty

The internal shunt has restored cerebral blood flow during meticulous endarterectomy and closure. We use this patch angioplasty for secure closure of all arteriotomies of the internal carotid or other arteries of this size. For secure closure, a large bite of the arterial wall is required, including adventitia 1 to 2 mm. from the edge of the arteriotomy. This may appear to be crude externally, but when the suture is pulled so that it is snug, the inside is very smooth. The wide cuff necessary for a secure closure narrows the lumen of the internal carotid artery unless a patch is interposed between the edges of the arteriotomy.

1. Irrigate and remove all debris and clots from the arterial lumen.

2. For the first stitch, pass one of the needles out of the superior end of the arteriotomy, and secure the stitch by tying it with a square knot to hold the apex of the patch in place (Fig. 13-5, *D*).

3. Sew the patch to the posterior edge of the arteriotomy, proceeding from above downward with an over-and-over stitch passing from the prosthesis to the artery. The assistant must hold the suture so that is taut in order to pull up the edges for ready access and rapid placement of the sutures. The second assistant pulls the inferior edge of the patch downward with the previously attached silk suture, holding it steady and in place.

4. Trim the patch to correct size and shape as the posterior suture line is completed.

5. Begin the anterior closure by continuing the posterior row around the bottom of the patch, ascending on the anterior side of the arteriotomy, and then sewing downward from above with the other limb of the double-armed suture. Do not complete suturing of the inferior end of the anterior edge of the patch. Leave an aperture for removal of the shunt (Fig. 13-5, *E*).

Removal of internal shunt and completion of patch angioplasty

1. Suture the portion of the patch on the internal carotid artery, leaving an aperture inferiorly for removal of the internal shunt tube (Fig. 13-5, *E*). This aperture should be on the common carotid inferior part of the arteriotomy.

2. Irrigate with heparin in saline solution so that no shreds or threads of clot or detritus remain inside the artery.

3. Loosen the clamps or tapes holding the shunt in the internal carotid artery, and withdraw the tip of the shunt and cross-clamp the internal carotid artery for a few moments while removing the shunt and flushing the artery. Pinch or cross-clamp the shunt. Also, remove it from the common carotid artery and cross-clamp the common carotid artery.

4. Flush the internal, external, and common carotid arteries and check the back bleeding in these arteries, and reapply the occluding clamps momentarily.

5. Apply the small tangential occluding clamp to the unclosed edge (Fig. 13-5, *F*). Then release the external carotid artery clamp and note any bleeding from the

patch or suture line; cover it with Gelfoam later. Next release the common carotid artery clamp so that blood flows into the external carotid artery for a few moments in case there are any minor emboli. Lastly, unclamp the internal carotid artery and restore flow to the brain.

6. Complete the patch angioplasty (Fig. 13-5, G). Apply a pad of Gelfoam soaked in topical thrombin to the patch if it oozes or leaks at suture holes.

7. Tie the final suture, release the tangential clamp, and apply the Gelfoam sponge to the remainder of the Dacron patch for complete hemostasis.

Closure of incision

1. Suture the carotid sheath over the vessels and the patch.
2. Close the cervical fasciae, platysma, and skin in layers.
3. No drain is needed.

Postoperative care

It is essential to maintain systolic blood pressure 10 to 20 mm. Hg higher than the patient's normal blood pressure. Vasopressors may be needed.

Antibiotics are given preoperatively and postoperatively when a Dacron patch is used. The use of anticoagulants is unnecessary unless the occlusion was embolic. A liquid diet during the first few days will prevent undue discomfort during swallowing. Hypotension and hypertension should be treated or prevented.

Neurological complications of carotid artery operations

The choice of patients is highly important in avoiding neurological complications. The surgeon should wait five to eight weeks after an acute stroke before attempting to restore flow, or hemorrhage may occur in the infarct. Hazards of operation for bilateral stenoses can be minimized with the use of good anesthesia and internal shunts. Both sides are never done simultaneously.

Endotracheal general anesthesia is preferable to the regional block that we formerly used. The anesthesiologist can and must maintain the blood pressure 20 to 30 mm. Hg above the patient's normal systolic pressure before carotid artery clamping and during the shunting. The systolic pressure can be maintained with vasopressors if it is unstable or low. The value of hypercarbia is debatable, but it is clearly unnecessary to ventilate the patient vigorously.

Blood pressure must be well maintained in the recovery room and monitored closely for several days. Some patients will require vasopressors. Hypotension and hypertension are dangerous.

Meticulous technique has already been discussed. Intimal flaps must be prevented. The arteriotomy must be lengthened so that the edge of intima is seen and can be sutured if it is loose. In some patients, especially diabetics, thin intima is loose and extends far up the internal carotid artery. This should be reattached with mattress sutures tied outside the artery. The intima may be soft. The sutures must not be pulled so tight that they tear through the soft intima.

The bulb of the carotid artery must not be palpated or manipulated in the region of the plaque until the internal carotid artery is clamped. Ulcerated plaques cannot be recognized until the artery is opened, and debris is easily dislodged.

In expert hands, neurological complications will occur in no more than 5% of the cases, and most of these complications will be minor.

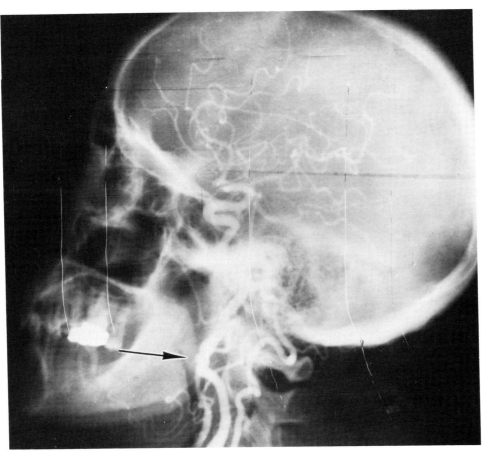

Fig. 13-6. Arteriogram showing fibromuscular dysplasia of internal carotid artery. Arrow points to area of dysplasia. Some irregularity is also seen in artery near base of skull.

FIBROMUSCULAR DYSPLASIA OF INTERNAL CAROTID ARTERY

Fibromuscular dysplasia is a rare cause of internal carotid artery stenosis and transient ischemic attacks in young people (Fig. 13-6). The pathological appearance and the arteriographic appearance have been discussed on p. 298 as they apply to the renal arteries. The arteriographic appearance is unique. Multiple areas of stenosis and dilation give a beaded appearance (Fig. 12-4). The stenoses are not always apparent at operation, but the appearance of the thin-walled tiny aneurysms is dramatic (Fig. 13-6).

Fibromuscular dysplasia presents a formidable technical challenge because the process frequently extends high up into the internal carotid artery near the base of the skull. Morris, Lechter, and DeBakey (1968) introduced the technique of internal dilation of the strictures, and this appears to be of lasting value. The natural history of the disease is unknown, but the disease is correctable by this method and does not appear to be progressive. Fibromuscular dysplasia usually occurs in long segments and/or zones that are frequently inaccessible. The only feasible operation on these is dilation. The dilation appears to be highly successful but must be done carefully, since fragile artery can be torn.

Lateral approach to internal carotid artery

Exposure of the upper part of the internal carotid artery is easier when the incision is made posterior to the sternocleidomastoid muscle. Incision along the posterior border of the sternocleidomastoid muscle gives easier access to the upper part of the internal carotid artery because it is unnecessary to divide the structures that cross the artery anteriorly and particularly because the hypoglossal nerve does not need to be lifted and retracted and dissected free of the troublesome veins that accompany the nerve.

The sternocleidomastoid muscle and the jugular vein are retracted anteriorly. The vagus nerve lies lateral to the carotid artery. The accessory nerve lies posteriorly. Both are well out of the way.

The common carotid artery is accessible over a longer length than with the anterior approach. The bifurcation lies in the middle of the operative field. Sufficient length of the external carotid artery can be uncovered to control it.

Procedure for dilation of artery in fibromuscular dysplasia

1. Prepare a graded series of Bakes common duct dilators by grinding a No. 3 dilator to 2 mm. in diameter.

COMMENT: *The Bakes dilator's malleable handle can be shaped to conform and to permit accurate manipulation of the tip of the dilator.*

2. Incise the skin along the posterior border of the sternocleidomastoid muscle. Retract it and the jugular vein anteriorly. Expose the full length of the internal carotid artery so that the dilator may be passed with the use of direct vision. Dissect along the posterior border of the artery to avoid the hypoglossal nerve.

3. Make a small transverse arteriotomy in the normal proximal portion of the common carotid artery where the arterial wall is sturdy and the arteriotomy can be sutured without causing stenosis.

COMMENT: *The other steps of obtaining control proximally and distally need not be detailed here. In this discussion, we are presuming a working knowledge of the basic principles and anatomy (Fig. 3-4).*

4. Pass the dilators with the use of direct vision. A finger behind the internal carotid artery is helpful in steadying it so that the dilator can be directed accurately.

5. The artery is thin and redundant in the involved segment. Blood may be seen swirling inside thin-walled dilated segments. The dilator encounters resistance at the septa, and a distinct give is felt as the dilator is passed through these septa or diaphragms. The dilator is passed until it impinges on the carotid foramen.

COMMENT: *If a slight rent is made, suture the defect with fine sutures, using the dilator as an internal stent.*

6. Occasionally, to complete the operation, endarterectomy may be required because of a plaque at the origin of the internal carotid artery, or reimplantation may be required because of redundancy or kinking (Fig. 13-7).

TORTUOSITY OR KINKING OF INTERNAL CAROTID ARTERY

Tortuosity, which is sometimes a complete loop, usually causes no symptoms and is probably a congenital anomaly (Fig. 13-7, *A*). Kinking is rare and may be accompanied by plaque formation (Fig. 13-7, *B*). Tortuosity or kinking may be a cause of minor stroke or transient ischemic attacks. Since it is difficult to see *intermittent* kinking in arteriograms taken in only one view of the head and neck,

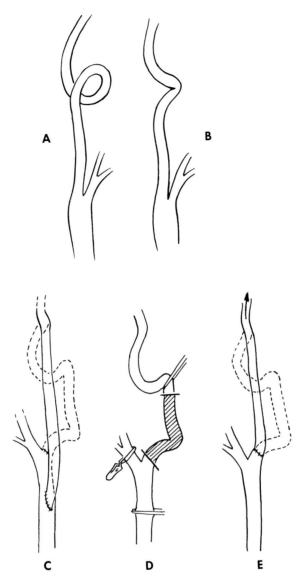

Fig. 13-7. Operations for tortuosity or kinking of internal cartoid artery. (Redrawn from Najafi, H., Javid, H., Dye, W. S., Hunter, J. A., and Julian, O. C.: Kinked internal carotid artery: clinical evaluation and surgical correction, Arch. Surg. **89**:134-143, 1964. Copyright 1964 by American Medical Association.)

arteriographic findings of tortuosity are sufficient indication of kinking unless another cause of the symptoms is found. Najafi (1964) has given a good review of the clinical and technical problems encountered.

The procedure of shortening the artery, straightening it, and reimplanting it is usually best (Fig. 13-7, *C*). Reimplantation of the redundant artery lower on the common carotid artery may not be sufficient; resection may be required as well because of plaque or other lesion (Fig. 13-7, *D* and *E*). Use of the internal shunt is advisable during occlusion of the internal carotid artery for these anastomoses

321

(Fig. 13-3). Other operations have been improvised to relieve or prevent kinking, such as the use of slings, lysis of adhesions, and division of bands.

ANEURYSMS OF EXTRACRANIAL PORTION OF INTERNAL CAROTID ARTERY

Aneurysms of the extracranial portion of the internal carotid artery are rare but challenging lesions. They may be traumatic or atherosclerotic. Aneurysmorrhaphy may be the only feasible treatment when the aneurysm is high and distal resection or anastomosis is not feasible. The procedure of resection and restoration of continuity with prostheses is preferred when feasible. The external carotid artery should be preserved or reimplanted and not ligated; reimplantation is facilitated when you save a flare or cuff of the aneurysm to use as the cuff (Figs. 6-9, B and 6-10, B,).

It is possible to obtain distal control above a high aneurysm near the base of the skull only inside the aneurysm. A No. 2 or 3 Fogarty balloon catheter can be passed up to the siphon and inflated to stop the back bleeding. However, the use of the internal shunt is always preferable to long occlusion times. We have used the tapered flexible vinyl catheter for this purpose (Fig. 13-3, E). This Travenol vinyl catheter tapers from 14 to 5 Fr. in outside diameter. It can be cut wherever the size is correct. In the case illustrated in Fig. 13-8, the tapered tip of the catheter was wedged into the orifice of the internal carotid artery at the base of the skull, and the proximal end was held in the common carotid artery with the Javid clamp. In this case, no resection or anastomosis was feasible at the upper end. The lining of this aneurysm was smooth intact endothelium; therefore, endoaneurysmorrhaphy was performed (Fig. 13-8, B and C).

BASILAR ARTERY INSUFFICIENCY
Diagnosis and indications

Basilar artery insufficiency is manifested by visual disturbance, cerebellar symptoms, and bilateral mixed cranial nerve and spinal nerve motor and sensory symp-

---

Fig. 13-8. High internal carotid aneurysm. A, Tapered internal shunt wedged into internal carotid artery at base of skull. B and C, Restoration of arterial continuity by Matas' endoaneurysmorrhaphy. We quote from Matas as follows: B, "Shows a possible but not yet tried method of restoring the large lumen of the parent artery in favorable cases of fusiform aneurism with two openings in which the healthy and flexible character of the sac will permit the restoration of the arterial channel by lifting two lateral folds of the sac and bringing them together by suture over a soft rubber guide. The principle of this operation is precisely like that adopted in a Witzel gastrostomy. The figure shows the soft rubber catheter lying on the floor of the sac and inserted in the two orifices of communication. The sutures are placed while the catheter is in position acting as a guide." In our case, A, the vinyl catheter was an internal shunt. C, "This shows a more advanced step of the procedure described in B. The sutures are nearly all tied, and the new channel is completed except in the centre. The two middle sutures are hooked and pulled out of the way while still in position, and the catheter is withdrawn. The obliteration of the sac and final steps of the operation are carried out precisely as previously described." See Fig. 6-13. (Quotes from Matas, R.: An operation for the radical cure of aneurism based upon arteriorrhaphy, Ann. Surg. 37:161-196, 1903.)

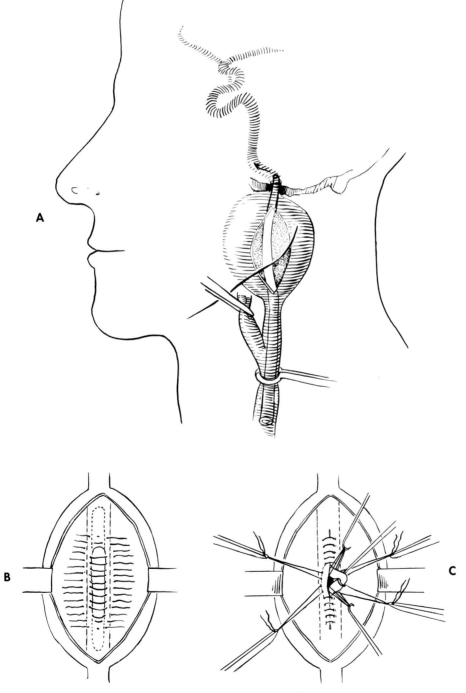

Fig. 13-8. For legend see opposite page.

toms. It may result from stenosis or atherosclerosis at the origin of the vertebral artery from the subclavian artery. Unilateral occlusion is seldom symptomatic; therefore, repair of only one artery is an adequate surgical procedure. Sometimes restoration of flow in a stenotic carotid artery relieves basilar symptoms. When carotid artery stenosis is associated with symptoms of basilar artery insufficiency, surgical relief of carotid artery stenosis may, at times, be all that is possible or necessary. Since increase of cerebral circulation in the circle of Willis may relieve basilar symptoms, surgery correcting carotid occlusions is usually helpful.

In the subclavian steal syndrome, the vertebral artery is open, and symptoms of basilar insufficiency are due to cerebrifugal or retrograde flow down the vertebral artery, which supplies collateral circulation to the arm around an occluded subclavian artery (Fig. 13-9, *A*). Symptoms due to the subclavian steal may be more severe than those from occlusion of the vertebral artery. Occasionally, the same syndrome is due to occlusion of the innominate artery. Bypass operation to perfuse the obstructed subclavian artery is the best method by which to restore normal pressure and flow (Fig. 13-9, *B*).

In all patients, a preoperative radiographic survey, including transbrachial-cerebral arteriography on the right and common carotid arteriography on the left, should be made (see Fig. 13-10).

Surgical approach to vertebral artery

Usually the origin of the vertebral artery may be approached through an incision along the upper border of the clavicle. Rarely, extended exposure is necessary for dangerous lesions such as traumatic aneurysms or arteriovenous fistulas. For these, subperiosteal resection of the clavicle or splitting of the upper part of the sternum in the midline and extension of the incision into the third intercostal space on the

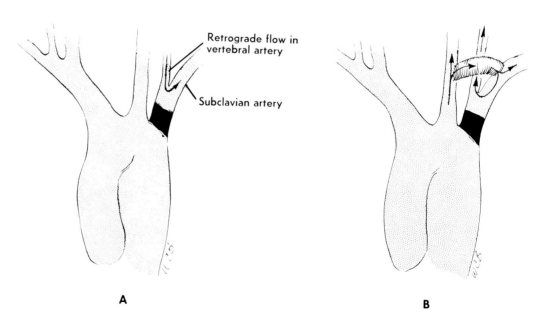

A

B

Fig. 13-9. A, Subclavian steal syndrome. Retrograde flow of blood from subclavian artery occlusion. **B,** Carotid-subclavian artery bypass for subclavian steal.

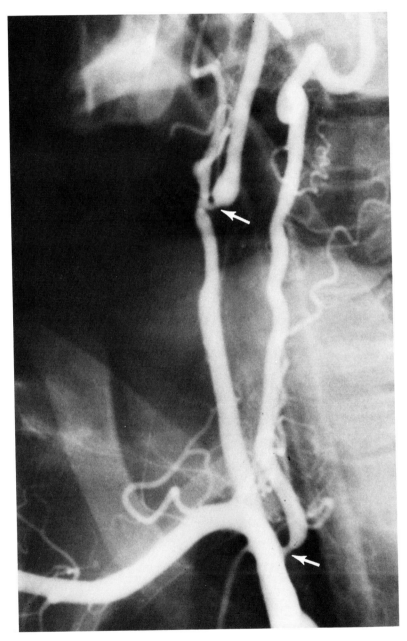

Fig. 13-10. Right transbrachial arteriogram. Top arrow shows marked stenosis at origin of internal carotid artery. Bottom arrow shows stenosis at origin of vertebral artery.

affected side may be required. The vertebral artery is visualized during the approach to the stellate ganglion, which is described as a portion of supraclavicular cervical sympathectomy (Fig. 15-4). The origin of the vertebral artery and other branches of the first portion of the subclavian artery may be visualized by a continuation of this procedure and blunt dissection downward along the medial side of the subclavian artery. To expose the vertebral artery, the deepest layer (prevertebral or prescalene layer) of the cervical fascia must be divided medial to the anterior scalene muscle and the phrenic nerve. It is necessary to divide the anterior scalene muscle. The phrenic nerve, the recurrent laryngeal nerve, and the thoracic duct are contiguous structures that must be protected. Extended exposure of the vertebral artery is seldom necessary. Descriptions of the surgical approaches to the upper portions of the vertebral artery in its extracranial course can be found in other publications.

Choice of operative procedure

For localized plaques at the origin of the vertebral artery, local endarterectomy with or without patch angioplasty is the best treatment. No operative procedure is indicated for partial occlusion of only one vertebral artery, since the collateral supply to the basilar artery is excellent.

Anesthesia

Because the pleura may be inadvertently opened, general endotracheal anesthesia is advisable.

Procedure—vertebral endarterectomy

1. Place the patient in the supine position, with the neck extended and slightly rotated away from the side to be operated on.
2. Make a supraclavicular incision (Fig. 13-11, *A*).

Exposure

For more details and drawings of the following steps, see Fig. 15-4.
1. Divide the clavicular head of the sternocleidomastoid muscle if the cervical approach is employed. Divide the entire insertion of the sternocleidomastoid muscle if the cervicothoracic incision is employed.
2. Divide the omohyoid muscle.
3. Retract the prescalene fat pad laterally.
4. Retract the jugular vein and carotid artery medially.
5. Identify the phrenic nerve or nerves on the anterior surface of the anterior scalene muscle.
6. Divide the anterior scalene muscle. Retract the phrenic nerve medially. The prevertebral layer of deep cervical fascia is divided in the direction of the phrenic nerve and is retracted medially, holding this and the other structures in the carotid sheath medially.
7. Identify and spare the thoracic duct on the left. If the duct is injured, ligate it to avoid the development of a troublesome lymph fistula.
8. Ligate and divide the thyrocervical trunk at its origin from the subclavian artery.
9. Dissect along the subclavian artery bluntly, using a finger or small dissecting sponge, until the innominate artery is reached on the right or the aortic arch on the left.

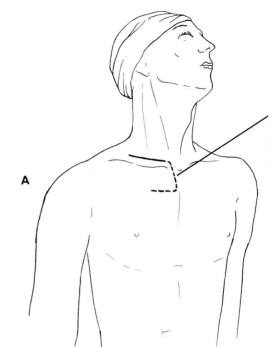

Sternal and intercostal extension for proximal control of aneurysms

A

Fig. 13-11. Vertebral artery—patch angioplasty. **A,** Usual incision. Dotted line shows sternum-splitting incision for patients with thick necks or low origin of vertebral artery. **B,** Patch angioplasty completed.

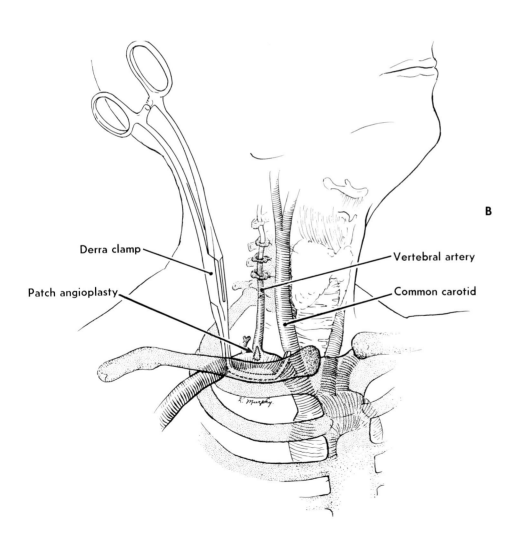

B

Derra clamp

Patch angioplasty

Vertebral artery

Common carotid

10. Divide the vertebral vein if necessary. Inferiorly, this lies anteriorly and laterally, but near the entrance of the vertebral artery into its foramen in the transverse process of the sixth cervical vertebra, the vertebral vein covers the artery.

11. Depress the pleura. It need not be freed laterally or anteriorly.

COMMENT: *The internal mammary artery may be visualized anteriorly with the phrenic nerve close behind or anterior to it.*

Proximal and distal control

1. Select a single deeply curved partially occluding clamp. The Derra clamp is ideal. This will serve as a handle and permits traction upward on the subclavian artery, allowing ample room for the arteriotomy (Fig. 13-11, *B*).

2. Inject 30 mg. of heparin in 30 ml. of normal saline solution into the subclavian artery while the clamp is held in position ready to be closed.

3. Close the Derra clamp to obtain proximal and distal control of the subclavian artery as illustrated in Fig. 13-11, *B*.

4. Obtain distal control of the vertebral artery just proximal to the sixth cervical vertebra with a delicate clamp. Separate and ligate the fragile vein if necessary.

Arteriotomy and endarterectomy

1. Make a vertical arteriotomy in the proximal vertebral artery, and extend it upward distal to the vertebral plaque and also into the subclavian artery.

2. Momentarily release the distal clamp to check for back bleeding.

3. Remove only a circumferential or ulcerated plaque. If endarterectomy proves to be unnecessary, only enlargement of the arterial lumen by patch closure (below) is done.

4. Suture the intima in the vertebral artery if it seems to be loose and might occlude the lumen.

5. Irrigate the area and flush out clots.

Patch closure of arteriotomy

The technique of patch angioplasty is described in detail on p. 317 and illustrated in Fig. 13-5, *D*. Interposition of a triangular patch between the edges of the arteriotomy permits secure placement of sutures in the adventitia 1 to 2 mm. from the edge of the arteriotomy and enlarges the lumen of the vertebral artery. It is simple to place a prosthetic patch. Vein patches may dilate in vessels of large diameter.

Closure of incision

Lungs and pleura are reexpanded with positive pressure and by aspiration. For details, see the closure after cervicothoracic sympathectomy in Fig. 15-4. Complete expansion of the lung is obtained by suction on an *extra*pleural catheter.

OPERATIONS FOR OCCLUSIVE DISEASE OF AORTIC ARCH AND ITS BRANCHES
Signs, symptoms, and indications

Various bypass procedures are useful when occlusive disease involves the aortic arch and the origins of the major branches to the head and arms. Occlusion may be complete or incomplete, and multiple sites of involvement are frequently found. A nonspecific arteritis (Takayasu's disease, pulseless disease) occurs in young women, with obliteration of the subclavian artery or innominate artery or both. Otherwise, the cause of obstructive lesions is usually atherosclerosis. Signs and symptoms referable to interference with blood supply to the brain are discussed on p. 306. Murmurs are audible in the neck or above the clavicle, differences of blood pressure and pulses in the two arms are noted, and occasionally weakness or pain in the arm occurs after exercise.

In special instances, attacks of basilar artery insufficiency are induced by exercise of the arm; this is a type of the subclavian steal syndrome. In patients with this condition, occlusion of the subclavian artery or, on the right, the subclavian or innominate artery may be found. Exercise involving the arm of the affected side causes retrograde flow in the vertebral artery on that side, inducing the cerebral symptoms. The simplest solution, if the innominate artery is not involved, is ipsilateral common carotid–subclavian arterial shunt with a Dacron prosthesis. (See Fig. 13-9, B.)

Corrective surgery can usually restore pulsatile pressure and normal flow with bypass prostheses from an uninvolved common carotid or subclavian artery. It is usually unnecessary to assume the risks of thoracotomy to attach the origin of the graft on the aorta. Fig. 13-12 shows a variety of bypass operations at the root of the neck. Physiological measurements and clinical experience have proved that flow increases and may double in the parent artery proximal to the bypass, so that the bypass does not steal blood from the brain or the normal arm in order to perfuse its outflow vessels.

Choice of operation

In most patients, bypass from carotid artery to carotid artery or from subclavian artery to carotid artery may be accomplished in the neck without resecting the clavicle and without entering the chest. We have done a few operations via the small right anterior thoracotomy, as described in the second edition. It was unnecessary to split the sternum, and the operation was well tolerated. However, this operation or endarterectomy in the branches close to the aortic arch is more difficult, requires wider exposure, and carries a higher mortality than the bypass procedures in the neck.

The general plan of all these bypass procedures is much the same. The proximal end of the prosthesis is sutured to the side of a normal common carotid or subclavian or axillary artery on the same side or on the opposite side. The distal end is implanted past the obstruction. End-to-side anastomoses are always feasible.

Endarterectomy of vessels with obliterative panarteritis should not be attempted. Endarterectomy should be employed only for very localized and readily accessible plaques.

Bypass to carotid or subclavian artery
Surgical exposure
Lateral approach to carotid artery

Incision along the lateral edge of the sternocleidomastoid muscle gives easy access to both the carotid artery and the apex of the subclavian arch. For exposure of the carotid artery, retract the sternocleidomastoid muscle and jugular vein anteriorly. The vagus nerve is lateral to the artery. A longer length of the proximal part of the common carotid artery is accessible than with the anterior approach, and

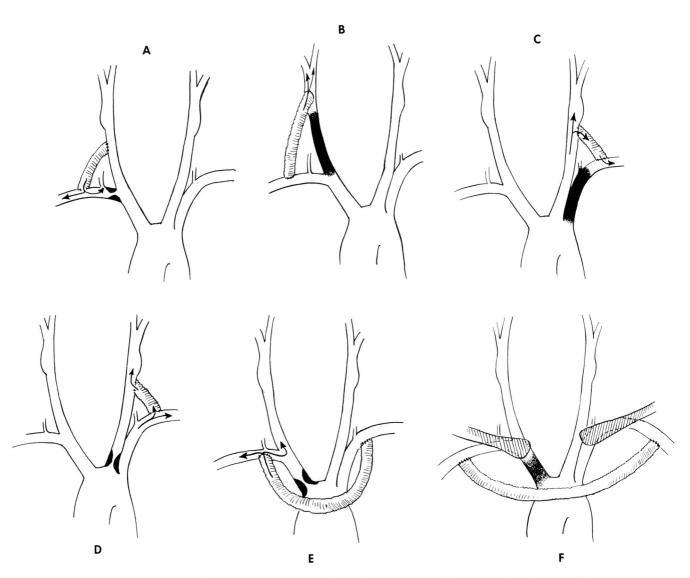

Fig. 13-12. Various bypass operations in neck. **A,** Bypass on right from carotid artery to subclavian artery for stenosis. **B,** Bypass on right from subclavian artery to carotid artery for stenosis. **C,** Bypass on left from carotid artery to subclavian artery for occlusion of subclavian and vertebral arteries. **D,** Bypass on left from subclavian artery to carotid artery. **E,** Bypass from left subclavian artery to right subclavian artery for innominate artery stenosis or occlusion. **F,** Axilloaxillary bypass (infraclavicular).

330

it is unnecessary to divide or displace the veins, the omohyoid muscle, and the other structures encountered anteriorly.

Supraclavicular approach to subclavian artery

The supraclavicular approach to the subclavian artery is described on p. 370 and illustrated in Fig. 15-4. The transverse incision above the clavicle gives excellent exposure.

Procedure

The proximal anastomosis is made to the side of a normal common carotid or subclavian artery on the same or opposite side of the neck. The distal anastomosis is made past the obstruction or stenosis. Sometimes two obstructed arteries can be bypassed with a Y graft fashioned from a 10 mm. and an 8 mm. tube sutured together. Prostheses 8 mm. in diameter function well in these locations because the outflow is large. The grafts are short and need not bend much or kink. The patient's veins should be saved for other purposes. The angle of takeoff or of attachment should not be a concern. The turbulence from acute angles of anastomoses is well tolerated.

1. Attach the proximal anastomosis first, preclot the prosthesis under pressure, and restore flow through the parent artery by clamping only the prosthesis until the second anastomosis is finished.

2. For anastomosis to the subclavian artery, use the most accessible protion, that is, the top of the arch of the subclavian artery, and sew the posterior row of sutures from inside the lumen of the subclavian artery.

3. For anastomosis to the common carotid artery, retract the jugular vein anteriorly after dividing or retracting the clavicular head of the sternocleidomastoid muscle. Review the lateral approach to the carotid artery (p. 320). Suture the posterior row of sutures from inside the lumen of the common carotid artery. Long occlusions of the common carotid artery can be bypassed by attaching the graft at the bifurcation of the carotid artery. A local endarterectomy may be needed, and an internal shunt should be used if the internal carotid artery will be temporarily occluded.

4. Avoid compression in the neck. Grafts from one subclavian artery to the opposite side of the neck can cross the manubrium subcutaneously instead of crossing the sternocleidomastoid muscles. No pain or erosion of the bone has been caused by the overlying grafts.

5. Review the anatomy. Beware of the phrenic and vagus nerves and the brachial plexus.

6. Review the general principles of flushing, irrigation, and other procedures. Prevent embolism to the head.

Aortic arch bypass
Indications

It will be a rare case in which the origin of the bypass cannot be attached to an open subclavian or common carotid artery in the neck or to the axillary artery just below the clavicle. Occasionally, however, the graft must originate in the chest. This transthoracic procedure can be performed without splitting the sternum. The graft is attached to the ascending aorta via a short right intercostal incision.

Preoperative preparation

Satisfactory arteriograms are necessary. Serial films are helpful after selective catheterization of the various branches of the aortic arch. Neurological consultation and medical evaluation of the cardiopulmonary status are very helpful. Preoperative digitalization is advisable.

Anesthesia

Since the chest will be opened, general endotracheal anesthesia must be employed. Blood pressure and adequate oxygenation must be maintained to ensure adequate cerebral blood flow during the short period of occlusion.

Choice of incision

The ascending aorta is exposed through an incision in the right third intercostal space (Fig. 13-13, *A*). The subclavian arteries are exposed through supraclavicular incisions, rarely aided by subperiosteal resection of the clavicle. A vertical incision along the posterior border of the sternocleidomastoid muscle offers ready access to the carotid artery (Fig. 13-13, *A*). At times a larger transverse cervical incision or a combination incision may be necessary. Exposure of the vertebral artery is discussed on pp. 324 and 326.

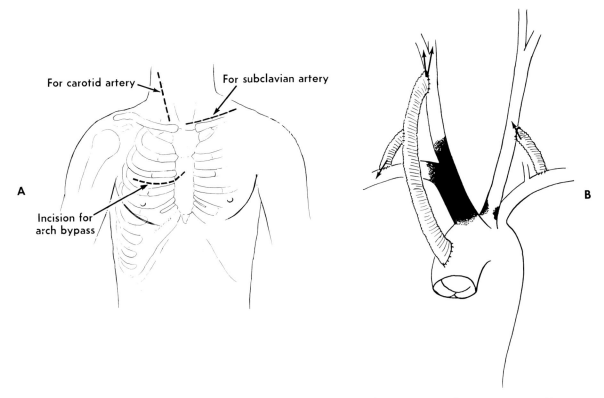

Fig. 13-13. Arch bypass. **A,** Incisions. **B,** Bypass from ascending aorta to right common carotid and right subclavian arteries. Bypass from left subclavian artery to left common carotid artery.

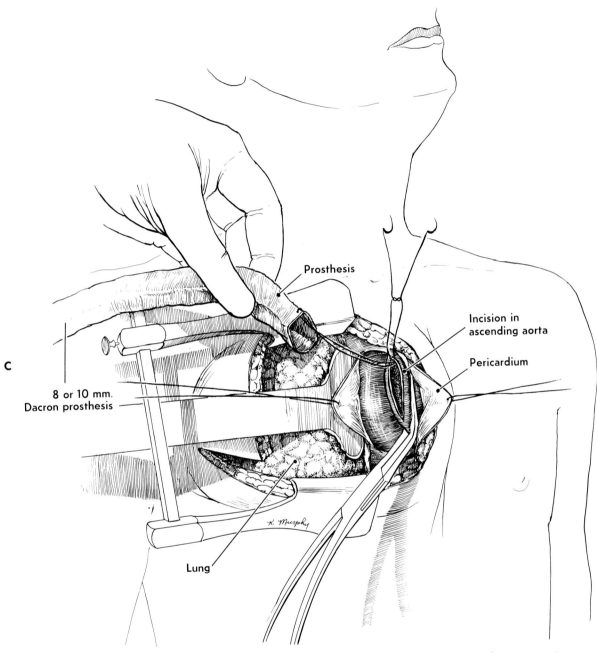

Prosthesis

Incision in
ascending aorta

Pericardium

C

8 or 10 mm.
Dacron prosthesis

Lung

K. Murphy

Fig. 13-13, cont'd. Arch bypass. **C,** Exposure of ascending aorta for proximal anastomosis of arch bypass.

Procedure

Exposure of ascending aorta

1. Make an incision in the right third intercostal space extending from the lateral border of the sternum laterally to the anterior axillary line (Fig. 13-13, *A*). Split the pectoralis major muscle. Divide the cartilages of the third and fourth ribs. Splitting the sternum is not necessary. Tilt the table to the patient's left, and enlarge the incision with the aid of a rib spreader (Fig. 13-13, *C*).

2. Retract the apex of the lung inferiorly.

3. Identify the superior vena cava and the phrenic nerve nearby beneath the parietal pleura.

4. Incise the pleura anterior to the superior vena cava, and clean the subpleural fatty tissue from the underlying pericardium.

5. Incise the pericardium longitudinally over the ascending aorta, and retract the cut edges of the pericardium with sutures (Fig. 13-13, *C*).

6. Identify the right lateral edge of the innominate artery arising from the aorta.

Selection and suture of prosthesis

Bifurcation prostheses used in the abdomen are too large and might compress the great veins in the upper mediastinum. Any type of bypass prosthesis can be fashioned from knitted Dacron tubes. The Y-shaped prosthesis is made by suturing a 10 mm. tube to an 8 mm. tube to form the necessary Y with an appropriate angle and shape. The fine-knitted prosthesis is preclotted with blood drawn from the superior vena cava or the surgical field.

Aortic anastomosis

1. Select a tangential occlusion clamp for the aorta. The jaw must be long enough to isolate a sufficient length, wide enough to hold the pulsating aorta securely, and deep enough to provide edges to attach the graft (Fig. 13-13, *C*).

2. Apply the clamp to the anterolateral surface of the ascending aorta, just proximal to the innominate artery. The back edge of the clamp must be readily accessible, and there must be an ample edge for anastomosis.

3. Incise the aorta with a scalpel, and complete the aortotomy with Potts angled scissors. The aortic wall is 2 to 3 mm. thick.

4. Cut the 10 mm. stem of the Y-shaped graft obliquely at the correct length (Fig. 13-13, *C*).

5. Begin the anastomosis with a mattress suture placed at the superior end of the aortotomy, using 3-0 arterial Dacron suture material with a needle at both ends (Fig. 13-13, *C*).

6. Start the posterior row with a very snug over-and-over continuous suture, sewing from prosthesis to aorta and placing the needle 3 mm. from the edge of the aortotomy.

7. Continue the posterior row of sutures around the inferior end of the aortotomy, and carry it superiorly along the anterior side of the anastomosis.

8. Complete the anterior row of sutures in the middle, joining the suture lines begun both inferiorly and superiorly.

9. Loosen the clamp *slightly* to preclot the prosthesis again, this time under pressure. Tighten the clamp immediately, and empty the prosthesis of any clotted blood. Apply a clamp to the prosthesis very close to the anastomosis, and release the aortic clamp.

Cervical incision and exploration of outflow tract

Make the appropriate neck incision to expose the carotid or subclavian artery or both distal to the occlusion.

Substernal tunnel

Use the tip of a finger to bluntly dissect between the great veins and the sternum. Pass the fingers both from below upward and from above downward. Draw the prosthesis through the tunnel without twists or kinks.

Distal anastomosis to subclavian or common carotid arteries

The lateral approach to the common carotid artery also gives access to the apex of the subclavian arch when bypass is needed to both. This is described on p. 320.

Appropriate arterial clamps with jaws and handles of a convenient size and shape should be on hand, and every possible detail should be prepared in advance to minimize carotid artery occlusion time. The principles and technique of end-to-side anastomosis are identical to those described in detail for bypass grafting of the abdominal aorta, with insertion of the distal limb of the prosthesis into the side of the iliac artery (Fig. 4-5). Occlusion time for the cerebral circulation should not exceed ten to fifteen minutes.

Restoration of circulation

Check for back bleeding, and expel air and clots before completing the distal anastomosis.

Closure

1. Employ an anterior chest tube attached to water-seal drainage.
2. Close the intercostal incision with pericostal sutures of No. 1 chromic catgut.
3. Close the cervical incision without drainage.

Postoperative care

No anticoagulants are used. Digitalization is continued. The chest tube is removed when the lung has reexpanded and oscillations have ceased, usually one or two days postoperatively.

F.B.H.

References

Cohen, A., and Manion, W. C., et al.: Occlusive lesions of the great vessels of the aortic arch. Surgical and pathological aspects, Arch. Surg. 84:628-642, 1962.

Morris, G. C., Jr., Lechter, A., and DeBakey, M. E.: Surgical treatment of fibromuscular disease of the carotid arteries, Arch. Surg. 96:636-643, 1968.

Najafi, H., et al.: Kinked internal carotid artery: clinical evaluation and surgical correction, Arch. Surg. 89:134-143, 1964.

14
Portal hypertension

The creation of Eck's fistula is one of the oldest deliberate vascular operations known. It was originally done experimentally on dogs as a side-to-side anastomosis of the portal vein and vena cava to settle the theoretical question of whether the portal vein could be ligated. The theory had been posed that with the portal vein ligated, experimental animals would die of hepatic failure. Eck ligated the portal vein centrally, that is, close to the liver, and then devised a distal fistula between the portal vein and the vena cava. He thus proved that the portal vein could be ligated provided that splanchnic blood flow was shunted into the systemic circulation. Soon a reversal of this procedure was devised, and historically, every conceivable variation has been devised. Eck did not divide the portal vein, but this was soon done, as were side-to-side anastomoses without interruption of the portal vein at all. From 1877 until 1945, when Whipple applied portacaval shunt in human beings, the operation was only an experimental procedure in laboratory animals. Since then, numerous variations have been devised.

Several procedures have been devised for the treatment of portal hypertension. Usually the portal vein or a large tributary such as the splenic vein is anastomosed to the inferior vena cava or the left renal vein. Anastomosis of the inferior vena cava to the superior mesenteric vein may also be accomplished. In extreme cases the omphalomesenteric vein may be dilated and anastomosed to a vein of the systemic circulation.

The main purpose of the venous shunts is relief of pressure in esophageal varices and prevention of bleeding from esophageal varices. Ascites caused by hepatic outflow block may also be decreased by relieving the intrahepatic pressure. The shunt procedures do not improve liver function and, indeed, may impair it in some patients.

Portal hypertension in children is usually the consequence of thrombosis of the portal vein. The block is extrahepatic, the liver function is usually normal, and the surgical approaches are quite different.

PERCUTANEOUS SPLENOPORTAL VENOGRAPHY

Splenoportal venography is useful in the diagnosis of bleeding of the upper gastrointestinal tract and in choosing an operation to relieve portal hypertension. Rarely, the portal vein is occluded and splenorenal anastomosis is performed. If splenic pulp pressure is not elevated and venograms show no gastroesophageal collateral circulation, bleeding from esophageal varices is unlikely, and at laparotomy a peptic ulcer or other cause for bleeding will be found. If there is portal cirrhosis, the venogram will show numerous collateral channels. In patients with obstruction of the extrahepatic portion of the portal vein, no contrast medium enters the portal

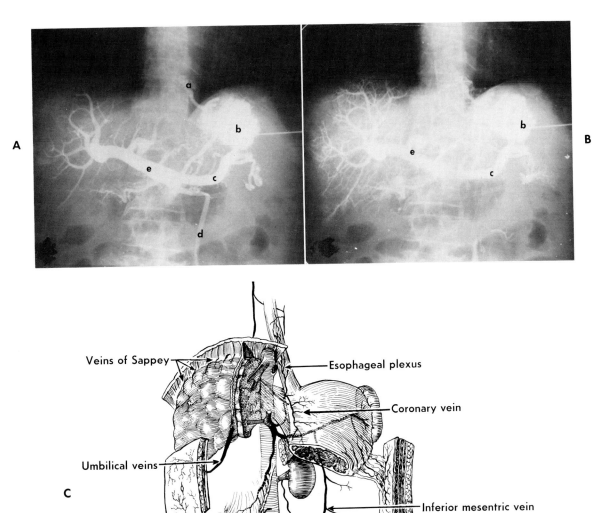

Fig. 14-1. Splenoportogram with early film, **A,** and late film, **B,** showing **a,** esophageal varices; **b,** deposit of media in splenic pulp; **c,** splenic vein; **d,** inferior mesenteric vein; **e,** portal vein. **C,** Artist's drawing of portal-systemic connections.

vein, and the abundant collateral circulation arising from the spleen or the splenic vein is the main feature of the splenoportogram. Fig. 14-1, *A,* depicts an early stage in the filling of the portal system, and Fig. 14-1, *B,* depicts the flow of contrast medium into collateral channels six seconds later. The splenic vein is large, and esophageal varices are seen. Portal-systemic connections are diagrammed in Fig. 14-1, *C.*

Splenic puncture is contraindicated in patients who have a bleeding tendency, thrombocytopenia, or prothrombin times of under 50%. After splenic puncture, slight intraperitoneal hemorrhage is common, but copious hemorrhage is rare. When portacaval shunt is contemplated, it is our custom to perform splenoportography on the morning of surgery. At exploration we have noted no unusual bleeding from the spleen. Splenoportography may be omitted provided that the clinical diagnosis is certain.

Anesthesia

The best procedure is to use adequate preoperative sedation and local anesthesia. If the patient is at all apprehensive or is to be operated on at once, light general anesthesia is preferable. Hepatotoxic anesthetic agents or those potentially hepato-toxic should be avoided.

Preparation

The large bowel is prepared by preliminary enemas and by the administration of 1 Gm. of neomycin every four hours for twenty-four hours. The patient should be tested with a small intravenous dose of contrast medium to determine the possibility of hypersensitivity. If the use of local anesthesia is contemplated, pre-medication should include sodium phenobarbital.

Procedure

1. Place the patient in the supine position on the x-ray table. A sandbag under the left upper quadrant may be helpful in elevating the spleen (Fig. 14-2, *A*).
2. Prepare and drape the skin of the lower left lateral chest wall.
3. Insert a 6-inch needle with a Teflon catheter snugly fitted over a needle in the midaxillary line of the ninth or tenth intercostal space at about the level of the xiphoid process, depending on the size of the spleen and the depth of the costophrenic sinus (Fig. 14-2, *B*). A sensation of firmness will be discerned as the needle enters the splenic pulp. Direct the needle approximately in the direction of the umbilicus and somewhat backward.
4. Before plunging the needle farther into the spleen, instruct the patient to make a maximum expiratory effort and to hold his breath. If general anesthesia is employed, the anesthesiologist maintains an apneic state.
5. Advance the needle into the spleen. A slow flow of dark blood will drip from the needle. Withdraw the metal needle, leaving the flexible plastic sheath in the splenic pulp. The patient can then be permitted to breathe lightly.
6. Inject a trial dose of 5 to 10 ml. of Conray (60%) and take a survey x-ray film to confirm the position of the needle.
7. Measure the splenic pulp pressure to confirm the diagnosis of portal hypertension: (a) First, inject 1 or 2 ml. of normal saline solution to flush the plastic tube. (b) Connect the spinal manometer, a three-way stopcock, and a syringe filled with

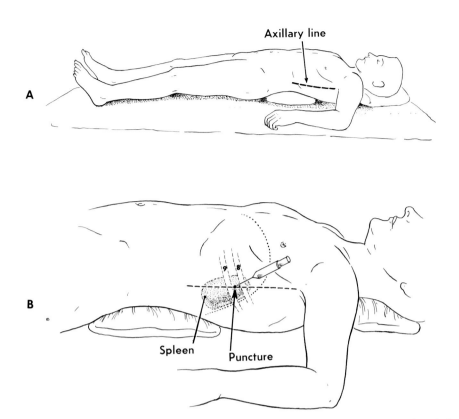

Fig. 14-2. Splenoportography. **A,** Position of patient. **B,** Position of skin wheal and direction of needle.

saline solution. (c) Fill the manometer with saline solution and turn the stopcock to connect the manometer and spleen. If the patient has portal hypertension, the column of saline solution will not fall and the pressures will usually exceed 250 mm. of water. Normal pressures are usually 40 to 80 mm. of water. Three readings are taken while the scout film is being developed. The zero point for calculation of the portal pressure is the level of the right atrium, which is 10 cm. from the table.

8. Inspect the scout film. If the needle is lodged correctly in the spleen, a small irregular radiopaque spot will be seen at the needle tip. Frequently the proximal part of the splenic vein may be seen faintly. If the tip is close to the capsule, a thin dense curved subcapsular line of radiopaque medium can be noted. If the needle is not in correct position, a repeat puncture with another needle may be made. Multiple punctures are not desirable. If the colon is punctured, discontinue the procedure to avoid contamination of a subdiaphragmatic hematoma.

9. Connect a 50 ml. syringe filled with Conray (60%) to the needle. Inject the contrast medium forcibly over a period of five to six seconds. Proportionately less contrast medium is used for children.

10. Take the first film at the end of the injection, and withdraw the needle. The collateral veins and portal vein fill more slowly. Therefore, multiple films are necessary. The cassette changer should be loaded to take six to eight exposures at the rate of one per second. Film cassettes may be changed by hand every few seconds if there is ample help and good teamwork.

Interpretation of splenoportograms

Various patterns of venous collateral circulation may be seen. In bleeding varices due to portal hypertension, the varices will always be seen, and abundant collateral circulation via the coronary and azygos veins will be apparent in the upper abdomen. These collateral pathways will be seen to fill before or at least simultaneously with the portal vein. This confirms the diagnosis. Visualization of large portal and splenic veins gives the surgeon a choice of operation.

Nonvisualization of the portal vein is rare but occasionally misleading. "Streaming artifacts" or "fading phenomena" in the opacification of the portal vein occur at the entrance of large tributaries, almost always the superior mesenteric vein. Complete thrombosis of the portal vein is rare. The ground-glass appearance of the vein on the films is sometimes due to delay and dilution of the dye in patients with severe portal hypertension in whom there is reduced blood flow into the liver. If at laparotomy the foramen of Winslow is open to the palpating finger, the portal vein is open, or rare thrombi are small and nonoccluding.

Portal venograms during laparotomy

Portal venograms can be made during laparotomy by injecting contrast medium through a small polyethylene catheter fastened into any accessible and sufficiently large vein that drains into the portal system. This is an extremely useful procedure if information is necessary at the time of operation or if the spleen has been previously removed. When splenectomy has been performed, portovenography is done through a small incision into which a loop of jejunum or the omentum is delivered for the procedure.

Complications

Complications of splenic puncture for x-ray visualization of the portal system include untoward amounts of bleeding from the spleen, infection in the subdiaphragmatic space, false puncture with extravasation of the contrast medium, pleuritis, referred pain in the left shoulder, and allergic response to the contrast medium. For the most part, it should be possible to avoid these complications by observing adequate precautions, that is, administration of a test dose of contrast medium, careful aseptic technique, use of the Rochester or similar plastic needle, and avoidance of excessive motion and consequent laceration of the spleen after the puncture.

OPERATIONS FOR PORTAL HYPERTENSION

The end-to-side portacaval shunt may be the only operation feasible when the portal vein is very short (Fig. 14-3, *A*). The side-to-side shunt (Fig. 14-3, *B*) is now preferred by some surgeons. Recently so-called double-barrelled shunts have been introduced; these consist of two end-to-side anastomoses. The procedure is difficult and does not seem to offer any advantage over a more simple side-to-side shunt.

The side-to-side shunt is chosen when the pressure on the hepatic end of the portal vein rises with temporary occlusion of the pancreatic side of the portal vein. After side-to-side shunts are made, the pressure in the liver and the hepatic end of the portal vein does not increase, as it may after the end-to-side shunt is made, in which the hepatic end of the portal vein is ligated and divided proximally. The hemodynamics in patients with cirrhosis of the liver with portal hypertension and esophageal varices is not completely understood, and the mechanism of ascites in

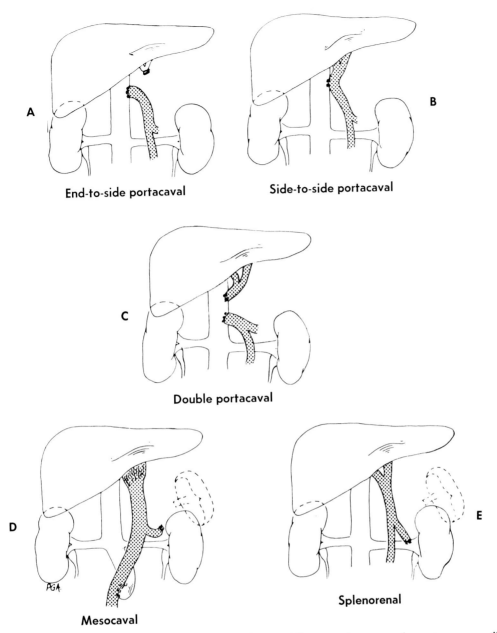

End-to-side portacaval

Side-to-side portacaval

Double portacaval

Mesocaval

Splenorenal

Fig. 14-3. Common types of portal-systemic shunts. All types of portacaval anastomoses will decompress collateral circulation and esophageal varices, lessening the danger of fatal esophageal hemorrhage. Recently, various investigators have compared the merits of end-to-side versus side-to-side shunts. The arguments revolve about the problem of decompression of the hepatic outflow tract. If flow in the portal vein is toward the liver, then all agree that end-to-side shunt is best. Side-to-side anastomosis is advocated when there is hepatofugal flow in the portal system, because side-to-side anastomosis decompresses the portal system on the hepatic side. An hepatic artery-portal-systemic shunt is thus preserved. The question arises of whether such decompression benefits hepatic function, improves or reduces hepatic blood flow, or relieves ascites or whether it is better that such flow be excluded by end-to-side anastomosis. There is little data on the effect of these two shunts on liver function in human beings with disease. Our present policy is to use small (1.5 cm.) side-to-side shunts when portal pressure measurements indicate hepatic outflow (centrifugal flow) block. (From McDermott, W. V., Jr.: Surgery of the liver and portal circulation. In Welch, C. E., editor: Advances in surgery, vol. 1, Chicago, 1965, Year Book Medical Publishers, Inc.)

these patients likewise is complicated. When the ascites is due to outflow block in the cirrhotic liver, the hepatic decompression with the side-to-side portacaval shunt is helpful, but the presence of ascites without portal hypertension and esophageal varices is usually a contraindication to operation.

For emergency shunts, the Valdoni midline approach is quickest and best (Fig. 14-7). Splenorenal shunts are usually possible. They decompress the liver like a small side-to-side portacaval shunt if the portal vein is open, but these splenorenal anastomoses are small and distal (Fig. 14-3, *E*). Warren has proposed a selective splenorenal shunt to decompress esophageal varices without diverting the superior mesenteric venous flow from the liver. He leaves the spleen in situ but divides the splenic vein and implants the splenic end of the vein into the left renal vein. He ligates the hepatic side of the splenic vein so that the rest of the portal flow is barred from the shunt. The vasa brevia are preserved and decompress the esophageal varices. The right gastric artery is also preserved, but the rest of the stomach is devascularized and the coronary vein is ligated to decrease inflow into the esophageal varices. We have had no experience with this ingenious but rather drastic operation. If the splenic vein is small or thrombosed or if there has been a previous splenectomy, a shunt of the proximal part of the inferior vena cava to the superior mesenteric vein should be considered (Fig. 14-3, *D*). The inferior vena cava is divided just about the iliac veins, and a section several inches in length is mobilized so that the superior end of the inferior vena cava can be implanted into the side of the superior mesenteric vein through a tunnel in the mesentery. Various other procedures have proved to be unsatisfactory. The procedure of division of the superior mesenteric vein and implantation into the inferior vena cava is not advisable because it is difficult and provides a small shunt. Ischemia or gangrene of the small bowel may result. Side-to-side anastomosis of the superior mesenteric vein and vena cava in the retropancreatic area is extremely difficult technically. Experimentally, synthetic grafts for portal-systemic shunts exhibit a high rate of thrombosis. The side of the portal vein may be joined to the vena cava with a short sleeve of prosthesis or of the jugular vein.

Indications

The usual indication for surgery is bleeding from esophageal varices. Varices, ascites, and enlargement of the spleen are a common triad of findings. These appear with cirrhosis of the liver, usually in men, and are associated with chronic alcoholism. The diagnosis may be made on a clinical basis alone, particularly when ascites is present. It should be confirmed by the visualization of esophageal varices either by esophagoscopy or by roentgenography. Once the patient has had hemorrhage from esophageal varices, the bleeding usually follows a relentless, recurrent course, and the varices should be decompressed surgically if it is at all possible.

While the patient is being prepared for surgery, hemorrhage is stopped by employment of the Sengstaken-Blakemore tube. The precipitating factors in portal hypertension are not well known. It is said, but obviously cannot be scientifically confirmed, that hemorrhage is lessened or does not occur when the patient is sitting upright in bed.

Portal hypertension may also result from thrombosis of the portal vein, which is usually a disease of infancy and childhood. In these patients, the liver is not diseased as it is in cirrhosis; however, decompression is much more difficult. The portal vein is obviously not available; either the small splenic vein must be employed, or a shunt from the superior mesenteric vein to the inferior vena cava must be employed. When this cannot be done, a drastic alternative is esophageal resection with interposition of the colon.

Because of the poor liver function of patients with portal hypertension, elective operation is to be preferred to an emergency procedure. In patients who are bleeding, operative mortality is high, and improved methods of controlling the bleeding are urgently needed. Possibly intragastric hypothermia may be useful. A twelve- to twenty-four-hour trial use of a Sengstaken-Blakemore tube is advisable and may arrest the hemorrhage.

Operative mortality, in general, is closely related to liver function, and the best surgical results are obtained in patients with good liver function evidenced by serum albumin of 4 gm. per 100 ml., Bromsulphalein retention of less than 35%, and no clinical jaundice.

Contraindications

Contraindications to elective surgery are jaundice, poor or deteriorating liver function, hypoprothrombinemia that does not respond to administration of vitamin K, ammonia intoxication, and other forms of hepatic coma.

Preparation for portacaval anastomosis

Preoperative preparation includes medical treatment to improve liver function and preparation of the intestine with intestinal antibiotics such as succinylsulfathiazole (Sulfasuxidine) or neomycin. The use of nasogastric tubes should be avoided to prevent possible abrasion of varices. At least six units of blood should be available.

Splenoportography is done the day before or on the morning of surgery to establish the patency of the portal vein and to measure portal pressure.

Preoperative bleeding parameters should be investigated. Low fibrinogen levels and fibrinolysis are occasional hazards during the operation. It is our policy to routinely use ϵ-aminocaproic acid (Amicar) to prevent fibrinolysis during surgery. This complication is usually irreversible and fatal when it occurs.

In patients who have bled massively, an elevated blood urea nitrogen level is not uncommon. Since it does not involve poor renal function, it is not an alarming finding. Laxatives and enemas are employed to remove as much blood as possible from the gastrointestinal tract. The serum levels of glutamic-oxalacetic transaminase, lactic acid dehydrogenase, and ammonium ion should be monitored routinely preoperatively and postoperatively in order to evaluate the status of hepatic function. The serum ammonium ion level is closely correlated with confusion and hepatic coma.

Anesthesia

Light general anesthesia should be employed. Hepatotoxic anesthetic agents should be avoided. Ample oxygenation and removal of carbon dioxide should be ensured. The dosage of Pentothal and muscle relaxants should be kept small. When the chest is open, a cuffed endotracheal tube is necessary. If the patient is actively bleeding or has recently bled, there is some danger of vomiting and aspiration during the induction period. To avoid this, the endotracheal tube should be inserted with the use of topical anesthesia with the patient awake. Once inserted, the cuffed tube prevents aspiration of blood, clots, or other gastric contents.

Incision

Either an abdominal or thoracoabdominal approach may be employed. Each incision is illustrated with one of the procedures that follows, and either incision may be used. The long subcostal abdominal incision is best for most patients. If the liver is very large, the thoracoabdominal incision is needed to displace the liver into the chest. In the presence of ascites, incision through the diaphragm invites the complication of pleuroperitoneal fistula.

Postoperative care

The diseased liver must receive maximum postoperative supportive care. A central venous pressure catheter inserted via the subclavian vein is used during surgery and postoperatively as a monitor and also is used for continuous administration of a 10% to 25% glucose solution to support liver function in the immediate postoperative period. The patient's head is elevated in bed. A gastrostomy is preferable to a nasogastric tube for decompression and for supplemental feedings but apparently is not essential. Our practice in the past was to use arginine glutamate (Modumate) or similar ammonium-detoxifying agents daily for the first few days, since the serum ammonium level is monitored daily. Vitamins are added to the infusion. Glutamic acid and arginine glutamate are no longer available on the commercial market; therefore, except for monosodium glutamate (MSG) administered orally or rectally,* this route of therapy has effectively been closed by the Food and Drug Administration in the United States. If large amounts of dextrose appear in the urine, fructose or invert sugar may be used in place of an all-glucose infusion, or small amounts of insulin may be added to the infusion. Therapy with ε-aminocaproic acid is started preoperatively and continued for a few days to prevent fibrinolysis.

During the immediate postoperative period and during the longer-term postoperative period, ascites should be removed or prevented by the administration of spironolactone (Aldactone) or removed by paracentesis. It is possible for the pressure of ascites to physiologically defunctionalize the low-pressure portacaval shunt, and we believe that in some cases this is a cause of recurrent bleeding.

End-to-side portacaval anastomosis
Preparation and anesthesia

See discussion on p. 343.

Procedure

1. Place the patient in the supine position with a small pillow under the right shoulder and another under the right hip.
2. Apply a strap across the hips and a brace under the opposite axilla.
3. The position may then be further improved by tilting the operating table to the patient's left (Fig. 14-4, A).

Exposure—thoracoabdominal approach

1. Commence the incision at the costal margin at the tenth intercostal space. Carry it downward and obliquely across the abdomen toward the umbilicus. Occa-

---

*Unapproved by Food and Drug Administration for this use.

344

sionally the rectus sheath must be divided anteriorly and posteriorly, but it is not necessary to divide the rectus muscle. (See Fig. 14-4, *B*.) Explore the abdomen.

COMMENT: *The porta hepatis, gastrohepatic ligament, foramen of Winslow, and other landmarks should be identified. Dense adhesions in the foramen of Winslow suggest old or recent portal thrombosis. If the precaution of splenoportography has not been taken, portal venography may now be done. Bleeding from the splenic puncture for the recent splenoportography is seldom more than a few hundred milliliters. In patients with portal hypertension of the intrahepatic type, there may be mild ascites. The posterior peritoneum and liver capsule are frequently edematous and thickened and appear to be whitish gray or frosted. Examine the pancreas, the pyloric area, the stomach, and the gallbladder.*

2. Extend the incision between the tenth and eleventh ribs. It is not always necessary to divide the costal margin.

3. Divide the diaphragm between medium-sized Pean clamps. Horizontal mattress sutures of 2-0 silk are placed, tied, held, and later tied together to close the diaphragmatic incision (Fig. 14-4, *B*).

COMMENT: *When the liver is small, a radial incision as far as the central tendon of the diaphragm may be sufficient and does not denervate too much of the diaphragm. Do not divide the triangular ligament. Larger livers can be tilted upward into the chest only after more extensive division of the diaphragm. For patients with larger livers, divide the diaphragm in a circumferential fashion, about 1 inch from the costal margin, and continue the incision until the liver can be displaced into the chest with the anterior edge of the liver above the costal margin. The undersurface of the liver and the hilum are than readily accessible.*

4. Mobilize the duodenum and head of the pancreas using the Kocher incision (Fig. 14-4, *C*). Obtain access to the vena cava by retracting the duodenum and head of the pancreas anteriorly and medially with a Deaver or Harrington retractor.

COMMENT: *There is an abundant venous collateral circulation, not normally seen, in the peritoneum in this area and in the omental adhesions. In uncovering the inferior vena cava and in exposing the portal vein, divide the surrounding peritoneum and connective tissue between clamps and obtain hemostasis with suture-ligatures of catgut on atraumatic needles.*

5. Dissect the front of the inferior vena cava free, and expose it from the level of the renal vein inferiorly to a point high up beneath the liver. Mobilize the hepatic flexure of the colon if necessary.

Dissection and exposure of portal vein

The portal vein lies posterior and slightly medial to the common bile duct and the hepatic artery. The posterior approach keeps the surgeon away from these structures. The vein is concealed by a mass of fat and lymph nodes in the edge of the gastrohepatic ligament. Rarely, an anomalous hepatic artery originating from the superior mesenteric artery is encountered.

1. Define the foramen of Winslow. Have the operating table tilted 30 degrees to the patient's left, and palpate the tense portal vein posteriorly. Pick up the peritoneal reflection at the posterior edge of the gastrohepatic ligament and incise it (Fig. 14-4, *D*). The vein lies just beneath the peritoneum posteriorly, and this approach avoids lymph nodes and collateral veins. It is not necessary to identify the common duct or the hepatic artery, which lie anteriorly and medially. Do not divide any large

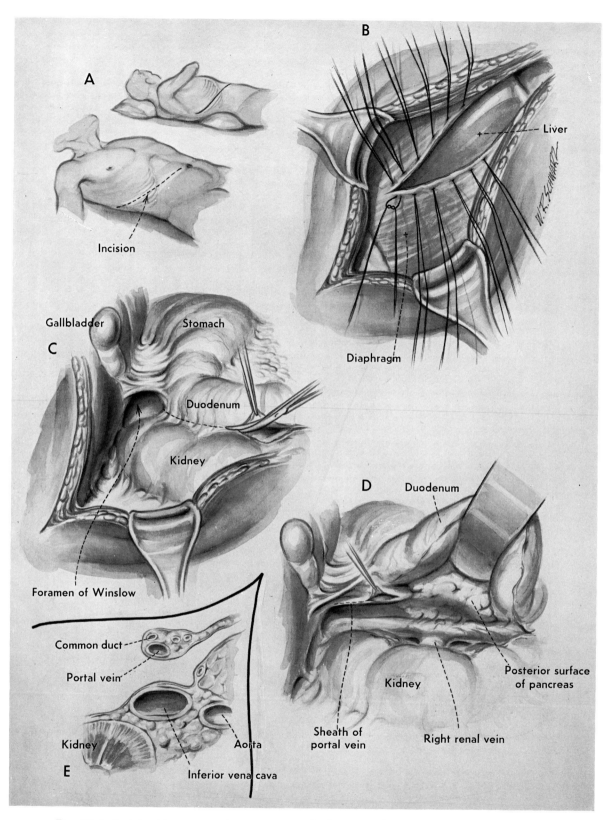

Gallbladder

Stomach

Liver

Diaphragm

Duodenum

Kidney

Duodenum

Foramen of Winslow

Common duct

Portal vein

Posterior surface
of pancreas

Kidney

Aorta

Kidney

Sheath of
portal vein

Right renal vein

Inferior vena cava

Incision

Fig. 14-4. End-to-side portacaval anastomosis. **A,** Position of patient for thoracoabdominal incision. **B,** Thoracic part of incision showing traction sutures in diaphragm. **C,** Liver tilted up into chest. Incision in peritoneum to mobilize duodenum. **D,** Duodenum lifted to gain access to portal vein and inverior vena cava. **E,** Cross section of gastrohepatic ligament.

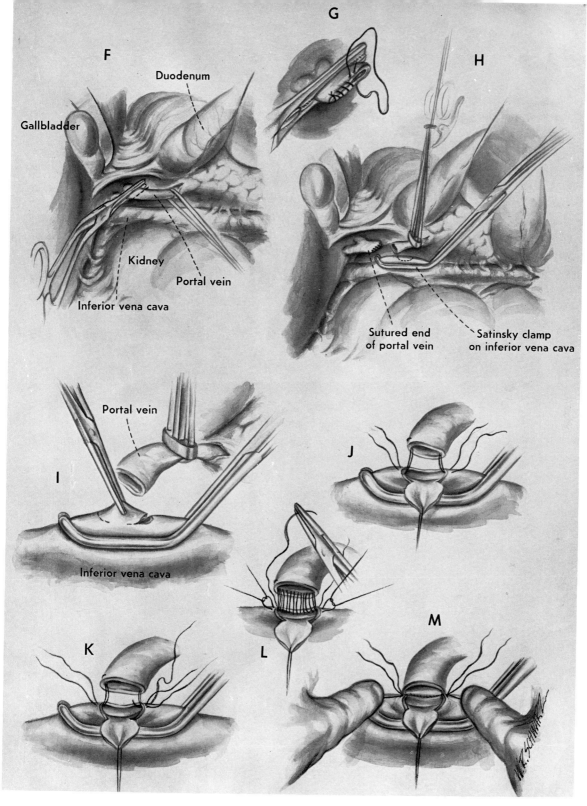

Continued.

Fig. 14-4, cont'd. End-to-side portacaval anastomosis. **F,** Patent ductus clamp at site of division of portal vein. **G,** Suture hepatic end of portal vein. **H,** Site of anastomosis to inferior vena cava. **I,** Cut ellipse from inferior vena cava. **J,** Everting mattress sutures at each end of anastomosis. **K,** Begin back row of continuous everting mattress sutures. **L,** Complete back row of continuous everting mattress sutures. **M,** Draw edges of back row of sutures together.

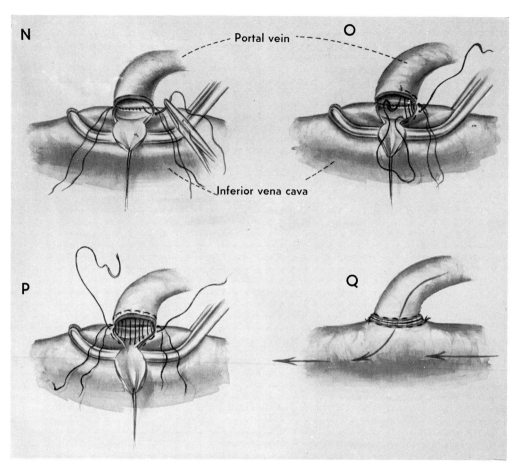

Fig. 14-4, cont'd. End-to-side portacaval anastomosis. **N,** Begin anterior row of sutures. **O** to **Q,** Completion of anterior row of sutures. A simple over-and-over suture pulled snugly with each stitch can also evert the edges easily and quickly.

artery in this region. The hepatic artery may be anomalous and may lie directly in front of the portal vein.

2. The portal vein lies in a tunnel of loose areolar tissue and is relatively sturdy and thick walled. Carefully work around it and pass a $^1/_4$-inch umbilical tape around it. Draw the vein laterally and posteriorly, and continue mobilization with small "peanut" sponge dissectors or with the suction tip. Mobilize the vein for a distance of 4 to 5 cm. between the pancreas and the liver. The first distal tributary is the pyloric vein (rarely seen). The first proximal tributary on the hepatic side is a small anteromedial branch to the caudate lobe.

3. Measure the portal pressure. A free connection through a No. 18 needle is satisfactory. Measurements are made with the inferior vena cava level as a zero or reference point, first with the vein occluded between the manometer and the liver and then with the vein occluded between the manometer and the pancreas. A rubber-shod bulldog clamp is useful for occlusion. If the portal pressure on the hepatic side of the bulldog clamp remains high after occlusion, side-to-side anastomosis is preferred.

Resection of caudate lobe

At times a large caudate lobe is interposed between the portal vein and the inferior vena cava. A wedge of the caudate lobe of the liver must be resected to gain access to the inferior vena cava in some cases.

1. Place a large No. 1 chromic catgut mattress suture through the liver substance along the proposed line of excision, using a swaged-on atraumatic needle. Cut the liver as far as the ligature will permit. The fibrous liver holds sutures well. Rarely, oxidized cellulose (Surgicel) is also needed.

2. Place a second mattress suture overlapping the first and continue the resection in order to uncover sufficient inferior vena cava for anastomosis.

COMMENT: *Resection of the caudate lobe is unnecessary with the Valdoni approach for side-to-side portacaval shunt (pp. 355-359).*

Anastomosis—end-to-side

Side-to-side shunts are preferred whenever they are technically feasible. Although the side-to-side shunt may be the universally preferred procedure, there are times when it is technically difficult. Then the surgeon resorts to end-to-side shunt, particularly if there is no ascites and if there is no pressure measurement indicating hepatofugal flow in the portal vein.

1. Divide the portal vein. Apply a patent ductus clamp transversely to the portal vein near the hilum of the liver (Fig. 14-4, *F*) and apply a modified Bethune clamp or a Potts right-angled forceps about 1.5 cm. proximally, placing the jaw parallel to the inferior vena cava. Divide the portal vein about 2 mm. below the hilar clamp, oversew the cuff with 4-0 arterial silk (Fig. 14-4, *G*), and remove the clamp. This maneuver conserves the full length of the portal vein to reach the inferior vena cava.

2. Apply the tip of a fine Adson hemostat to the site selected for anastomosis on the anterior and medial aspect of the inferior vena cava. Place the stoma close to the liver so that the portal vein will not be kinked when the anastomosis is completed. With slight traction on the hemostat, place a toothed Satinsky clamp on the inferior vena cava (Fig. 14-4, *H* and *I*), occluding one fourth to one third of the lumen.

3. Excise a window in the inferior vena cava (Fig. 14-4, *I*). This should be elliptical in shape. Cut the back side of the ellipse no longer than one-half the circumference of the portal vein. Leave the lateral side of the ellipse attached for traction (Fig. 14-4, *J*). Place a fine arterial suture for traction on the ellipse and for holding the edges of the inferior vena cava apart.

4. Place an everting mattress suture at each end of the anastomosis (Fig. 14-4, *J* and *K*). The sutures are 4-0 Tevdek or monofilament polyethylene and are double armed. These sutures should be closely placed, about 1 mm. apart and 1 to 2 mm. from the edge of the stoma. Hold but do not tie the ends.

COMMENT: *Do not attempt to approximate the portal vein and inferior vena cava until the row of sutures has been completed (Fig. 14-4, L) unless the portal vein is long and reaches the vena cava without tension. In such cases the back row is a single over-and-over stitch pulled snugly each time the needle is passed through the vein.*

5. Place the back row of everting mattress sutures from within the lumen. While you place the back row of sutures, an assistant holds the portal vein about 1 cm. from the inferior vena cava so that the back edge of the vein can be manipulated for accurate placement of the sutures. Start the back row by passing the needle from

the outside into the lumen of the inferior vena cava about 1 mm. from the end mattress suture. Pass the needle and suture inside the lumen to the back edge of the portal vein, and pierce the portal vein from within outward next to the end mattress suture. Reenter the portal vein from without inward 1 to 2 mm. farther along the lumen. Cross to the caval side within the lumen. Repeat the everting mattress suture on the caval side.

To complete the back row, end the suture outside the lumen on the side of the inferior vena cava. Hold the inferior vena cava and portal vein in approximation with clamps. Draw the suture straight so that it is snug and seals the posterior edges. The suture should be correctly placed and be pulled straight with the tips of the index fingers (Fig. 14-4, M). Tie the mattress sutures, and tie the ends of the posterior row to one of the ends of the mattress suture at each end.

6. Use one of the ends of the mattress sutures to close the anterior portion of the anastomosis. Fig. 14-4, N to P, shows an everting mattress suture similar to that used in the posterior row. However, a simple over-and-over stitch gives equally good results and can be done more rapidly because the edges of the portal vein and inferior vena cava are now in close approximation.

7. Slowly release the Satinsky clamp. There is seldom any bleeding or leakage. Remove the occluding clamp on the portal vein and measure pressure in the portal vein and the inferior vena cava.

COMMENT: *The aggravating high-pressure capillary oozing from the operative field stops promptly after the anastomosis is completed and the clamps are released. Do not waste time attempting capillary hemostasis. Complete the anastomosis.*

Closure

1. Close the diaphragm by tying the previously placed silk mattress sutures. Large suture material (No. 2) should be used so that the sutures do not tear the diaphragm.

2. A chest tube is brought out in the midaxillary line in the seventh or eighth interspace and connected to water-seal drainage. If the lung is expanded under positive pressure before closure, an anterior tube is unnecessary.

3. Dovetail the costal margins and close them with No. 24 steel wire sternotomy suture. This is not necessary when the costal margin has not been divided. Close the intercostal incision with pericostal sutures of No. 1 catgut.

4. Perform a Stamm gastrostomy using a No. 24 Hurwitt gastrostomy catheter in the fundus of the stomach along the greater curvature before closing the abdominal incision. Draw the tube out through a hole in omentum, suture the anterior wall of the stomach to the peritoneum, and snub the catheter to the skin with a sturdy silk suture in order to prevent leakage of ascitic fluid. The gastrostomy tube can be used for feeding later as well as for decompression in the early postoperative period.

Side-to-side portacaval anastomosis
Introduction

Side-to-side anastomosis is preferred for most patients with portal hypertension, since the liver is also decompressed by this procedure. Side-to-side anastomosis can be accomplished if the veins can be mobilized and held in serrated arterial clamps as illustrated in Fig. 14-5, *C.* The ideal size for side-to-side shunts is still unknown. Present policy is 1.5 to 2 cm.

The purposes, indications, anesthesia, and preoperative and postoperative care are given on p. 338.

The subcostal approach is illustrated with this procedure. This incision may be used for either type of shunt and is most satisfactory when the costal arch is not too narrow. Thoracoabdominal incisions should be avoided in patients with ascites because of the possibility of pleuroperitoneal fistulas through the diaphragmatic suture line. See the preceding discussion of end-to-side anastomosis for details of the thoracoabdominal incision, as well as greater detail concerning abdominal exploration, isolation of the inferior vena cava and portal vein, and resection of the caudate lobe.

Procedure

1. Place the patient in the supine position with sandbags under the lower right thorax and right hip (Fig. 14-5, *A*).

2. Make a long subcostal incision extending from far out in the right flank upward, across both rectus muscles (Fig. 14-5, *A* and *B*). Divide the round ligament between clamps and ligatures.

3. Mobilize the duodenum and head of the pancreas using the Kocher incision. Detach the hepatic flexure of the colon if necessary. Retract the duodenum and pancreas medially and inferiorly.

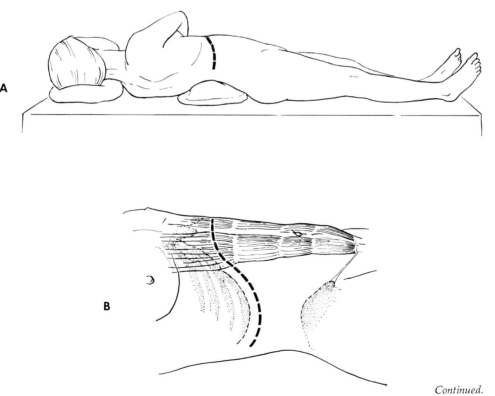

Continued.

Fig. 14-5. Side-to-side portacaval shunt. **A,** Position of patient. **B,** Subcostal incision.

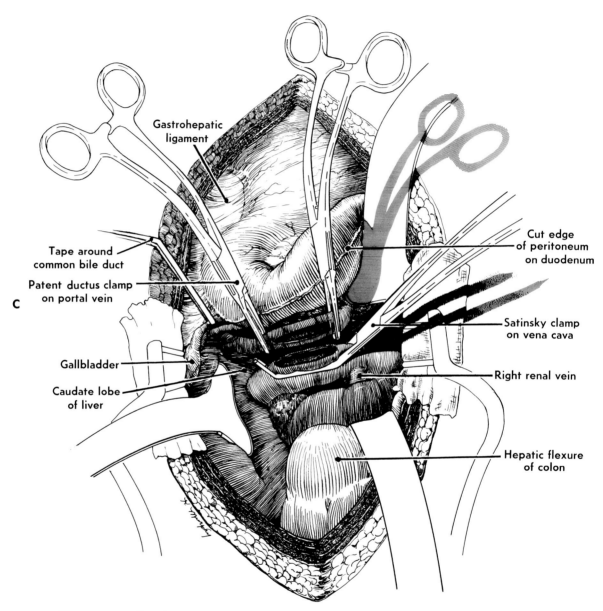

Labels on figure:
- Gastrohepatic ligament
- Tape around common bile duct
- Patent ductus clamp on portal vein
- Gallbladder
- Caudate lobe of liver
- Cut edge of peritoneum on duodenum
- Satinsky clamp on vena cava
- Right renal vein
- Hepatic flexure of colon

C

Fig. 14-5, cont'd. Side-to-side portacaval shunt. **C,** Exposure for side-to-side portacaval anastomosis. Shunt is unnecessarily large in this drawing. From 1.5 to 2 cm. is sufficient. Extra large shunts appear to impair liver blood flow. **D,** Place everting mattress sutures at each end. **E,** Hold veins together with clamps. Begin posterior row of sutures. **F,** Posterior row of continuous over-and-over sutures. **G,** End posterior row. **H,** Begin anterior row. **I,** Complete anterior row.

352

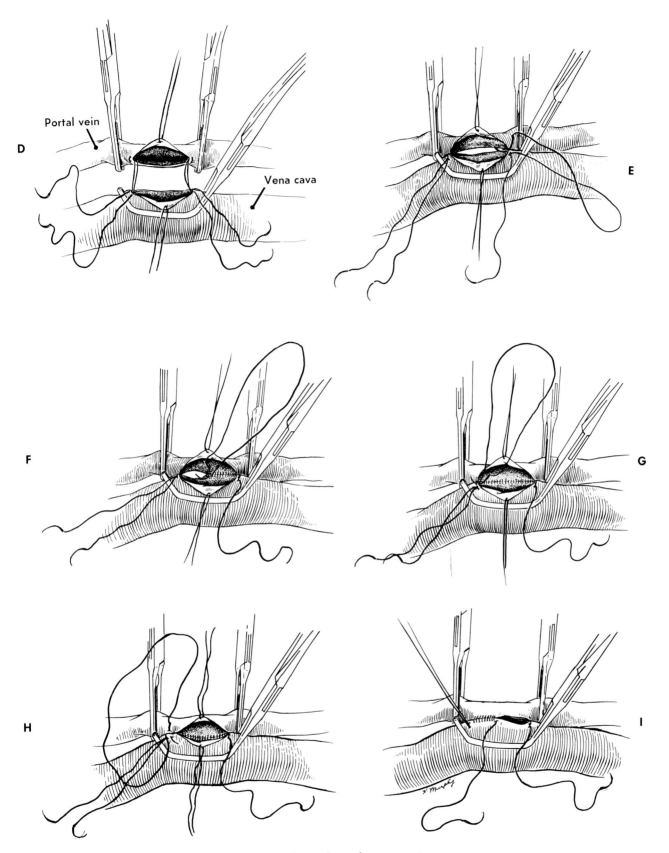

Portal vein

Vena cava

D

E

F

G

H

I

Fig. 14-5, cont'd. For legend see opposite page.

353

COMMENT: *There is an abundant venous collateral circulation, not normally seen, in the peritoneum in this area and in the omental adhesions. In uncovering the inferior vena cava and in exposing the portal vein, divide the surrounding peritoneum and connective tissue between clamps and obtain hemostasis with suture-ligatures of catgut on atraumatic needles.*

4. Locate the common bile duct. Retract it anteriorly and medially. Tilt the table to the left. Incise the peritoneal reflection over the posterolateral aspect of the portal vein at the foramen of Winslow. Pass an umbilical tape about the portal vein, and with traction on the tape, carefully dissect the portal vein so that it is free. Avoid dissection of the vascular lymphatic tissue in the free edge of the gastrohepatic ligament.

5. Free the portal vein from the hilum of the liver to the pancreas, visualizing the tributary to the quadrate lobe. Divide the pyloric vein and the pancreaticoduodenal vein so that the portal vein can be mobilized from its tunnel in the pancreas. Measure the portal venous pressure.

6. Expose the anterior surface of the inferior vena cava, and apply the toothed Satinsky clamp (Fig. 14-5, *C*). Apply patent ductus clamps to the portal vein, the distance between them being slightly longer than the proposed length of the anastomosis. These clamps are applied at a 60-degree angle to the sagittal plane and are rotated toward the sagittal plane to gain access to the posterior row of sutures.

COMMENT: *The three-bladed clamp is useful also. The clamp and the technique of anastomosis are similar to those in the description and drawings of the Valdoni technique (pp. 355-359).*

Resect a wedge of caudate lobe if it prevents close approximation of clamps and an ample length of vein.

If necessary, cut the posterior portion of the pancreas between the portal vein and the vena cava in order to approximate them.

7. Cut the openings in the portal vein and inferior vena cava (Fig. 14-5, *C*). Do this by first tenting the vein with a fine-pointed Adson forceps. The opening in the portal vein is on the posterior side and that in the inferior vena cava on the anteromedial side. The Potts 90-degree scissors is employed to excise a narrow ellipse from each vein, the length of the opening being 1.5 to 2 cm.

COMMENT: *The size of the shunt in the drawing is larger than necessary. A size from 1.5 to 2 cm. is adequate.*

8. Lift the inferior vena cava with the Satinsky clamp. Push the clamps on the portal vein toward the inferior vena cava. Place a retracting suture (Fig. 14-5, *D*) on each side of the anastomosis in order to visualize the posterior row of sutures. Place a mattress suture across the anastomotic site on each end, using a double-armed 4-0 monofilament or Tevdek arterial suture.

9. Tie the mattress sutures. Enter the inferior vena cava posteriorly and from the outside with one of the sutures (Fig. 14-5, *E*). Suture the back side of the anastomosis with a running over-and-over-stitch placed 1 to 2 mm. from the edge and 1 to 2 mm. apart (Fig. 14-5, *F*).

10. At the hepatic end of the anastomosis, pass the needle outside the inferior vena cava and tie the suture to one end of the adjacent mattress suture (Fig. 14-5, *G*).

11. Use the remaining mattress suture to suture the front row of the anastomosis with an over-and-over continuous stitch. Hold the suture taut to evert the edges

(Fig. 14-5, *H* and *I*). Bring the suture up next to the first mattress suture and tie it to one limb of the mattress suture.

12. When the anastomosis is complete, release the caval clamp first. There is usually little bleeding. Release the clamps on the portal vein. Measure the postoperative portal pressure, and close the abdomen without drainage. Insert a gastrostomy tube through a separate stab wound in the left upper quadrant of the abdomen. Because of ascites, special care must be taken to seal the gastrostomy with omentum and to suture the stomach to the peritoneum around the tube.

Emergency portacaval shunt through midline incision—medial approach to portal vein and inferior vena cava

Preoperative control of hemorrhage

Patients bleeding from esophageal varices require an emergency operation if the Sengstaken-Blakemore tube (Fig. 14-6) does not stop the hemorrhage or if hemorrhage recurs when the tube is decompressed or removed in twenty-four to forty-eight hours. If the tube does not control the hemorrhage, varices may not be the source of the bleeding. Obviously, patients who were denied elective shunts because of poor liver function cannot survive emergency operations.

Traction must be applied to the Sengstaken tube in order to draw the gastric balloon up and compress varices at the esophageal hiatus as well as compress them with the esophageal balloon. The Preston traction helmet* is the most satisfactory device for maintaining alignment of the tube. Two constant-tension spring devices on the lightweight padded helmet maintain $^3/_4$ or $1^1/_2$ pounds of traction as selected.

If special apparatus is not available for traction on the Sengstaken tube, an ordinary orthopedic traction apparatus may be set up at the foot of the bed. The amount of traction necessary is only 1 or 2 pounds, and even this amount is quite uncomfortable.

The tubes available now no longer require the manometer and connections shown in Fig. 14-6 and may be inflated with a predetermined amount of air and then sealed by clamping. Once inserted, the tube should not be neglected. Irrigation of the stomach is carried out at least hourly to determine if bleeding continues. At least once on every shift, that is, every eight hours, the nurse must check the pressure in the esophageal and gastric balloons to make certain that the tube is functioning properly.

Ammonia intoxication results from the deamination of blood proteins in the bowel. Prevention and treatment of this and other aspects of preoperative and postoperative care have been discussed previously.

Introduction

For the emergency portacaval shunt through a midline incision, the portal vein and the inferior vena cava are mobilized medial to the hepatic artery after the gastrohepatic ligament is opened at this site. The veins are very close to each other, and the caudate lobe does not intrude. The dissection is less extensive; therefore, the blood loss is small and operating time is short. The special three-bladed Valdoni clamp is essential. It fits nicely into the small operative field. We have still had little experience with this technique, but it appears so promising that we include it here (Valdoni, 1962 and 1963).

---

*Manufactured by E. J. T. Industries, 8439 W. Sunnyside Ave., Chicago, Ill. 60631.

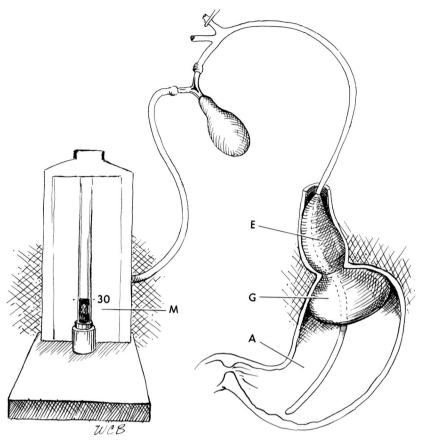

Fig. 14-6. Sengstaken tube to arrest hemorrhage from espophageal varices. **E,** Esophageal balloon. **G,** Gastric balloon. **A,** Aspirating or feeding tip in stomach. **M,** Manometer used to set pressure in balloons.

Procedure

1. Make a midline incision from the xiphoid process to below the umbilicus (Fig. 14-7, *A*). Explore the abdomen. Palpate the foramen of Winslow.

2. Open the gastrohepatic omentum widely, and palpate the hepatic artery at the superior border of the pancreas and its ascending portion overlying the portal vein. Divide the right gastric artery to free the pyloric end of the stomach and retract it inferiorly (Fig. 14-7, *B*).

3. Expose the ascending portion of the hepatic artery, pass an umbilical tape about it to lift it, and retract it laterally (Fig. 14-7, *C*).

4. Expose the portal vein beneath the hepatic artery, and resect the lymphatic tissue and fat along its medial border. The vein is thick walled and lies in a tunnel of areolar tissue. Pass a tape around the portal vein to lift it (Fig. 14-7, *C*).

5. Expose the front of the inferior vena cava directly posterior by incising and excising the peritoneum that overlies it (Fig. 14-7, *D*).

6. Prepare the portal vein and inferior vena cava for anastomosis by resection of intervening lymphatic tissue. This is not an extensive dissection. Measure the portal pressure.

356

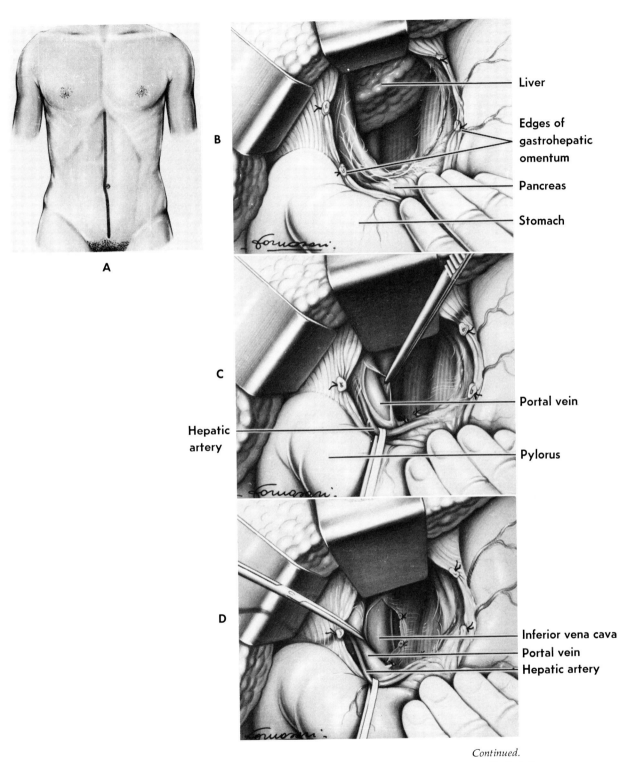

Liver

Edges of gastrohepatic omentum

Pancreas

Stomach

Hepatic artery

Portal vein

Pylorus

Inferior vena cava
Portal vein
Hepatic artery

Continued.

Fig. 14-7. Emergency portacaval shunt—medial approach (Valdoni). **A,** Incision. **B,** Relationship of hepatic artery, portal vein, and inferior vena cava after opening the gastrohepatic omentum. **C,** Retracting the hepatic artery and exposing the portal vein. **D,** Exposing the inferior vena cava.

357

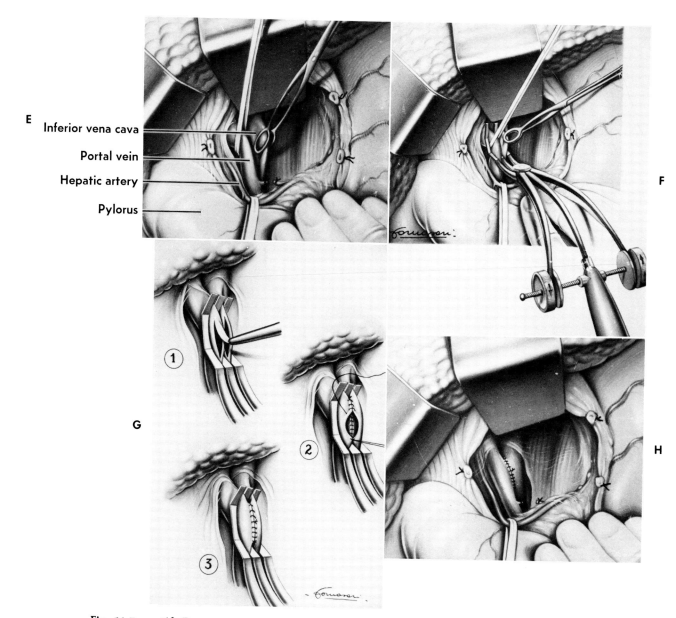

E — Inferior vena cava
Portal vein
Hepatic artery
Pylorus

F

G

H

Fig. 14-7, cont'd. Emergency portacaval shunt—medial approach (Valdoni). **E,** Portal vein and inferior vena cava at site of anastomosis. **F,** Three-bladed clamp (Valdoni) applied. **G,** Side-to-side portacaval anastomosis: **1,** excision of ellipse; **2,** posterior anastomosis completed and anterior anastomosis begun; **3,** completed anastomosis. **H,** Clamp removed. (Courtesy Prof. Pietro Valdoni, Surgical Clinic, University of Rome, Rome, Italy.)

358

7. Apply the three-bladed Valdoni clamp to the posteromedial aspect of the portal vein by seizing that part of the wall of the vein with a fine-pointed long hemostat and tenting it up anteriorly to place and close the clamp. This is the part of the vein that lies close to the front of the inferior vena cava.

COMMENT: *The instrument that we use is not identical to that illustrated in Fig. 14-7, F and G; it has been improved so that the handles have rings similar to those of a hemostat. Because of the limited space, a special instrument is still necessary. It has the disadvantage of providing only a small (approximately 1 cm.) area for anastomosis.*

8. Pick up the center of the intended anastomotic site on the inferior vena cava with another long fine-pointed hemostat and apply the other side of the Valdoni clamp (Fig. 14-7, *F*).

9. Excise an ellipse from both veins (Fig. 14-7, *G, 1*). Save at least a 2 mm. edge in the clamp for secure anastomosis. Place retracting sutures in the outside edges of the veins to hold them apart.

10. Start the anastomosis at the most accessible end (that is, inferior end), and tie the knot of the double-armed Tevdek or polyethylene monofilament suture outside (Fig. 14-7, *G, 2*). Pass the needle inside and suture the edges of the veins snugly together with an over-and-over suture, progressing superiorly.

11. At the superior end of the anastomosis, pass the needle outside, and suture the anterior edges together with an over-and-over suture or everting mattress sutures as shown in Fig. 14-7, *G, 2*, progressing inferiorly.

12. Complete the anastomosis by tying the two sutures together outside (Fig. 14-7, *G, 3*, and *H*).

13. Release the portal vein from the three-bladed clamp, and then release the inferior vena cava. Depress the clamp posteriorly, and then slide the middle blade out from behind the anastomosis carefully.

14. Measure postoperative portal pressures.

15. Perform a Foley or Hurwitt catheter gastrostomy to decompress the stomach and to avoid the use of a tube in the esophagus. Place the tube through a purse-string suture high on the greater curvature of the stomach. Draw the tube out through a hole in the omentum and a separate snug stab incision in the left upper quadrant. Suture the stomach wall to the parietal peritoneum. The tube may be useful for supplementary feedings in the postoperative period or for antacid medication.

Extrahepatic portal block—mesocaval shunt

For extrahepatic portal block, mesocaval shunt may be the only operation feasible. The portal system is decompressed by attaching the divided end of the inferior vena cava to the side of the superior mesenteric vein (Fig. 14-3, *D*). It is most useful in children with the extrahepatic obliteration of the portal vein, since many of them have had splenectomy, or the splenic vein is small. It has been used in adults not only for extrahepatic block, but also for portal hypertension due to cirrhosis of the liver.

The inferior vena cava is divided at the confluence of the iliac veins, and sufficient tributaries up to the renal veins are divided to permit the vena cava to reach the superior mesenteric vein, and a terminolateral anastomosis is made. The inferior end of the inferior vena cava is sutured shut (Fig. 14-3, *D*).

The papers of Gliedman, (1965); Clatworthy, Wall, and Watman (1955); and Marion (1958) furnish further detail and illustrations.

CRITIQUE OF CURRENT RESULTS

Collected results from 1963 to 1971 of portacaval or portal-systemic venous shunt for portal hypertension secondary to cirrhosis of the liver are available in the report of the Inter-Society Commission for Heart Disease Resources. This series totals 783 cases, but undoubtedly a great many more have been done and either were not included in this series or were simply never reported.

With cirrhosis of the liver, which is more or less a standard situation, operative mortality has ranged from 2% to 29%. Of the lowest mortality series, the 2% mortality is for prophylactic shunts, and the mortality is given at thirty days. It rose to 10% at ninety days. The mortality figure of 10% or 12% seems to be reasonable throughout the decade covered, and higher mortality figures seem to be at least in part related to the inclusion of urgent as opposed to elective operations. Prophylactic portacaval shunts in persons with cirrhosis and esophageal varices prevent hemorrhage, but long-term follow-up shows that longevity in such persons is no better than in persons in the control group who were not operated on.

The results are poor and the mortality higher with extrahepatic portal venous obstruction, usually due to thrombosis of the portal vein.

C.H.C.

References

Clatworthy, H. W., Jr., Wall, T., and Watman, R. N.: New type of portal-to-systemic venous shunt for portal hypertension, Arch. Surg. **71**:588-596, 1955.

DeWeese, J. A.: Report of the Inter-Society Commission for Heart Disease Resources, Circulation **46**:A-305–A-324, 1972.

Gliedman, M. L.: The technique of the side-to-end superior mesenteric vein to inferior vena cava shunt for portal decompression, Surg. Gynecol. Obstet. **121**:1101-1103, 1965.

Marion, M. P.: Anastomose spléno-rénale, anastomose mésentérico-cave, pour obstructions portales extra-hépatiques, J. Chir. **76**:698, 1958.

Valdoni, P.: Complementary surgical technique in portal caval anastomosis, J. Cardiovasc. Surg. **3**:26-31, 1962.

Valdoni, P.: Portal hypertension. Personal experience of the surgical treatment, Proc. R. Soc. Med. **56**:261-263 (section of surgery pp. 9-11), 1963.

15
Sympathectomy

INTRODUCTION

Sympathectomy will release vasomotor tone and will increase blood flow through collateral arterioles. Therefore, it has been widely used in the treatment of patients with occlusive and vasospastic diseases of the extremities. The dilation of collateral vessels is helpful when arterial insufficiency is not very severe and when ischemic lesions are superficial. Dilation of collateral arterioles is never sufficient to save extremities with established gangrene caused by major arterial occlusions. The dilation or development of collateral vessels is seldom sufficient for an adequate arterial supply during exercise, although the intermittent claudication may be lessened. The new techniques of arterial reconstruction are the only effective ways to restore normal or nearly normal flow in such patients.

Sympathectomy is, however, a very useful procedure. Over the last ten years we have seen many patients with failure of their arterial reconstructive procedures who continue to thrive because of sympathectomies done either before or after definitive reconstruction. Morbidity and mortality of sympathectomy are, in general, low. When there is a problem of extremely poor runoff, such as frequently occurs in the older age group, sympathectomy should be done with or shortly before a reconstructive procedure. At times the result is pleasing, and no further surgery is necessary.

Since the medical course of diffuse vascular disease in a limb is difficult to predict, one cannot say with complete certainty in any particular case that a good result will eventuate. Lumbar sympathetic block may be used as a diagnostic procedure, as may the various potent vasodilators now available. In patients who have marked vasospasm, an initial clue can sometimes be obtained by simply observing the circulation in the feet and the warmth of the skin of the feet after the induction of general anesthesia. If vasospasm is a marked component of the disease, general anesthesia usually relieves it.

The usual situation, however, is that the blood vessels of the lower limbs are completely occluded, perhaps from the popliteal or even the femoral region on down. Distal bypass is impossible. The patient may not have improved with routine walking or vasodilators and may indeed have had a sudden turn for the worse and have color changes on the foot that suggest imminent gangrene. Vascular surgery has little else to offer such patients aside from adequate sympathectomy.

The proper selection of patients increases the number of good results. Good results are expected in intermittent claudication, superficial and localized necrosis of the toes frequently, and severe pain at rest occasionally. However, ischemia of the entire forefoot and atrophy of the skin or muscle or other signs of severe arterial insufficiency cannot be arrested solely by sympathectomy. Doppler measurement of the systolic pressure in the posterior tibial or dorsalis pedis artery may be useful in selecting patients for sympathectomy. Yao and Bergan in 1973 reported that forty-three patients who had a good response to sympathectomy had a pressure index (ratio of ankle pressure to arm pressure) greater than 0.30, whereas twenty-two of thirty-one patients whose index was less than 0.2 required amputation. The success of sympathectomy has long been recognized as being related to the severity of the ischemia, and this appears to be an objective measurement to supplement clinical observation.

We recommend denervation of the entire extremity, releasing vasomotor tone in the thigh as well as in the leg. This requires removal of the sympathetic chain from the twelfth dorsal to the fifth lumbar vertebra. Unless the first lumbar ganglion is preserved on one side, there may be difficulty with ejaculation in men. The high sympathectomy is more certain to interrupt the aberrant pathways that occasionally occur. An extended sympathectomy is also advisable for the arm (pp. 368-375).

Shortly after operation, the extremity will be warm and dry. A few days later the vasodilation decreases temporarily and then stabilizes, but the extremity seldom regains its initial warmth and color. Failure to achieve significant vasodilation generally means that the patient was not a suitable subject or the operation was inadequate. Inadequate denervation may occasionally result from the anomalies and variations in the sympathetic system, particularly from crossover of nerve fibers from the other side and from ganglionic cells and sympathetic outflow in the ventral nerve roots and spinal nerves. Patients have been observed in whom bilateral sympathectomy was necessary before maximum effects of denervation appeared on the first side.

Long-term survival or limb survival may be frustrated by progression of the underlying occlusive disease in the visceral arteries as well as in the limbs. Patients with diffuse arteriosclerosis in the affected limb or in the heart, kidneys, or brain have a poor prognosis. Diabetic patients likewise have a poor prognosis. Frequently the main arteries to their legs are open, but they have arteritis of the terminal blood vessels. Some have sufficient peripheral neuritis to have already destroyed sympathetic innervation, particularly below the knee. There is little evidence for regeneration of the nerves, sensitization to norepinephrine, and the like. There is one important exception to this observation: that is, the not infrequent improvement of patients with Raynaud's disease when they are medically treated with reserpine after a sympathectomy that was proved to be adequate. Presumably this is a peripheral effect, but the exact mechanism is not completely understood.

Sympathectomy is helpful for Buerger's disease if the patient stops smoking. It is useful for Raynaud's disease and other vasospastic diseases that do not respond to medical therapy. It is of no value as treatment for varicose ulcers unless they are accompanied by arterial insufficiency. It aggravates lymphedema. It is recommended for acute frostbite only if performed early, that is, before twenty-four to forty-eight hours.

Sympathectomy may also be used to relieve disabling hyperhidrosis or causalgia caused by major nerve injury. Except in children, we favor the use of sympathectomy early when causalgia or reflex sympathetic dystrophy is diagnosed. The diagnosis must be made carefully, since reflex sympathetic dystrophy is a difficult diagnostic and therapeutic problem. Posttraumatic pains and other conditions that are sometimes confused with it are amputation neuroma, phantom limb, postsympathectomy neuralgia, erythromelalgia, and cauda equina injuries or other conditions affecting somatic nerve roots in a rather obvious way. In spite of the separation of causalgia from posttraumatic sympathetic dystrophy, both conditions seem to have an initial traumatic origin, although the trauma is very slight. Almost always one has the impression of poor peripheral circulation with coldness of the limb, sweating, and bluish discoloration. Confirmation of the diagnosis can be made by the appropriate sympathetic block: the stellate ganglion block is used for the arm, and multiple blocks of the appropriate lumbar areas are used for the leg. The condition progresses, of course, to Sudeck's atrophy but should be treated long before this.

When the condition is found in children, it is best to relieve it by repeated sympathetic blocks rather than to risk the differential growth effect of the limbs that may be brought about by the changing blood supply secondary to surgical sympathectomy.

Evaluation of the extent of sympathectomy

From time to time a patient is seen with a previous sympathectomy, and it is of some importance to ascertain whether or not the sympathectomy has been complete. This is true in both the upper and lower extremities.

The starch iodine sweat test to see if perspiration can be provoked in the ostensibly sympathectomized limb is carried out as follows:

1. Prepare an iodine solution as follows:

Castor oil	25 ml.
Mild iodine tincture	112 ml.
Absolute alcohol	56 ml.
Distilled water	56 ml.
	249 ml.

2. Paint the extremities to be tested with iodine solution.

3. Dust powdered cornstarch liberally over the prepared limb or limbs after the iodine solution has dried.

4. Stimulate perspiration by draping hot moist packs or towels over extremities that are not to be tested or over the trunk. The patient must be made warm enough to produce perspiration in an obviously unsympathectomized area. Leave test extremities exposed. After a suitable period of time, usually about thirty to forty minutes, you can outline fairly well the areas of the skin that are not denervated, for they are able to perspire and produce a blue color as the iodine is dissolved in perspiration and carried up into the cornstarch.

The physiotherapy department is an excellent place in which to carry out this procedure, and the Polaroid camera provides an instant record of the results.

LUMBAR SYMPATHECTOMY

The lumbar portion of the sympathetic chain, like the rest of the vegetative nervous system, is subject to great anatomical variation. In the lumbar area, the surgeon may find one or several nerve strands and from one to three or four ganglia. The chain may lie conveniently anterior to the lumbar veins or may go beneath them partially or completely; in the latter case the veins may be divided and ligated. In some cases the strands of sympathetic nerve are unbelievably thin; in others a strong prominent strand several millimeters in diameter is found. Because of the structural variation and interconnections and because some sympathetic fibers are probably contained in the spinal nerves and do not traverse the sympathetic chain or its ganglia, it is probably impossible to do an anatomically complete sympathectomy.

Uhrenholdt and associates (1971) studied in human subjects the subcutaneous ^{133}Xe clearance before and after sympathetic blockade. They found a definite increase in patients suffering only from intermittent claudication and a paradoxical decrease in those suffering from gangrene. They suggested that sympathectomy was contraindicated in patients with severe arterial obliteration and that this might be the cause of so-called paradoxical gangrene that at times follows sympathectomy.

It should be pointed out that this work was based on lumbar sympathetic block, which was not always successful, and, furthermore, that we have not been able to confirm any such effect clinically. It is, however, worthy of further investigation. The notion that gangrene can be precipitated by sympathectomy is an old one; we have always been hesitant to ascribe further progression of arteriosclerotic gangrene to sympathectomy. New thrombosis is the usual cause.

For clinical purposes, however, removal of the sympathetic ganglia does seem efficacious. Functional tests of skin resistance and sweating ability, if done routinely, will usually establish the fact of sympathetic interruption, which persists for many years.

Lumbar sympathectomy need not affect sexual function. When sympathectomy is unilateral, no complication is anticipated. When sympathectomy is performed bilaterally, it is advisable to preserve the first lumbar ganglion on one side. Otherwise, ejaculation may not be normal.

Plan of operation

The plan of operation is to remove the lumbar sympathetic ganglionated nerve from at least the first to the fifth lumbar vertebra, including afferent and efferent rami to the chain and the terminal portion of the sympathetic trunk. If sympathectomy is to be bilateral, the first lumbar ganglion should be removed on only one side.

Anesthesia

General endotracheal anesthesia is desirable, since there is some chance of entering the pleural cavity superiorly.

Position

Place the patient in the lateral position with the side to be operated on upward. The area between the twelfth rib and the pelvic crest should be centered over the break in the operating table or over the kidney rest. The lower leg is flexed for stability, and the upper leg is half flexed to provide relaxation of the psoas muscle (Fig. 15-1, *A*). For muscle-splitting incisions, it is advantageous to rotate the patient's hips toward the operator. Otherwise, no rotation is necessary.

The muscle-splitting incision is not illustrated. It has the disadvantages of being more difficult to work through and requiring more light, more retraction, more assistance, and more instruments. Nevertheless, in a rather thin person, this may prove to be an ideal incision in experienced hands. If the surgeon attempts it, he must

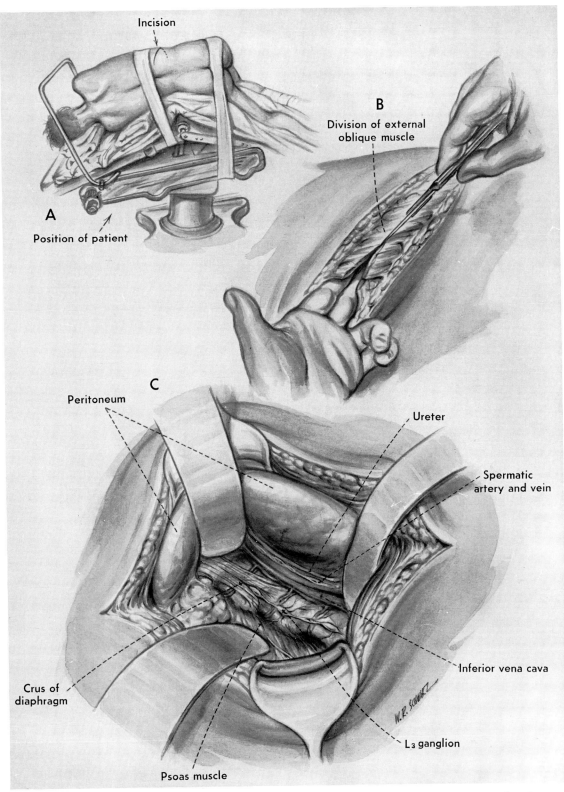

Fig. 15-1. Lumbar sympathectomy. **A,** Incision. **B,** Division of external oblique muscle. **C,** Exposure of lumbar sympathetic ganglia.

365

always be ready and willing to change his mind and to divide all the muscle layers of the abdominal wall as illustrated in Fig. 15-1, B. This may be necessary for exposure or because of severe bleeding. The only advantage of the muscle-splitting incision is the diminished risk of hernia.

The following method includes division of all the muscles of the abdominal wall and provides unparalleled exposure for wide lumbar sympathectomy.

Procedure

1. Begin the skin incision at the tip of the twelfth rib (Fig. 15-1, B). Carry it downward and medially to meet the lateral border of the rectus sheath at a point approximately 2 cm. below the umbilicus, or roughly at the level of the anterior superior spine. If the distance between the twelfth rib and the iliac crest is relatively short, the incision should include 3 or 4 cm. of the tip of the twelfth rib, which will be resected. If the space between the twelfth rib and the iliac crest seems ample, the incision may be brought 1 or 2 cm. below the twelfth rib without removing it.

2. Incise the external oblique and internal oblique muscles in the direction of the skin incision. This will require cutting across the fibers of these structures.

3. The transversus abdominis muscle may usually be incised in the direction of its fibers. Properitoneal fat and peritoneum are found directly under the transversus muscle anteriorly. In the lateral part of the incision, the retroperitoneal fat is encountered.

4. Retract the edges of the divided transversus abdominis muscle, and bluntly dissect the peritoneal sac and its contents medially. As this dissection is performed, the psoas muscle and other structures in the retroperitoneal area will come into view (Fig. 15-1, C). Avoid the groove behind the quadratus lumborum muscle.

5. Identify the anatomical landmarks. The sympathetic chain is identified by palpating the chain with its characteristic ganglia in the position indicated on the vertebral bodies. For visualization of the chain, frequently division of the prevertebral fascia is required, although in many patients this is not a particularly strong structure.

6. Hold the sympathetic chain taut with the nerve hook, and trace it upward and downward. Divide rami as they are encountered. Remember that the chain has many anatomical variations (Fig. 15-2, A to C). As the chain is traced upward, the tendinous arc of the diaphragmatic crus must be divided and the muscle fibers separated at the first lumbar vertebra or beyond (Fig. 15-2, F and G). Tilt the patient's head down, and spread the crus with the dissecting scissors before dividing it. The crus may be inserted as low as the third or fourth lumbar vertebra (Fig. 15-2, D). When the top of the sympathetic chain is reached, apply several silver clips for identification, and divide the chain (Fig. 15-2, G). The nerve runs behind the pleural reflection at this level, but a small nick need not be sutured and is covered when the retracted crus is released.

7. Grasp the superior portion of the sympathetic chain with a hemostat. Trace the chain downward. One or more lumbar veins are encountered. They are usually posterior to the chain, which is gently dissected from them. If the chain goes behind the veins, it may be easier to isolate and divide the veins. The inferior portion of the sympathetic chain lies under the iliac vessels and should be carefully dissected out. On the left side, take advantage of this opportunity to palpate the distal portion of the aorta and the left iliac artery. It is unnecessary to attempt to follow the chain

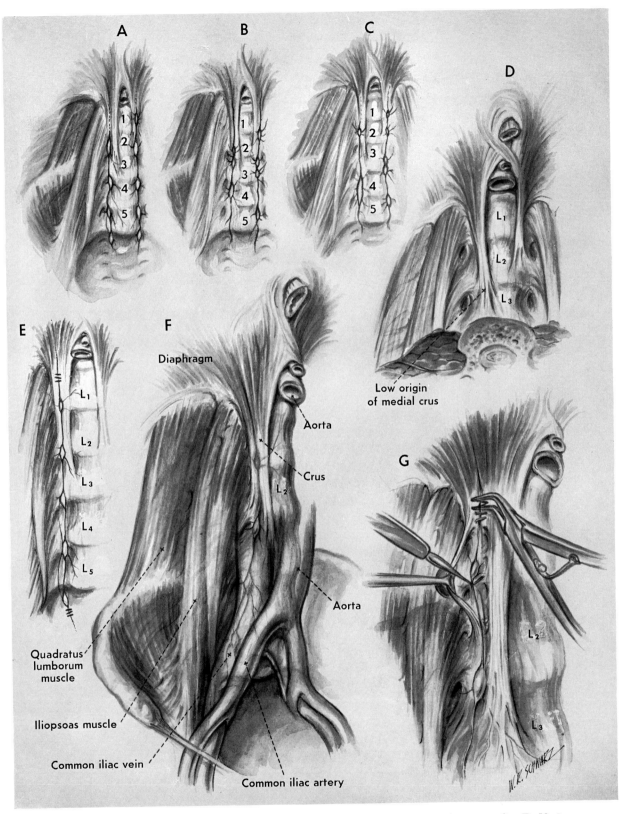

Fig. 15-2. Lumbar sympathectomy. **A** to **C,** Variations of lumbar sympathetic ganglia. **D,** Variations in origin of crus of diaphragm. **E,** Extent of resection of ganglionated nerve marked with silver clips. **F,** View of retroperitoneal structures in relation to sympathetic ganglia. **G,** Crus split to show upper limit of resection marked with clips.

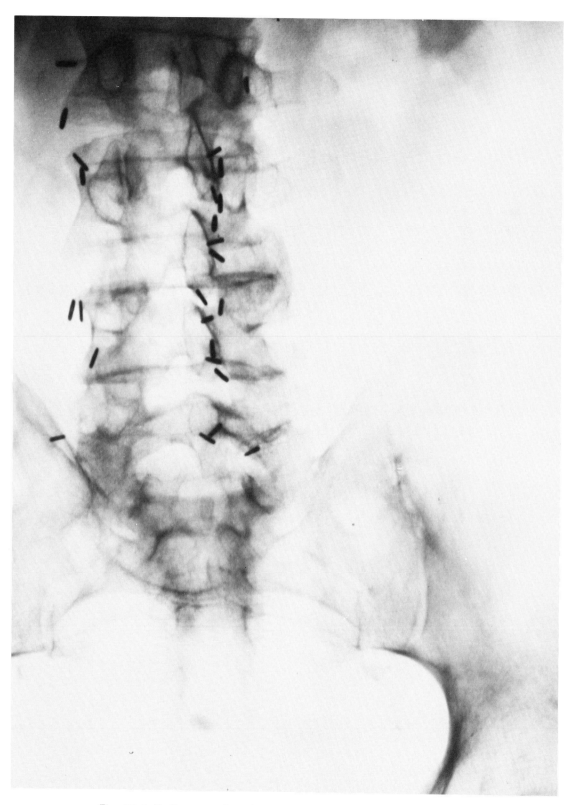

Fig. 15-3. Radiopaque clips showing extent of lumbar sympathectomy.

beyond this level, since usually it then divides into two or three terminal branches. Apply silver or tantalum clips to these branches, and divide the chain inferiorly (Fig. 15-2, *E*). Oozing from this dissected area may be minimized by using a strip of oxidized cellulose gauze (Surgicel) as a hemostatic agent.

8. Close the incision in layers.

Postoperative care

As a rule, the skin of the sympathectomized extremity will become warm and dry almost immediately. The use of a supporting binder for several weeks postoperatively adds comfort during the postoperative period.

Complications

Aside from the ordinary complications of wound healing, those complications peculiar to lumbar sympathectomy can, for the most part, be avoided. The ureter and the genitofemoral nerve must not be mistaken for the sympathetic chain.

After lumbar sympathectomy, the complications of nausea and ileus are rare even when the peritoneal cavity has been opened.

Troublesome neuritis usually referred to the area of the ilioinguinal or genitofemoral nerve may occur. It has been reported that the incidence of this is much greater when the sympathetic chain is avulsed and the remaining ends are not clipped or tied. We do clip the ends with metallic clips, and we rarely encounter the complication. When it does occur, it is manifested by pain in the ilioinguinal region and the anterior or anteromedial part of the thigh. The condition is self-limited, and the pain disappears in three to six weeks.

CERVICODORSAL SYMPATHECTOMY BY SUPRACLAVICULAR APPROACH

Vasospastic disease of the upper extremities that does not respond to medical treatment may be treated by cervicodorsal sympathectomy. The cervicodorsal sympathetic chain is removed from the level of the sixth cervical vertebra inferiorly to the fourth thoracic ganglion. The supraclavicular approach as described provides a more extensive sympathectomy than the ordinary dorsal sympathectomy performed extrapleurally after resection of the proximal portions of the third rib.

Patients who have had a sympathectomy by the supraclavicular approach on one side and by one of the various extrapleural or transpleural approaches on the other are almost unanimous in recommending the supraclavicular route. The transaxillary approach can also be used to gain access to the upper thoracic ganglia, but this is rarely necessary unless it is in conjunction with an operation for thoracic outlet syndrome.

The Horner's syndrome that results from this sympathectomy is of cosmetic significance only, and the more conservative operations that avoid it are less satisfactory.

The diseases requiring cervical sympathectomy differ from those requiring lumbar sympathectomy in that arteriosclerosis is hardly ever the consideration. The operation is of no lasting value to patients with collagen disease such as scleroderma. Intractable and disabling hyperhidrosis of the hands requires only stellate ganglionectomy. The extended operation we describe is advisable for other peripheral vascular diseases such as Raynaud's disease, Buerger's disease, and causalgia or reflex sympathetic dystrophy involving the arm. It is also advisable for improving the blood sup-

369

ply of the arm and hand after occlusion of the brachial artery; this condition is becoming more common as cardiac catheterization becomes more widespread.

Anesthesia

Because the pleural cavity may be entered, endotracheal general anesthesia with a cuffed tube is essential.

Procedure

Incision and surgical approach

1. Place the patient in the supine position with the head turned away from the side of the incision and the neck somewhat hyperextended. Make the incision above and parallel to the clavicle from the midportion of the sternocleidomastoid muscle laterally to the anterior edge of the trapezius muscle (Fig. 15-4, *A*).

2. Divide the platysma and the clavicular head of the sternocleidomastoid muscle (Fig. 15-4, *B*).

3. Divide the omohyoid muscle near its clavicular origin (Fig. 15-4, *C*).

4. Retract the prescalene fat pad laterally, retract the jugular vein medially, and identify the phrenic nerve overlying the anterior scalene muscle.

Dissect out the phrenic nerve, leaving an abundant amount of perineural connective tissue about it. Pass a tape around the phrenic nerve, and retract it medially. Divide the anterior scalene muscle close to its attachment at the first rib (Fig. 15-4, *D*).

COMMENT: *Dissection and retraction of the phrenic nerve should be gentle. Otherwise hiccup or partial phrenic paralysis may occur. The operator may encounter and should spare any accessory phrenic nerves. Bilateral operation at one stage is not advisable because of possible interference with phrenic nerve function.*

Identification of stellate ganglion and cervical sympathetic trunk

1. Identify and expose the subclavian artery, and ligate and divide the thyrocervical arterial trunk (Fig. 15-4, *E*). Beware of the thin vertebral vein that lies along the vertebral column and adjacent to the sympathetic chain. Palpate the stellate ganglion as it lies on the neck of the first rib lateral to the vertebral artery and in close proximity to the vertebral vein. Keep in mind the variations of the stellate ganglion. The dumbbell-shaped ganglion may be fused into one large ganglion or divided into two. It may be displaced upward or downward from the textbook anatomical location.

2. Lift the stellate ganglion with a nerve hook, and with gentle, blunt, and sharp dissection, identify its dumbbell shape and its various rami. Trace the sympathetic chain upward as far as is convenient, usually to the transverse process of the sixth cervical vertebra, where the vertebral artery dips posteriorly to enter the foramen in the transverse process. Fig. 15-4, *F*, represents the relationships of the stellate ganglion and shows the relationship of the sympathetic chain to the vertebral artery and vein, the cervical plexus, the cupola of the lung, and the subclavian vessels.

Exposure and removal of sympathetic ganglia—first to third dorsal inclusive

1. With sharp and blunt dissection, mobilize the pleura from the entire circumference of the first rib. Posteriorly, the attachments are more dense (Sibson's fascia). Detach the apical pleura from the upper dorsal vertebras and the subclavian artery,

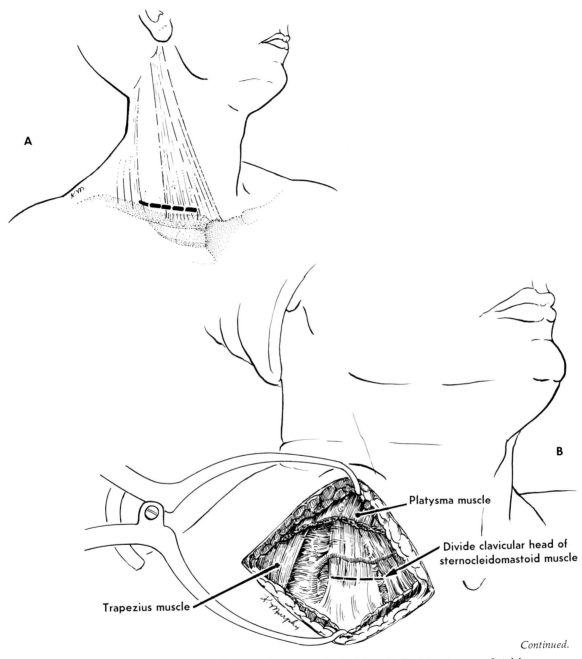

Continued.

Fig. 15-4. Supraclavicular cervical sympathectomy. **A,** Incision. **B,** Incision in superficial layer of deep cervical fascia and sternocleidomastoid muscle.

371

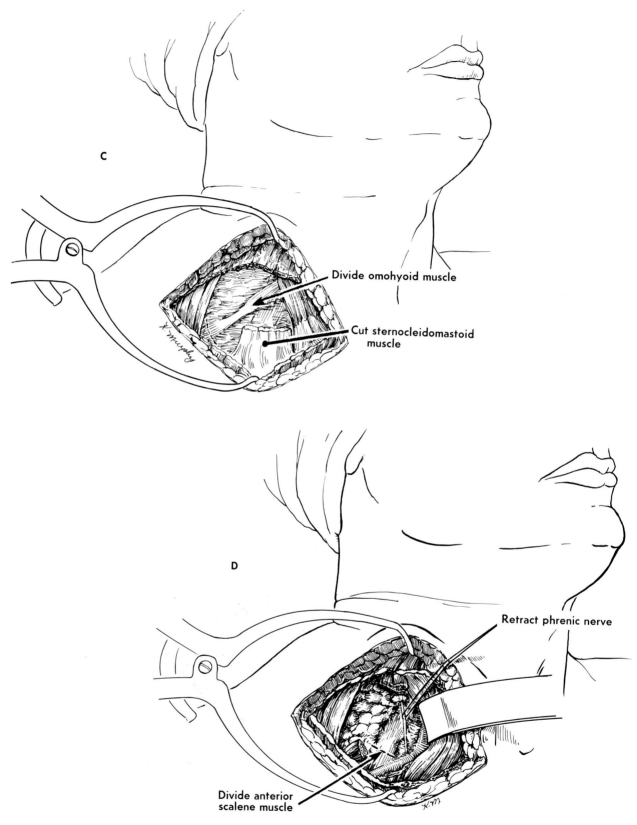

C

Divide omohyoid muscle

Cut sternocleidomastoid muscle

D

Retract phrenic nerve

Divide anterior scalene muscle

Fig. 15-4, cont'd. Supraclavicular cervical sympathectomy. **C** and **D**, Successive steps in surgical approach to cervical sympathetic chain.

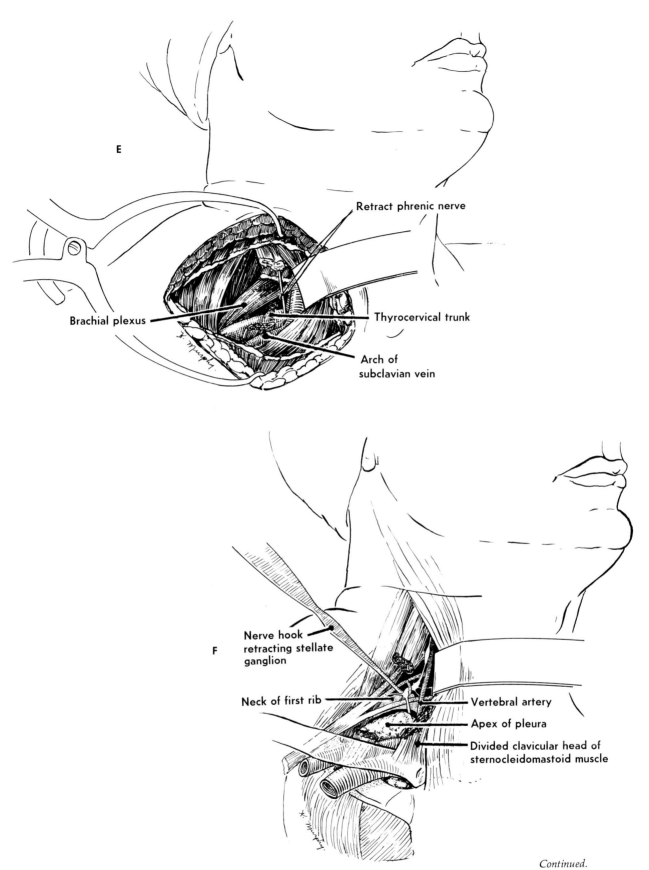

E

Retract phrenic nerve

Brachial plexus

Thyrocervical trunk

Arch of
subclavian vein

F

Nerve hook
retracting stellate
ganglion

Neck of first rib

Vertebral artery

Apex of pleura

Divided clavicular head of
sternocleidomastoid muscle

Continued.

Fig. 15-4, cont'd. Supraclavicular cervical sympathectomy. **E,** Step in surgical approach to stellate ganglion and cervical sympathetic chain. **F,** Diagram showing relationships of stellate ganglion.

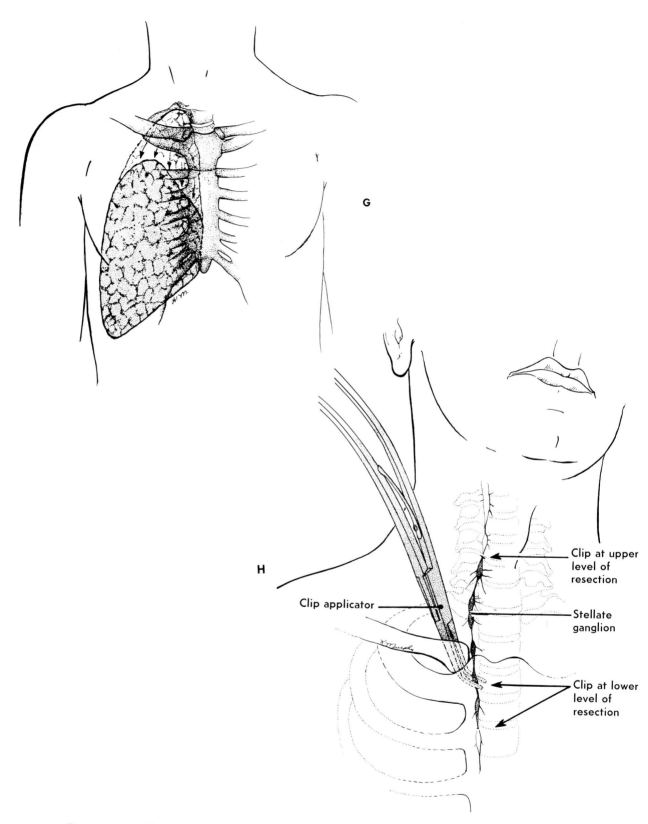

Fig. 15-4, cont'd. Supraclavicular cervical sympathectomy. G, Diagram of mobilized pleura dropping inferiorly. H, Diagram of extent of sympathectomy.

and push it downward (Fig. 15-4, *G*). Dissection is done in the extrapleural space.

Divide the highest intercostal artery if it is present. The artery crosses the thoracic inlet after the pleura over the cupula of the lung has been pushed downward. Hold the pleura laterally with a narrow Deaver or a narrow malleable retractor, and continue extrapleural dissection, peeling the pleura away from the dorsal vertebras and the necks of the first four ribs. If the thoracic inlet through the circle of the first rib is large, the pleura can be mobilized as far as the azygos vein on the right side and the fourth or fifth dorsal vertebras on the left side. Divide the insertion of the posterior scalene muscle if necessary to enlarge the thoracic inlet.

2. Place a nerve hook under the sympathetic chain, and lift it from the vertebras. Identify and clip the various rami with silver clips. At the lower end of the resection,

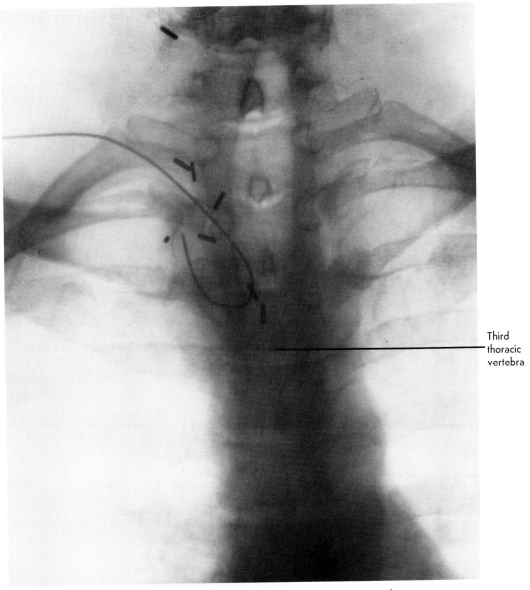

Third thoracic vertebra

Fig. 15-5. Radiopaque clips showing extent of cervical sympathectomy.

375

place several clips across the chain to mark the inferior limit of the resection. (See Fig. 15-4, *H*.)

Divide the chain inferiorly below the third dorsal ganglion or lower when feasible, then trace it superiorly, dividing the rami of the stellate ganglion, and mark the upper extent of the resection with silver clips.

Closure

1. Leave a No. 20 catheter in the extrapleural space along the spine until closure of the skin is airtight.

2. Suture the clavicular head of the sternocleidomastoid muscle. Do not attempt suture of the scalene or the omohyoid muscle.

3. Suture the platysma with fine silk.

4. After a correct sponge count, close the skin so that it is airtight around the catheter.

5. Apply suction to the catheter while the anesthesiologist applies positive pressure to the lungs. This inflates the lung and prevents dead space.

6. Withdraw the catheter slowly while applying continuous suction.

COMMENT: *The morbidity of the extended cervicothoracic sympathectomy by this approach is very low.*

Adequate exposure, careful hemostasis, and the precautions emphasized in the text will prevent disturbances of the phrenic nerve or opening of the pleural cavity. The various rami of the sympathetic chain are clipped before they are divided, and hemostasis is ensured. Endotracheal anesthesia ensures that an inadvertent perforation of the pleura will cause no serious difficulty. The vertebral vein is frequently fragile and may have to be ligated. To divide the anterior scalene muscle, a small curved clamp is carefully passed behind it, and the fibers are incised a few at a time in order to identify and ligate several small blood vessels that course in the substance of the muscle. The operation described will result in Horner's syndrome with anhidrosis of the affected side of the face and neck, the entire upper extremity, the upper part of the chest, and part of the axilla.

UPPER DORSAL SYMPATHECTOMY BY ANTERIOR TRANSTHORACIC APPROACH

Indications and choice of operation

Sympathectomy by the transthoracic route removes the dorsal sympathetic chain, usually from the first to the fifth dorsal vertebra, including the cardiac rami or nerves. The upper part of the stellate ganglion is not accessible by this approach and is usually left or incompletely removed, depending on whether or not it is fused with the first dorsal ganglion. Indications for the transthoracic approach are vasospasm or arterial insufficiency of the upper extremity that relapses after stellate or cervical ganglionectomy, angina pectoris (Palumbo, 1956), or paroxysmal auricular tachycardia refractory to all medical therapy (White, Smithwick, and Simeone, 1952). In general, the anterior approach through the thorax has a lower morbidity and produces better exposure than the dorsal extrapleural method through the beds of the second and third ribs as advocated by White, Smithwick, and Simeone. Although the extended cervical thoracic sympathectomy by the supraclavicular approach (pp. 369-376) is probably best for vasospastic disease of the arm or causalgia, this procedure must occasionally be supplemented by the anterior transthoracic approach.

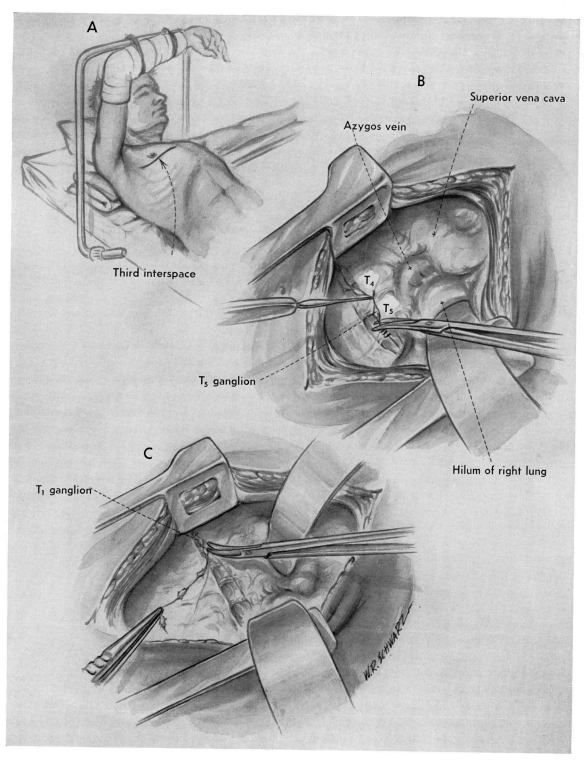

A

Third interspace

B

Azygos vein

Superior vena cava

T₄

T₅

T₅ ganglion

Hilum of right lung

C

T₁ ganglion

W.R.SCHWARZ

Fig. 15-6. Anterior transthoracic sympathectomy. **A,** Position of patient and incision. **B,** View of sympathetic ganglion at inferior limit of resection. **C,** View of sympathetic ganglion T₁ at superior limit of resection.

Anesthesia

General endotracheal anesthesia is necessary.

Procedure

1. Place the patient in the supine position with the arm elevated and supported (Fig. 15-6, *A*). Tilt the table away from the side to be operated on.

2. Make a long incision in the third intercostal space, extending from the sternum laterally to the anterior axillary line (Fig. 15-6, *B,* which shows the operation on the right side).

3. Incise the pectoralis major muscle in the direction of its fibers.

4. Incise the intercostal muscles and pleura widely to permit spreading of the ribs. Rarely it may be necessary to divide the second costal cartilage. Insert the rib spreader.

5. Free the lung if necessary, and retract it inferiorly, holding it in place with a Harrington retractor.

6. Tilt the table to the left about 15 degrees, and visualize the superior vena cava and phrenic nerve. The mediastinal structures will be retracted medially (Fig. 15-6, *B*). On the left side, the aorta and subclavian artery are seen.

Removal of sympathetic nerve and ganglion

1. Identify the ganglionated chain beneath the parietal pleura on the vertebral bodies close to the necks of the ribs.

2. Incise the pleura overlying the sympathetic chain, and place three metallic clips on the chain (Fig. 15-6, *B*) to mark the distal end of the resection for roentgenographic identification at a later date. This will be at the level of the hilum of the lung, normally about the level of the fifth dorsal vertebra.

3. Remove the sympathetic chain from below upward, dividing the rami connecting it to the spinal nerves as they are encountered (Fig. 15-6, *C*).

4. Identify the neck of the first rib and the first dorsal ganglion, that is, the lower part of the stellate ganglion. The upper part of the stellate ganglion will not be completely visualized from this approach.

5. Mark the upper extent of the resection with a metallic clip, and divide the chain between the ganglia on the neck of the first rib. Measure and diagram the specimen.

COMMENT: *Anatomically, exposure is excellent, and the underlying intercostal veins usually cause no difficulty. Comparisons of anatomy on the right and left are shown in Fig. 15-7, A and B. The large cardiac rami course anteriorly. The nerve of Kuntz may occasionally be noted. Sometimes the first intercostal vein passes anterior to the sympathetic chain in the upper portion of the thorax. The first thoracic ganglion may be independent or fused to the inferior cervical ganglion to form the stellate ganglion. The latter arrangement is more common. The second thoracic ganglion may be similarly fused. Below the second thoracic level, the ganglia of the thoracic chain are rather regularly segmental, with less variation than is encountered in the lumbar chain. The highest (greater) splanchnic nerve arises from about the level of the fifth to the ninth thoracic segments. With regard to cardiac innervation, the preganglionic sympathetic fibers either terminate in the upper thoracic chain ganglia or ascend to synapse in the cervical ganglia. Thus, upper thoracic sympathectomy, if it extends to the first dorsal vertebra, interrupts the preganglionic fibers to the heart. Afferent fibers, not part of the sympa-*

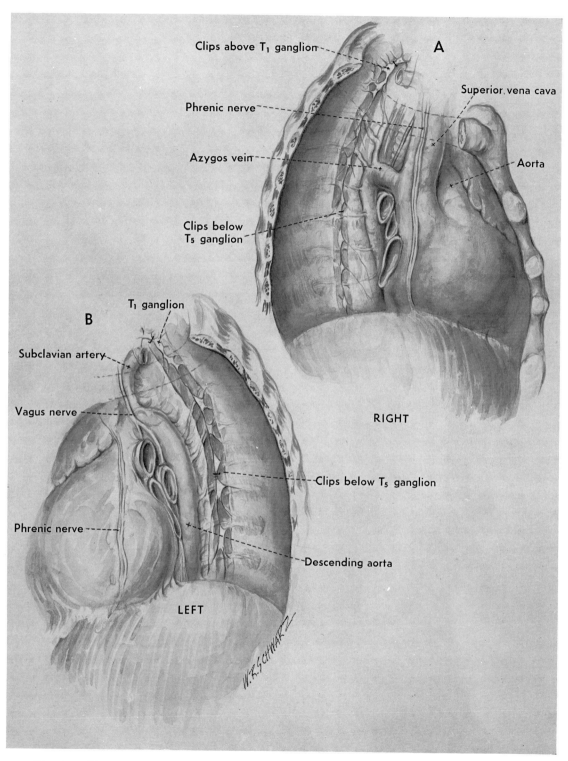

Clips above T₁ ganglion

A

Phrenic nerve

Superior vena cava

Azygos vein

Aorta

Clips below
T₅ ganglion

RIGHT

B

T₁ ganglion

Subclavian artery

Vagus nerve

Clips below T₅ ganglion

Phrenic nerve

Descending aorta

LEFT

W.R.SCHWARZ

Fig. 15-7. Thoracic sympathectomy. **A,** Lateral view of mediastinum and sympathetic ganglia (right). **B,** Lateral view of mediastinum and sympathetic ganglia (left).

thetic system, may run in any of the so-called cardiac nerves, however. As in sympathectomy elsewhere, interruption of the sympathetic chain will not affect any sympathetic fibers that lie within the somatic nerves. Sympathetic denervation of the heart for treatment of angina has not received the attention that it deserves.

Closure

1. Place an anterior chest tube in the fourth intercostal space through a small separate stab incision.
2. Approximate the ribs with pericostal sutures.
3. Close the pectoral fascia, superficial fascia, and skin in layers.

Complications

Morbidity is as low as that of operations with less satisfactory exposure. Horner's syndrome does not occur unless the upper portion of the stellate ganglion or its rami are disturbed.

C.H.C.

References

Bergan, J. J., and Conn, J., Jr.: Sympathectomy for pain relief, Med. Clin. North Am. **52**:147-159, 1968.

Edwards, E. A.: Evaluation of arterial reconstruction and sympathectomy by direct stimulation ergometry, Arch. Surg. **76**:200-209, 1958.

Palumbo, L. T.: Anterior transthoracic approach for upper thoracic sympathectomy, Arch. Surg. **72**:659-666, 1956.

Shaw, R. S., Austen, W. G., and Stipa, S.: A ten year study of the effect of lumbar sympathectomy on the peripheral circulation of patients with arteriosclerotic occlusive disease, Surg. Gynecol. Obstet. **119**:486-494, 1964.

Uhrenholdt, A., et al.: Paradoxical effect on peripheral blood flow after sympathetic blockades in patients with gangrene due to arteriosclerosis obliterans, Vasc. Surg. **5**:154-163, 1971.

White, J. C., Smithwick, R. H., and Simeone, F. A.: The autonomic nervous system, New York, 1952, The Macmillian Co.

Yao, J. S., and Bergan, J. J.: Predictability of vascular reactivity relative to sympathetic ablation. Paper presented at twenty-first meeting of the International Cardiovascular Society, Toronto, June 21, 1973.

16

The upper extremity, superior mediastinum, and thoracic outlet

This chapter describes for most diseases only the surgical anatomy and approaches to the arteries of the upper extremity. Other common conditions such as injury, embolism, and more rarely, aneurysm are treated according to principles discussed in previous chapters.

Additional diseases peculiar to the upper extremities are arterial entrapment syndrome or thoracic outlet syndrome of the upper extremity, Raynaud's disease, and Buerger's disease. All three of these are more commonly seen in the upper extremity, and indeed, by definition, the thoracic outlet syndrome is confined to the upper extremity.

For a number of these conditions and for reflex sympathetic dystrophy, sympathetic denervation of the upper extremity is more widely applicable than arterial reconstruction. Sympathectomy of the upper extremity is described in Chapter 15.

EXPOSURE OF BRACHIAL ARTERY IN ANTECUBITAL FOSSA

Exploration of the brachial artery and its bifurcation in the antecubital fossa may be necessary after trauma about the elbow joint. Exploration should not be delayed when the signs and symptoms indicate interference with the circulation to the forearm. Delay in decompression of the forearm by a fasciotomy and in attempts to reopen the brachial artery may result in ischemia and irreversible fibrosis in the muscles of the forearm (Volkmann's ischemic contracture).

Exploration and decompression of the brachial artery alone may not restore circulation if distal thrombotic occlusion has taken place. Arteriography prior to or during surgical exploration is helpful. Thrombi are removed by arteriotomy and, if there has been distal propagation, with a small Fogarty balloon catheter or by retrograde flushing via the radial artery at the wrist. Patch angioplasty is essential in small arteries such as the distal brachial (Fig. 13-5, *D* to *G*). In these small arteries, the best patch is a piece of vein because of its smooth intimal lining and flexibility.

Procedure

1. Place the arm in the outstretched position.
2. Begin the incision on the medial side of the arm about 10 cm. above the elbow. Locate the position of the brachial artery there by palpation of the groove between

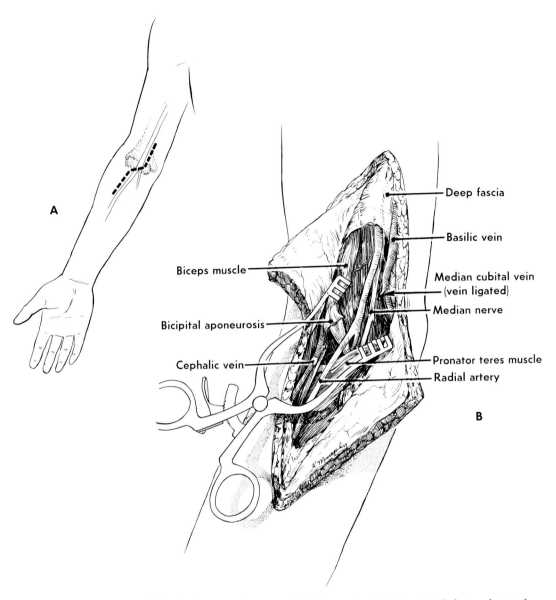

Fig. 16-1. Exposure of brachial artery in antecubital fossa. **A,** Incision. **B,** Relationships of brachial artery.

the biceps muscle and the long head of the triceps muscle. Carry the incision downward to the crease of the antecubital fossa and then across the skin crease to the lateral side of the arm. Then carry the incision again downward and slightly medially, following the medial border of the brachioradialis muscle and other flexors of the forearm. (See Fig. 16-1, *A*.)

3. Reflect the skin flaps superiorly and inferiorly.

4. Divide the median cubital vein.

5. Divide the deep fascia over the brachial artery just medial to the biceps muscle. Follow the artery to the midpoint of the antecubital fossa, and divide the thick

insertion of the biceps tendon into the deep fascia of the forearm (bicipital aponeurosis) (Fig. 16-1, *B*).

6. Reflect the brachioradialis muscle laterally to expose the distal portion of the brachial artery.

EXPOSURE OF BRACHIAL ARTERY IN UPPER ARM

Introduction

A frequent indication for exposure of the brachial artery in the upper arm is retrograde injection for vertebral arteriograms or retrograde catheterization for arteriograms of the aortic arch. The details of retrograde catheterization with the Seldinger technique are given in Chapter 2. The percutaneous route using the brachial artery at the antecubital fossa is preferable for arteriography.

The brachial artery may be needed for retrograde flushing of propagating thrombus from emboli in the axillary region if balloon catheters are ineffective. Such "tail" thrombus may be removed by inserting a large (No. 15) cannula into the exposed artery and flushing the vessel in a retrograde direction with warm heparin in saline solution (10 mg. or 1,000 units of heparin per 100 ml.).

The brachial artery in the upper arm may be exposed either by the method shown, which allows a fairly wide exposure, or through a small transverse incision over the artery in the antecubital fossa. The latter approach is frequently used for retrograde catheterization and is quite satisfactory. Those expert in its employment are frequently able to do percutaneous puncture of the brachial artery at the antecubital level.

Anesthesia

Local anesthesia, brachial plexus block, and general anesthesia are all satisfactory.

Procedure

1. Place the arm in the outstretched position with the palm turned upward. If retrograde catheterization of the artery is the purpose of exposure, wide draping should be employed.

2. Identify the groove between the biceps muscle and the long head of the triceps muscle.

3. Make an incision approximately 6 to 8 cm. long (Fig. 16-2, *A*) in the midportion of the arm over the groove just identified. Deepen the incision through the skin, subcutaneous tissue, and superficial fascia. When the deep fascia is reached, the brachial artery can be identified by its pulsations (Fig. 16-2, *B*).

4. Carefully incise the deep fascia over the groove between the long head of the triceps muscle and the biceps muscle. Retract the basilic vein and medial cutaneous nerve of the arm posteriorly to expose the artery (Fig. 16-2, *C*).

5. If local anesthesia has been employed, identify and infiltrate the median nerve.

6. Dissect carefully around the brachial artery. Exposure is improved by a small self-retaining retractor (Fig. 16-2, *B* and *C*). At about the midportion of the forearm, the median nerve crosses superficial to the brachial artery but is easily retracted anteriorly. Occasionally there is a high division of the brachial artery into two branches, and sometimes the median nerve lies behind the brachial artery.

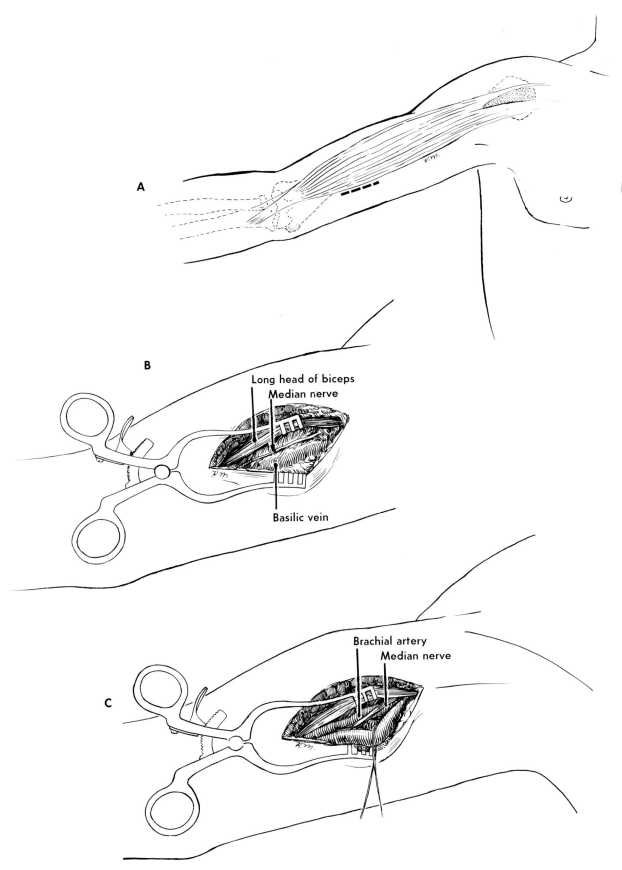

Fig. 16-2. Exposure of brachial artery in arm. **A,** Incision. **B,** Exposure of neurovascular bundle in midportion of arm. **C,** Exposure of brachial artery in midportion of arm.

Discussion

The arteries of the arm seem to be susceptible to spasm. Therefore, unnecessary dissection or excessive stretching should be avoided. Of course, sufficient lengths of artery should be exposed for satisfactory control of bleeding. If the purpose of the operation is insertion of a needle or catheter for arteriography, access to the front of the artery is sufficient, and bleeding after withdrawal of the needle is controlled by gentle pressure or perhaps by a single stitch in the adventitia. For arterial injuries, however, control is obtained proximally and distally before the injury is approached, and a sufficient length of brachial artery is readily mobilized for end-to-end anastomosis or vein graft reconstruction.

EXPOSURE OF AXILLARY ARTERY

Anesthesia

Because of the proximity of numerous large nerve trunks of the brachial plexus, the use of general anesthesia is recommended.

Procedure

1. Place the arm in an abducted position with the palm upward.
2. Make an incision beginning in the arm along the medial side of the deltoid muscle and extending upward along the deltopectoral groove to the lateral border of the clavicle and along the clavicle for a short distance (Fig. 16-3, A).
3. Reflect a moderate-sized skin flap in the arm.
4. Incise the insertion of the pectoralis major muscle over the short head of the biceps muscle, and reflect the origin of the pectoralis major muscle medially and inferiorly to bare the contents of the axilla (Fig. 16-3, B).
5. Usually the tendinous insertion of the pectoralis minor muscle must be divided on the coracoid process. If at this time, it is necessary to follow the axillary artery into the neck, the midportion of the clavicle is resected subperiosteally with a Gigli saw. The anatomy is amply illustrated by Henry (1958). The clavicle need not be replaced, but the periosteum may be closed loosely and the tendons resutured.

Wide exposure of axillary and subclavian vessels

When extensive exposure of the axillary artery and distal subclavian artery is required, Lexer's approach may be suitable. With this method, the incision starts at the midportion of the clavicle and extends medially to the sternoclavicular junction, then downward over the costal cartilages of the second and third ribs, and again laterally toward the apex of the axilla (Fig. 16-4, A). The clavicle is divided or disarticulated medially and divided in its midportion with the Gigli saw but remains attached. The incision is then deepened through the subcutaneous fascia, the deep fascia, and the pectoralis muscles. The entire flap, including the pectoralis major and minor muscles and the medial one half to two thirds of the clavicle, is lifted up and reflected laterally to expose the upper portion of the axillary artery and the subclavian artery (Fig. 16-4, B).

Useful variations are resection of the clavicle and a short sternum-splitting incision with resection of a portion of the first rib to widen exposure of the subclavian vessels (Mannsberger and Linberg, 1965).

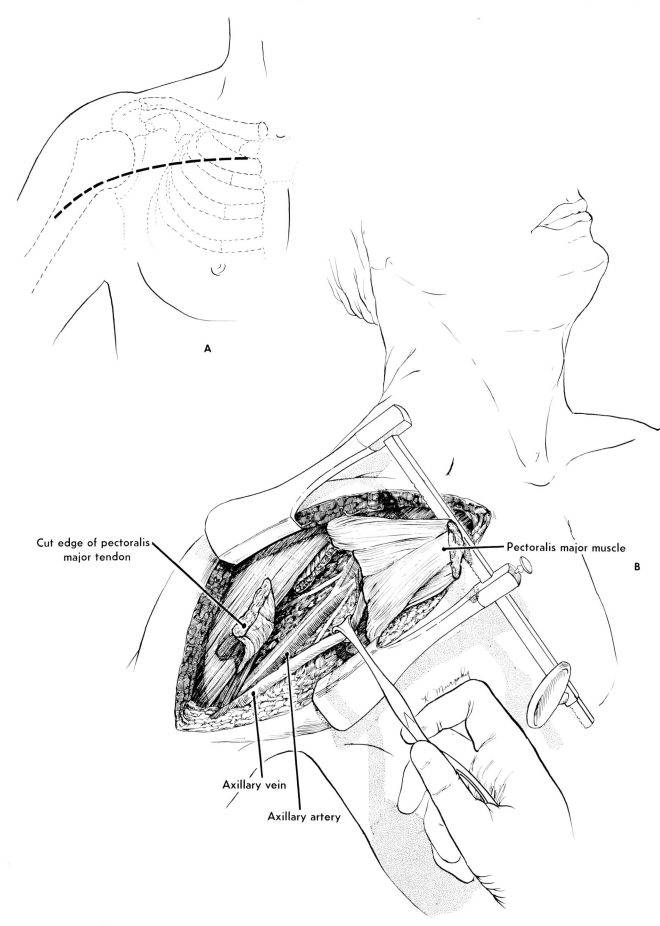

A

Cut edge of pectoralis
major tendon

Pectoralis major muscle

B

Axillary vein

Axillary artery

Fig. 16-3. Exposure of axillary artery. **A,** Incision. **B,** Relationships of axillary artery.

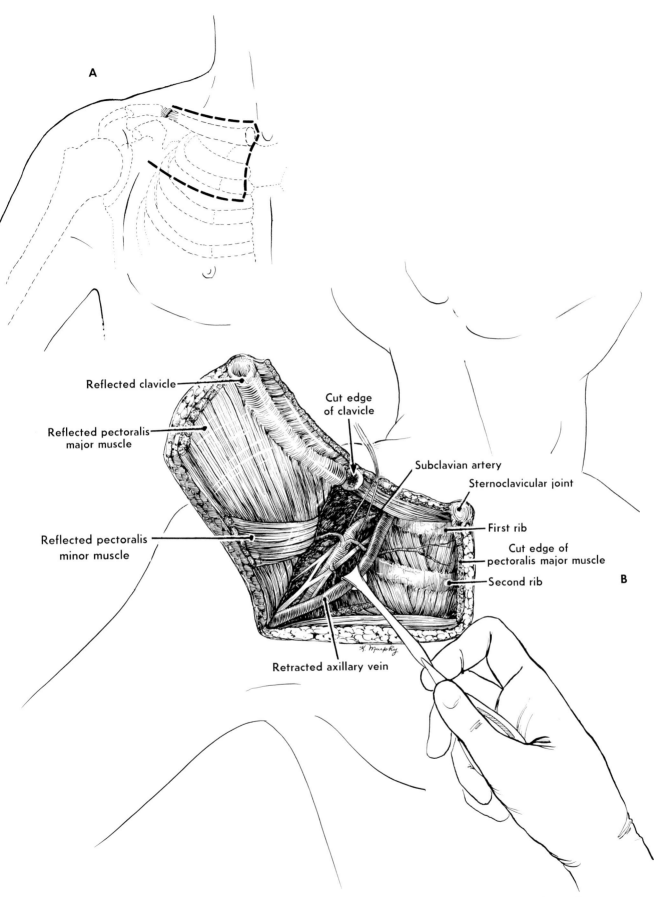

Fig. 16-4. Wide exposure of axillary and subclavian vessels. **A,** Incision. **B,** Relationships of axillary and subclavian arteries.

EXPOSURE OF SUPERIOR MEDIASTINUM

Introduction

Splitting the sternum gives access to the superior mediastinum for operations on the innominate artery, the proximal end of the carotid artery, or the right subclavian artery and for operations on the vertebral artery in a person who has a short neck. Arterial injuries, aneurysms, and lacerations of the great veins are rare but all require surgical treatment.

Proximal control of the origin of the left subclavian artery or of the innominate artery is readily obtained by an anterolateral approach through the third interspace. This incision may be extended easily by splitting the sternum transversely or vertically as needed. Sternal incisions are seldom needed for treating occlusive diseases of the great vessels in the superior mediastinum, since the bypass procedure described in Chapter 12 is preferable to endarterectomy.

Study of the following description of the approach must be supplemented by reference to anatomy textbooks.

Procedure

1. Begin the incision at the midpoint of the sternal notch, and continue it vertically downward to the third intercostal space and then laterally through the appropriate intercostal space. Superiorly, the incision may follow the upper border of the clavicle or may be extended upward along the sternocleidomastoid muscle in the neck (Fig. 16-5, *A*) according to the distal exposure needed.

2. Reflect the skin flap laterally.

3. Incise the deep cervical fascia between the sternal heads of the sternocleidomastoid muscles in a transverse direction. Continue this incision to the side, and divide the insertions of the sternocleidomastoid muscle. Isolate and divide the sternothyroid and sternohyoid muscles. Beware of the great veins beneath.

4. Separate the contents of the upper mediastinum from the posterior surface of the sternum, using careful blunt dissection.

5. Begin the sternum-splitting incision with the Lebsche knife in the space of Burns. When the third intercostal space has been reached, carry the incision into it in a slanting direction. When necessary, the sternum can be split into the left third interspace also. The sternal closure is more stable if the transverse incision is V shaped (Fig. 16-5, *A*).

6. When the sternal incision has been made, spread the cut edges of the sternum by inserting a self-retaining sternum retractor (Fig. 16-5, *B*). For further exposure, divide the clavicle with a Gigli saw or divide the ribs attached to the flap. A portion of the first rib may be resected. These procedures allow the sternal edge to be moved farther laterally.

7. After the operation, the sternum must be reapproximated with stainless steel wire, since even the stoutest silk may fray and break. The stout needles and attached wires supplied for sternotomy closure are most useful for this.

COMMENT: *The fourth or even lower interspaces may be used for the lateral limb of the skin and sternum-splitting incisions to obtain lower exposure. If exposure remains difficult, either the first rib or the clavicle, both of which effectively brace the sternum, may be divided as noted previously.*

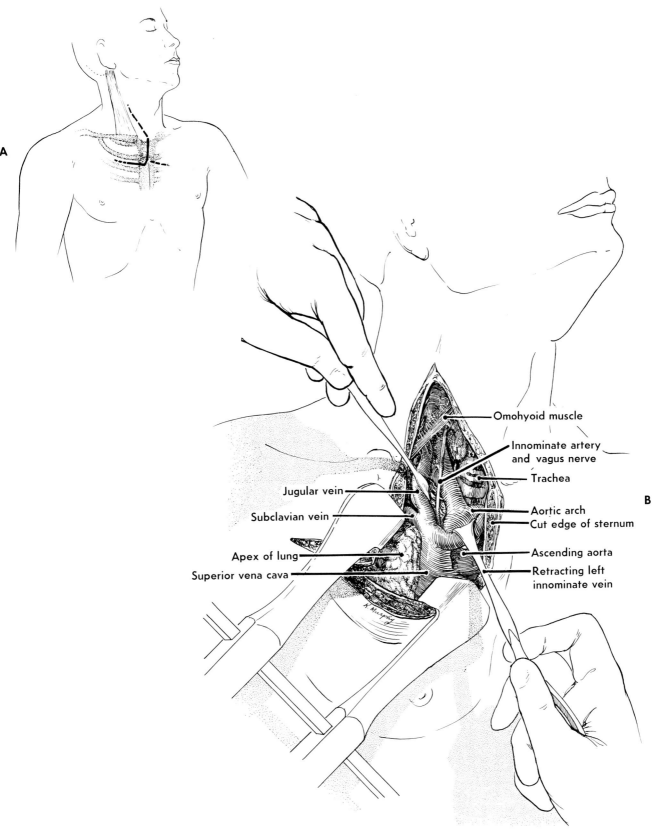

Fig. 16-5. Exposure of innominate artery. **A,** Incision. **B,** Anatomy of right anterior superior mediastinum.

Omohyoid muscle

Innominate artery and vagus nerve

Trachea

Aortic arch

Cut edge of sternum

Ascending aorta

Retracting left innominate vein

Jugular vein

Subclavian vein

Apex of lung

Superior vena cava

B

EXPOSURE FOR TREATMENT OF SUBCLAVIAN STEAL SYNDROME

The subclavian steal syndrome has recently been of extreme interest, to the extent that papers describing the disease and its treatment almost exceed the number of actual cases reported. The known history of observation of subclavian artery occlusive disease is a long one, the clinical picture of combined brachial and cerebrovascular insufficiency having first been described in 1944 and the first successful subclavian reconstruction having been done by Davis and associates in 1956.

As a rule, the subclavian steal syndrome can be treated through a supraclavicular incision after an accurate localization of the occluded area by roentgenography.

The method of exposure follows all the steps for cervical sympathectomy, including division of the scalene muscle so that the entire arch of the subclavian artery is exposed. If adequate exposure can be obtained by this method, then further flaps and sternal splitting are unnecessary. The area to be treated can usually be isolated between tapes and vascular clamps; then an endarterectomy of a short portion of the subclavian artery can be done through a short arteriotomy, and the arteriotomy can be closed quickly.

If careful cervical exposure does not succeed, then sternum splitting and the incisions given previously must be used to achieve exposure of the subclavian artery more proximally.

EXPOSURE FOR TREATMENT OF PULSELESS DISEASE

Takayasu in 1908 first described blockage of the branches of the aortic arch in Japanese women, which has, in addition, been reported as pulseless disease and is usually referred to by that name.

This condition is rare in both the Oriental and the Occidental worlds; tends to be more proximally situated, that is, at the arch level; and may be seen affecting the circulation to one or both arms or to the brain.

The disease is managed by thromboendarterectomy or by bypass from the aortic arch. If as shown by arteriography, the disease is located proximally, as it should be, the best surgical approach is probably through a lateral thoracotomy with the use of a subscapular incision and excision of the fourth rib on the affected side.

In any case, when there is combined subclavian and common carotid artery occlusion, priority should be given to the restoration of circulation to the brain.

THORACIC OUTLET SYNDROME

Thoracic outlet syndrome includes a number of rather ill-defined complaints relating to the arm and the anterior chest wall that come about as a result of interference with the blood flow through the subclavian artery or as a result of pressure on the great nerves to the arm; in all cases this is the result of these structures passing through the narrow thoracic outlet. Occasionally this same anatomical arrangement results in thrombosis of the subclavian vein; thrombosis or actual occlusion of the subclavian artery is less frequently seen.

The syndrome has received numerous other names in the past, although it is probably best described by the term *neurovascular compression at the superior thoracic aperture.* However, the terms *scalenus anticus syndrome, cervical rib syndrome, costoclavicular compression syndrome,* and *hyperabduction syndrome* are used to describe it in various forms. All these names give a fairly clear picture of the varied etiology of the compression syndrome.

Making an exact diagnosis is somewhat more difficult, particularly since patients affected may have puzzling signs and symptoms and since many normal patients have compression of the subclavian artery with perhaps loss of the radial pulse when even an otherwise normal symptomless arm is placed in hyperabduction.

Signs and symptoms of thoracic outlet syndrome

Pain even though ill defined is the most common symptom. It is related to the arm and sometimes to the anterior chest wall. In addition, paresthesia, usually described as a feeling of numbness or pins and needles, is present in almost all patients, frequently in the hand alone but sometimes in the arm and hand or the shoulder, arm, and hand.

Motor symptoms are rare and are perhaps seen in about 25% of patients. They are ill defined and do not involve complete paralysis. Venous compression symptoms of edema and vein distension are unusual but happen from time to time. In these instances, venous thrombosis should be easily eliminated by venograms of the arm.

In the physical examination, the result of Adson's test is usually positive, and obliteration of pulses with hyperabduction also usually occurs. It is quite puzzling when symptoms are unilateral and physical findings are the same bilaterally; nevertheless, this situation is not unusual.

Besides being given physical examinations, these patients should be examined by roentgenography for cervical rib and also for arthritis of the cervical spine. Occasionally, special studies such as electromyography and myelography are necessary.

Procedures

Two surgical procedures are possible. The older and more widely known approach is through a supraclavicular incision. In this procedure, the scalene muscles are sectioned in order to free the subclavian artery. The cervical rib is removed if it is known to be present. Fibrous bands representing the cervical rib may not appear on the x-ray film but may be found on exploration, and when these further narrow the thoracic outlet, they should be carefully sectioned. At the end of the operation, the subclavian artery should be completely free. We have frequently found the subclavian artery, when it is involved, to be enmeshed in the scalene muscle or in fibrous bands of insertion of the scalene muscle.

Murphy in 1910 first designated the condition of brachial neuritis caused by pressure of the first rib. It is obvious that the first rib forms the underlying floor for all the compression syndromes, so that resection of the rib should provide fairly complete relief for almost all types of neurovascular compression. Resection of the first rib formerly involved a fairly difficult operation from above. Roos in 1966 described an operation using the transaxillary approach to the first rib that is fairly easy and that can also be easily combined with upper thoracic sympathectomy through the same incision.

Superior approach (scalenectomy)

The operation using the superior approach is quite similar to the operation for cervical sympathectomy. The scalene muscles must be carefully divided, and the possibility of any pressure by fibrous bands or cervical rib on the brachial plexus or on the subclavian artery must be eliminated surgically. All fibrous bands are sectioned as well as the scalene muscles. Frequently, this procedure results in relief. It is easier and gives better visualization than resection of the first rib. However, all compressive factors may not be removed in this manner.

First-rib resection through transaxillary approach

1. Position the patient with the affected side up on the operating table. The use of endotracheal anesthesia is necessary. Although the entire forequarter should be prepared and draped, it is desirable to leave the arm somewhat free so that is can be moved by a nonsterile assistant as necessary.

2. Make a transverse incision approximately 4 to 5 inches long just below the hairline in the axilla, and carry it down through the subcutaneous tissue until you identify the lateral edge of the pectoralis major muscle. Free the edge of the pectoralis major muscle, and retract it to expose the pectoralis minor muscle. If compression from the pectoralis minor muscle is a valid diagnostic consideration, follow the muscle upward and divide it at its insertion, high in the axilla, on the coracoid process of the scapula.

3. Dissect upward along the thoracic wall, identifying the ribs one by one until you reach the first rib.

4. It is next necessary to protect the neurovascular structures that lie just above the first rib. To do this, several measures are required: (1) provision of excellent light in the now fairly deep wound; (2) manipulation of the arm and shoulder upward, lifting the axillary vessels and the brachial plexus away from the first rib as much as possible; and (3) insertion of a special narrow retractor developed by Roos to further retract these important structures.

5. Next carefully divide the scalene muscles and intercostal muscles as they attach to the first rib superiorly, and leave the periosteum attached to the rib. The area of greatest danger is that superior to the rib, and this should be well visualized. A first-rib shears, which is a special instrument, may be used to divide the rib posteriorly, or a suitable small rongeur may be used to divide it piecemeal. Usually posterior sectioning can be done within 2 cm. of the transverse process. Anterior sectioning of the rib poses no great problem.

6. Dorsal sympathectomy may be combined with the rib resection, and as a rule, the dorsal sympathetic chain can be picked up extrapleurally again with good retraction, good lighting, and good exposure. As much of the chain as is accessible should be removed; usually the segments from the lower portion of the stellate ganglion to the third dorsal ganglion are accessible and can be removed.

7. After surgery, the subcutaneous and skin incisions are closed in layers. A suction drain is inserted before closure and brought out through a separate stab wound. The arm is placed in a sling for a few days.

Complications are unusual. The most distressing, of course, is injury to the brachial plexus, which can result simply from the pressure of a retractor. This is usually quickly reversible. Surgical injury is, of course, disastrous. Occasionally the intercostobrachial cutaneous nerve, or nerve of Kuntz, which supplies the inner aspect of the upper arm and the axilla, is injured in the axilla, but the only result is some numbness in this area.

COMMENT: *The thoracic outlet syndrome is protean in its manifestations. Even though first-rib resection is designed to relieve most of the symptoms without an accurate diagnosis, it should be used as carefully as any other surgical procedure. If hyperabduc-*

tion syndrome is the main concern, the tendon of the pectoralis minor muscle must be released. It is impossible from the axillary approach to completely release the subclavian artery from fibrous bands that may also compress it. For this reason and because of the better exposure of structures other than the first rib, we prefer to approach this condition primarily through a supraclavicular incision, exploring the structures in the neck that may be responsible for neurovascular compression. If no cause is found or if no relief results, then the surgeon should resort to resection of the first rib through the transaxillary approach. Usually the cases that are not relieved by the superior approach are those in which compression of the brachial plexus is the predominant factor.

EXPOSURE FOR TREATMENT OF OTHER COMPRESSION SYNDROMES

Although the thoracic outlet syndrome is by far the most common neuromuscular compression syndrome in patients referred to vascular surgeons, the general situation is present in a number of other areas. Two that the surgeon should be aware of are the carpal tunnel syndrome, compressing the median nerve at the wrist, and the rare but similar tarsal tunnel syndrome, compressing the posterior tibial nerve on the medial side of the heel. In both instances, relief is obtained by dividing the overlying retinaculum. Ulnar tunnel or compressive ulnar neuropathy may also occur in the hand where the nerve is compressed in its tunnel at the wrist. Vascular surgeons are brought in for consultation in cases of these compression syndromes because circulation is thought to be involved.

C.H.C.

References

Adams, J. T., et al.: Intermittent subclavian vein obstruction without thrombosis, Surgery 63:147-165, 1968.

Brickner, W. M.: Brachial plexus pressure by the normal first rib, Ann. Surg. 85:858-872, 1927.

Cohen, A., Manion, W. C., et al.: Occlusive lesions of the great vessels of the aortic arch. Surgical and pathological aspects, Arch. Surg. 84:628-642, 1962.

Davis, J. B., Grove, W. J., and Julian, O.: Thrombic occlusion of branches of the aortic arch, Martorell's syndrome: report of case treated surgically, Ann. Surg. 144:124-126, 1956.

Ferguson, T. B., et al.: Neurovascular compression at the superior thoracic aperture. Surgical management, Ann. Surg. 167:573-579, 1968.

Henry, A. K.: Extensile exposure, Baltimore, 1958, The Williams & Wilkins Co.

Hill, R. M.: Vascular anomalies of upper limbs associated with cervical ribs; report of case and review of literature, Br. J. Surg. 27:100-110, 1939.

Kleinert, H. E., et al.: The ulnar tunnel syndrome, Plast. Reconstr. Surg. 47:21-24, 1971.

Lang, E. K.: Roentgenographic diagnosis of the neurovascular compression syndromes, Radiology 79:58-63, 1962.

Law, A. A.: Adventitious ligaments simulating cervical ribs, Ann. Surg. 72:497-499, 1920.

Mannsberger, A. R., and Linberg, E. J.: First rib resection for distal exposure of subclavian vessels, Surg. Gynecol. Obstet. 120:578-579, 1965.

Martorell-Otzet, F., and Fabre, T. J.: El sindrome de obliteración de los troncos supra-aorticos, Med. Clin. 2:26-30, 1944.

Murphy, T.: Brachial neuritis caused by pressure of first rib, Aust. Med. J. 15:582, 1910.

Roos, D. B.: Transaxillary approach for first rib resection to relieve thoracic outlet syndrome, Ann. Surg. 163:354-358, 1966.

Takayasu, M.: Case of queer changes in central blood vessels of the retina, Acta Soc. Ophthalmol. Jap. **12:**554, 1908.

Urschel, H. C., Jr., et al.: Thoracic outlet syndrome, Ann. Thorac. Surg. **6:**1-10, 1968.

Wright, I. S.: The neurovascular syndrome produced by hyperabduction of the arms, Am. Heart J. **29:**1-19, 1945.

17

Surgery of the veins and thrombophlebitis

DIAGNOSTIC PROCEDURES FOR VARICOSE VEINS

The surgeon must determine if varicosities are secondary to other diseases or conditions such as deep phlebitis, pregnancy, pelvic tumor, or arteriovenous fistula. The diagnosis is usually made solely on the basis of history and physical examination, although phlebography may be helpful. If the varicosities result from diseases of the deep veins or other causes, the prognosis and treatment are different. Varicosities may accompany multiple congenital arteriovenous fistulas. These are noted in young persons. The varicosities may have an unusual distribution, are often unilateral, and cause the affected limb to grow larger than the normal one. The anomalies may involve skin, muscle, or bone. Port-wine stains or cutaneous nevi are frequent manifestations. Various combinations of these signs and symptoms have various eponyms such as the Klippel-Trenaunay syndrome. We prefer to call these rarities *congenital angiodysplasias* without further subclassification. Multiple tiny arteriovenous fistulas are found.

Phlebography has been helpful in diagnosis and in guiding the surgery, and we perform it in almost all cases before surgery on varicose veins.

Postphlebitic syndrome

The symptoms of the postphlebitic syndrome are edema, pigmentation and induration, dermatitis, ulcer, enlarged superficial veins, and congestive leg pain. The patient suffering from severe complications of phlebitis of the deep veins of the leg usually gives a history of pregnancy, a fracture, or a serious illness. The original episode of acute phlebitis may have been overlooked, and complications are frequently not severe for many years. Phlebography and the injection of radioactive fibrinogen have revealed unsuspected thrombi in 20% to 40% of patients hospitalized for elective surgery or for trauma. Recanalization of the acute thromboses usually occurs gradually. Valves may be damaged, however, and the final result is valvular incompetence, reflux, and stasis. Superficial veins may dilate early to serve as venous collateral vessels. Later they may become varicose as pressure is transmitted to the superficial system via incompetent communicating veins.

If the phlebitis is mild, only a few perforating veins may be incompetent, and stasis ulcer may appear without superficial varicosities.

Rarely, when there is occlusion of the deep veins, recanalization does not occur, and the complications of stasis appear early and are unusually troublesome. For patients with such obstruction, surgical excision of the superficial venous collateral vessels is useless and even hazardous. Phlebography shows these deep-vein obstructions.

Physical examination

The physical examination should be conducted in good light with the patient standing erect. Visible varicosities are marked with gentian violet. When the continuation of a vein is not obvious from visual inspection, palpation will usually reveal its location. Nests of varicosities are, as a rule, the wormlike tortuosities of a single vein rather than several veins. The short saphenous vein should always be sought by palpation, since this vein is frequently not visible in the upper one half or two thirds of the lower leg.

Incompetency of greater saphenous system

The Trendelenburg test is performed to test the function of the venous valves.
1. The patient lies down and elevates the affected leg.
2. A tourniquet is applied high on the thigh.
3. The patient stands.
4. Interpretation is as follows:
   a. If the varicosities fill rapidly, blood is flowing into them through incompetent communicating veins.
   b. If the varicosities do not fill within about thirty seconds, release the tourniquet. Sudden filling of the varicosities from the greater saphenous vein above the tourniquet demonstrates that the valves of the greater saphenous system are incompetent and reassures the examiner that there are probably no seriously incompetent communicating veins. Incompetence of some perforating or communicating veins is difficult to localize without phlebography.

Incompetent communicating veins

Incompetent communicating veins are one of the most frequent causes of recurrent varicose veins and are an important cause of stasis dermatitis and ulceration. Most incompetent communicating veins are found below the knee, important locations being just above the ankle, medially and laterally, and at the lower end of the adductor canal. The more advanced the varicose veins have become, the more likely it is that incompetent veins will be communicating between the deep and superficial systems. In some patients, the location can be apprehended without a dynamic test, by observing a nest of varicosities and palpating a small defect in the deep fasica at the site of perforation. Many of these perforating veins have only a tortuous or indirect superficial communication with the saphenous system. The modified Trendelenburg procedure is the usual test for localizing communicating or perforating veins. Now we use phlebography in most cases.

Modified Trendelenburg procedure

1. Elevate the leg.
2. Apply three tourniquets: one below the knee, one just above the knee, and one about the thigh.
3. Have the patient stand.
4. Observe and palpate the filling of the superficial veins and varices. Rarely,

all segments will fill independently. First, release the most distal tourniquet. If filling that was not previously observed is noted, the assumption is that the lesser saphenous vein is incompetent. Next, release the middle tourniquet. Filling of superficial veins that were previously empty will occur if there are incompetent veins communicating between the deep and superficial systems in the thigh. The purpose of the highest tourniquet is to prevent downward reflux of blood in an incompetent greater saphenous system. By repeating the test and varying the position of the middle tourniquet or by placing a tourniquet around the calf, more precise localization of incompetent perforating veins can be attained.

Perthes' test

Perthes' test is the standard examination for determining the state of deep venous return. It may be difficult to interpret.

1. Collapse the superficial varices with a snugly applied elastic bandage.
2. Have the patient walk for five to thirty minutes.
3. If the patient suffers from increasing discomfort or cramplike pain during the period of exercise, he will not be materially benefited by stripping of the superficial veins.

Modified Perthes' test

A modification of Perthes' test is performed by having the patient elevate the leg and applying a tourniquet around the thigh. The patient is instructed to walk with the tourniquet applied. If the superficial veins collapse and remain empty, it is assumed that deep venous return is adequate. If superficial veins under these conditions remain engorged, the cause may be either obstruction in or reflux from the deep veins via incompetent communicating veins.

Venous pressures

Measurement of venous pressure while the patient walks (walking erect venous pressure) is a quantitative demonstration of the tests just described. It is seldom needed but occasionally useful in difficult diagnostic problems. The venous pressure in the saphenous system is measured with a long manometer connected to a Rochester needle or plastic catheter in the saphenous vein or one of its tributaries. Pressures are compared while the patient is standing and walking in the erect position with and without occlusion of the saphenous vein.

When venography is done, the walking venous pressure test is conveniently done through the same vein as the venography. Actual ambulation is unnecessary, for the patient may perform walking movements of the foot and calf in an almost upright position on the fluoroscopic table footrest.

By this method, the venous pressure in the foot when the patient rests in the erect position is almost identical with the distance from the foot to the right auricle. In a normal person, the pressure falls about 50 cm. when he walks without saphenous occlusion. In a person with simple varicose veins, the fall in pressure is only 25 cm., but the decrease in pressure is normal when he walks with digital or tourniquet occlusion of the saphenous vein. When the valves in the deep veins are incompetent or obstructed, there is little or no fall in the venous pressure when the patient walks, and the pressure may even increase.

The method of measuring venous pressures while the patient walks furnishes physiological data in evaluating patients who have had deep phlebitis.

Discussion

If varicose veins fill from above only, no further examination is necessary, and the surgeon may assume that this is a case of primary varicose veins and that there is no involvement of the deep circulation. If filling occurs through incompetent veins connecting the deep and superficial systems, you must localize those veins. The value of Perthes' test is limited. Phlebography is recommended for all patients with previous phlebitis or previous vein surgery. It reveals perforating veins in unusual locations, permits ligation of them with small incisions, and has made the subfascial exploration and ligation of perforating veins unncessary in most cases.

For the ordinary case of varicose veins, the diagnostic value of numerous dynamic tests has been overemphasized and overrated, and the simple procedures of inspection and palpation have not been sufficiently emphasized.

PHLEBOGRAPHY OF LEG
Introduction

Phlebography is needed for visualization of the deep veins, whose condition can otherwise only be inferred. We have found phlebography helpful in providing a guide in varicose vein surgery. It may reveal a normal saphenous vein in the thigh that can be preserved for use later in coronary or peripheral arterial reconstruction. Also, the phlebogram may reveal (1) a doubled saphenous vein, (2) extension of the short saphenous vein up the posterior part of the thigh, (3) varicosities that might be overlooked in a fat leg, (4) unsuspected incompetent perforating veins, and (5) signs of old phlebitis that may suggest the need for prolonged elastic support after vein surgery. Phlebography is most useful in distinguishing between obstruction and incompetence of the deep veins of the leg.

Injection is usually made into a vein of the foot, and passage of the opaque medium into the superficial veins is prevented by a tourniquet at the ankle. The patient is in the semierect position to prevent layering of the dye and to keep the dye in the legs until the films are made. Phlebography is also used for the more precise diagnosis and localization of acute phlebitis.

Clear visualization of the iliac veins is easily obtained by injection of a vein on the foot. Partial obstruction of the iliac veins is frequently revealed and evidenced by crossover of the dye to the opposite iliac vein or by visualization of collateral channels up along the spine. For visualization of the iliac vein by injection at the foot, larger volumes (90 to 120 ml.) of more concentrated radiopaque medium such as Conray (60%) are injected while the patient is tilted with his feet down. After the films of the leg are obtained, the table is flattened, and a film of the abdomen is taken after the leg is elevated three or four seconds to empty the leg and fill the iliac vein.

The newer contrast media such as Conray are safer and less irritating, and complications are rare even during acute phlebitis.

Tilting (ascending) phlebography of leg

The ascending phlebogram furnishes a map of the deep and superficial veins and supplies functional information about the venous pump of the lower leg. We perform it in all cases of varicose veins or when we suspect that there is thrombophlebitis unless there is some contraindication, such as allergy to the radiopaque medium.

Position and anesthesia

No anesthetic is necessary. Place the patient in a supine position on the tilting fluoroscopic x-ray table with the feet 30 to 40 degrees lower than the head. Place a tourniquet about the ankle. An ordinary piece of rubber tubing or Penrose drain will do.

Choice of site of injection—intracalcaneal or dorsal vein of foot

A dorsal vein on the foot is usually accessible for injection, and intraosseous injection is rarely needed.

The intracalcaneal injection is useful for patients with edema that obscures the foot veins. We used this intraosseous injection in more than fifty patients, but it caused more discomfort and offers no advantages for most patients. Rarely, osteomyelitis has been reported after intraosseous injections.

Technique of intracalcaneal phlebography

1. With the patient in the supine position, prepare and drape the foot. Inject 1% lidocaine (Xylocaine) 1 inch distal to the tip of the *lateral* malleolus and $^3/_4$ inch posterior to it so that a dermal wheal is formed. Infiltrate the subcutaneous tissue and periosteum.

2. Introduce a No. 17 Rosenthal needle or a Turkel sternal biopsy needle through the skin and to the periosteum. The needle can then be turned like a drill and advanced into the marrow $^1/_2$ to $^3/_4$ inch.

3. Aspirate blood freely from the marrow. Then inject 3 to 4 ml. of 1% lidocaine slowly. Inject 5 to 10 ml. of Conray (60%), and take one film to ascertain the position of the needle and to be certain that there is no extravasation.

4. Tilt the table 40 to 60 degrees from the verticle, with a footrest attached. Take a series of x-ray films or cinephlebograms as described later. Inject slowly over a three- to four-minute period so that pain is not excessive. A tourniquet above the malleolus will be necessary only if there is an incompetent perforating vein in the foot. To detect other incompetent perforating veins higher in the leg, the dye must be kept out of the superficial veins by the tourniquet.

5. Withdraw the needle on completion of the procedure, apply a pressure bandage over the foot with an elastic bandage, and keep the foot elevated for several hours to avoid extravasation.

Technique of intravenous ascending phlebography

1. Enter any prominent vein on the foot percutaneously with a No. 21 scalp vein or "butterfly" needle and tubing, and tape the needle in place. Inject saline solution slowly to be certain that there is no extravasation, and connect the bottle of saline solution while you load syringes with 90 to 120 ml. of Conray (60%).

2. The foot of the table should be 30 degrees lower than the head. The patient stands with his feet on a pile of folded towels on the footboard attached to the x-ray table.

3. Inject 30 ml. of Conray (60%) slowly during one minute, and take the first film to show the veins in the calf and the popliteal area.

4. Take a film of the anteroposterior view centered at the patella after you slowly inject another 30 ml. of Conray (60%). Then turn the patient in order to get films of a lateral view of the lower leg and lower thigh, or shoot the lateral view across the table top, holding the film by hand.

COMMENT: *While the patient is tilted, the dye remains in the leg and films and position can be changed by hand without special tables or tunnels. Less dye can be used for patients with slender legs or few varicosities.*

5. Take a film of the anteroposterior view of the upper thigh and groin after slowly injecting another 30 ml. of Conray (60%).

6. Visualize the iliac veins and vena cava by the following method. In patients with large legs or with many varicosities, another 30 ml. of dye should be injected. Everything must be ready before the table is leveled, since the dye then begins to move up.

7. After the casette is loaded and in position, the x-ray tube is in position, and the Bucky tray is cocked, level the table, raise the leg for a slow count of three or four seconds, and then expose the film of the abdomen and pelvis.

COMMENT: *The veins of the entire leg have been filled with dye, and when the leg is elevated, the radiopaque medium opacifies the iliac vein very nicely or reveals collateral veins, indicating iliac vein obstruction. Rarely, injection of contrast medium at the groin may be needed to reveal full details of the pelvic and iliac veins.*

8. Infuse 500 ml. of saline solution to clear the contrast medium from the veins, and in five minutes take another film for an intravenous pyelogram.

COMMENT: *If there is any clinical indication suggesting the need for detailed pyelograms or if the five-minute film shows any clues, the full sequence of films is taken in order to complete the intravenous pyelogram.*

Venous pressure determination in foot

Determination of walking erect venous pressures in the foot may be done in conjunction with phlebography in the leg to demonstrate the physiological changes.

Purpose

The procedure is performed to test competence of function of the "venous pump" of the leg and the valves of the superficial veins of the leg.

Indications

Determination of venous pressure in the foot is an excellent physiological demonstration for the students but is seldom needed in clinical practice. The phlebograms reveal the mechanism and sites of reflux and are more useful.

Technique

1. Use a No. 19 or 20 plastic cannula or needle that has been inserted into a foot or leg vein. This is larger than the needle used for phlebography.

2. Connect it to a plastic venous pressure monitoring set with manometer tube and infusion bottle.

3. Tape the venous pressure manometer and centimeter ruler to the side of the intravenous stand with the top slightly higher than the level of the heart. It can be lowered if necessary to keep the pressures on the scale.

4. Fill the manometer and tubing while the patient is standing.

5. Open the connection of the manometer to the foot and permit the fluid to rise in the manometer until the level is stationary. Repeat several times and record the pressure as the SVP (standing venous pressure) in centimeters of water. Consider zero to be at the floor level.

6. Measure and record the WVP (walking venous pressure) by having the patient rise up on tiptoes, repeating once per second for ten seconds.

These walking motions may conveniently be done in place on the foot board of the tilted fluoroscopic table and do not require actual walking. Measure the decrease in pressure by observing the manometer, and record the decrease as a percentage of the standing venous pressure. Use the percentage decrease instead of the actual decrease in centimeters in order to take into account the variation that might otherwise be induced in the figures by differences in the patients' heights.

Interpretation of ascending phlebograms

The ascending phlebogram performed as just described furnishes a map of the veins and some functional information about the venous pump of the lower leg. Tilting ascending phlebograms as described on p. 399 have been helpful as guides in operations for varicose veins.

Superficial veins should not be visible when blood flow has been directed into the deep circulation by the tourniquet. The valves of normal communicating veins allow flow into the deep system but not in the reverse direction. Communicating veins may be visualized above the tourniquet. If communicating veins are incompetent, reflux into superficial veins is seen. Retrograde filling of communicating veins as far as the fascia is normal. Occlusion of the deep veins is evident by collateral circulation around the obstructions. Nonvisualization of the anterior tibial veins may result from tight tourniquets at the ankle.

Phlebography assists the surgeon in locating incompetent perforating veins and in determining the patency of deep veins. In phlebograms of good technical quality, saccular dilations representing the valves of the deep system can be readily discerned. When recanalization of the deep system takes place after deep thrombophlebitis, these valves appear abnormal or are absent from the roentgenogram. Clearing of contrast medium from the leg after repeated contraction of the calf muscles suffices to demonstrate valvular competency below the knee, but the competency of valves in the femoral vein is not so readily demonstrated. Do not, however, rely on roentgenographic findings without knowing exactly how the procedure was performed. Phlebograms should be performed frequently to learn proper technique and interpretation.

Cinephlebography (ascending phlebography) with image intensifier

When a television monitor with a 12-inch screen is available, cinephlebography is the most satisfactory technique with which to localize the incompetent communicating veins. The observation of the flow and the use of the television tape and spot films furnish information that other methods do not. Cinephlebography supplies additional information about the venous pump and the perforating veins. Loose tourniquets or other errors are seen and corrected immediately, and spot films can be repeated to verify doubtful findings. The leg can be emptied by raising it, and injections can be made with various views. The exit of the incompetent communicating vein is marked on the skin while it is viewed on the screen.

Preparation of leg for cinephlebography

1. The dorsal vein of the foot has been cannulated.
2. Tape lead numerals on the skin of the anterior aspect of the leg 3, 6, 9, 12, and 15 cm. superior to the tip of the lateral malleolus.

3. Tape a lead marker on a cotton ball over the center of any ulcer or indurated area.

4. Incline the table 45 to 60 degrees from the vertical after the footrest is attached. The patient will bear weight on the opposite leg so that the leg being examined can be rotated.

Injection of dye and identification of communicating veins

1. Place a Penrose drain tourniquet tightly about the ankle below the malleoli to prevent filling of the superficial veins. If the tourniquet fails to prevent direct filling of the superficial veins, stop the injection and remove the unwanted dye by exercise or elevation of the leg. Reapply the tourniquet more tightly and continue the injection. It may be necessary to reapply the tourniquet just above the malleolus or at the top of an ulcer.

2. Inject Conray (60%) at a rate as slow as 5 to 10 ml. per minute.

COMMENT: *Avoid overfilling of the superficial veins in the early part of the examination. Otherwise, superimposition of many superficial veins confuses the identification of deep veins.*

3. View the contrast material flowing in the deep veins by observing the television monitor, and govern the volume and rate of injection by the abnormalities observed. Watch for retrograde flow from the deep into the superficial veins via the communicating veins.

COMMENT: *Normal communicating veins may fill at rest. The communicating veins are abnormal only when retrograde flow into the superficial veins is observed. This is revealed by the cine technique. Series of static films at intervals can be used for records of the flow, or the cine recording or video tape can be used if this equipment is available.*

4. Rotate the leg internally and externally so that any opacified superficial veins do not overlie the deep veins and so that they may be more readily distinguished.

COMMENT: *Sometimes transverse or circumferential skin veins appear to connect the deep and superficial systems, but rotation of the leg identifies these readily. The deep veins are displaced very little during rotation of the leg. By referring to the anterior lead markers, one can readily distinguish posterior veins because they move in the opposite direction during rotation.*

5. Mark on the skin with a ballpoint pen the location of any incompetent communicating vein. The films during rotation of the leg show that the vein and the tip of the pen coincide, and pressure with the tip of the pen partially empties the vein being marked.

6. Take spot films for reference in the operating room. The level of each perforating vein is seen on the films because of the lead markers. Fill the deep veins slowly but adequately in order not to overlook any incompetent perforating veins.

COMMENT: *Note if deep veins are obliterated. The anterior tibial vein may not fill readily, and another tourniquet below the knee may be needed for making certain that nonvisualization signifies occlusion.*

7. When dye is plainly visible in the popliteal and femoral veins, inspect these for the presence of valves. For filling all the veins, 50 ml. of Conray (60%) may be needed.

8. To test the function of the valves of the deep system, remove the tourniquet

402

and have the patient stand on tiptoes five to ten times; observe the clearing of dye from the leg and film it if cine equipment is available.

COMMENT: *When the deep veins are normal, the dye moves upward rapidly and clears in a few minutes. Several abnormalities of flow may be noted:*

a. The normal veins empty, but dye remains pooled in varicosities.

b. Dye may move up the leg with exercise but reflux down again when muscle contraction stops. The Valsalva maneuver may force dye back down the popliteal or femoral vein.

c. Reflux into the superficial system at rest may be followed by flow from the superficial to the deep system during exercise.

Interpretation of cinephlebograms

As in all phlebography, good technique is essential. The main advantage to the surgeon is the identification of the perforating or communicating veins so that incompetent perforating veins can be ligated. The tourniquet test of Trendelenburg does not localize these veins as well as the films.

The location of indirect perforating veins is quite variable. The direct perforating veins described by Cockett are fairly constant, but there may be others, particularly if the leg has been operated on before. The lowest perforating vein medially is posterior to the malleolus, and if it is incompetent, the tourniquet may have to be placed above the malleoli to prevent flooding of the superficial system via this lowest perforating vein.

Perforating veins causing stasis or reflux are also noted far above the area of the induration or ulceration. Dye may be observed flowing up the deep veins, out the perforating vein, and down the superficial vein toward the ulcer. With the use of the cine technique, the localization of incompetent perforating veins will not require the exploratory long incision in the fascia and subfascial ligation procedures of Cockett or of Linton.

STRIPPING OPERATION FOR VARICOSE VEINS

Completeness of operation

The operation described has supplanted previous techniques. Removal of the varices prevents stasis, relieves symptoms, and improves the appearance of the leg. Varicosities may recur after incomplete operations or because an underlying disease is not recognized and treated. For example, varicosities may develop or recur in tributaries of untreated, incompetent perforating veins.

Varicosities of the lesser saphenous system are difficult to detect but often appear within a few years unless these veins are stripped also. The overlooking of a tributary in the groin or an accessory saphenous vein is a preventable cause of recurrence.

Deep phlebitis with incompetence of the deep veins does not contraindicate removal of the superficial varices for cosmetic and functional reasons. Obstruction in the deep system, however, contraindicates removal of the superficial veins that can be regarded as collateral circulation. With or without stripping, patients with severe postphlebitic changes require lifelong attention to prevent edema of the leg. In difficult cases, support with a pneumatic boot is advisable.

Preoperative care

When there is ulceration, marked swelling, induration, or dermatitis, a preliminary period of bed rest is desirable. Great improvement will follow bed rest and adequate elastic support of the limb. Disappearance of the dermatitis and edema and healing of small ulcers before operation improve postsurgical healing and prevent many complications.

Choice of procedure

The most complete procedure is the best procedure. Two teams can work simultaneously. Adequate operation includes the following aspects:
1. Ligation of the greater saphenous vein at its entrance into the femoral vein with interruption and ligation of all tributaries near the fossa ovalis
2. Stripping of the greater and lesser saphenous systems
3. External stripping of the accessory saphenous vein or other large tributaries at the groin
4. Local ligation or interruption of incompetent communicating veins
5. Local excision of large nests of varicosities through which the stripper cannot be passed

Anesthesia

Spinal or general anesthesia is suitable.

Other preparations

Prior to the operation, examine the patient in the erect position. Mark visible and palpable veins of the long and short saphenous systems and other large varicosities with gentian violet or ferric chloride–pyrogallic acid solution or by superficial scratches. Small varices may not be seen when the patient is recumbent. Instruct the patient to lather himself thoroughly with antiseptic soap such as pHisoHex and to blot the legs dry without rinsing to leave an antiseptic film on the skin. The patient should renew any marks that have faded.

Procedure
High ligation of greater saphenous vein

1. Place the patient in the supine position.
2. Suspend the leg so that the leg and foot can be cleansed and prepared completely.
3. Drape the legs so that they may be lifted or flexed at the knee.
4. Make a groin incision over the fossa ovalis and parallel to the inguinal ligament.

COMMENT: *The fossa is easily palpated as a depression just medial to the femoral pulse and close to the inguinal ligament. In fat people, the crease of the groin is low. The incision need not be long in slender persons. One third of the incision is lateral, and two thirds is medial to the fossa.*

5. Deepen the incision through the subcutaneous fat and the subcutaneous fascia. This fascia is the first landmark. Any of the tributaries encountered beneath the fascia will lead to the greater saphenous vein. Do not search for the vein until you have incised the superficial fascia (Fig. 17-1, *A*).
6. Trace the saphenous vein upward, and as branches are encountered, carefully free, ligate, and divide them. The number of tributaries may vary from a few to six, seven, or eight.

COMMENT: *The medial accessory saphenous vein, a large tributary that drains the*

404

upper medial thigh, frequently connects with tributaries on the posterior part of the thigh and with the short saphenous vein in the popliteal region. The external strippers devised by Doyle* permit removal of long lengths of this and other veins without extra incisions. The external strippers are also useful when a large tributary is found coursing down the anterior part of the thigh toward other varicosities. When there are varicosities in these regions, make a special effort to identify and strip these large tributaries.

7. Lift the saphenous vein sufficiently to tent up the saphenofemoral junction slightly. Enlarge the fossa ovalis by incision of the femoral sheath 2 cm. superiorly and inferiorly. Indentify the common femoral vein, and make sure that there are no additional subcutaneous tributaries entering the saphenous or femoral veins.

8. Divide and ligate the saphenous vein flush with the femoral vein with transfixion suture. Irrigate and cover the incision.

Stripping of greater (long) saphenous veins

Make a short transverse incision anterior to and just below the medial malleolus (Fig. 17-1, *C*). Isolate the greater saphenous vein. If the vein is prominent on the dorsum of the foot, it may be identified and stripped from there. Tie the vein distally with 2-0 or 3-0 plain catgut, divide it, and pass the flexible intraluminal stripper upward through the veins. In many patients, the stripper reaches the groin at once. However, sometimes the stripper is arrested by large and tortuous varicosities, and accessory incisions are necessary. Through the accessory incision, a perforating vein may often be found and ligated, and the same or another stripper can be passed up the rest of the saphenous vein to the groin.

COMMENT: *Transverse incisions are preferred in the leg because they are under less tension and heal as a thinner scar than vertical incisions.*

Make short transverse incisions to excise varices that are (1) too tortuous for the stripper to pass through them, (2) too far off the course of the stripper to be disconnected, or (3) too large to be fulgurated with the Vein Eraser (p. 410).

External stripping of large tributaries

The elegant external strippers of small diameter with longer and sharper barrel-shaped heads and short handles devised by Doyle can be passed over the flexible internal strippers inserted in the lumen of large tributaries. The flexible cable of the internal stripper guides the external stripper until it is stopped by a large tributary. Thrusting the external stripper forward cuts off the vein at that site so that a section many inches in length can be withdrawn through the proximal incisions without a counter incision's being made at the distal end of the cable stripper. This is very useful for large tributaries in the thigh, those of the short saphenous vein, and occasionally, those on the foot.

COMMENT: *Do not confuse Doyle's external strippers with the antique and crude external strippers that were retired forty years ago.*

Selection of small vein retractors of various widths and depths helps to make the exposure better in small incisions on the lower leg or foot.

Stripping of lesser (short) saphenous vein

1. The lesser saphenous vein is approached by tilting the table, flexing the knee, and rotating the thigh. It is cumbersome and unnecessary to turn the patient unless

---

*Custom-made by Storz Instrument Co., St. Louis, Mo.

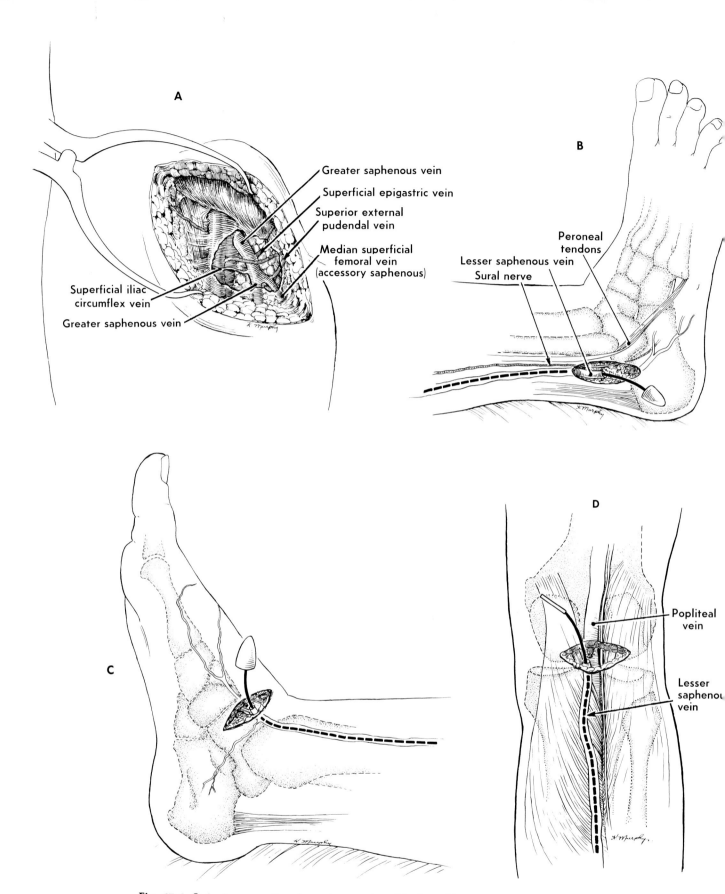

Fig. 17-1. Stripping operation for varicose veins. Thigh and leg incisions should be transverse and *shorter than illustrated.* **A,** Groin incision and exposure for high ligation of greater saphenous veins. **B,** Ankle exposure for stripping of lesser saphenous vein. **C,** Foot incision and exposure for stripping of greater saphenous vein. **D,** Popliteal incision and exposure for ligation and stripping of lesser saphenous vein.

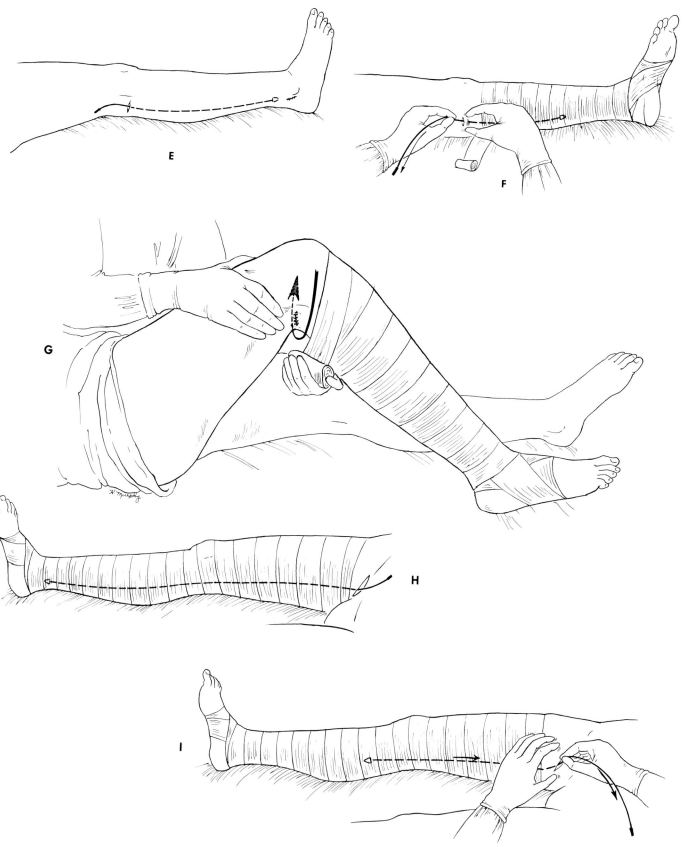

Fig. 17-1, cont'd. Stripping operation for varicose veins. **E,** Vein strippers in place and incisions closed below knee. **F,** Lower leg wrapped and stripper withdrawn from lesser saphenous vein. **G** and **H,** Entire leg wrapped. All incisions closed below groin. **I,** Stripper withdrawn from greater saphenous vein.

prominent popliteal varicosities require wider exposure. The patient can be prepared and draped so that it is unnecessary to turn or redrape him.

2. Make an incision just behind the lateral malleolus (Fig. 17-1, *B*). The lesser saphenous vein is located in the groove between the tendo Achillis posteriorly and the tendons of the peroneus longus and brevis muscles anteriorly. The sural nerve lies deep to the vein. Divide the vein and ligate it distally with fine catgut. There are numerous tributaries that also should be ligated.

3. Pass the stripper upward to the popliteal fossa, and palpate the stripper with the patient's knee flexed. Keep in mind the following anatomical variations of the lesser saphenous system if the stripper follows an unusual course:

a. The lesser saphenous vein may penetrate the deep fascia in the midcalf.

b. The lesser saphenous vein penetrates the deep fascia in the popliteal fossa, and the branch of varying size (accessory saphenous) ascends subcutaneously into the medial portion of the thigh.

c. The lesser saphenous vein may continue beyond the popliteal fossa into the medial part of the thigh, joining the greater saphenous system at a higher level. There is a communicating branch to the popliteal vein in the popliteal fossa.

4. With the patient's thigh and knee flexed and the thigh externally rotated, make a small incision in the popliteal fossa (Fig. 17-1, *D*). A sitting position is advantageous for the surgeon. Palpate the stripper. Ligate and divide either the lesser saphenous vein or its branch entering the popliteal vein at this site.

COMMENT: *Longer popliteal incisions are necessary in patients with many popliteal tributaries and large lesser saphenous varices. The longer incision permits meticulous ligation and interruption of these tributaries in the popliteal fossa. If the long popliteal incision is necessary, the legs should be draped so that the patient can be turned on his side. Annoying herniation of fat will occur unless the popliteal fascia is carefully closed.*

Treatment of residual varicosities

Thorough stripping removes most of the varicosities and disconnects others from the incompetent communicating veins. However, other varicosities may be found along the course of large tributaries in the thigh or in the lower leg, and these must be treated before the legs are wrapped and the strippers removed. The following methods are available: (a) removal of large and tortuous varices through multiple transverse incisions, (b) fulguration of smaller veins as described on p. 410, and (c) internal or external stripping of other varicose tributaries through which the flexible cable will pass.

Further eradication of smaller veins that are not removed at a stripping operation may be requested by women who desire treatment of varicose veins for cosmetic purposes. Sodium tetradecyl sulfate (Sotradecol) is injected into small residual veins segmentally and carefully in the office after operation. This method is applicable only to small veins and must not be used on the major veins of the leg.

Closure of incisions

1. Excise any large nests of varicose veins locally. Ligate any previously located incompetent perforating or communicating veins. Below the knee all ligations should be accomplished with fine plain catgut. Close these incisions.

2. Place the appropriate-sized olive tips on the distal ends of the vein strippers.

Start withdrawing them under the skin for a short distance (Fig. 17-1, *E*). Close the distal incisions with continous sutures of 4-0 nylon. Apply sterile dressings, and pad the ankle, dorsum of the foot, and subcutaneous edge of the tibia. Wrap the leg with a sterile foam rubber–coated elastic bandage or with a sterile self-adherent (Peg*) elastic bandage (Fig. 17-1, *F*).

Withdraw the stripper from the lesser saphenous vein, and close the popliteal incision (Fig. 17-1, *G*), when the wrapping has reached the knee.

COMMENT: *Hematoma at the site of stripping is the cause of most postoperative pain. It is avoided by withdrawing strippers with the gentle pressure bandage in place over the incisions.*

3. Wrap the remainder of the leg so that the compression dressing is in place when the stripper is withdrawn at the groin; this reduces extravasation, swelling, and hematoma formation. Protect the knee with padding. Continue wrapping the leg with the elastic bandages until other incisions or the groin is reached (Fig. 17-1, *H*). Withdraw the strippers (Fig. 17-1, *I*), closing and dressing the incisions as you proceed with the wrapping.

The lower leg and ankle incisions as well as the patella, Achilles tendon, and front of the foot should be padded.

The elastic foam rubber and the self-adhering elastic bandages do not slip or wrinkle easily and minimize postoperative hematoma, swelling, and discomfort.

4. Close the groin incision in layers, using catgut for the subcutaneous fascia.

COMMENT: *The following method is expeditious when there are several assistants to work on both legs simultaneously.*

Place the appropriate-sized olive tip on the proximal end of the strippers, and withdraw them under the skin a short distance.

The surgical team simultaneously closes all incisions except at the ankle, where the ends of the strippers emerge. Place skin stitches in these ankle incisions, but do not tie them until the legs are wrapped and the strippers are withdrawn.

Apply sterile dressings and pad all pressure points so that the leg can be wrapped snugly with sterile elastic bandages. Use the bandage with the 6-inch width to wrap the thigh and knee after the patella is padded. Use the 4-inch bandage to wrap the lower leg to the ankle after the tibia and Achilles tendon are padded.

Withdraw the strippers at the ankle. Tie the stitches previously placed. Then pad the dorsum of the foot and continue wrapping the bandage down over the ankle and foot.

Postoperative care

On the following day the patient should walk five minutes every hour. Sitting is not allowed. When not walking, the patient must lie in bed with the foot of the bed elevated.

Groin sutures are removed after three or four days and other skin sutures after one week. However, incisions lower in the leg, particularly if made through edematous and pigmented skin, heal more slowly. Elastic bandages or elastic stockings are worn until edema and discomfort have ceased.

Foam rubber–lined or self-adhering elastic bandages provide better support than

*Becton, Dickinson & Co., Rutherford, N. J.

ordinary elastic bandages because they do not slip. In wrapping the leg with the foam rubber–lined bandage, care must be taken to avoid excessive tension. These bandages may easily be applied too tightly by those accustomed to applying stretchable cotton bandages. Because of the degree of pressure exerted, padding, as indicated in the preceding description, is essential beneath the bandage.

Complications

The most common complication of vein stripping is hematoma. External pressure obtained by wrapping the legs prior to stripping, as previously described, prevents troublesome subcutaneous hemorrhage.

Phlebitis in the deep veins is relatively rare if the postoperative regimen of early and frequent ambulation, snug wrapping, and elevation of the legs is followed. For the first few postoperative weeks, the patient is cautioned against long periods of sitting with the legs in a dependent position.

Complications in the groin incision are unusual. Careful preoperative cleansing, hemostasis, irrigation, and careful closure of the incision in layers prevent the collections of serum and lymph that predispose to infection.

FULGURATION OF VARICOSE VEINS
Purpose

Fulguration is used during vein operations to obliterate small varicosities and small perforating veins and to avoid multiple incisions.

Principle

Both saphenous trunks are stripped and large perforating veins are ligated by the usual method. The remaining smaller veins can be reached and fulgurated with the special probe* through a few tiny stab incisions.

Procedure

1. The vein strippers are in place. The varicose veins and perforating veins have been marked. The patient is in the Trendelenburg position so that the veins are empty, and all veins to be obliterated by this method must therefore be carefully marked in advance.

2. Choose the site of the incisions so that the probe can be passed in several directions to reach the veins. Make a small stab incision with a No. 11 blade to pass the 11-gauge fulgurating probe beneath the skin. The incision should be at least 2 cm. from the first point of electrocoagulation.

3. Pass the probe subcutaneously along the vein, and coagulate the vein at 1 cm. distances by pressing the trigger on the probe handle. Depress the handle so that the tip of the probe elevates the skin lightly.

COMMENT: *The duration of current is preset for 0.7 second. Set the current output at 8.5 for the larger electrode and 3 for the smaller electrode. There will be an audible sound with each "shot." The tip of the probe must not be too superficial, or a blister and small burn will appear. Use caution in coagulating veins overlying bone, since periosteal and cortical bone necrosis may result when the tip of the probe is too close to the bone.*

---

*Vein Eraser, Medtronic Inc., Minneapolis, Minn.

4. The smaller electrode (16-gauge) is used where the skin and subcutaneous tissue are thin (for example, on the feet or popliteal area, over bone, at the ankle, and over the tibia) and also for the cosmetic eradication of small intradermal angiectases or venules. The probe can also be passed inside the lumen. The generator output is set at 3.0.

5. The stripping is completed as previously described. The fulguration incisions need no closure, only Steristrips or butterfly bandages.

6. Postoperative care is the same as that given following stripping. An occasional blister or burn needs no special treatment, but the small eschar may persist several weeks. If a few veins remain they may be fulgurated under local anesthesia on an outpatient basis. Fulguration is far superior to the sclerosing injections sometimes used for this purpose.

Some numbness or paresthesia may occur and remain several months. However, such peripheral neuritis is not troublesome.

SUBFASCIAL LIGATION OF COMMUNICATING VEINS FOR POSTPHLEBITIC SYNDROME

A small proportion of patients with numerous varicose veins and many incompetent perforating veins require a more extensive incision with ligation of the perforating veins beneath the deep fascia. These patients have usually had previous operations, recurrent varicosities, and ulceration from old thrombophlebitis. The advantages of subfascial ligation are better visualization of the perforating veins and better healing of the skin than after multiple incisions or more superficial skin flaps. Some of the patients will have had many previous incomplete operations. This extensive procedure should be reserved only for patients with severe recurrent varicose veins, ulceration, and postphlebitic syndrome.

Phlebography is indicated to ensure patency of the deep veins of the calf before subfascial ligation is performed. Ulcers superior to one or both malleoli may be fed by incompetent perforating veins just above the malleoli, but in some cases the cinephlebograms show reflux from incompetent perforating veins higher up in the leg or on the opposite side of the leg. Sometimes superficial varicosities are minimal.

Anatomy

Communicating veins connect the superficial and deep systems of veins in the legs. The usual sites of penetration of the deep fascia are (1) just medial to the subcutaneous border of the tibia, connecting to the long saphenous system, (2) the calf on the posterolateral aspect of the leg, and (3) the anterior portion of the calf just lateral to the anterior tibial muscle.

Preoperative preparation

Bed rest with elevation of the leg, skin grafts, and preliminary vein stripping must all be employed as indicated so that cellulitis, dermatitis, and ulceration have either healed or improved greatly before subfascial ligation is undertaken. For details of the stripping procedure, refer to p. 403. For skin grafting, refer to p. 413.

Procedure

1. Prepare and drape the leg so that the thigh and knee can be flexed.
2. Make a longitudinal incision along the course of the long saphenous vein from

just below the knee toward the medial malleous. Incise the fascia in a longitudinal direction.

3. Elevate the anterior flap of skin, subcutaneous tissue, and fascia to the edge of the tibia.

4. Ligate and divide all veins penetrating the fascia.

5. Elevate the posterior flap of skin, subcutaneous fat, and fascia as far as the midline posteriorly, and ligate all other veins penetrating the fascia.

6. If it still remains, identify the subfascial portion of the lesser saphenous vein in the popliteal fossa. Ligate this vein near the popliteal vein. The anatomical variations of the lesser saphenous vein have been reviewed in the preceding pages.

7. Identify the sural nerve as it accompanies the lesser saphenous vein and penetrates the deep fascia somewhat lower than the vein. Incise the deep fascia on both side of the lesser saphenous vein. Exposure is obtained by flexing the knee and retracting the calf muscles. Remove a strip of fascia $1/2$ to 1 inch wide from the popliteal space to well down the posterior aspect of the calf. The strip may be narrowed toward the ankle.

COMMENT: *Linton has advised that this fasciectomy be done to remove a possible barrier to future communications between the deep and superficial lymphatic vessels of the leg. It is probably better to allow the fascia to remain intact. The envelope of deep fascia about the calf muscles is an integral part of the venous pumping mechanism of the leg. It has been suggested that when the fascia is loose, venous return may indeed be restored by tightening the fascial compartments, but we have had no experience with the procedure. Firm elastic support should accomplish the same end.*

8. Subfascial dissection can extend laterally as far as the fibula. Ligate the incompetent communicating veins.

9. Complete any stripping, local excisions, and similar procedures that have been done. Close the medial incision in the deep fascia with 3-0 chromic catgut. Close the skin incision with nonabsorbable suture material. Splint the foot, ankle, and leg with a well-padded compression dressing.

Distal subfascial ligation of communicating veins

A less extensive subfascial ligation is sufficient for some cases. The incision may not have to extend the full length of the leg, and the subfascial dissection need not extend around to the fibula.

1. Make a longitudinal incision 1 inch posterior and parallel to the posterior border of the tibia. The incision starts 1 to $1^1/2$ inches above the medial malleolus and 1 inch posterior to it and is extended superiorly as far as necessary.

2. Divide the deep fascia.

3. Identify the perforating veins beneath the deep fascia. With small ulcers there are usually only two or three perforating veins. Incompetent perforating veins are larger than normal veins and may be 3 to 10 mm. in diameter.

4. Divide and ligate these veins.

5. Close the fascia and skin with interrupted sutures.

6. Elevate the leg and apply elastic dressing snugly from toes to knee.

COMMENT: *This operation is most suitable for small ulcers, particularly if there are no superficial varicosities. In patients with such ulcers, stripping of the superficial veins or the more radical excision and grafting are unnecessary. Occasionally, stasis ulcers anterior to the lateral malleolus are fed by veins that course inferior to the malleolus and enter the lesser saphenous system posterior to the lateral malleolus.*

Postoperative care

Healing tends to be prolonged. The leg is kept elevated for seven to ten days, and the dressing is changed when necessary. Walking and weight bearing are allowed when the incisions are well healed and the limb is not edematous. A stout knee-length, open-toe, closed-heel elastic stocking is worn for six to twelve months after the operation or as long as necessary to prevent edema.

EXCISION AND GRAFTING FOR STASIS ULCER
Indications and preoperative preparation

Ulcers that cannot be healed by more conservative measures should be excised, and a skin graft should be applied. A preliminary period of bed rest lasting for several weeks, with elevation of the legs and frequent change of dressings, helps to clear local infection, relieve edema, and ensure rapid healing. Many stasis ulcers are colonized by *Pseudomonas, Proteus,* and other resistant organisms. Compresses dampened or soaked with 0.5% silver nitrate solution are very effective in such cases. The silver nitrate compresses can be reapplied at the end of the grafting operation just as in treatment of burns. Many ulcers can be healed by a regimen of conservative treatment consisting of bed rest followed by external elastic support.

When stasis in superficial varicosities is the main etiological factor, the veins should be stripped. If there has been a previous stripping, it is likely that incompetent communicating veins have been overlooked. Excision of the ulcer may reveal underlying veins, and it permits ligation and interruption of some of them. A search for other incompetent perforating veins should also be made by phlebography. The fascia beneath the ulcer is also affected by stasis and must be removed to furnish a healthy bed for the skin graft.

Some leg ulcers have an avascular base, especially those over bone, those occurring after compound fractures, and those from previous radiation treatment. Muscles can be transplanted as described by Ger (1972) to form a healthy base to heal and nourish the skin grafts, which are applied five to seven days later. (See Ger's descriptions and drawings for full details.) The muscles shifted vary according to the site of the ulcer. In the midportion of the leg, flaps of the soleus muscle can be detached from their distal insertion and turned or folded anteriorly. In the lower leg, a few minor muscles are transplanted, and the distal ends of divided tendons are sutured to other nearby tendons with similar actions. The skin graft is performed five to seven days later on the healthy muscular base.

Differential diagnosis

Other types of leg ulcers must be considered in differential diagnosis, including the ulcers associated with arteriosclerosis, blood dyscrasias, and hypertensive ischemic ulcer and leg ulcers associated with rheumatoid arthritis and erythrocyanosis. Carcinoma may develop in chronic stasis ulcers.

Anesthesia

Local anesthesia, spinal anesthesia, or general anesthesia may be employed.

413

Procedure

1. Prepare the entire leg on the affected side or both legs if the procedure is to be bilateral.

2. Drape the leg. Remove a split-thickness skin graft from the lateral part of the thigh, where the skin is somewhat thicker. This should be taken with the dermatome set at 0.015 to 0.02 inch. Dress the donor site. Preserve the graft in a sponge dampened with Ringer's solution.

3. Outline the area on the leg to be excised with gentian violet or some similar marking fluid. The extent of exicision is determined not by the area of ulceration but by the area of induration and dermatitis still surrounding the ulcer after a period of elevation or elastic support. Lymphatic vessels have not regenerated in indurated areas. Such areas must be excised. Otherwise, edema will prevent satisfactory take of the graft. The incision may be made through pigmented skin but not through the indurated area. (See Fig. 17-2, A.)

4. Incise down to and through the deep fascia. The skin may be beveled. Along with the skin, remove the deep fascia. The bed for the graft is the areolar tissue overlying the periosteum and muscle. Do not follow fascia into the muscle septa.

5. Ligate the perforating veins as they are exposed.

6. Apply the split-thickness graft. Sew the edges of the graft to the fresh skin edges (Fig. 17-2, B). Continuous sutures are suitable for this procedure. The graft may overlap normal skin and may be held securely in many cases with only a few stitches and a snug dressing. Make a few small holes in the graft to allow drainage of any serum that may accumulate beneath it.

7. Cover the graft with Xeroform or petrolatum gauze topped by a generous bulky pressure dressing of machinist's waste. Apply an elastic bandage. A splint for the foot may be needed to prevent undue motion of the bed of the graft.

Postoperative care

The leg must not be dependent at any time during the immediate postoperative period. If it is, the skin graft will not adhere. Bed rest must be encouraged for the

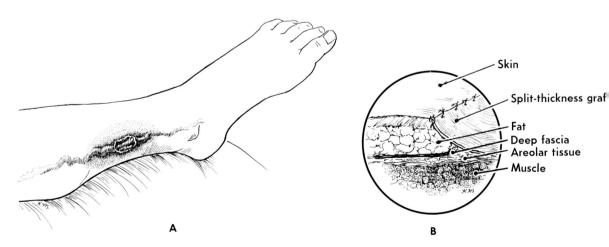

Fig. 17-2. Excision and grafting of stasis ulcer. **A,** Stasis ulcer above medial malleolus. **B,** Cross section of edge after excision and graft of stasis ulcer.

first ten to fourteen days. If 0.5% silver nitrate compresses were needed preoperatively for resistant infections, they can be applied over the skin grafts for a few days.

Dress the wound on the fifth day or before. Remove the old dressing carefully in order not to disturb the graft. Trim any dead skin at the edge of the graft. At the first dressing, some areas of the graft will appear pink and healthy, whereas others may be darkly colored. Darkly colored areas should not be removed, since they are usually viable. The superficial layers of skin will peel off; this condition should not be mistaken for death or loss of the graft. Make a tiny hole in the graft over any small blister or accumulation of blood or fluid that may have appeared. Reapply a bulky pressure dressing. Remove the sutures between seven and ten days after operation.

After the initial period of bed rest for seven to ten days has passed and after take of the graft seems ensured, observe the appearance of the graft while the leg is dependent. Allow ambulation for five to ten minutes each hour, but only with strong elastic support. The 4-inch elastic foam bandages are less likely to slip than the usual Ace bandage. Gradually increase the periods of dependency and increase ambulation. Change the dressing and inspect the graft daily until the patient leaves the hospital. The patient must wear an elastic support and must have careful supervision for three months or until there is no edema in the limb. In patients with venous obstruction, lymphatic obstruction, or severe edema, the Aeropulse pneumatic legging* may control edema and maintain healing of the graft when all other forms of elastic support fail.

THROMBOPHLEBITIS

Thrombophlebitis may involve the superficial or the deep veins or both. If the superficial veins are involved, the diagnosis is obvious. In the deep veins of the calf, the diagnosis of thrombophlebitis is difficult when the onset and initial symptoms are insidious. The clinical manifestations may be so mild that they pass unnoticed. Indeed, the first manifestation can be pulmonary embolism.

Thrombophlebitis in the legs is far more common than any of us have realized. Phlebography and the ^{131}I-labeled fibrinogen test have detected clots in 20% to 40% of routine postoperative cases, and few of these have clinical signs or symptoms.

The physician must be watchful and suspicious of fever, pain, or discomfort in the legs of patients during early postoperative periods or in patients with fractures or other illnesses or injuries requiring bed rest. Slight distension of the pretibial vein, slight cyanosis, or edema may develop when the clots become obstructive. Pain and tenderness appear when the thrombosis excites inflammation or vasospasm. Homans' sign is helpful in differentiating phlebitis in the deep veins and other causes of calf tenderness. Phlebograms show that clots are more extensive than suspected.

Saphenous phlebitis

Although minor episodes of saphenous phlebitis are managed conservatively, extensive cases can be quickly cured by excision of the affected vein. Conservative treatment is prolonged and is followed by recurrence and varicosities.

When the patient has had varicosities prior to the attack of phlebitis, high ligation of the saphenous vein, together with excision of the thrombosed segment, or strip-

---

*Surgical Research Corporation, c/o Turner Bellows Co., 165 N. Waters St., Rochester, N. Y. 14604.

ping can be performed. The saphenous vein should be opened before the ligation because unsuspected thrombus may extend into the femoral vein and should be removed with the techniques and precautions described for iliofemoral thrombectomy. The use of anticoagulants is unnecessary. Ambulation is begun the day after operation, and postoperative care is the same as for elective stripping of varicose veins. Incisions for removal of the inflamed and clotted saphenous vein may be quite long, but the period of disability is short.

Septic thrombophlebitis

Infected clots cause septicemia and metastatic abscesses to the lungs, brain, liver, or other organs. Septic thrombophlebitis is uncommon; but it may result from inlying plastic catheters or pelvic inflammatory disease, and it is frequently seen in drug addicts. The treatment is ligation of the veins and the use of appropriate antibiotics. Rarely, fever remains until the septic vein is excised. The use of anticoagulants is no substitute for operation in the treatment of septic thrombophlebitis.

Nonoperative management of phlebitis of deep veins

The following measures are beneficial to patients with acute phlebitis of the deep veins:

1. Elevate the foot of the bed. Phlebograms show that this prevents venous stasis in the small pockets just behind the valves of the deep veins.

2. Begin anticoagulation therapy with heparin. Heparin is given intravenously at six-hour intervals, usually at 8 A.M., 2 P.M., 8 P.M., and 2 A.M., in doses sufficient to maintain the partial thromboplastin time (PTT) at twice the normal value when obtained five hours after the heparin dose is given. The use of a small scalp vein infusion needle with attached tubing and a rubber cap avoids multiple venipunctures.

COMMENT: *Lee-White clotting times are unreliable for clinical laboratories. The PTT is reproducible, sensitive, and accurate and is the only reliable guide to heparin therapy outside the research laboratory. The PTT can be obtained at 7 A.M. daily, that is, one hour before the 8 A.M. dose is given. The usual dosage is 7,000 to 10,000 units every six hours.*

3. Maintain bed rest. This prevents edema, congestion, and stasis. Loosely attached thrombi are less likely to be dislodged. Later the patient may walk for a few minutes each hour.

4. Apply hot packs to the leg for the first few days. Application of heat as hot wet packs enhances blood flow in the extremity and helps prevent the extension of thrombosis. Ambulation has been advocated to achieve this same result but is undesirable for patients with pain or edema. Elastic bandages are applied to divert venous return into the deep system after the use of hot packs is discontinued.

5. Begin warfarin sodium (Coumadin sodium) therapy on the fifth day while heparin therapy is continued for ten to fourteen days from onset.

COMMENT: *Even though therapeutic antiprothrombin activity may be rapidly attained, the full antithrombotic effect of warfarin is not attained for four or five days. Therefore, the overlapping of the heparin therapy and warfarin therapy is essential.*

While the patient is being given heparin, 10 mg. daily is sufficient for the first few days. Do not give large "loading" doses of warfarin to patients who are also receiving heparin.

6. Regulate the warfarin dosage with daily Orrin prothrombin and proconvertin

(P and P) tests while the patient is also being given heparin. Try to attain a P and P time of 5% to 10% of normal. Rarely, it may be necessary to give 12 to 15 mg. of warfarin daily for a few days. After three or four days, less will be needed.

COMMENT: *Heparin prolongs the usual prothrombin time (PT), so that it is useless to obtain the PT until heparin therapy is stopped.*

7. Decrease the heparin dosage gradually each day after the Orrin P and P time is in the therapeutic level, which is 5% to 10% of normal.

COMMENT: *The PTT may remain twice the normal value even after the heparin dosage has been halved because warfarin also increases the PTT.*

8. Stop heparin therapy twelve to fourteen days after onset when P and P time is in the therapeutic range. Begin obtaining PT daily after heparin therapy has been stopped, and maintain warfarin dosage sufficient to keep the PT at twenty to thirty seconds.

COMMENT: *Give some warfarin daily, even if only a few milligrams; otherwise, the P and P times swing over a wide range and it is harder to adjust the dosage to a steady level.*

9. Vigilant and frequent observation is essential. Small emboli may give no sign at all or only increases in pulse, temperature, and respiration (Allen's sign). Pleuritic pain, chest pain, cough, and hemoptysis signify pulmonary infarction.

10. The patient begins to walk a few minutes each hour after five to ten days if the leg is not painful. Elastic wrapping is essential.

Discussion

Conservative treatment has failed if pulmonary embolism occurs. Embolism may occur despite improvement of the legs. In such situations, interruption of the inferior vena cava must be considered, as discussed in Chapter 18.

Techniques for enzymatic dissolution of clots are under investigation and may be practicable in the future.

Currently dextran for the treatment of phlebitis is under investigation, but we have had little experience with it. Dextran, which alters the physical and flow properties of blood, is no substitute for anticoagulants, particularly heparin, as outlined previously.

We routinely advise a low-fat diet because of the effect on coagulation of small fat globules in the bloodstream.

Bypass operation for venous obliteration

When permanent common femoral or iliac vein occlusion has occurred, the collateral flow around the obstruction can be improved and some relief obtained surgically. The saphenous vein in the opposite leg is divided low in the thigh, and the end is brought subcutaneously across the pubis to the affected femoral vein below the site of obstruction, where it is anastomosed and will now function as a cross-leg femorosaphenous vein bypass. Since the ulceration that follows phlebitis of the deep veins frequently takes years to appear, some time must pass before the long-term end results of this new procedure are evident. As criteria for the operation, we recommend edema or discomfort of the affected limb persisting for over six months and roentgenographic evidence of competent unaffected valves in the deep veins of the calf along with a demonstrated obstruction at the common femoral level or above.

Massive venous occlusion (phlegmasia cerulea dolens)
Signs and symptoms

The onset of massive venous occlusion may be slow, following a smoldering phlebitis, or it may develop rapidly even in an ambulatory patient. The symptoms are massive tense edema, severe pain, and bluish discoloration of the leg, thigh, and even the buttock. The limb becomes cold. Peripheral pulses may diminish and disappear in the involved extremity. Gangrene may result even though the arteries are patent. Venous pressures in the affected leg are very high, ranging from 40 to 100 cm. of water compared to pressures of under 10 cm. in the normal extremity (with the patient supine).

Nonoperative treatment

Medical treatment and large intravenous doses of heparin give rapid relief of pain and such rapid improvement that operation or sympathetic nerve block is seldom necessary. Conservative treatment includes elevation of the legs, anticoagulation with large doses of heparin, and prompt intravenous replacement of the extracellular fluid lost into the massively swollen leg. Many of the clinical manifestations of venous thrombosis of this degree are caused by vasospasm of both the arterial and the venous systems. Edwards (1958) observed a consistent and gradual decline in venous pressure after sympathetic block by spinal anesthesia.

If symptoms do not improve rapidly, thrombectomy should be performed before the clot becomes adherent (that is, within twelve to forty-eight hours after onset). Thrombectomy has also been advised for phlegmasia alba dolens to restore normal flow and to prevent the long-term aftereffects of phlebitis of the deep veins and destruction of the valves. However, postoperative phlebograms almost always show occlusion of the vein and loss of the valves, so that the operation is seldom performed.

The syndrome may be a complication of some grave underlying disease.

FEMORAL VEIN THROMBECTOMY FOR ILIOFEMORAL THROMBOSIS
Preoperative preparation

The clotting time is determined preoperatively. Heparin and several pints of blood should be available in the operating room. The operator should be prepared to encounter variations in the anatomy of the femoral veins (Fig. 17-3). The entire leg should be prepared and draped.

Anesthesia

Local anesthesia is preferred. Spinal or general anesthesia is also suitable.

Procedure
Exposure

1. Make a vertical incision beginning at the midportion of the inguinal ligament or at the point where femoral pulsation can be palpated. Extend the incision 4 or 5 inches downward and medially, following approximately the medial border of the sartorius muscle (Fig. 17-4, *A*).

2. Incise the deep fascia medial to the sartorius muscle, and retract the muscle laterally (Fig. 17-4, *B*). The tissue is edematous.

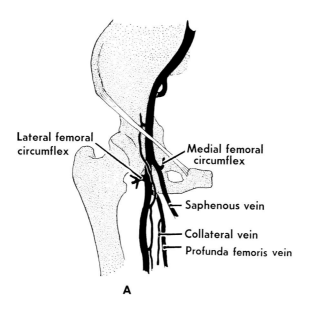

A

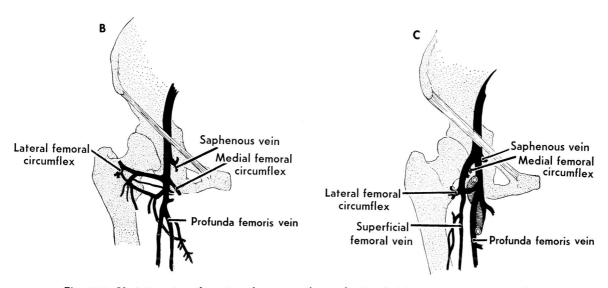

Fig. 17-3. Variations in tributaries of common femoral vein. **A,** Most common pattern of veins at groin. **B** and **C,** Other variations. Note the progressively increasing size of the profunda femoris branch and the corresponding decrease in size and importance of the superficial femoral vein in the changing patterns **A** to **C.** (Redrawn from Edwards, E. A., and Robuck, J. D.: Surg. Gynecol. Obstet. **85**:547, 1947; by permission of Surgery, Gynecology & Obstetrics.)

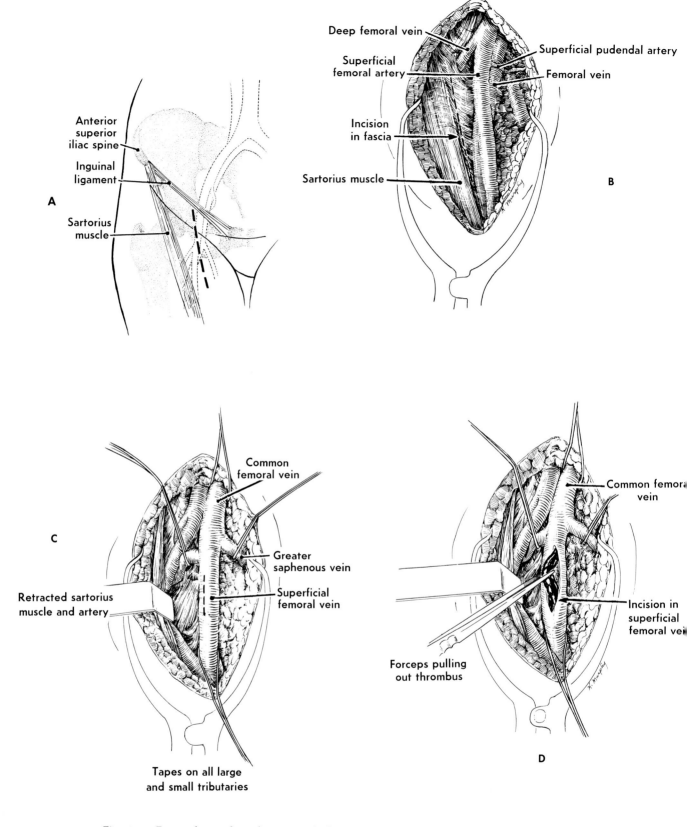

Fig. 17-4. Femoral vein thrombectomy. **A,** Incision. **B,** Exposure of veins and artery. **C,** Tapes in place for control of all tributaries during phlebotomy. **D,** Clot is extruded spontaneously under pressure.

420

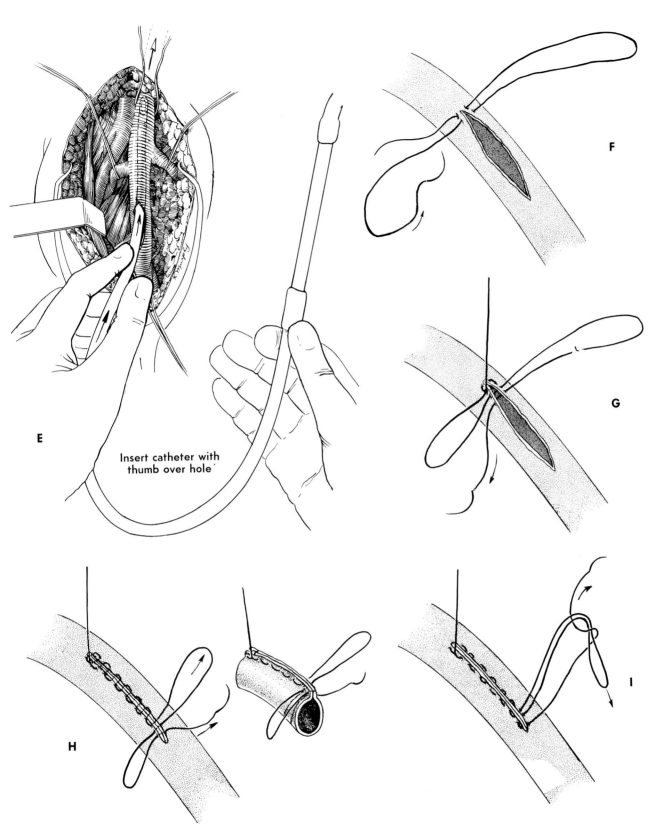

Insert catheter with
thumb over hole

E

F

G

H

I

Fig. 17-4, cont'd. Femoral vein thrombectomy. **E,** Removal of iliac thrombus with suction catheter. **F** to **I,** Closure of phlebotomy with continuous everting mattress suture.

3. Incise the femoral sheath, beginning proximally, and carefully and gently isolate the femoral artery and vein. The diagnosis is confirmed by the tense bulging femoral vein, which appears to be thick walled, pale, and dull. Divide the superficial external pudendal artery as it crosses the femoral vein.

Proximal and distal control

Pass tapes about the common femoral vein proximally, about the saphenous vein, and about the common or superficial femoral vein distally (Fig. 17-4, *C*). The common femoral vein is preferable if the deep femoral vein is difficult to isolate. Variations in the anatomy of tributaries of the common femoral vein are illustrated in Fig. 17-3. All tributaries must be isolated and some provision (tape or clamp) made for their occlusion, or troublesome bleeding occurs after the incision in the vein.

Phlebotomy and thrombectomy

1. Traction on the tapes placed proximally and distally on the femoral vein and other tributaries controls bleeding. Tilt the operating table to elevate the patient's head.

2. Make a longitudinal incision about 1 to 1.5 cm. long in the vein, and the black gelatinous thrombus will be extruded under pressure. The anesthetist should give 50 mg. of heparin intravenously at this time.

3. Now remove the peripheral portion of the thrombus by a combination of pressure and massage of the leg and thigh, suction, and introduction of Fogarty balloon catheters. These procedures should be continued until back bleeding is rather brisk.

COMMENT: *Vigorous massage begun distally is essential. Wet the leg so that your hands can slide on the skin.*

4. The proximal portion of the thrombus can usually be removed by Fogarty balloon catheters or a combination of suction with a long thin tip and forceful abdominal straining on the part of the patient. The suction tubing must have a side hole near the proximal end so that suction is controlled by the operator's thumb (Fig. 17-4, *E*). A rubber or plastic open-ended catheter is suitable. If general anesthesia has been used, the surgeon may apply manual pressure on the lower part of the abdomen. Also, particularly if the patient is under general anesthesia, the Fogarty catheters may be employed for proximal thrombectomy. These procedures should be continued until blood flows freely from the vein proximally.

5. Hemostasis is obtained by elevation of the tapes rather than by application of clamps to the vein.

6. Irrigate the venotomy with dilute heparin solution.

7. Begin the closure with a mattress suture of 5-0 silk on an atraumatic needle (Fig. 17-4, *F*).

8. Continue the suture with small bites approximately 1 mm. apart as a horizontal running mattress suture, everting the edges of the vein until the end of the venotomy is reached (Fig. 17-4, *G* to *I*).

9. Close the fascia, subcutaneous layers, and skin carefully to avoid hematoma and lymph fistulas.

Postoperative care

Heparinization is continued for seven to ten days, during which time the administration of bishydroxycoumarin (Dicumarol), warfarin, or a similar anticoagulant is commenced. Details of the anticoagulant regimens and other aspects of postoperative care, such as elevation and wrapping of the legs, are described earlier in this chapter.

Prolonged follow-up will be needed for appraising the long-term results. The prompt relief of pain and edema after operation is gratifying.

Postoperative phlebograms are helpful in visualizing the results of thrombectomy. Phlebograms taken after several months usually show occlusion of the iliac vein even though the patient may have few symptoms.

British researchers are hoping to improve the long-term patency after thrombectomy by using (1) intraoperative venograms to ascertain that all clot has been removed from the iliac veins and (2) treatment with fibrinolysin as well as heparin during the early postoperative period to prevent the re-formation of thrombi.

F.B.H.

References

Edwards, W. S.: Observations on the pathogenesis and management of massive venous occlusion, Surgery 43:153-163, 1958.

Ger, R.: Surgical management of ulcerative lesions of the leg, Curr. Probl. Surg., pp. 1-52, March 1972.

18

Surgical prevention of pulmonary embolism

INTRODUCTION

Thromboembolism continues to kill many persons after operations, trauma, and various illnesses. The emboli arise in almost all cases from the lower half of the body, and when the use of anticoagulants fails or is contraindicated, surgical interruption of the inferior vena cava may be necessary. Partial interruption with plastic clips or filters blocks all dangerous emboli and appears to cause fewer complications in the legs than ligation of the inferior vena cava; however, ligation of the vena and ovarian veins continues to be necessary in cases of septic pelvic thrombophlebitis.

New information from lung scans and pulmonary angiograms has improved the diagnosis and treatment. Phlebography and the use of ^{131}I-labeled fibrinogen have revealed unsuspected venous thrombosis and potential emb/li in the legs of 30% of postoperative and injured patients, as discussed in the previous chapter.

Large emboli cause dramatic signs and symptoms, but small ones offer no reassurance since catastrophic emboli may follow. Prompt and adequate heparinization or surgical interruption of the vena cava is essential. Angiograms and lung scans reveal that numerous emboli have preceded or accompanied the first recognizable pulmonary infarct.

Routine chest x-ray films are rarely diagnostic, since pulmonary emboli, even large ones, rarely cause infarction of the lung. Many emboli do not cause complete occlusion. Furthermore, the lung tissue is also supplied by the bronchial arteries, which arise from the aorta. This supply of arterial blood maintains viability and prevents necrosis of the lung tissue in most cases.

Diagnosis of pulmonary embolism

New information from lung scans, pulmonary angiograms, and phlebograms has improved the diagnosis and treatment and explains the variety, manifestations, difficulties of diagnosis, and clinical course.

Lung scan

The lung scan is the most important advance in the diagnosis. It is now available in most community hospitals and is convenient, rapid, and safe even when the patients are very sick. The scintillation counter supplies a map of the distribution of

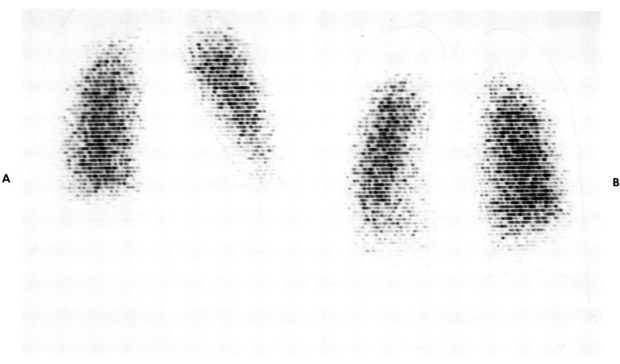

Fig. 18-1. Normal lung scan. A, Anteroposterior view. B, Posteroanterior view.

the radioactive colloid lodged in the capillaries of the lungs (Fig. 18-1). Cold areas in the scan signify poor perfusion and may be diagnostic of pulmonary embolism. There are no harmful effects, since only a fraction of the capillaries of the lungs are blocked; furthermore, the colloid is removed in a few hours by the reticuloendothelial phagocytes.

Even when a patient has had only one known episode of embolism, the scan always shows multiple perfusion defects that are bilateral, peripheral, and frequently crescent shaped (Fig. 18-2, A). Such a scan is diagnostic if the ordinary chest x-ray film is normal (Fig. 18-2, B). The classic pulmonary infarct with pleurisy, hemoptysis, and a peripheral wedge-shaped density on the chest x-ray film is a rare manifestation of pulmonary embolism. In some patients with the localized pulmonary consolidation that only suggests infarction, the scan may be diagnostic and reveal multiple areas of decreased perfusion (Fig. 18-3).

Routine chest x-ray films are rarely diagnostic in pulmonary embolism, since most emboli do not cause infarction or other changes in density of the lung. Furthermore, the changes in the chest film are delayed twelve to twenty-four hours after embolism occurs. However, simultaneous chest films are essential for interpretation of the scans, since various pulmonary diseases may decrease regional perfusion and therefore cause abnormalities of the lung scan. In such cases, pulmonary angiography may be helpful. However, the lung scan is the best screening test. Unless the scan demonstrates a pattern of poor regional perfusion, pulmonary angiography is unnecessary; and if the scan is typical, angiography is not needed. Emboli that are too small to show on the lung scan are rare and probably of no clinical importance, with only one important exception—septic emboli.

425

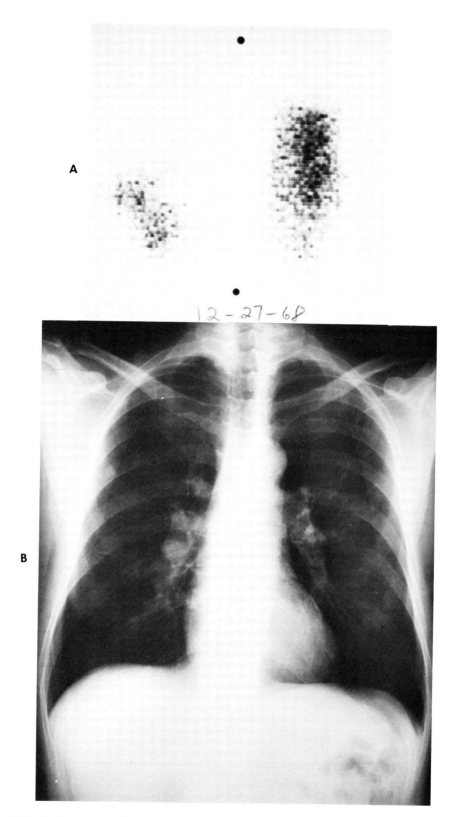

Fig. 18-2. A, Lung scan. Posteroanterior view showing multiple pulmonary emboli. B, Chest x-ray film.

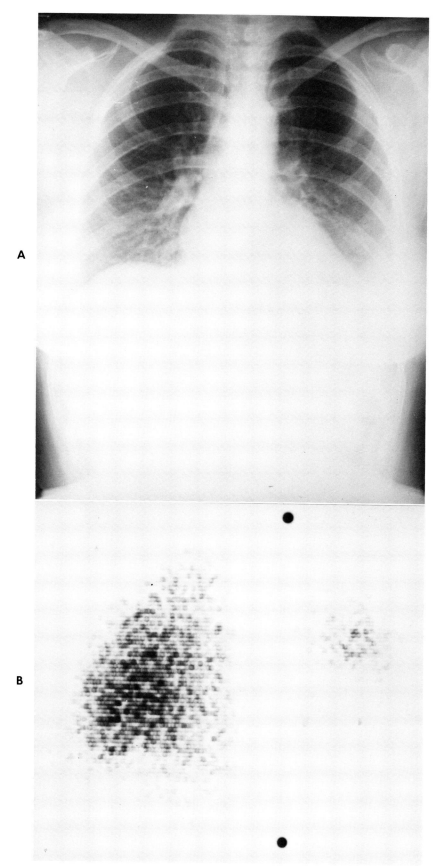

Fig. 18-3. A, Chest x-ray film showing small left pleural effusion. **B,** Anteroposterior view of lung scan showing multiple perfusion defects due to multiple emboli.

Pulmonary angiography

Pulmonary angiography is the most accurate and the most specific method of diagnosis. Lung scans may be difficult to interpret in patients with preexisting pulmonary diseases. The new ventilation scans may be helpful by showing poor ventilation in an area of poor perfusion, but only the pulmonary angiogram shows the emboli in the pulmonary arteries.

A simple technique for critically ill patients is an adaptation of angiocardiography. Insert a large-bore needle or cannula into veins in both arms. Inject 100 ml. of Angio-Conray (80%) rapidly by hand and take a series of films at half-second intervals for ten seconds in the anteroposterior projection. Make a second injection after rotating the patient to the right posterior oblique position if it is necessary to see more detail of the left pulmonary artery. Opacification of the heart in the frontal view obscures some of the details in the adjacent lung.

The technique of pulmonary arteriography preferred for semielective cases is selective catheterization and separate injection of the opaque material into the right and left pulmonary arteries in several positions. Cut down on the basilic vein, and advance a suitable catheter into the main pulmonary artery under fluoroscopic control. Suitable catheters can be directed into the right or the left pulmonary artery. Inject 30 ml. of Angio-Conray (80%) in two to three seconds with a pressure injector. Films taken at half- to one-second intervals for ten seconds visualize the arterial capillary and venous phases of the pulmonary circulation of one lung. Repeat the procedure for the other side.

The angiographic catheter can be left in place and the pressures monitored so that the trend or the results of treatment can be seen. This type of data may clarify the indications for pulmonary embolectomy.

COMMENT: *Pulmonary embolectomy is rarely needed and should never be attempted unless the diagnosis of massive emboli is proved by pulmonary angiography. Most patients who are critically ill with massive emboli improve rapidly. The problem is to select for operation only those patients who will not survive without it.*

A normal pulmonary angiogram shows rapid symmetrical filling of the pulmonary arteries and branches that gradually taper. The signs of embolism are as follows:

1. Pruning. Major branches appear to be cut off because of obstruction.
2. Filling defects. Irregularities within the lumen of the pulmonary arteries may be of various types. Globular or stingy filling defects that are constant in several successive films are the shadows of fresh clots, or emboli may form plaques or cushions at one branch while obstructing the adjacent one.
3. Asymmetry and delayed arterial filling in various parts of the lung. These are frequently seen but difficult to interpret unless obstruction or filling defects accompany them. Slow or irregular opacification of the lower lobes occurs in heart failure or in mitral stenosis with pulmonary congestion. Unilateral delay in the filling of a lower lobe suggests embolism. Absence of the blush of the opaque medium in parts of the peripheral lung field occurs with embolism but is not diagnostic.

In summary, multiple emboli in 2 to 3 mm. arterioles are hard to detect by any method. Pulmonary angiography is the most accurate diagnostic test. However, pulmonary angiography is not needed if the lung scan is normal, and it is not needed

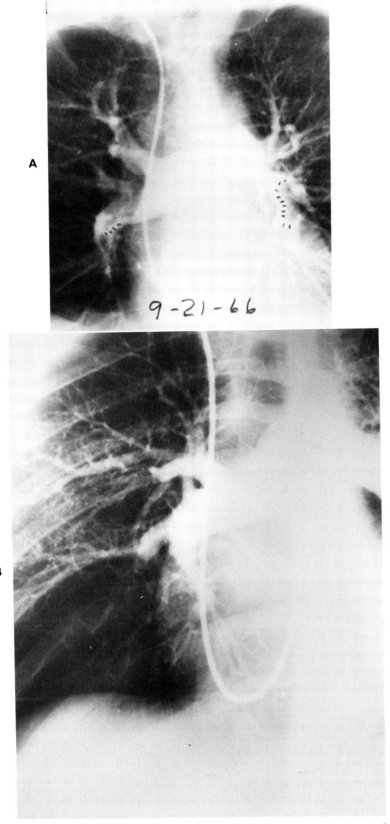

Fig. 18-4. Pulmonary arteriograms. Frontal view of, **A,** early and, **B,** late arterial phases. **A,** Filling defects in both main pulmonary arteries are outlined. **A** and **B,** Note also the pruning, that is, absence of vascular markings in right upper and lower lung fields.

if the lung scan is typical. When associated heart or lung disease confuses the interpretation of the scan, pulmonary angiograms may be diagnostic.

Indications for surgical operation to prevent embolism

Anticoagulation with heparin is usually sufficient to prevent further emboli and to permit resolution of the thrombophlebitis; however, the use of anticoagulants is not safe after recent major trauma, brain surgery, urological operations, or operations that require extensive dissection.

Interruption of the inferior vena cava will be needed if (1) the use of anticoagulants is contraindicated, (2) hemorrhage develops during anticoagulant treatment, or (3) anticoagulant treatment has failed to prevent embolism. Because anticoagulant treatment sometimes fails, we advise operation for patients who are so ill that they may not survive a second embolism. Also, for some patients with cardiac disease who will be at risk from embolism for the remainder of their lives, the long-term use of anticoagulants is less effective and may not be as safe as the implantation of a filter in the inferior vena cava under local anesthesia.

Choice of operation

Almost all emboli arise from the pelvic or leg veins, so that the most certain prevention is the interruption of the inferior vena cava.

For poor-risk patients, the safest operation is the transjugular implantation of the Mobin-Uddin umbrella filter. This requires only local anesthesia and may be performed in patients who are short of breath and unable to lie flat on the operating table.

Other operations on the inferior vena cava require general anesthesia and a retroperitoneal or transabdominal approach.

Emboli can be stopped without completely obstructing the vena cava, by narrowing or compartmenting it with the Miles or the DeWeese-Adams Teflon clip. These are highly effective in filtering emboli. Although it is unproved that these methods of partial interruption are less harmful to the legs than ligation of the inferior vena cava, it is already clear that unless the clips are plugged by emboli or thrombi, they cause little difficulty.

Ligation of the inferior vena cava is essential only for the treatment of septic emboli, which usually originate from pelvic thrombophlebitis after a septic abortion. These septic emboli are so small that partial interruption by clips or filters is not effective. The septic course, the fever, and emboli are not controlled until both ovarian veins and the inferior vena cava are ligated.

Relapses of thrombophlebitis may occur after any form of interruption of the inferior vena cava. This is the main cause of postoperative difficulties and therefore must be prevented and controlled. The collateral circulation around a ligature or an occluding clip is probably better if the ligature or clip is placed just below the renal veins. The different approaches and sites of ligation or caval interruption are described and compared later.

Ligation of the femoral veins with the use of local anesthesia is a safe operation that was once in vogue for prevention of pulmonary emboli. However, most surgeons have abandoned this procedure because embolism so frequently recurs from thrombi elsewhere or from new thrombi above the ligatures.

430

PARTIAL INTERRUPTION OF INFERIOR VENA CAVA WITH MOBIN-UDDIN FILTER

The technique of partial interruption of the inferior vena cava with the Mobin-Uddin filter is safe and effective. It is preferred for poor-risk patients who cannot tolerate general anesthesia for an abdominal operation. The usual indications are failure of heparin therapy, hemorrhage, or other contraindications to heparin treatment.

The filter is introduced with the patient under local anesthesia, via a right internal jugular venotomy. The long applicator containing the compressed filter is passed into the inferior vena cava under fluoroscopic control. There the filter is extruded

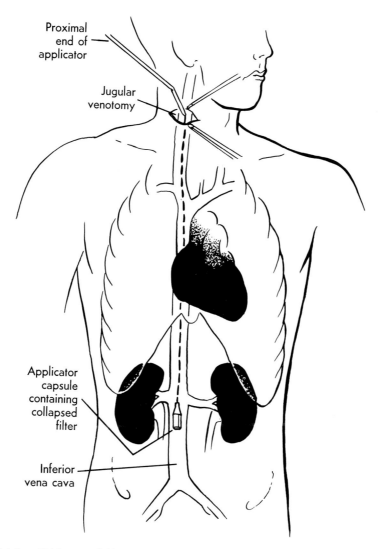

Fig. 18-5. Mobin-Uddin caval filter. Diagram showing applicator introduced via right internal jugular venotomy and hollow applicator capsule containing collapsed umbrella filter in place below renal veins.

431

and fixed in position below the renal veins and above the confluence of the iliac veins (Fig. 18-5). Errors of implantation have been reported, but these are avoidable if proper precautions are taken and if the surgeon reads, understands, and remembers the details of the technique. The technique is not difficult, but the details are very important.

Heparin therapy is discontinued four to six hours preoperatively for elective cases. It may be resumed postoperatively if not otherwise contraindicated. Antibiotics are administered preoperatively.

The operation is performed in the x-ray department under fluoroscopic control with television amplification. All sterile precautions, drapes, and the like are essential.

Procedure

1. Place the patient in the supine position (Fig. 18-6, *A*), or prop him up if orthopnea or dyspnea is troublesome. Turn his head to the left. An anesthesiologist should be present during operations on poor-risk patients to assure patency of the airway and to render supportive treatment.

2. Make a vertical incision above the clavicle over the sternocleidomastoid muscle; and separate the clavicular and sternal heads, or just split the sternocleidomastoid muscle in the direction of its fibers. Divide the omohyoid muscle as it crosses the internal jugular vein. Insert a self-retaining retractor (Fig. 18-6, *B*).

COMMENT: *The cosmetic advantages of transverse incisions are irrelevant in this operation. Vertical incisions are easily extended upward to uncover as much of the jugular vein as necessary. If the thyroid gland is large, make the incision in the upper part of the neck.*

3. Expose the jugular vein lying immediately beneath the fascia behind the sternocleidomastoid muscle. Uncover at least 4 cm. of the vein. Loop or divide and ligate the middle thyroid vein if it enters at this level. Pass umbilical tapes around the jugular vein at the upper and lower extent of the incision (Fig. 18-6, *C*).

COMMENT: *The tapes are essential for controlling the vein during insertion and manipulation of the applicator and during fluoroscopy. Air embolism will occur if the assistant is distracted and loosens the lower tape.*

Jugular venotomy

Apply bulldog or other fine-toothed vascular clamps, and incise the vein longitudinally for 1.5 to 2 cm. (Fig. 18-6, *D*).

COMMENT: *Do not extend the incision so that it is too close to the clavicle. The vein is deeper there. Excessive traction or manipulation has caused the vein to contract and become snug around the applicator.*

Transverse venotomy offers no advantages, and when the patient is dyspneic, it gapes and may permit air embolism.

Assembling of applicator and filter

The filter and applicator are shown in Fig. 18-7, and the parts are labeled in the diagram in Fig. 18-8, *A*. Good illustrations accompany the equipment when it is delivered. *Follow the directions precisely.* An experienced assistant can assemble the equipment during the exposure of the jugular vein; however, an inexperienced assistant is more safely employed making the incision than assembling the device.

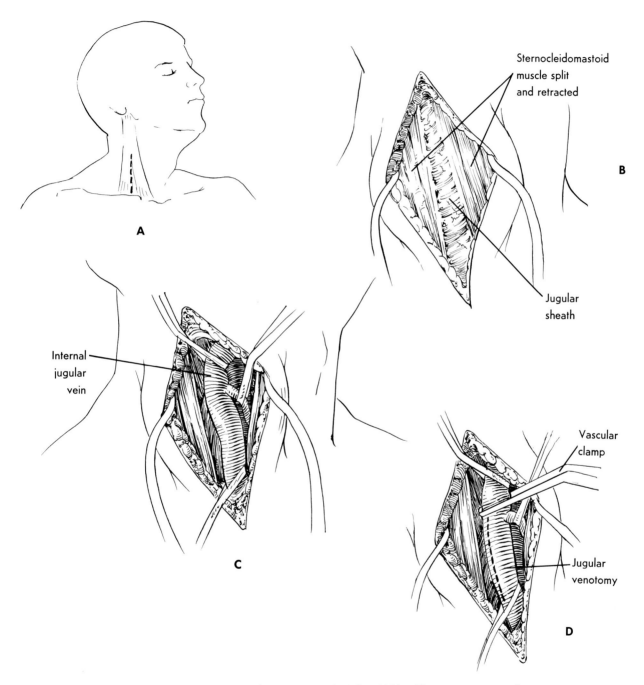

Fig. 18-6. Transjugular venotomy for insertion of Mobin-Uddin filter to interrupt inferior vena cava. **A,** Position of neck and incision. **B,** Sternocleidomastoid muscle split and retracted to reveal jugular sheath. **C,** Internal jugular vein isolated and controlled with tapes. **D,** Jugular venotomy. It should not be as long as illustrated.

433

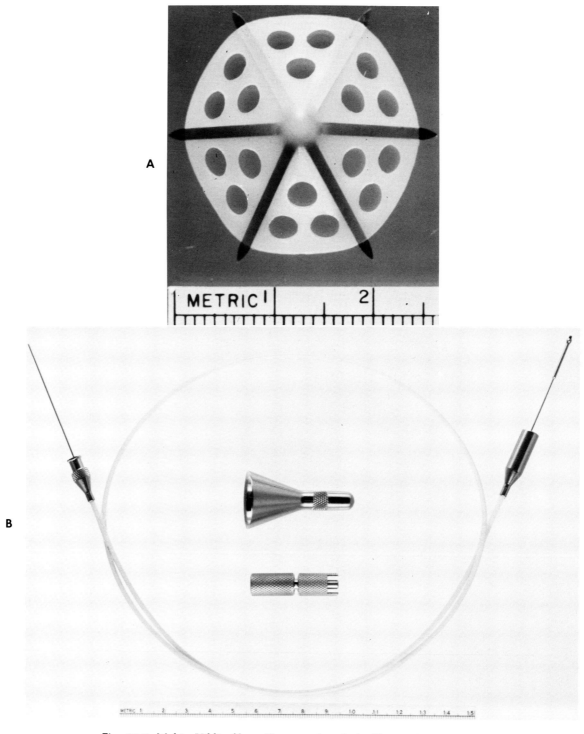

Fig. 18-7. Mobin-Uddin filter. Photographs of, **A,** filter and, **B,** applicator.

434

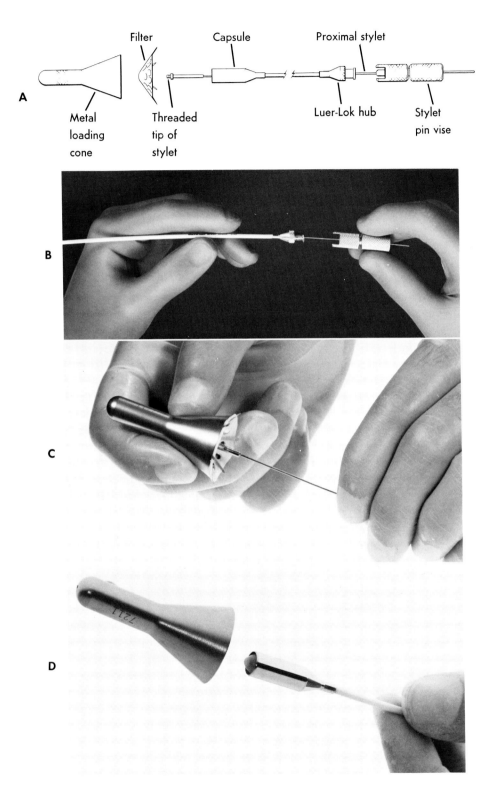

Fig. 18-8. Diagram of components of applicator for Mobin-Uddin filter. **B,** Luer-Lok hub and stylet pin vise. **C,** Filter advanced into loading cone. **D,** Collapsed filter withdrawn into hollow applicator capsule.

1. Loosen the stylet pin vise and slide it away from the Luer-Lok hub; then tighten the vise again to grip the stylet (Fig. 18-8, *B*).

2. Advance the stylet through the applicator until the stylet pin vise joins the Luer-Lok hub. Now the threaded tip of the stylet protrudes from the capsule.

3. Thread the filter onto the stylet. Do not force the delicate threads. To be certain that the threads are not crossed or stripped, unscrew or back off the filter one turn before loading it into the cone. This assures you that the filter can be released when it is in the inferior vena cava.

4. Collapse the filter in the metal loading cone as follows: Lubricate the filter and the loading cone with several milliliters of blood or local anesthetic. The assistant steadies the upper end of the applicator and stylet. The surgeon sits, rests his wrists on the sterile table, and holding the loading cone and stylet in a single straight axis, pushes the filter into the lubricated loading cone as far as it can go. This procedure folds and collapses the umbrella filter in the loading cone (Fig. 18-8, *C*).

5. Withdraw the collapsed filter into the capsule on the end of the applicator. This requires teamwork. Advance the capsule into the loading cone, and hold them firmly in a straight line while your assistant at the other end of the applicator pulls the stylet back through the applicator, thus pulling the compressed and folded umbrella into the applicator (Fig. 18-8, *D*).

COMMENT: *Before going back to the patient, repeat steps 4 and 5, eject the umbrella to check the tines, and make sure that the threads permit it to unscrew readily. So that the capsule may pass under the clavicle easily in the vein, allow the round end of the collapsed filter to protrude slightly at the end of the capsule to form a bullet-shaped nose.*

6. Fasten the stylet and applicator so that they advance together and so that the umbrella cannot accidentally be ejected or unscrewed. To hold the collapsed umbrella in the applicator capsule, first loosen the stylet pin vise at the upper end and advance it to the Luer-Lok hub and then tighten the vise again.

Intraoperative pulmonary arteriograms or cavagrams

If the diagnosis of pulmonary embolism is in doubt, catheters can now be passed via the jugular vein to obtain pulmonary arteriograms. The technique of pulmonary angiography is described on p. 428. However, the morbidity and mortality from insertion of the umbrella filter are so low that liberal interpretation of the indications is permissible. A diagnostic lung scan is sufficient indication.

A catheter in the inferior vena cava or one or both iliac veins can be used for phlebography when caval thrombi or anomalies of the vena cava are suspected of being present. A nonoccluding caval thrombus was found in one of our cases; after the cavagram was obtained, the umbrella was inserted somewhat higher than usual, above the clot but below the renal veins.

Anomalies of the vena cava and renal veins are suspected of being present when there are abnormalities of the intravenous pyelogram. If these films are not already available, dye is injected and a few films are obtained that reveal the position of the kidneys. When the kidneys and renal pelves are seen in normal position, the filter is inserted at the lower border of the third lumbar vertebra. This site is safely below the renal veins and above the confluence of the iliac veins.

Advancement of applicator into inferior vena cava

1. Place a small vascular clamp across the vein proximal to the venotomy (Fig. 18-9, *B*). Insert the capsule end of the applicator into the jugular venotomy, and advance it slowly as far as the occluding tape. Maintain tension on the umbilical tape with the right hand to prevent entrance of air or loss of blood (Fig. 18-9, *C*). Manipulate the applicator with the left hand.

COMMENT: *Air embolism is a real hazard, especially in dyspneic patients. After the applicator is passed under the clavicle, the distal tape is controlled by the assistant. The assistant must not become distracted from this essential task.*

2. Advance the applicator under fluoroscopic control. The jugular vein is large, but occasionally a minor obstruction is encountered under the clavicle, possibly a

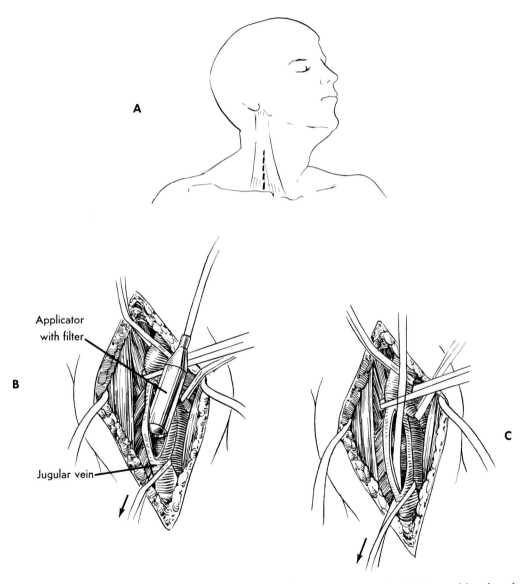

Fig. 18-9. Insertion of Mobin-Uddin filter into inferior vena cava. **A,** Position of head and incision. **B,** Applicator inserted into jugular venotomy. **C,** Traction on tape prevents leaking while applicator is advanced.

web, cushion, or partial septum. In two cases, we were unable to advance the applicator because of dilated or tortuous subclavian or innominate arteries beneath the clavicle.

If the capsule appears to enter the heart or moves synchronously with the heart, withdraw it slightly, and turn the patient toward the right side so that the heavy capsule falls to the right and is easily advanced down the vena cava.

The capsule may enter the right renal vein as evidenced by deviation to the right and stoppage at the level of the first or second lumbar vertebra. Withdraw the applicator from the renal vein, and tilt the patient somewhat to the left before advancing the applicator further.

3. Advance the applicator until the tip of it is at the lower border of the third lumbar vertebra (Fig. 18-10, *A*). Deviation to the right at a lower level signifies entry into the iliac vein, and the applicator must be withdrawn slightly.

COMMENT: *The exact location at the lower border of the third lumbar vertebra is important, and the surgeon and the radiologist must be certain of the location. Placement in the iliac vein is embarrassing to the surgeon, but it may be corrected by insertion of another filter proximally in the correct position. At the confluence of the iliac veins, the vena cava is too wide for the spokes of the umbrella to impinge on and be fixed in the wall of the vena cava. At the site recommended, namely, the lower border of the third lumbar vertebra, the filter fits and is readily fixed in position.*

A slightly larger filter, 28 mm. in diameter, is now available and under trial. It requires a larger loading cone and slight modification in technique.

Ejection of umbrella filter

During the next maneuvers of ejecting the umbrella filter (Fig. 18-10, *B*), the assistant holds the applicator at the correct level and snubs the tape around the applicator in the vein to prevent egress of blood or aspiration of air.

1. Loosen the stylet pin vise at the upper end of the stylet (Fig. 18-8).
2. Slide the vise proximally 2 cm. and tighten it again.
3. Have your assistant advance the stylet and eject the filter while you hold the catheter and applicator firmly. Watch the television screen to see the filter emerge from the capsule and spring open (Fig. 18-10, *B*).

Fixing filter in place

1. Pull up on the stylet gently and firmly to embed the sharp prongs of the filter in the wall of the inferior vena cava (Fig. 18-10, *C*).

COMMENT: *The prongs are sharp; therefore, to avoid hemorrhage, neutralize heparin with protamine or discontinue administration of it four to six hours before operation. Several cases of retroperitoneal hemorrhage have been reported.*

Fig. 18-10. Ejecting and fixing filter in place. **A,** Capsule containing collapsed filter in position in inferior vena cava. **C,** Eject filter by advancing stylet. **D,** Pull up on stylet. **E,** Unscrew umbrella and withdraw applicator. **B,** Fluoroscopic view of applicator and capsule containing folded umbrella filter. **F,** Fluoroscopic view of umbrella filter in inferior vena cava.

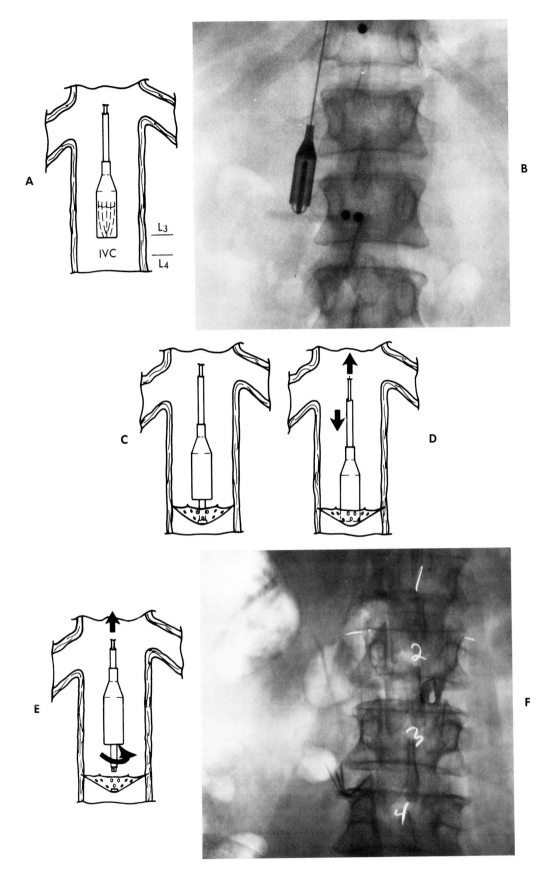

Fig. 18-10. For legend see opposite page.

2. While pulling up on the stylet, slide the applicator down to spread the ribs of the umbrella further (Fig. 18-10, *D*).

3. Watch the fluoroscopic screen. The filter should not tilt during traction and should move up very little until you feel firm resistance while pulling on the stylet.

COMMENT: *Tilting of the filter signifies that the tilting side of the filter is not embedded and that the filter will migrate to the lung if released. This has occurred when the older (and smaller) filter was ejected too low, where the vena cava widens at the confluence of the iliac veins. If tilting occurs, push the umbrella down into the femoral vein at the groin and remove it later with the use of local anesthesia after inserting another filter correctly.*

Releasing filter and withdrawing stylet and applicator

Release the filter and withdraw the stylet and applicator as follows:
1. Pull up gently on the stylet (Fig. 18-10, *D*).
2. Simultaneously rotate the stylet counterclockwise (Fig. 18-10, *E*), maintaining gentle traction, until it is free. Withdraw the apparatus from the jugular vein, and close the venotomy with a continuous suture of 4-0 or 5-0 vascular suture. Vascular clamps applied below and above the venotomy at the site of the tapes prevent bleeding or air embolism.

Closure of incision

Suture the fascia, platysma, and skin.

Postoperative care

Antibiotics are administered for five days. They have been helpful in preventing infection around various other prostheses. Antibiotics should also be given before tooth extractions or at other times when bacteremia might occur. No infections have been reported yet, but this is a potential hazard with any intravascular prosthesis.

Heparin may be given for treatment or prevention of thrombophlebitis if it is not otherwise contraindicated. The neck incision is no contraindication to the administration of moderate doses of heparin, and a hematoma is easily detected if it occurs.

Elastic wrapping of the legs is essential. It prevents stagnation and thrombosis in the superficial veins, and elastic stockings should be worn for six months or longer if there is any tendency toward edema. Long-term anticoagulation therapy with warfarin may be needed to prevent relapse of thrombophlebitis.

Complications

The procedure is safe and effective, and complications are exceedingly rare. Most complications are avoidable by careful attention to the details of the technique. It is a delicate operation, not a difficult one.

In our experience with more than fifty cases, the complications have been air embolism (one case), migration of filter (one case), and inability to pass the applicator through the jugular vein (two cases). None of our patients died as a result of the operation. The new 28 mm. filter may be advantageous for the few patients with chronic congestive heart failure and unusually large vena cava. Several cases have been reported in which massive emboli dislodged the smaller filter. One of our patients died from embolism after implantation of the filter; this occurred from a mural thrombus in the right atrium. Small emboli will doubtless arise above the filter or via collateral veins around the filter in rare cases after this or after any other method of caval interruption.

Edema and thrombophlebitis of the legs have not been a problem as yet, but they should be managed and treated if they occur and prevented whenever possible. Elastic stockings are worn for three months or as long as any edema occurs in the feet. Anticoagulation with warfarin is continued for three to six months after an episode of thrombophlebitis and continued indefinitely if a second episode appears.

It remains to be seen whether or not the filters will stay patent, but it is proved that they are safe and effective. Patients who have serious underlying diseases will always have an increased rate of thrombophlebitis after any procedure and embolism and occlusion of a filter or clip will be more likely to occur.

ABDOMINAL APPROACH TO INFERIOR VENA CAVA

If the patient is a reasonable risk for general anesthesia and there are no contraindications, the abdominal approach may be elected instead of the transjugular approach described earlier for partial interruption of the inferior vena cava.

The indications are pulmonary emboli recurring despite anticoagulant therapy or pulmonary emboli in patients in whom the use of anticoagulants is contraindicated.

The traditional approach to the vena cava below the renal veins is the retroperitoneal approach through the right flank (similar to that for lumbar sympathectomy). This retroperitoneal route is preferred for obese persons and for those who have had recent intra-abdominal operations or infection. This right flank retroperitoneal approach gives easy access to the vena cava just above the confluence of the iliac veins. For access to the ovarian veins, which must be ligated in cases of septic pelvic thrombophlebitis, the transperitoneal anterior midline or the right subcostal approach may be used according to the circumstances.

The use of plastic clips or intraluminal plastic filters is not advisable in the presence of infection, and partial interruption does not block the tiny septic emboli. Therefore, the vena cava and both ovarian veins are ligated for prevention of septic pulmonary

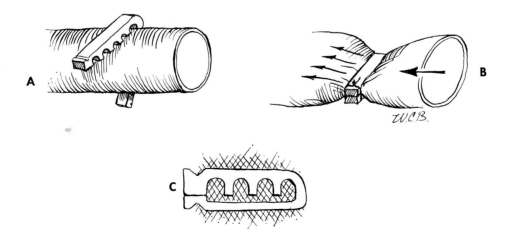

Fig. 18-11. Partial occlusion of inferior vena cava with DeWeese-Adams clip, which filters lethal emboli. **A,** Teflon clip applied to inferior vena cava. Smooth lower limb slips easily underneath vein. **B,** Flow continues, but significant emboli are "strained" from venous system. **C,** Drawing of clip.

embolism. Partial interruption of the inferior vena cava by use of a plastic clip is preferred to ligation for all other cases (Fig. 18-11).

The best level at which to interrupt the vena cava is just below the renal veins. This is proposed for the following reasons:

1. The collateral circulation would be better because of the abundant connections between the lumbar veins below the ligature and tributaries of the left renal vein and the ascending lumbar veins.

2. There is no blind cul-de-sac above the clip or ligature, and the large inflow from the left renal vein would prevent stasis and possible thrombosis above the ligature or above an occluded clip.

The vena cava at this level must be approached anteriorly as in the midline exposure of the abdominal aorta, which is illustrated in Fig. 3-1, or by a right subcostal incision and reflection of the duodenum and pancreas with the Kocher maneuver, which is discussed and illustrated later.

Retroperitoneal approach to inferior vena cava

The retroperitoneal approach via the right flank is the traditional approach to the inferior vena cava. The supine position and a short transverse muscle-splitting incision gives good exposure for thin patients. However, the surgeon should not hesitate to divide the external oblique muscle, and if the patient is obese, the left lateral decubitus position, that is, the kidney position, improves the exposure. In the surgical procedure described as follows, the lateral approach is used.

Anesthesia

Endotracheal general anesthesia is employed.

Procedure

1. Place the patient in the left lateral decubitus position, which is similar to that employed for lumbar sympathectomy. Employ the kidney rest to widen the space between the twelfth rib and the iliac crest. Flex the lower (left) leg, but extend the upper (right) leg. The left leg serves to stabilize the patient, and extension of the right leg puts tension on the psoas muscle, drawing it out of the operator's way. Place a pillow between the legs. This position is not identical to the position recommended for lumbar sympathectomy. (See Fig. 18-12, A.)

2. Make a transverse skin incision beginning 2 or 3 cm. to the right of the rectus muscles and at about the level of the umbilicus. The umbilicus is a landmark for the bifurcation of the iliac arteries and the confluence of the iliac veins. Carry the incision backward and slightly upward toward the twelfth rib. (See Fig. 18-12, A.)

3. Split the external oblique muscle, cutting directly across its fibers (Fig. 18-12, B).

4. The internal oblique muscle may be split in the direction of its fibers (Fig. 18-12, C). More ample exposure is obtained by dividing the muscle.

5. Split the transversus muscle in the direction of its fibers (Fig. 18-12, D).

6. Retract the edges of the wound widely (Fig. 18-12, E). In the plane of the properitoneal fat, roll the peritoneum and its contents anteriorly, using blunt dissection with gauze pads and sponge holders. The inferior vena cava is easily visualized deep and medial to the psoas muscle in the depths of the incision.

COMMENT: *Beware of thrombus in the inferior vena cava. In two patients, we have*

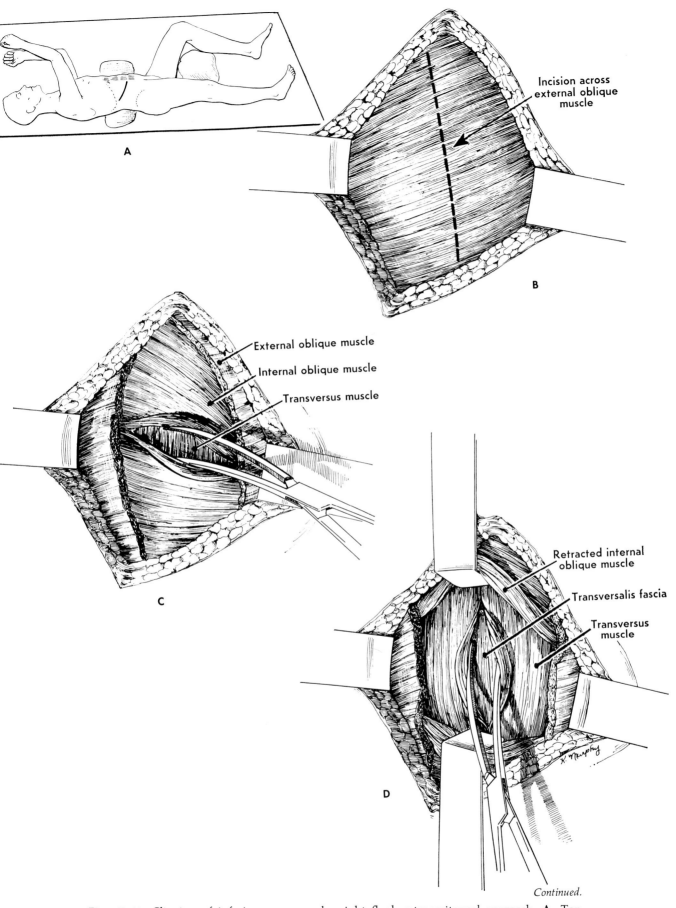

Incision across
external oblique
muscle

A

B

External oblique muscle

Internal oblique muscle

Transversus muscle

C

Retracted internal
oblique muscle

Transversalis fascia

Transversus
muscle

D

Continued.

Fig. 18-12. Clipping of inferior vena cava by right flank retroperitoneal approach. **A,** Top view of position of patient on his side over kidney rest. **B** to **D,** Successive muscular layers in incision.

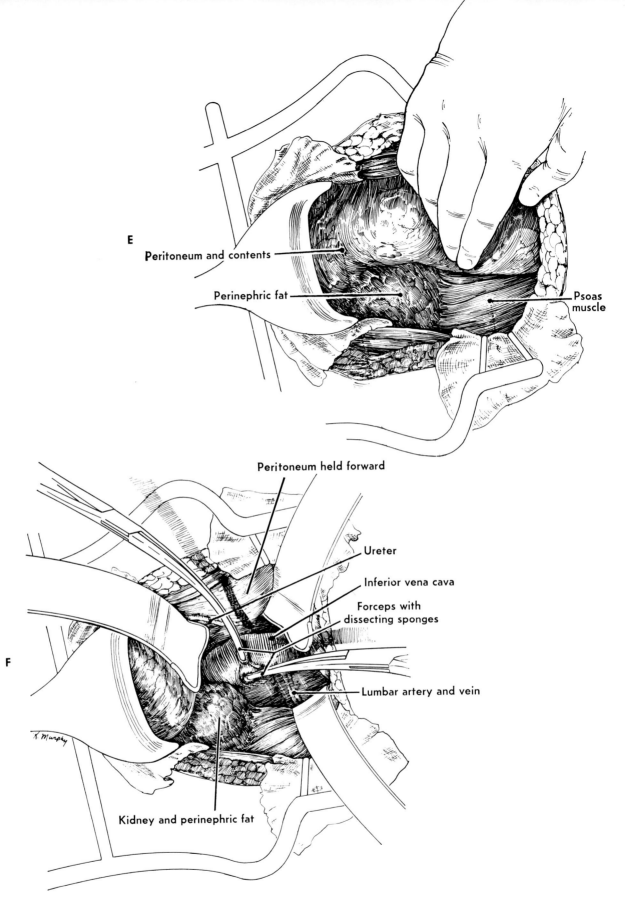

E

Peritoneum and contents

Perinephric fat

Psoas muscle

Peritoneum held forward

Ureter

Inferior vena cava

Forceps with dissecting sponges

Lumbar artery and vein

F

Kidney and perinephric fat

R. Murphy

Fig. 18-12, cont'd. Clipping of inferior vena cava. **E,** Peritoneum rolled forward to expose psoas muscle. **F,** Exposure and dissection of inferior vena cava.

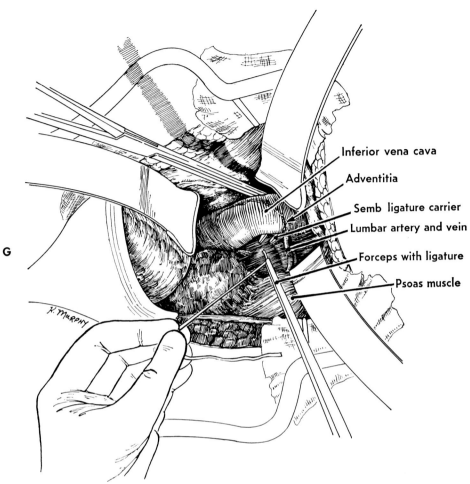

Inferior vena cava

Adventitia

Semb ligature carrier

Lumbar artery and vein

Forceps with ligature

Psoas muscle

G

Fig. 18-12, cont'd. Clipping of inferior vena cava. **G,** Pass ligature as illustrated here or apply DeWeese-Adams clip (Fig. 18-11).

found and removed thrombi that extended above the level of intended interruption and might have been torn away or released by manipulation. The thrombectomy can be performed with the Fogarty venous thrombectomy catheter. In one instance, the resident used a Foley urinary catheter with the 30 ml. bag.

7. Choose a convenient point on the inferior vena cava just above the iliac veins. Use two long clamps holding small rolls of umbilical tape as dissectors. Hold the vein to one side with one dissector, and with the other, carefully roll the loose perivascular tissue away from the vein. Observe and avoid the lumbar veins; they are fragile and easily torn. A small pack of oxidized cellulose may be needed. (See Fig. 18-12, *F.*)

8. When the inferior vena cava is free, pass the clip around it. The DeWeese-Adams or Miles clips have a smooth limb posteriorly, and this slides under the vena cava very nicely. Pass a large gallbladder clamp, renal pedicle clamp, or other curved long-handled clamp under the vena cava to grasp the tip of the open clip.

9. Tie the clip securely with a Dacron suture.

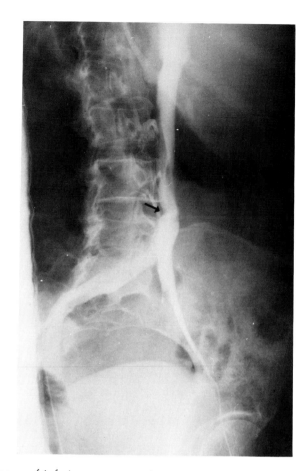

Fig. 18-13. Angiogram of inferior vena cava. Arrow points to open clip that permitted recurrent pulmonary embolism.

COMMENT: *A patient was referred to us because of recurrent emboli after application of a clip. At our exploration, the clip was found open (Fig. 18-13), and no remnant of a silk suture could be identified.*

10. Irrigate the operative field, and close the incision in layers.

Postoperative care

The main postoperative problem after ligation of the vena cava is edema. Prevention begins immediately by wrapping both thighs and legs with foam rubber–coated or self-adherent elastic bandages before the patient leaves the operating room. Postoperatively, the foot of the bed must be constantly elevated 15 or 20 degrees. Ambulation is begun early and is gradually increased unless swelling is troublesome. Prolonged elastic support* is necessary for several months or as long as there is any edema of the feet. Intermittent use of heparin is advised for seven to ten days if there has been phlebitis before the operation, and anticoagulation with orally administered warfarin may be needed if there is any later sign of relapse of the thrombophlebitis.

---

*Supports for both legs to the waist are obtainable from the Jobst Institute, 1803 Jefferson Ave., Toledo, Ohio.

Midline transabdominal approach to infrarenal vena cava and its tributaries

Introduction

The midline transabdominal approach is the best for wide exposure of the infrarenal vena cava. The vena cava is situated alongside the abdominal aorta and can be approached by the same route, lifting the transverse colon superiorly and reflecting the duodenum and small bowel to the right. For injuries of the vena cava and, of course, injuries of the suprarenal vena cava, reflection of the overlying viscera to the left side is required as discussed and illustrated in Chapter 10.

Indications

The midline transabdominal approach is used for exploration and interruption of the inferior vena cava and its tributaries when wide exposure is needed. Following are situations in which this approach is indicated:

1. When septic embolism from pelvic thrombophlebitis necessitates ligation of the ovarian veins as well as the vena cava and when the pelvis must also be explored.
2. When prophylactic interruption of the inferior vena cava during various abdominal operations is required in patients with high risk from phlebitis and embolism.
3. When you wish to avoid the other routes because of previous surgery or infection.
4. When anomalies of the infrarenal vena cava are suspected of being present. When anomalies are present, wider exposure is required than is possible with the alternate subcostal or retroperitoneal routes. In one of our first patients, the vena cava ligated via the right-flank retroperitoneal approach seemed small, but the significance of this was not appreciated until she died of another embolism and was found to have a double vena cava, with branches on each side of the aorta joining at the level of the left renal vein. Anomalies such as retroureteric vena cava may be confusing and dangerous without wide exposure. The presence of anomalies elsewhere, unusual findings at operation, or unexpected findings on venograms are important clues.
5. When embolism follows previous ligation or clipping. In one instance, we found that a clip was open. The ovarian veins may dilate tremendously after ligation, and a few emboli apparently travel this route until the ovarian veins are also ligated.
6. When you suspect that a clot is present in the inferior vena cava. Bilateral edema of the legs and thighs is highly suggestive. A venogram also may suggest the presence of a clot in the vena cava. Exposure and control of the vena cava for thrombectomy of the vena cava or of the iliac veins are feasible by this route, and the clip can also be applied to prevent new embolism.

Procedure

1. Make a long midline abdominal incision from the xiphoid process to a point a few inches below the umbilicus (Fig. 18-14, *A*).
2. Explore the abdomen and pelvis.

Exposure of abdominal aorta and inferior vena cava

Uncover the abdominal aorta, using the following maneuvers:
1. Deliver the small bowel out of the incision and lay it on a moist towel on

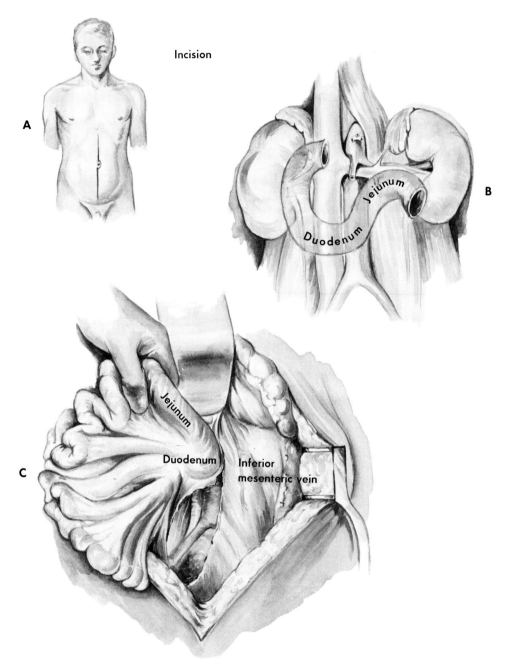

Fig. 18-14. Midline transabdominal ligation or clipping of inferior vena cava. A, Incision. B, Anatomical relationships of structures overlying renal veins and infrarenal vena cava. C, Peritoneal incision and division of ligament of Treitz.

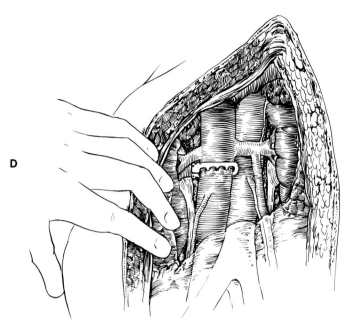

Fig. 18-14, cont'd. Midline transabdominal ligation or clipping of inferior vena cava. **D,** Plastic clip in position to partially interrupt inferior vena cava.

the right side of the abdomen and cover it with another moist towel. Lift the transverse colon up and out of the abdomen superiorly. This and the small bowel are easily held with wide Deaver retractors. The duodenum, aorta, and inferior mesenteric vein can readily be seen (Fig. 18-14, *B*).

2. Incise the peritoneum in front of the distal portion of the aorta and the left edge of the duodenum, and incise the peritoneal fold called the ligament of Treitz, marking the junction between duodenum and jejunum and suspending the origin of the jejunum from the mesocolon (Fig. 18-14, *C*).

3. Divide the inferior mesenteric vein where it crosses the aorta from the left side and passes under the inferior border of the pancreas. This step is not always necessary but frequently permits more ready access to the left renal vein and left ovarian vein by permitting lateral retraction of the left mesocolon.

4. Uncover the aorta, inferior vena cava, and left renal vein by reflecting the few intervening lymph nodes and lymphatic trunks lying in front of the aorta (Fig. 18-14, *D*).

Exposure of left renal vein

Rarely, the left renal vein may pass behind the aorta. Ligation or clipping of the vena cava just below the left renal vein avoids a blind pouch above the ligature and leaves three pairs of lumbar veins as outflow below the ligature.

Ligation or clipping of inferior vena cava

Palpate the inferior vena cava carefully to make sure that there is no thrombus in it at the site of the intended ligation.

COMMENT: *We have encountered thrombus in the inferior vena cava in three cases. In one case, our resident extracted clot dangling above the renal veins by inserting a*

449

Foley urinary catheter, inflating the balloon above the clot, and withdrawing the catheter and balloon to extract the clot before tying the ligature.

Exposure and ligation of ovarian veins

Exposure and ligation of the ovarian veins are necessary only for septic emboli or for the rare cases of emboli recurring after ligation. The left ovarian vein arises from the inferior border of the left renal vein. The right ovarian vein arises from the front of the vena cava near the right renal vein. Ligate the ovarian veins at any convenient place, or if one contains thrombus, ligate it at its termination at the inferior vena cava or renal vein.

Right subcostal intraperitoneal approach to inferior vena cava

Purpose

The right subcostal intraperitoneal approach is used for exposing the renal veins and inferior vena cava just below the renal veins.

Indication

The intraperitoneal approach is an excellent route by which to apply the plastic clip or to ligate the vena cava and the ovarian veins at the preferred level, namely, just below the left renal vein.

Advantages

1. This approach avoids intraperitoneal adhesions or infection from earlier lower abdominal or midline incisions.

2. The clip or ligature is applied just below the left renal vein in order to avoid a blind pouch above it. The lumbar veins below the ligature have abundant connections with tributaries of the left renal vein and the ascending lumbar veins.

3. This is also the approach for transabdominal right nephrectomy. The surgeon can determine operability and control the renal pedicle at the beginning of the operation.

Contraindications

Because this subcostal incision cannot be extended and because associated injuries of other viscera are common, injuries of the vena cava or kidney should be explored through the midline incision described previously.

Procedure
Incision

1. Make a right subcostal incision (Fig. 18-15, *A*), divide the muscles, open the peritoneum, and divide the round ligament.

2. Divide the attachments between the hepatic flexure of the colon and the liver. Some blood vessels will need to be ligated. Retract the hepatic flexure inferiorly to uncover the second portion of the duodenum and the head of the pancreas (Fig. 18-15, *B*).

3. Mobilize the duodenum and head of the pancreas anteriorly and medially (Kocher maneuver) (Fig. 18-15, *C*). The plane between the vena cava and the overlying duodenum and pancreas is avascular.

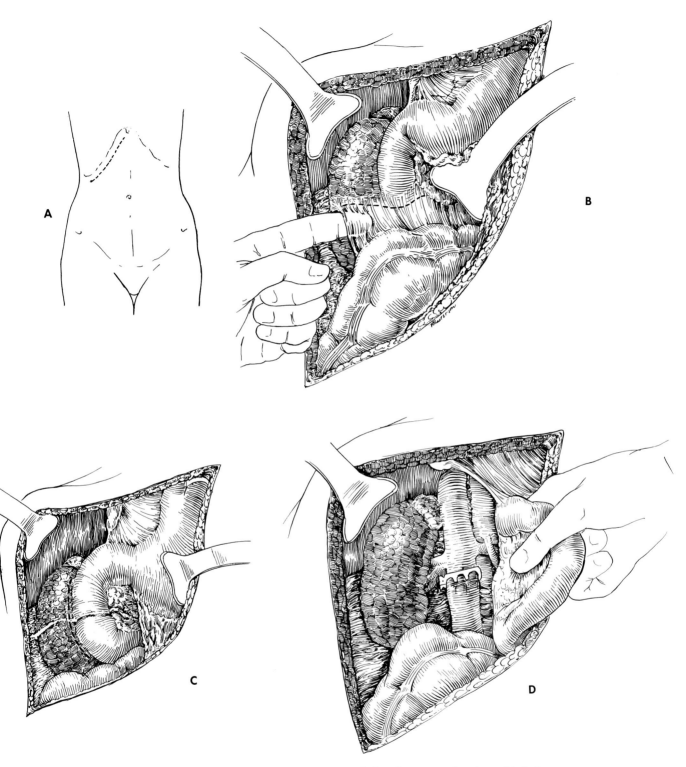

Fig. 18-15. Right subcostal transabdominal approach for clipping or ligation of inferior vena cava. **A,** Incision. **B,** Division of attachments of hepatic flexure of colon. **C,** Incision of peritoneum lateral to duodenum (Kocher maneuver). **D,** Clip around vena cava should be moved superiorly until it is closer to left renal vein.

451

4. Palpate the foramen of Winslow, and posteriorly note the vena cava. In thin patients, it is visible through thin peritoneum.

5. Incise the peritoneum to the lateral side of the duodenum and pancreas. This is avascular. (Do not try to separate the duodenum from the pancreas.) Use the finger in the foramen of Winslow to lift the duodenum and pancreas off the vena cava as you incise the avascular areolar tissue.

Exposure of vena cava and right renal vein

1. Dissect distally for a few centimeters to reveal the left renal vein.

2. Further mobilization of the inferior border of the head of the pancreas and duodenum uncovers a wider area.

Ligation or clipping of inferior vena cava

Ligate or clip the inferior vena cava as described previously (Fig. 18-15, *D*).

Postoperative care

Postoperative care is described earlier in this chapter.

F.B.H.

19

Amputations, infections, and gangrene of the lower extremity

GENERAL PRINCIPLES OF AMPUTATION FOR VASCULAR DISEASE

In civilian medical practice in the United States, over 800 legs are amputated each week because of chronic occlusive arterial disease. The disease is usually diffuse, involving arteries proximal to the proposed site of amputation. The sites and techniques of amputation therefore differ somewhat from amputations done for trauma or other reasons.

The surgeon must always keep in mind three principles in regard to amputation: First and foremost, the objective of amputation is restoration of function, that is, walking, as soon as possible after operation. The patient will not learn to walk again without the assistance of the rehabilitation therapists and the prosthetist. Second, the team is mobilized early, the patient evaluated, and the program planned. Preoperative consultation with the rehabilitation service, preoperative exercises, explanation, and motivation of the patient are helpful. Third, amputation is done at the level at which the most function can be conserved, that is, at the lowest level at which the wound will heal.

Only three levels of amputation need be considered for vascular disease in the lower limb. The low-thigh area is the best site for amputation to ensure healing when there is advanced arterial insufficiency. However, many knees are sacrificed unnecessarily, and in many large medical centers, above-the-knee amputation has become a rare operation. Amputation below the knee permits more rapid and more complete rehabilitation and a more normal gait. With the transmetatarsal amputation, no prosthesis is required, and the affected foot functions almost as well as a normal foot. After distal conservative amputations, healing may be slower, and some patients will subsequently require reamputation at a higher level. Syme, Lisfranc, and other similar foot amputations are not usually suitable for patients with vascular disease.

Most patients capable of rehabilitation can walk earlier than we expected when we wrote the previous edition of this book. The rigid plaster dressing and early fitting of the below-the-knee or above-the-knee prosthesis are prescribed on p. 455. Considerable flexibility is necessary in adapting the program to the individual patient, but we apply the rigid plaster dressing to most patients whom we expect to use a prosthesis. They will walk early even if weight bearing must await firm healing. Indeed, some surgeons such as Burgess believe that a properly fitting rigid plaster socket provides the optimum environment for healing.

The usual indications for amputation are gangrene, intractable infection, and severe intractable pain secondary to arterial insufficiency. More urgent problems, fortunately not too common, are uncorrectable arterial trauma or invasive infection that cannot be controlled by antibiotics or other conservative measures. The open amputations and drainage procedures for infections and gangrene of the neurotrophic feet of diabetic patients are special problems and are discussed on pp. 484 and 486.

Amputation as treatment for vascular disease is a semielective, definitive, closed, one-stage procedure. The aim is conservation of as much of the extremity as is consistent with good healing and rapid rehabilitation. The correct level for amputation is determined after consideration of the patient and his associated medical diseases as well as evaluation of the limb. The absence of both pedal pulses or the more proximal pulses is a definitive and reliable sign of arterial occlusion. However, estimation of collateral circulation requires observation and judgment of the nutritional state of the limb as reflected in the skin, nails, toes, hair follicles, and muscle mass. Collateral circulation in diabetic persons without peripheral pulses is frequently excellent, and transmetatarsal or below-the-knee amputation may succeed even when popliteal and distal pulses are absent. When arterial insufficiency is further advanced, atrophy and dryness of the skin, muscle atrophy, and atrophy of soft tissues in the toes will be found.

Continuous pain on rest, improved somewhat by a dependent position of the foot, results in edema, since the patient keeps the foot down almost constantly. Such a foot shows other signs of advanced arterial insufficiency, such as skin and muscle atrophy. Transmetatarsal amputation will fail when pain on rest and dependent rubor are observed. Below-the-knee amputations frequently fail and should not be elected unless the signs of trophic change are mild and distal.

Healing after amputation requires adequate collateral circulation. Special tests have not been helpful for evaluation of collateral circulation. Arteriograms occasionally reveal a correctable arterial block and are sometimes helpful in the selection of the amputation level. Inability to visualize the collateral circulation in arteriograms may be caused by technical factors in the examination and should not be discouraging. Collateral circulation does not register on the oscillometer. More sophisticated methods of measuring blood flow in the limb are not available outside the laboratory. Moore (1973) uses ^{133}Xe to determine skin blood flow at the site of the proposed amputation; this method appears to be promising. At the present, clinical observation, including evaluation of the local response to several weeks of conservative treatment, is probably the most useful and reliable method for choosing the level of elective amputation. At the time of operation, pulsatile bleeding in the skin incision is always a good sign. The degree and amount of bleeding from muscular collateral circulation are more difficult to judge.

Conservative treatment and preoperative preparation for amputation should include management of associated diseases, the use of antibiotics, rest, treatment and drainage of local infections, and skin preparation with an antiseptic soap (pHisoHex or similar preparation). The physiatrist should discuss and plan rehabilitation with the patient. The patient should not observe doubt or conflict among his physicians.

Careful and gentle surgical technique is essential, both to preserve blood supply and to minimize the opportunities for wound infection. Skin incisions are designed to conserve blood supply. The skin is elevated with the underlying fascia and is protected with moist packs. Crushing instruments and crude mass ligatures are avoided. Careful hemostasis will prevent hematoma. The incision may be closed without drainage. For the posterior portion of the amputation, a large sharp amputation knife is less traumatic than the small scalpel and prevents shredding of muscle tissue.

Many stump complications are prevented by careful closure of the wound. Irrigations with copious amounts of saline solution remove bone dust and debris. In the handling of the skin, tissue forceps are avoided. There should not be excessive tension on the skin flaps.

Postoperative care must include correct positioning of the limb to avoid the tendency toward contracture. Sutures are removed in stages after ten to fourteen days, except for excessively tight sutures that are cutting into the skin, which may be removed earlier. Exercise and rehabilitation should be begun as early as possible.

Mortality after amputations, particularly those necessitated by extensive gangrene, is rather high. Many of the patients are elderly and have advanced coronary and cerebral atherosclerotic diseases. Careful medical supervision is essential to reduce postoperative mortality.

Some of the complications of the surgical procedure in amputations are avoidable. Infection can usually be avoided by preliminary drainage, by local treatment, by preservation of the blood supply, and by avoidance of hematoma and excessive surgical trauma at the time of operation. Phantom limb pain rarely persists unless amputation is long deferred and the pain pattern is established. Contracture of the hip, the knee, or the Achilles tendon is avoided by preoperative and postoperative exercises and correct positioning. The rigid plaster dressing or early stump wrapping controls edema. Amputation neuroma is not symptomatic unless the lesion lies just under the skin or between skin and bone or is incorporated into the surgical scar. Progressive thrombosis sometimes necessitates reamputation at a higher level, and an occasional distal amputation will fail when collateral circulation is insufficient. Meticulous technique is necessary. Minor separation or infection may cause failure to heal when blood supply at the amputation site is barely sufficient.

The surgeon must evaluate the prospect of success and the expenses and hazards of failure in each individual patient when choosing the level of amputation. Unless a few of his conservative amputations fail, he is probably denying conservative amputation to some patients for whom a successful outcome might be anticipated.

IMMEDIATE POSTSURGICAL FITTING OF PROSTHESES FOR ABOVE-THE-KNEE AND BELOW-THE-KNEE AMPUTATIONS

Weiss in Europe and Burgess (1969) in the United States introduced methods that permit early ambulation with a temporary prosthesis. With these techniques, divided muscles are stabilized by being sutured to each other or to bone, a plaster dressing is applied at the completion of the amputation, and this plaster dressing serves as a socket for a temporary prosthesis (Fig. 19-1). Early ambulation has many important advantages. The rapid physical rehabilitation and ambulation improve morale. A properly fitting plaster socket decreases postoperative pain and allows normal wound healing without the usual edema and induration.

The methods require close teamwork by the physiatrist and prosthetist and the surgeon. Postgraduate courses are available at several centers.* Prosthetists trained in this method are now available in many parts of the country.

---

*New York University, Post Graduate Medical School, 317 E. 34th St., New York, N.Y.; Northwestern University Medical School, 401 E. Ohio, Chicago, Ill.; University of Southern California of Los Angeles Prosthetic and Orthotics Program, 1000 Veteran Ave., Los Angeles, Calif.

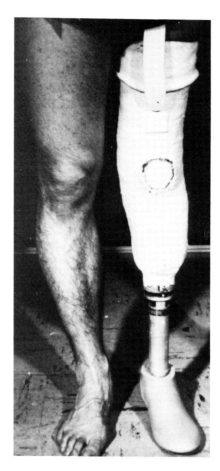

Fig. 19-1. Plaster dressing and temporary below-the-knee prosthesis.

Indications

Immediate fitting should be considered for any patient for whom a prosthesis is intended. Contraindications include mental and physical impairments that make it unlikely for rehabilitation and walking to be accomplished. Legs with contractures, stumps with doubtful blood supply, or those with increased risk of infection are not suitable. Immediate fitting should not be attempted unless satisfactory supervision and rehabilitation facilities are available and the prosthetist has had the necessary training.

The plaster dressing, which is applied after closure of the skin, is usually changed at weekly intervals, but the remainder of the rehabilitation schedule is flexible and adaptable. Patients with vascular disease are not permitted to bear weight on the stump for two to three weeks. Meanwhile the leg is fitted. After an interval, the patients stand or walk in the parallel bars or walker, wearing the leg and touching it down to the floor. In a few weeks, they bear weight partially in the parallel bars and, later, with crutches.

Preoperative preparation

Preparation of all patients for whom a prosthesis is intended must include (1) explanation, motivation, and discussion with the patient; (2) care of local lesions to prevent invasive infection or contamination at the operative site; (3) exercise to strengthen the muscles of the body and limbs in preparation for walking; and (4) measures to prevent contractures.

AMPUTATION BELOW KNEE

Indications and choice of level of amputation

Amputation below the knee succeeds in the great majority of patients with vascular disease if careful attention is given to detail. This is a major advance in surgical technique and prosthetic management. Even the short stumps can be fitted with the modern prostheses, but there is no satisfactory substitute for the patient's own knee. Loss of the knee is a severe handicap to older patients with peripheral arterial disease.

Below-the-knee amputation is performed when there is gangrene or arterial insufficiency distal to the ankle that is too severe to permit saving the foot.

Popliteal pulsation need not be present if collateral flow is adequate. In the operation described, the posterior flap is made long because the collateral flow is more abundant posteriorly from muscular branches of the peroneal arteries or the posterior tibial arteries when these are patent. Difficulty with healing almost always occurs at the center of the anterior flap, which should therefore be kept short and broad based. Circular incisions offer no important advantages in the calf, and placement of the scar is unimportant, although it should not adhere to the underlying bone. Other flaps and debridement of ischemic or damaged muscle, as described in orthopedic textbooks, are useful for acute occlusion of the popliteal artery, injuries, or other conditions in which cutaneous circulation is normal.

The technique of operation is different when immediate fitting of the prosthesis is intended.

Contraindications

Definitive elective closed amputation below the knee should not be done when there is (1) invasive infection, (2) unstabilized arterial insufficiency after acute arterial occlusion, (3) ischemic pain above the ankle, (4) other signs of severe arterial insufficiency, or (5) diabetic neuropathy with hypalgesia at the level of the skin flaps.

Anesthesia

Spinal or light general anesthesia is suitable.

Infracondylar amputation for immediate fitting of prosthesis*

The fundamental principles, preoperative care, and anesthesia for amputations are exceedingly important. These are discussed earlier in the chapter.

A 5- to 7-inch stump is ideal, but shorter stumps are useful and worthwhile. A shorter stump is advisable in patients with arteriosclerosis obliterans or arterial insufficiency; a stump including $4^{1}/_{2}$ to 5 inches of tibia (measured from the knee joint) or a stump extending 2 inches below the tibial tubercle is adequate.

---

*We are deeply grateful to Dr. Oblendo Cuento, who directed this project during his residency.

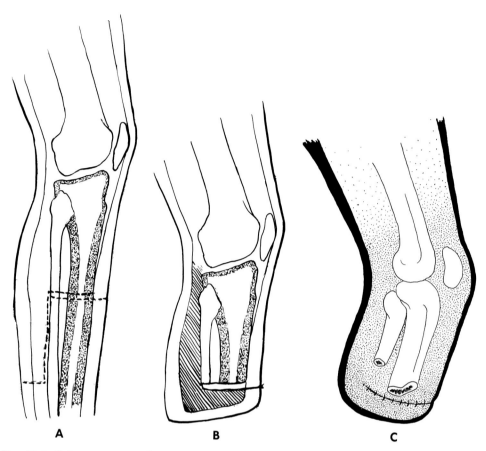

Fig. 19-2. Schematic view of incision and closure. Below-the-knee amputation for immediate prosthesis. **A,** Incision. **B,** Side view of myoplastic flap at closure. **C,** Skin closure. (Drawings by Polly Cullinane.)

Procedure

Incision

The incision is made in three directions, as diagrammed in Fig. 19-2, *A.* The blood supply to the skin is always sparse anteriorly, and therefore the anterior skin is not undermined. There is *no* anterior flap. Later the posterior musculocutaneous flap is folded up to cushion the end of the bone. The skin incision is cut deeply so that the fascia is cut at the same level as the skin.

1. Incise the anterior skin and deep fascia at the level at which you intend to saw the tibia. This anterior incision extends around two thirds of the circumference of the leg.

COMMENT: *Pulsatile bleeding from the skin edge is reassuring. Only experience teaches the surgeon how much bleeding is sufficient. Unless a few of these operations fail, you are denying the operation to some for whom it will be successful. If you are in doubt, do not apply the plaster socket at the end of the operation. If the bleeding is obviously too sparse, complete the operation above the knee. However, little is lost with an unsuccessful below-the-knee amputation if the second-stage above-the-knee operation is not delayed too long.*

458

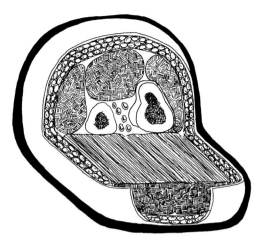

Fig. 19-3. Schematic view of below-the-knee amputation before myoplasty. (Drawing by Polly Cullinane.)

2. Incise the skin and deep fascia distally (at a 90-degree angle to the anterior incision) for a distance slightly longer than the diameter of the calf.

3. Incise posterior skin circumferentially, that is, transversely, to connect the lateral and medial incisions (Fig. 19-2, *A*).

Transection of muscles anteriorly, medially, and laterally

Transect the muscles anteriorly and laterally at the same level as the anterior skin incision, down to the interosseous membrane and the subjacent neurovascular bundle (Fig. 19-3). Ligate and divide vessels with 3-0 chromic catgut. Ligate the anterior tibial and superficial peroneal nerves under moderate traction, and allow the ligated ends to retract into the muscle. If the anterior tibial muscle is pale or ischemic, remove it and the fibula.

Transection of tibia and fibula

The tibia is cut vertically at the correct level 2 to 3 inches below the tibial tubercle, and the fibula is cut to a somewhat shorter length so that it can be padded with muscle. Short stumps can be fitted with modern prostheses, and the patient's own knee is superior to any prosthetic hinge because of the muscular attachments to the tibia.

1. Incise the periosteum of the tibia slightly distal to the level of the skin incision and elevate it proximally for $1/2$ inch. This periosteal flap will be sutured later to the posterior fascia in order to stabilize the muscles and to cushion the end of the tibia.

2. Pass a narrow ribbon retractor behind the tibia, and saw the tibia close to the periosteal flap, slightly proximal to the skin incision. Bevel the anterior edge of the tibia, and round the edge of the cortex slightly with the rasp.

3. Transect the fibula $1/2$ inch proximal to the tibia. The Gigli saw or bone cutter is useful for this.

COMMENT: *In short stumps, remove the fibula completely.*

459

Cutting of posterior musculocutaneous flap

1. Free the muscles from the posterior aspects of both bones as far as the distal transverse posterior incision.

2. Cut the muscles, skin, and fascia transversely at the level of the distal incision.

COMMENT: *The posterior flap muscle mass has abundant collateral circulation. Necrosis, if it appears, will always occur at the edge of the anterior skin. It is important not to fold the flap and not to separate skin, fascia, and muscle layers from each other.*

3. Ligate the posterior nerves with 3-0 silk after crushing the nerve with a hemostat at the site of ligation. Divide the nerve while it is drawn down under tension so that it retracts into the muscle proximal to the ends of the bone.

COMMENT: *Neuroma cannot be prevented by injecting alcohol into the nerve ends or by covering the nerve ends with plastic, silk, or tantalum. The method proposed involves confining the regenerating ends in the nonabsorbable ligature and cushioning the retracted ends with muscle.*

Myoplasty

Myoplasty is the preferred method below the knee. In preparation for either technique, the fascia and muscles have been sectioned so that they are longer than necessary, and now they are trimmed and sutured so that they form a well-shaped stump and pad the bone. Both techniques stabilize the muscles so that they develop some tone and supply neurological feedback and reflexes not generated by unattached muscles.

The fascial closure is made fairly snug, in order to shape the stump. Myodesis, that is, suturing of muscles to drill holes in bone, is not performed unless circulation appears to be adequate. The attachment of some muscles to drill holes in the tibia gives more stability but it appears to offer no advantage for amputation below the knee. Myodesis is more helpful in above-the-knee cases.

Burgess method of myoplasty. The posterior flap comprises the deep fascia and, in its midportion, the sturdy gastrocnemius fascia also. Anteriorly the periosteum of the tibia was saved over the medial cortex, and this is reinforced by incorporating the deep fascia into the same sutures that join the periosteum to the posterior flap.

1. Cut the posterior tibial and deep flexor muscles at the level of the tibia.

2. Fold the posterior flap forward and approximate it to the periosteum of the tibia and the adjacent deep fascia medially and laterally.

3. Trim or tailor the gastrocnemius and soleus muscles as needed to permit good approximation of the fascia and periosteum. The muscles must be tapered toward the end and sides of the flap.

4. Suture the posterior fascia and gastrocnemius fascia to the anterior fascia and periosteum with 2-0 chromic catgut, burying the knots as illustrated in Fig. 19-5, *H* and *I*.

Skin closure

1. Trim the skin corners so that the edges fit loosely and fit without folds or grooves or dog-ears. Drains should rarely be necessary and must not be sutured to skin. If there is concern about infection, abandon the plan for immediate fitting of the prosthesis. Drains that are left a little long and are not sutured to the skin are easily removed through a small window cut in the cast a few days postoperatively.

2. Suture the skin with monofilament suture such as fine nylon (Fig. 19-2, *C*). Handle the skin only with fingers. Do not pinch the skin with forceps. Sutures should not strangle skin or leave crosshatchings.

Plaster dressing and temporary socket

The prosthetist is present in the operating room and proceeds with the plaster dressing, which can also serve as a total contact socket for the prosthesis. The only contraindication is unexpected poor blood supply, causing concern for healing and need for inspection of the stump frequently. The rigid dressing is applied even if you do not intend to permit weight bearing early.

1. Cover the incision with Adaptic or other nonadherent gauze.

2. Place sterile lamb's wool over the end as an absorbent cushion that will not compress into a soggy hard wad.

3. Apply the sterile Lycra Orlon stump sock snugly to hold all this in place (Fig. 19-4, *A* and *B*). Hold tension on the sock sufficient to lift the stump and hold it off the operating table with 5- to 15-degree flexion of the knee.

4. Trim and bevel the felt or compressed urethane foam relief pads to fit around the patella and over the tibia (Fig. 19-4, *C*). These pads are glued to the sock. The medial felt relief pad is placed with the center of the posterior extension on the concave apex of the medial condylar flare and the beveled portion $^1/_4$ inch medial to the tibial crest throughout its length. This should extend distally $^3/_8$ inch beyond the cut end of the tibia. The lateral felt relief pad is placed opposite the medial pad with the beveled portion $^1/_4$ inch lateral to the tibial crest throughout its length. Cut and bevel the lateral felt pad distally in the same manner as for the medial pad. Next, a circumpatellar felt relief pad is placed around the patella.

Applying plaster dressing. Apply the plaster dressing over the end of the stump and the lower two thirds of the thigh (Fig. 19-4, *D*). The elastic plaster applies gentle compression over the end, and the compression diminishes gradually as the plaster ascends the limb in spiral fashion. It is elastic while wet, but it is firm when it has set.

1. Use the elastic plaster bandage wrapped fairly snugly to prevent medial displacement of the gastrocnemius muscle. Continue the wrapping distally over the stump area, pulling the plaster bandage so that it is snug at the lateral portion of the stump. Over the anterior margin, release the tension slightly; then continue the wrapping medially as well as posteriorly with a slight pull on the plaster bandage. Repeat this process of wrapping over more of the stump, and finish the first roll just below the knee (Fig. 19-4, *D*).

2. Start using a second roll of elastic plaster bandage just distal to the first roll, and wrap the limb to the midthigh level, applying less tension as you ascend the thigh until there is no tension at the brim. Proximal constriction must be avoided. The knee must be flexed slightly to keep the cast from slipping later when set.

3. Reinforce and cover the elastic plaster bandage with conventional plaster and incorporate a $1^1/_2$-inch suspension strap with safety buckle into the wrapping at the anteroproximal level of the rigid dressing, and fold the remaining distal portion of the strap back and wrap it in place with the remaining plaster bandage (Fig. 19-4, *E*).

Attaching suspension belt. After the cast has hardened sufficiently, cut a slot in the stump sock at the level of the safety buckle that corresponds to the size of the

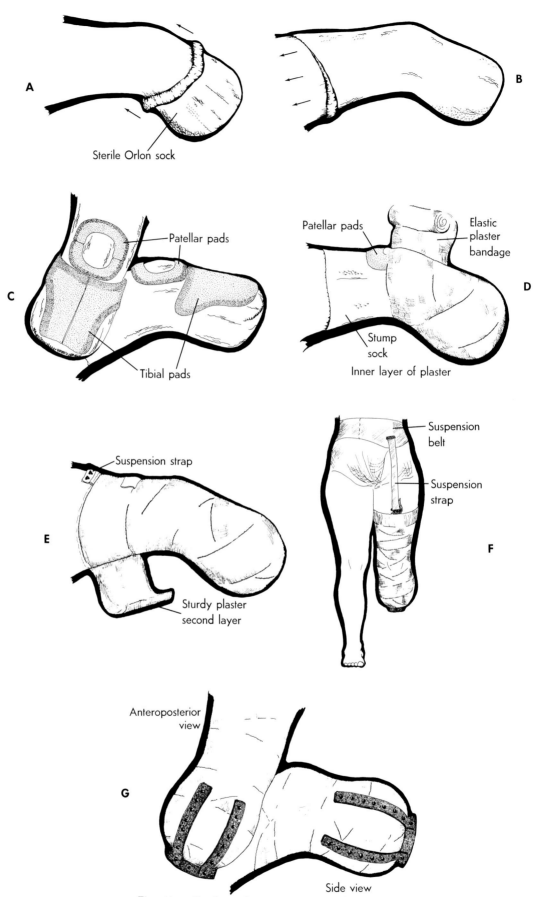

A

Sterile Orlon sock

B

C

Patellar pads

Tibial pads

D

Patellar pads

Elastic plaster bandage

Stump sock

Inner layer of plaster

E

Suspension strap

Sturdy plaster second layer

F

Suspension belt

Suspension strap

G

Anteroposterior view

Side view

Fig. 19-4. For legend see opposite page.

safety buckle, pull down the edge of the sock over the cast brim, and pass the buckle through the slot. Apply the suspension belt around the waist, and attach the elastic strap to the suspension strap buckle (Fig. 19-4, F).

Applying socket attachment plate. Apply the socket attachment plate so that it is held at a 90-degree angle to the table top when viewed laterally and set $1/_2$ inch medially from an imaginary line passing through the center of the knee and center of the stump when viewed anteriorly (Fig. 19-4, G). Fill the space between the back of the socket attachment plate and the cast socket with a double layer of plaster splints in order to fill any hollows. Secure the socket attachment plate to the cast wrapping with one roll of conventional plaster bandage.

Attaching prosthesis. Attach the adjustable prosthetic unit to the socket attachment plate by means of a quick disconnecting screw. Attach the measured pylon tube with the SACH foot in an approximate toe-out to the prosthetic unit with a screwdriver. Detach the complete assembly from the socket attachment plate by means of the quick disconnecting screw before the patient leaves the operating room. Later, when ambulation is begun, the prosthetic unit is attached again.

Postoperative management

The preoperative exercises of arms and legs are continued on schedule in bed. The bed has a trapeze or monkey bar. With assistance, the patient turns and lies on his face for short periods several times daily to prevent groin contracture.

Ambulation begins in the rehabilitation department during the first few days. The patient may stand with the prosthesis attached and rest the prosthesis on the floor. The rehabilitation time table must be flexible. Limited ambulation in parallel bars begins in a few days, but full weight bearing is not permitted for three to six weeks. Patients graduate from parallel bars to a walker and, finally, to crutches. The purpose of ambulation is to help the patient to develop tolerance for partial weight bearing and to begin the walking process in order to gain confidence and security. Although full weight bearing must await firm healing, the prosthesis should be worn and ambulation begun early. The patient may touch the the prosthesis down to the floor and begin partial weight bearing in a few weeks. The therapists supervise weight shifting, heel-toe exercises, and postural control from the onset.

For some older or feeble patients, ambulation may be delayed until the cast is removed and sutures are out, but ambulation need not await complete healing when the patient's general condition permits it.

The cast is changed every five to seven days, and the sutures are removed fourteen to twenty-one days after surgery. However, if there is unexplained fever, increasing pain, or even persistent pain more than usual, the cast should be removed forthwith. If there is any doubt about the condition of the stump, remove the cast. Unscheduled cast changes are inconvenient, but your only regret will be finding concealed or

---

Fig. 19-4. Plaster dressing for below-the-knee amputation. **A** and **B,** Apply sterile Orlon stump sock. **C,** Fit felt relief pads over patella and tibia. **D,** Apply elastic plaster dressing. **E,** Incorporate suspension strap into plaster. **F,** Attach suspension belt and strap. **G,** Incorporate socket attachment plate into plaster. (Drawings by Polly Cullinane.)

overlooked complications. Of course, replace any cast that becomes loose or ill fitting. Casts should be replaced within an hour, since swelling may increase very rapidly during the time the cast is off.

Complications

Any of the complications of the usual infracondylar amputation may occur. Wound complications may be concealed in the plaster socket, and of course, they will occur more frequently when the cast is not well padded or when weight is borne too soon on the healing stump. Complete healing of the stump is not required for ambulation; weight can be borne on the ischial tuberosity during ambulation with the temporary prosthesis for the below-the-knee amputation, and the healing stump can be left open for dressings.

Infracondylar amputation

Recent improvements in prostheses and in the preoperative and postoperative management allow successful amputation below the knee in the majority of patients who require a major amputation above the foot.

When the facilities and the team for immediate attachment of a prosthesis are not available, the operation proceeds as follows. It is a simple, but still a fastidious, meticulous technique.

Indications, contraindications, choice of level, preoperative preparation, and anesthesia are all described on pp. 453-454.

Procedure

1. Place the patient in the supine position with the knee extended throughout the operation.

2. Mark the level of division of the tibia at a point 10 to 12 cm. distal to the knee joint (Fig. 19-5, A). Measure the circumference of the calf at this level with a silk suture. Divide the circumference measurement in half by cutting the suture. This piece of thread may then be used to measure the length of the flaps, the anterior flap being one third and the posterior flap two thirds of the thread's length. The tibia should be divided slightly above the junction of the two flaps.

3. Make the skin incision as measured and indicated in Fig. 19-5, A. Divide the deep fascia at a level slightly above the skin level. Reflect the anterior flap of skin and fascia (Fig. 19-5, B) and cover them with moist gauze. Incise the anterolateral group of muscles down to the tibia and fibula. Evidence of stasis or lack of pulsatile bleeding from the muscle should suggest the need for amputation above the knee.

4. Retract and protect the soft tissues. Using the Gigli saw, divide the fibula at as high a point as possible (Fig. 19-5, C).

5. Dissect the muscles posterior to the tibia so that they are free. Pass a ribbon retractor beneath the tibia. Incise the periosteum at the level selected for division of the tibia, and elevate the periosteum distally. (See Fig. 19-5, D.)

6. Before sawing directly through the tibia, make the anterior bevel cut just above the proposed line of division. Divide the tibia. Use the rasp or rongeur to reduce bony spurs.

7. Hold the distal end of the divided tibia inferiorly. Use a sharp amputation knife to make a slanting cut through the posterior muscle mass of the leg (Fig. 19-5, E). Ligate the bleeding points in the posterior muscle flap.

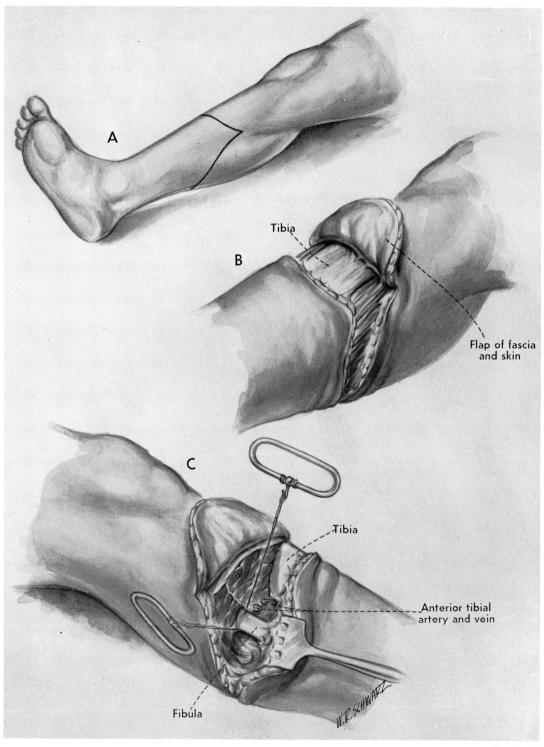

Tibia

Flap of fascia
and skin

Tibia

Anterior tibial
artery and vein

Fibula

W.R.SCHWARZ

Continued.

Fig. 19-5. Amputation below knee. **A,** Incision. **B,** Medial view of skin flap. **C,** Lateral view of division of fibula.

465

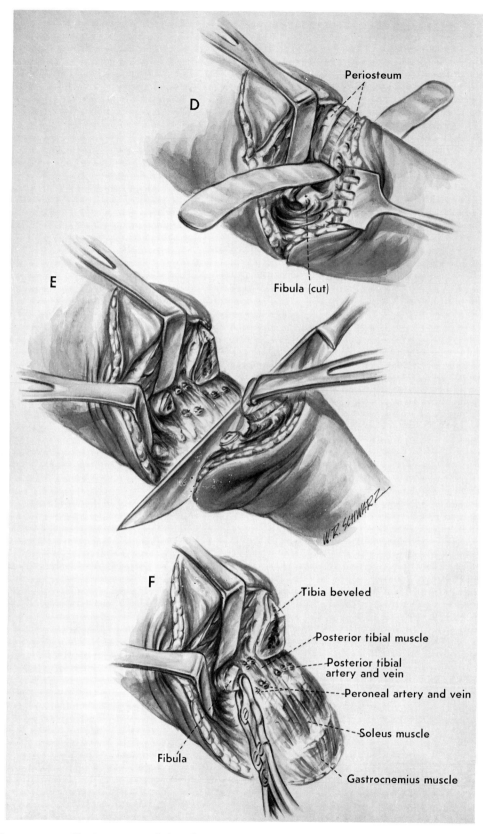

Fig. 19-5, cont'd. Amputation below knee. D, Site of division of tibia. E, Posterior muscles cut. F, Fibula shortened with double-acting rongeur.

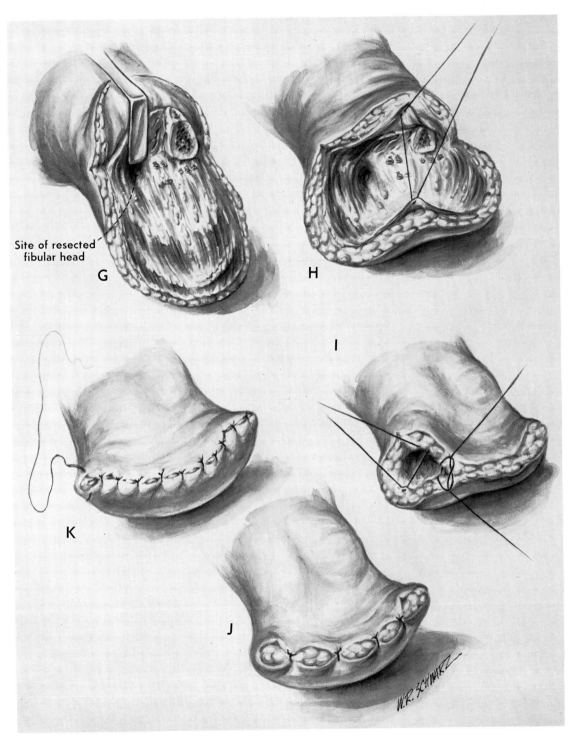

Site of resected
fibular head

G

H

I

K

J

W.R. SCHWARZ

Fig. 19-5, cont'd. Amputation below knee. **G,** Flaps prior to closure. **H,** Beginning fascial closure. **I,** Fascial closure completed. **J** and **K,** Skin closure.

8. Shorten the fibula by stripping periosteum away, retracting soft tissues upward, and dividing it so that it is at least an inch shorter than the tibia (Fig. 19-5, F).

9. Draw the nerves down with a hemostat, crush them proximally with three hemostats, ligate the crushed nerves with nonabsorbable suture, divide the nerves, and allow them to retract.

Closure

1. Irrigate the wound abundantly with saline solution, and inspect it for additional bleeding (Fig. 19-5, G). When amputation is done for vascular disease, bleeding is less than from limbs with a normal circulation. Hemostasis should be meticulous. Use no drains unless there is considerable oozing. If drainage is necessary, the drain should be removed within forty-eight to seventy-two hours.

2. Suture the fascia. Begin in the center (Fig. 19-5, H) and bisect the remaining sectors once or twice to ensure even distribution of tension (Fig. 19-5, I).

3. Place a few deep skin sutures rather far apart to close the skin and subcutaneous tissue (Fig. 19-5, J). Monofilament sutures such as 4-0 nylon are ideal. Complete the skin closure with fine sutures placed somewhat more superficially (Fig. 19-5, K). Avoid the use of tissue forceps on the skin. Skin closure should be accurate. Fig. 19-5, K, shows slight separation of the skin edges that we ordinarily would not tolerate.

Dressing and postoperative care

A small dry dressing is applied and held in place with a sock of sterile stockinette. Tincture of benzoin applied to the skin of the leg and thigh secures the dressing in place. A small posterior splint may be applied to keep the knee extended.

Some details of postoperative care are given on p. 463. If drains have been necessary, they are removed within the first few days. The first dressing should otherwise be done on the fifth day. A dusky anterior flap is usually a poor prognostic sign at this time. Stump wrapping is begun seven days after surgery. Stitches are removed twelve to fourteen days after the operation. Exercises and other rehabilitative procedures are commenced early when healing seems assured. (See p. 463.)

ELECTIVE AMPUTATION ABOVE KNEE
Indications and choice of level

Amputation is performed through the thigh when the circulation is too poor to save the knee joint or when there is persistent contracture or other disease of the joint. The knee will be of little use to patients who will be unable to use a prosthesis. If such patients have serious heart disease, cerebral atherosclerosis, severe arterial insufficiency in the opposite leg, or blindness, the amputation should be done above the knee when there is any doubt about the healing of a more distal amputation wound.

In the majority of patients requiring amputation above the foot, there is successful healing below the knee. The criteria for choice of level are not always clear, and some patients should sign permission for both above-the-knee and below-the-knee operations. The surgeon can decide after incision below the knee whether the operation should be completed at that level or above the knee.

The optimal level above the knee is just above the distal expansion of the femur provided that the common femoral and deep femoral arteries are open. The stump should be short enough that the knee hinge of the prosthesis can be placed at the level of the normal knee. Midthigh amputation, operation through the thicker portion of the thigh, is reserved for those limbs with less blood supply, that is, those in which the common femoral pulse is absent or weak and collateral circulation appears to be poor.

Preoperative care

Careful preoperative regulation and treatment of associated medical problems is mandatory, as is control of infection with drainage, antibiotic treatment, and other conservative measures as indicated. We recommend preoperative daily cleansing of the skin of the thigh and knee with an antiseptic soap (pHisoHex or similar preparation).

Rehabilitation and adaptation to a prosthesis are aided by preoperative consultation with the physiatrist. The patient is taught his exercises, crutch walking, and similar procedures.

The feasibility of immediate fitting of the prosthesis should be considered. If it is expected that the patient can and will wear a prosthesis and walk, the early fitting and the early ambulation program is outlined and the team is mobilized as discussed on p. 455. The technique of the operation for immediate fitting of the prosthesis is somewhat different from the traditional technique and is described first.

Anesthesia

Light general anesthesia or spinal anesthesia confined to the diseased limb is suitable.

Supracondylar amputations for immediate fitting of prosthesis

The technique for supracondylar amputation for immediate fitting of the prosthesis differs from the usual amputation at this level in that flaps are made so that the muscles may be sutured together (myoplasty) or to the bone (myodesis). They are attached with modest tension so that they are stabilized. If poor femoral pulse or poor flow in the profunda femoris artery requires midthigh amputation, myoplasty of the bulky muscles will be difficult. Either myoplasty or myodesis can be done in the lower thigh.

Amputation should not be performed closer than 4 inches above the knee joint. The knee hinge and contralateral knee should be at similar levels.

Procedure
Incision

Make short, equal anterior and posterior skin incisions, and cut the deep fascia at the same level as the skin. Each flap is made as long as two thirds of the diameter of the thigh (Fig. 19-6, *A*).

Division of tendons and muscles

Divide the tendons and muscle sharply, and cone or bevel the cut. In the low thigh, cut the deeper muscles at the level at which the femur will be divided. However, leave a long flap of the expansion of the quadriceps muscle anteriorly and a long tendon of the adductor magnus muscle medially. These sturdy structures are useful for the myoplasty reconstruction. The muscles are trimmed and tailored later as needed.

469

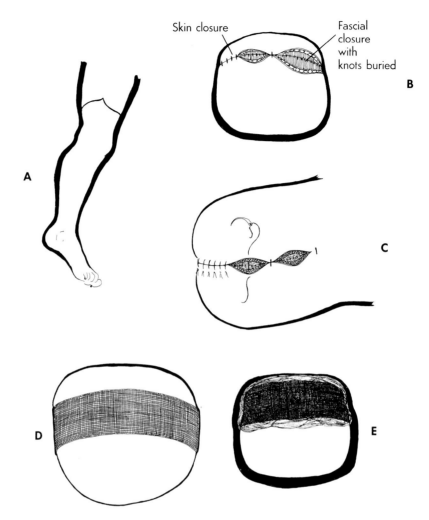

Fig. 19-6. Above-the-knee amputation for immediate prosthesis. A, Incision. B, End view of skin closure. C, Lateral view of skin closure. D, End view of nonadherent gauze over incision. E, End view of pad of sterile lamb's wool over incision. (Drawings by Polly Cullinane.)

Division of femur

Divide the femur at a point high enough to permit the anterior and posterior muscle flaps to be sutured together to cover the end. Cut the periosteum with a sharp knife, and scrape it distally; then divide the bare bone for a distance of a few millimeters distal to the living periosteum. Saw the linea aspera slowly and neatly, since cracks or chips here have a tendency to form exostoses.

Division of remaining structures

1. Divide the ligate the superficial femoral vessels.

2. Draw the sciatic nerve down under tension, crush it proximally with a hemostat, ligate it at the crushed section, and then cut it and allow it to retract up into the muscles.

3. Cut the posterior muscles obliquely with the sharp amputation knife, leaving the posterior flap long.

Myoplasty or myodesis

Myoplasty. Suture the tendons of the quadriceps muscle and anterior fascia to the posterior muscle and fascia in order to cover the end of the femur. Some muscle ends must be trimmed and thinned so that the fascial closure is snug but not tight. Use 0 chromic catgut and bury the knots inside.

COMMENT: *As in below-the-knee amputations, the stabilization of the muscle ends helps to shape the stump, and modest tension preserves muscle tone and decreases atrophy and stump shrinkage. The proprioceptive feedback from muscles with normal tension supplies the patient with a better sense of position and appears to favor ambulation and early gait training.*

Tension myodesis in low-thigh amputations. When there is no ischemia, the medial and posterior muscles can be sutured to drill holes in the end of the femur. This is a sturdier fixation of the muscles to the femur. This is feasible only in low-thigh amputations and is indicated only where there is ample blood supply.

Attach the adductor magnus muscle to the femur medially to try to prevent lateral drift of the end of the femur. Attach the hamstring muscles posteriorly to the femur. Attach the wide expansion of the quadriceps muscle anteriorly to the femur, and attach the medial and lateral expansions of the quadriceps muscle to the adjacent adductor magnus muscle medially and the adjacent hamstring muscle posteriorly and laterally. Laterally, you can use the fascia lata to cover the end of the femur, and you can suture the fascia lata to the adductor magnus muscle. Use a nonabsorbable monofilament suture with modest tension, and tie the knots in the marrow cavity.

The use of the fascia lata is important for preventing the drift of the femur to the lateral side of the stump. Drift of the femur is inevitable without myoplasty or myodesis, since these are total-contact, weight-bearing stumps, not the ischial weight-bearing sockets of the traditional above-the-knee amputation.

After myoplasty or myodesis, cover the end of the stump by suturing the anterior and posterior fasciae with 2-0 chromic catgut, burying the knots.

Closure of skin

Suture the skin with fine monofilament suture such as 4-0 nylon (Fig. 19-6, *B* and *C*). Trim the skin wherever it appears to be redundant. Approximate the edges without causing strangulation or tension. Do not pinch the skin with forceps. Avoid depressions or angulations or wrinkles of the skin, since this is a total-contact plaster fitting.

Plaster dressing for immediate fitting of prosthesis

A close-fitting nonbulky dressing and plaster are applied. No felt pads are necessary. A sheet of stockinette protects the perineum from contact with plaster. Various belts, straps, or cables are needed to keep the cast from slipping down. Various devices may be used to shape the plaster socket above the knee. It must not be forgotten that this socket differs from the former quadrilateral ischial weight-bearing socket in one important aspect. Some compression of the distal stump is desirable, there is full contact, and some muscle function and weight bearing by the healed stump are intended. Therefore, the socket need not be long, but it must be snug.

1. Cover the incision with a strip of Adaptic or Xeroform gauze, and pad the end with sterile lamb's wool (Fig. 19-6, *D* and *E*).

2. Roll on the sterile elastic Orlon stump sock up to the perineum, and cut the

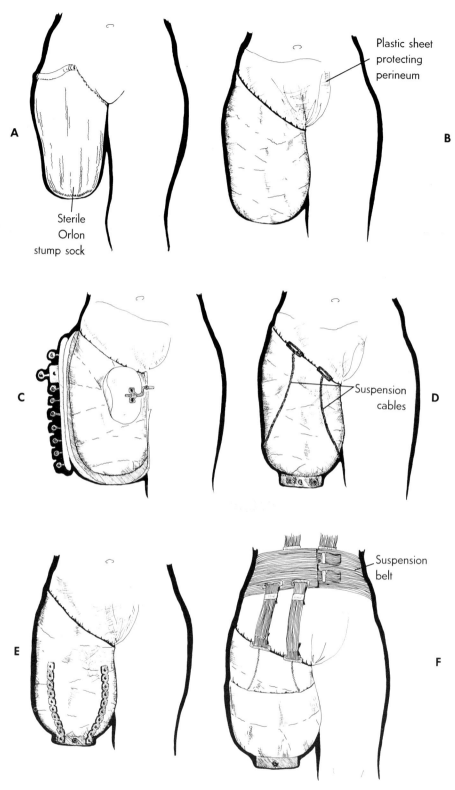

Fig. 19-7. Plaster dressing for above-the-knee amputation preparatory to early fitting of prosthesis. **A,** Sterile Orlon stump sock. **B,** Plastic apron protecting perineum during application of plaster. **C,** Casting fixture for molding plaster. **D,** Bowden suspension cables. **E,** Socket attachment plate. **F,** Suspension waist belt. (Drawings by Polly Cullinane.)

sock vertically over the origin of the adductor longus muscle (Fig. 19-7, *A*). The assistant elevates the stump and steadies it by traction on the stump sock.

3. Protect the perineum with the perineal apron; then begin the plaster dressing.

Applying plaster dressing

1. Apply the elastic plaster bandage distally over the end as well as circumferentially; then continue applying it proximally with firm, even, steady tension. Continue applying the second roll of elastic plaster proximally for $2^1/_2$ to 3 inches higher on the anterior, lateral, and posterior aspects and then on the medial side near the perineum. Apply less stretch or tension in the upper thigh and no tension at the brim and the upper third of the cast. Use enough plaster that the socket brim is smooth and well rounded, not thin or sharp.

2. While the plaster is wet, apply the casting fixture over the plaster with the handle down and open. This will shape the plaster into the proper quadrilateral shape and form Scarpa's bulge. Remove the casting fixture in a few minutes, and reinforce the cast with several rolls of the conventional nonelastic plaster bandages. Two layers are usually sufficient.

COMMENT: *Hand shaping or molding of the plaster is preferred by some prosthetists.*

Applying cables. Apply a pair of Bowden cables on the medial and lateral sides of the cast (Fig. 19-7, *D*).

COMMENT: *Suspensions other than the Bowden cables are also available. The trained prosthetist will use his own equipment and appliances well. We include this section mainly to provide principles for the surgeon, and the method we describe is one of the current ones.*

Drains are rarely needed and are a nuisance to take out. If a drain has been used, the apex of the cables must not cross the drain site or the intended window to be made later for removal of the drain.

Secure the cable housing with a layer of plaster bandage.

Applying socket attachment plate. Apply the socket attachment plate with its attachment straps (Fig. 19-7, *E*). Shorten the straps to one-half the length of the stump so that they are below the level of exposed cable housing. When viewed laterally, the socket attachment plate should be parallel to the foot edge of the table and posterior from the distal socket center in order to achieve the desired thigh-knee-ankle relationship. The plate should be perpendicular to the table top to accommodate the flexion angle in the cast socket. An imaginary vertical line drawn from the ischial tuberosity should bisect the medial border of the socket attachment plate.

COMMENT: *In short stumps, the socket attachment plate will not contact the end of the stump until the space between the plate and cast is filled with balsa wood or Styrofoam. The socket attachment plate must be far enough distal that the knee bend of the attached prosthesis is at a functional level. For maximum stability, with plaster, fill all spaces between the socket attachment plate and the distal end of the wood as well as any space between the wood and cast socket.*

Applying suspension attachments. Trim all excess stockinette from the perineal apron, retaining 1 inch of overhang after applying a roll of plaster bandage over the socket attachment straps. Apply the suspension waist belt, the distal border of which is resting just proximal to the iliac crest (Fig. 19-7, *F*). Attach the waist straps anteriorly, and tighten the two lateral adjustment straps so that the belt will not displace distally or rotate on the patient. Bring both shoulder straps over each shoulder after crossing them in the back for men and in front for women. Attach the shoulder straps to the anteroproximal attachment buckles. Place the felt apron between the cast socket and the exposed portions of the cables and housings. Thread both anterior suspension straps through the retainers of the Bowden cables, and fasten them to each corresponding safety buckle, exposing at this time all available cables to allow for 90 degrees of hip flexion when the patient is sitting up. Fasten the two posterior suspension straps to their corresponding safety buckles to maintain distal tissue support by suspending the cast socket and retaining it securely on the stump. Attach the adjustable prosthetic unit with all adjustments in the neutral position to the socket attachment plate, and attach the pylon tube to the SACH foot. Detach the completed assembly from the socket attachment plate by the quick disconnecting screw before the patient leaves the operating room.

Postoperative care

The plan of postoperative care is to establish ambulation early, as soon as the general condition of the patient and of the stump will tolerate it. Casts are changed at seven- to ten-day intervals or sooner if they are loose or if fever or pain is in any way unusual. Casts are reapplied immediately or at least within one hour after they are removed because swelling may develop quickly while they are off.

Physical therapy, exercises, and similar procedures begin early, as described for below-the-knee amputations (p. 463). The temporary prosthesis is attached, and early weight bearing begins gradually but is not complete until sutures are removed after fourteen days and the wound is healed. Results of ambulation, healing, and rehabilitation are classified separately. A patient is classified as having immediate ambulation success when walking one week postoperatively. Early ambulation success signifies that he is walking one month postoperatively. Rehabilitation success signifies that the patient is home and walking less than a month postoperatively. Some limbs will be successfully healed while the patients are not ambulatory or rehabilitated. Some patients can and must be ambulatory before healing is complete.

Supracondylar amputation

When immediate fitting of the prosthesis and the rigid plaster dressing is not feasible, the operation is simple because no myoplasty or myodesis is needed. The prosthesis will have the traditional quadrilateral ischial weight-bearing socket.

The lower thigh is the best level for amputation when the blood supply is adequate for healing. This and other introductory matters are discussed on pp. 454 and 455.

Procedure

Place the patient in the supine position with the leg extended. Perform the amputation from anterior to posterior, dividing successive layers as a cone (Fig. 19-8, B).

1. Make a circular incision in the skin several centimeters above the patella (Fig. 19-8, A).

2. The plan of operation, the coning of the successive layers, is shown in Fig. 19-8, B.

3. Divide the deep fascia, the patellar tendon, and the muscles anterior and lateral to the femur (Fig. 19-8, C).

4. Divide the tendinous attachments to the linea aspera. Pass a ribbon retractor

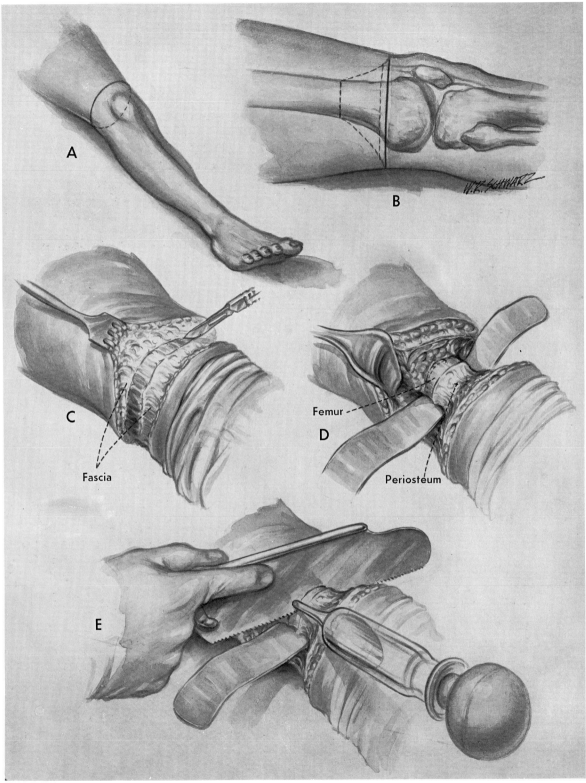

Continued.

Fig. 19-8. Elective amputation above knee. **A,** Circular incision. **B,** Lateral view of incision. **C,** Incision in deep fascia. **D,** Incision on femur. Periosteum stripped distally. **E,** Femur sawed.

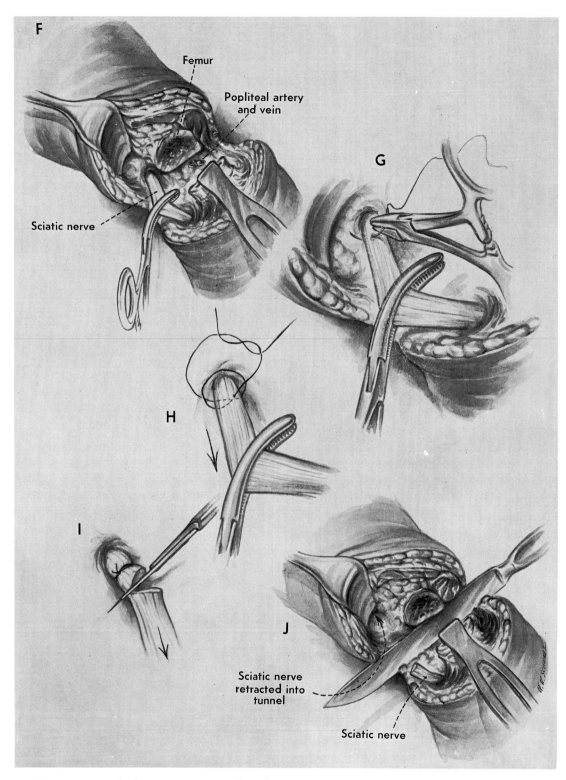

Fig. 19-8, cont'd. Elective amputation above knee. **F,** Sciatic nerve identified and drawn down. **G** and **H,** Suture ligature in sciatic nerve. **I,** Sciatic nerve divided under tension so that it retracts. **J,** Posterior muscles divided.

476

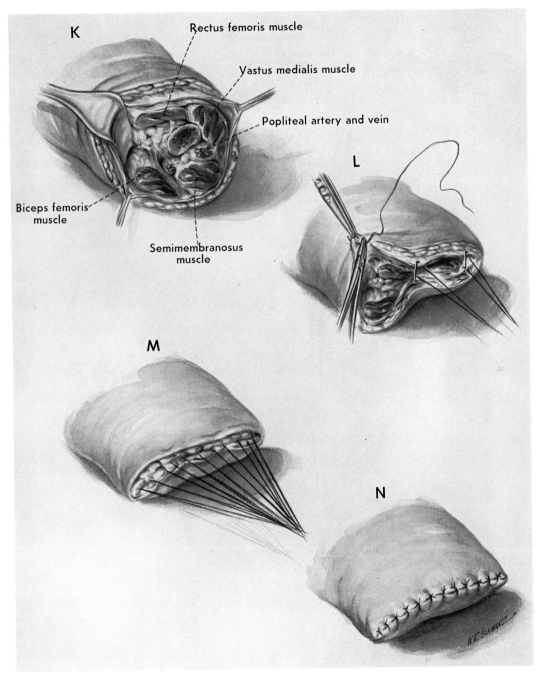

K — Rectus femoris muscle

Vastus medialis muscle

Popliteal artery and vein

Biceps femoris muscle

Semimembranosus muscle

L

M

N

Fig. 19-8, cont'd. Elective amputation above knee. **K,** Veins of open end of stump. **L,** Placement of sutures for closure of deep fascia. **M,** Closure of deep fascia completed. **N,** Closure of skin completed.

477

beneath the femur. Retract the soft tissues remaining lateral to the femur. Divide and elevate the periosteum, stripping it distally. (Fig. 19-8, *D*.)

5. Hold the vascular bundle posteriorly with the ribbon retractor, and saw through the femur (Fig. 19-8, *E*).

6. Retract the distal end of the femur with a small retractor. Identify the popliteal artery and vein in the fat of the medial side of the popliteal fossa (Fig. 19-8, *F*). Clamp and divide these structures, and ligate them with a suture ligature.

7. Identify the sciatic nerve in the lateral aspect of the popliteal space (Fig. 19-8, *F*). Clamp the nerve and draw it downward for a distance of several inches (Fig. 19-8, *G*). Tie the nerve with a suture ligature at as high a point as possible (Fig. 19-8, *H*).

8. Divide the sciatic nerve with a sharp knife, and allow it to retract a distance of several inches into the thigh (Fig. 19-8, *I*).

9. Straighten the leg. Place the amputation knife at the proximal end of the femur, and rapidly cut the muscles posteriorly (Fig. 19-8, *J*). Remove the amputated limb. Ligate the various bleeding points in the posterior muscle mass for complete hemostasis.

Closure

1. Inspect the stump carefully (Fig. 19-8, *K*). Meticulous hemostasis is important. Irrigate the wound with saline solution. Elevate the stump on an inverted basin or a pack of towels.

2. Suture the fascial layer with 2-0 silk or chromic catgut, inverting the sutures in order to place the knot beneath the fascia (Fig. 19-8, *L*).

3. Suture the skin with fine silk or nylon (Fig. 19-8, *N*). The placement of a drain is usually unnecessary.

4. Paint the skin of the thigh with tincture of benzoin. Apply dry gauze sponges over the end. Hold the dressing on the stump with stockinette rolled onto the stump. Avoid the use of adhesive tape on the nearby ischemic skin. Do not elevate the stump on a pillow, since this encourages flexion contracture at the hip joint.

Postoperative care

After five days the stump may be wrapped with an elastic bandage applied directly over the stockinette dressing. Redundant skin, the result of the circular incision, will shrink nicely. After the fifth day the patient must lie face down for short periods and hyperextend the stump. Later he may sit and may move around in a wheelchair. The physiatrist should visit before the operation and later, and exercises should be commenced as indicated. Patients may be trained with a temporary prosthesis without the intervening stages of crutch and wheelchair ambulation. However, temporary prostheses are an added expense.

Remove the sutures between the twelfth and fourteenth days.

TRANSMETATARSAL AMPUTATIONS
Indications

Transmetatarsal amputation is a useful conservative procedure when arterial insufficiency involves one or more toes proximal to a suitable level for transphalangeal amputations. Open transmetatarsal amputation is also useful for ulcerated or infected neuropathic feet and is described on p. 484. Considerable judgment is necessary in selecting patients for transmetatarsal amputation. However, the success of this procedure, which requires no prosthesis, is very rewarding.

Contraindications

Contraindications to transmetatarsal amputation are as follows:
1. Advancing infection in the foot
2. Necrosis or skin lesions proximal to the metatarsal-phalangeal joints
3. Insufficient collateral circulation for healing as evidenced by (a) pain on rest, (b) dependent rubor at the line of proposed skin incision, and (c) venous filling time of over one-half minute

Preoperative preparation

Preoperatively, a period of conservative treatment may be required to localize and stabilize necrosis, to arrest infection, and to encourage and evaluate collateral circulation. During this time, the patient should be treated with bed rest, elevation of the limbs, antibiotics, local surgical drainage, and Buerger-Allen exercises. A period of several weeks may be required for preoperative preparation.

Anesthesia

Either light general anesthesia or spinal anesthesia is suitable.

Procedure—transmetatarsal amputation of the forefoot

Perform the operation with the patient in the supine position.

1. Make a dorsal skin incision straight across the foot at the level of the proposed division of the metatarsals (Fig. 19-9, A). Do not undermine the skin proximal to the dorsal incision.

2. Hold the toes down, and cut through the tendons and soft tissues dorsally until you reach the bone (Fig. 19-9, B). Ligate the bleeding vessels with fine plain catgut.

3. Make a plantar incision of sufficient length to close the wound (Fig. 19-9, C).

4. Now hold the toes up so that the tendons of the flexor muscles will be stretched and, when incised, will retract proximally (Fig. 19-9, D). Leave all the soft tissue on the plantar flap, and do not trim the flap.

5. Dissect all soft tissue of the joints and metatarsal bones back to the proposed site of amputation (Fig. 19-9, E).

6. Divide the first metatarsal with the Gigli saw (Fig. 19-9, F). This bone is sturdy, and it fractures if divided with an ordinary bone cutter. Divide the first interosseous muscle with a sharp knife.

7. Divide the second metatarsal and the remaining metatarsals with the bone cutter (Fig. 19-9, G).

8. With a sharp knife, divide the remaining interosseous muscles without loosening the proximal periosteum (Fig. 19-9, H). Remove the specimen. Change gloves and irrigate the wound with copious amounts of saline solution. Then smooth the irregular ends of the metatarsals with a rongeur.

Closure

Close only the skin.
Approximate the plantar flap to the dorsal incision with fine nylon or fine stain-

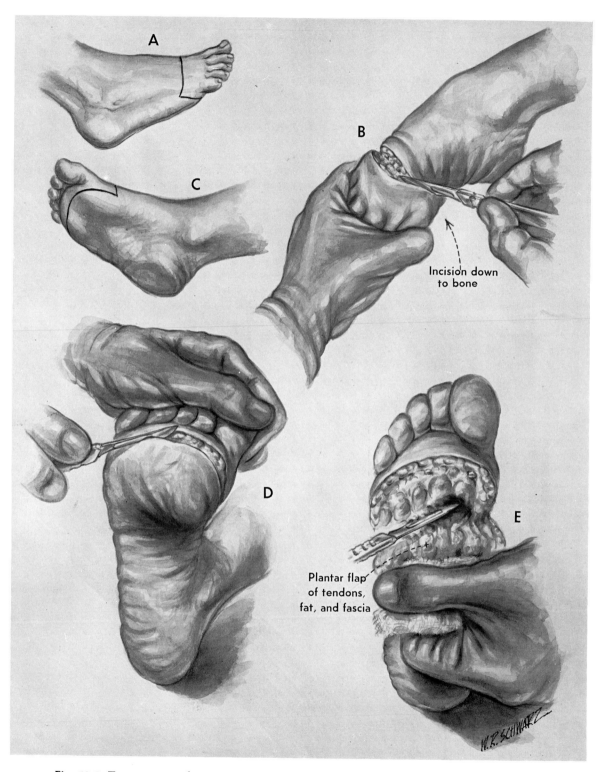

Fig. 19-9. Transmetatarsal amputation. **A,** Dorsal incision. **B,** Dorsal incision with toes flexed. **C,** Plantar incision. **D,** Plantar incision with toes dorsiflexed. **E,** Plantar flap, full thickness, dissected off metatarsal heads.

480

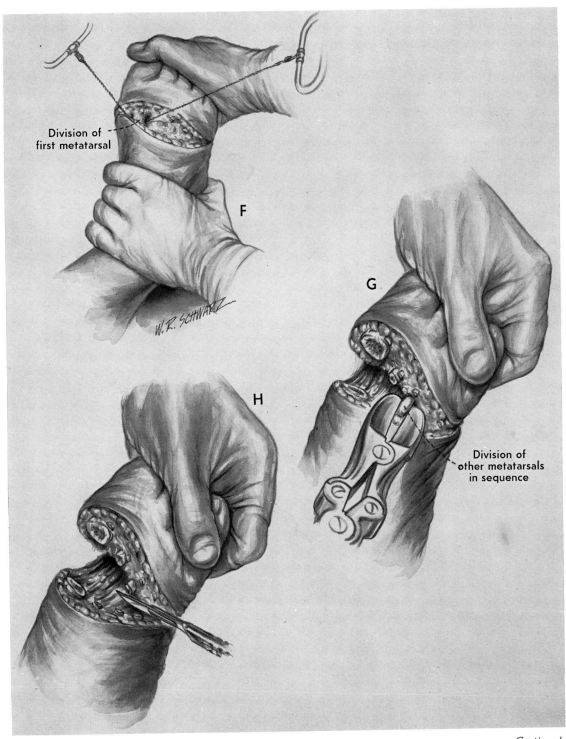

Division of
first metatarsal

F

W. R. SCHWARZ

G

H

Division of
other metatarsals
in sequence

Continued.

Fig. 19-9, cont'd. Transmetatarsal amputation. **F,** Division of first metatarsal with Gigli saw. **G,** Division of other metatarsal bones. **H,** Division of interosseous soft tissue.

481

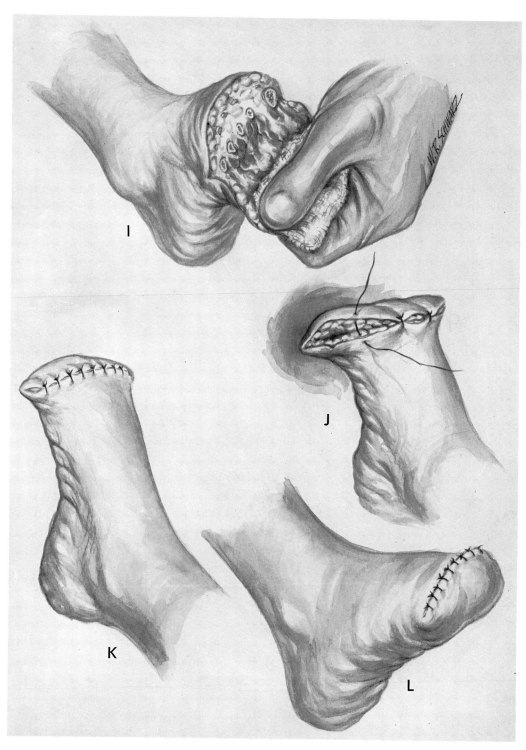

Fig. 19-9, cont'd. Transmetatarsal amputation. **I,** View of end of stump. **J,** Closure of skin flaps. **K** and **L,** Closure completed.

less steel wire. Be gentle. Do not use toothed forceps on the skin. Avoid an excessive number of sutures, and do not tie them too tightly. The placement of a drain is unnecessary (Fig. 19-9, *I* to *L*).

Postoperative care

Apply a loose dressing to support the plantar flap and to prevent tension on the sutures. Do not elevate the foot. You may elevate the head of the bed 6 inches to avoid blanching. If healing is in doubt, do not hesitate to splint the foot and the ankle.

Change the dressings on the fifth and tenth days. Remove the occasional suture that may have been place too tightly and is cutting into the flaps. Ordinarily you can remove the sutures on the fourteenth day.

Buerger-Allen exercises are begun on about the tenth day, and exercises for crutch walking may also be begun early. However, prolonged early dependency of the foot that has been operated on is avoided. Weight bearing is allowed after three to five weeks. When the patient is walking, the toe of the shoe is filled with lamb's wool.

ELECTIVE AMPUTATION OF TOES
Transmetatarsal amputation of fifth or first toe

Either the fifth or the first toe may be amputated at the metatarsal level through a racquet-shaped incision. Collateral circulation is abundant in the thick plantar skin; therefore, this flap is folded up to cover the end of the metatarsal bone. The operation is indicated for ischemic lesions or infections in the proximal phalanx but not if there is ischemia at the line of incision or in the interdigital creases. For lesions of other toes that extend to the interdigital creases complete transmetatarsal amputation of the front part of the foot is required. Open or drainage transmetatarsal amputation of the second, third, and fourth toes is discussed later and illustrated in Fig. 19-13, *A;* this operation is applicable only to neurotrophic feet in diabetic patients with relatively good circulation.

Preoperative care is the same as for other foot amputations.

Procedure

Make a racquet-shaped incision (Fig. 19-10, *A* to *C*) so that the plantar flap is long and may be folded up to cover the cut ends of the bone (Fig. 19-10, *D* and *E*). Do not undermine the dorsal skin incision. Leave all soft tissue on the plantar flap, and cut the metatarsal obliquely at the level of the dorsal skin incision. Since the second metatarsal joint is close, cut close to the first joint.

Postoperative care

The same principles of surgical technique and postoperative care apply as for more extensive amputations of the foot.

Transphalangeal amputation

Transphalangeal amputation is indicated for deformity, infection, or ischemia in the tips or midportions of the toes. More proximal amputations have been discussed previously. Open amputation for drainage is discussed later. For the first and fifth toes, transmetatarsal amputation (Fig. 19-10) is preferable, and as a rule, the wound heals with less difficulty.

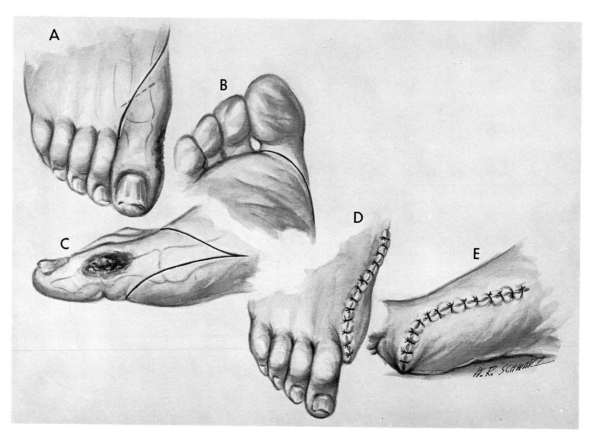

Fig. 19-10. Transmetatarsal amputation of fifth or first toe. **A** to **C,** Views of racquet-shaped incision. **D** and **E,** Views of closure.

Procedure

Incisions should be made so that the digital vessels are divided at the tips of the lateral flaps (Fig. 19-11). There is no need for plantar skin over the end of the toe. Anterior and posterior flaps have less blood supply and heal more slowly.

Make the incisions for the flaps down to the bone, and turn the flaps back. The site elected for division of the proximal phalanx is close to the metatarsal-phalangeal joint. Divide the bone at the base of the flap, leaving only a button of proximal phalanx without entering the joint. Close the incision with a few interrupted fine nylon sutures.

DRAINAGE AND DEBRIDEMENT FOR INFECTIONS AND GANGRENE IN FOOT ASSOCIATED WITH DIABETES

Metabolic abnormalities appear to make diabetic patients unusually susceptible to infections and gangrene. In some instances, arterial occlusion involves only smaller vessels, collateral circulation is good, and conservative treatment and minor amputations may be successful. The feet of diabetic patients are frequently affected by certain distinctive ulcers and infections that require surgical procedures. In each individual, the degree and admixture of atherosclerosis and diabetic neuropathy vary. Accompanying the diabetic neuropathy, there is analgesia of the limb. Various minor

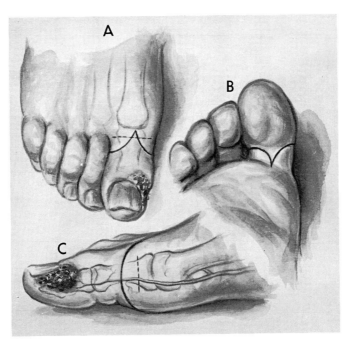

Fig. 19-11. Transphalangeal amputation. **A,** Dorsal view of skin flaps and site of division of bone. **B,** Plantar view of skin flaps. **C,** Lateral view showing digital artery at tip of flap.

infections can therefore proceed to abscess formation and osteomyelitis without causing warning of pain or discomfort.

Calluses, bunions, hammer toes, corns, blisters, and other minor foot disorders can lead to infection with major complications in the diabetic patient. Directions for care of the feet are included in the Appendix.

Infection of deep plantar space

Dangerous invasive infection deep to the plantar fascia and among the tendons of the flexor muscles of the foot can result from a break in the skin almost anywhere on the foot or toe. From a "corn" or a "hammer toe," infection travels via the lumbrical canal (Fig. 19-12) directly into the plantar space. Web space infection between the toes invades the plantar space between the digital extensions of the plantar fascia. The tendon sheaths of the flexor muscles lead infection into the plantar space from infected bunions, calluses, or ulcers over the heads of the metatarsals.

Sepsis in the deep plantar space is difficult to diagnose but must be suspected of being present when there is any infection of a toe or the front part of the foot, particularly when there is severe systemic reaction, difficulty in control of diabetes, edema of the dorsum of the foot, or edema behind the medial malleolus. On examination, the plantar surface of the foot is thick but frequently shows no redness or fluctuation. Pus is confined beneath the plantar fascia, which is a closed space. Sepsis in the plantar space may cause thrombosis of the digital arteries with moist gangrene of the toes.

The diagnosis of plantar space sepsis is made by thorough examination, including removal of eschar, trimming of infected calluses, and opening of the skin to appraise

485

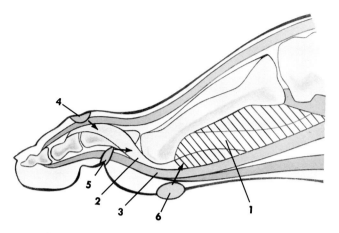

Fig. 19-12. Sources and routes of entry of plantar space abscess. **1,** Plantar space abscess. **2,** Lumbrical canal. **3,** Flexor tendon sheath. **4,** Infected callosity. **5,** Web space infection. **6,** Mal perforant. (Courtesy Smith, Kline & French, Philadelphia, Pa.)

the extent of infection and to permit probing of wounds. X-ray examination will occasionally reveal osteomyelitis that is not apparent on physical examination.

The operative treatment for plantar space sepsis is drainage and debridement. This is best accomplished by open amputation of the infected toe, drainage or debridement of the attached infected tendon, and incision extended into the plantar space for drainage. The required amputation may be transphalangeal, transmetatarsal, or wedge amputation, depending on the extent of debridement that is necessary.

Mal perforant

Mal perforant is a typical manifestation of diabetic neuropathy and is characterized by chronic painless ulcer on the plantar surface of the foot over a pressure point. As a rule, the ulcer appears over the first, third, or fifth metatarsal head. The initial manifestation is a callus, which soon becomes infected. When the feet are neglected, necrosis under the callus results in the characteristic ulcer with overhanging edges, which is painless. Infection spreads into the underlying joint and proximally into the plantar space. Such complications may be avoided by proper care of calluses and of the feet, early treatment of minor infections, and the use of corrective shoes or arch supports. Open amputation of the toe and metatarsal head may be necessary for debridement and drainage.

Suppurative thrombophlebitis

Suppurative thrombophlebitis is occasionally observed in diabetic patients. If it becomes subfascial, incision and drainage, including fasciotomy, are required in addition to proximal ligation of the involved vein and ligation of the perforating veins.

AMPUTATION FOR DEBRIDEMENT AND DRAINAGE

Guillotine amputation for debridement and drainage is occasionally necessary when incision and drainage and antibiotic treatment do not control the infection. The best level in the lower leg is just above the ankle. After the guillotine procedure,

486

a second definitive closed amputation below the knee is performed at a later date. When the guillotine amputation is required above the knee, it should be performed as low as possible or through the knee joint. Revision of the stump and secondary closure may be necessary later.

Open amputation above knee

Open amputation above the knee is rarely necessary. The procedure results in prolonged morbidity. However, healing by second intention will occur if adequate collateral circulation is available. Elective definitive amputation at a higher level may be impossible, but secondary closure in stages is occasionally helpful. Skin traction is difficult and uncomfortable and may even be hazardous to the skin in patients with diabetes or an ischemic limb. The procedure should be performed with a circular incision at as low a level as possible consistent with adequate blood supply and good healing. The amputation may be done below a sterile tourniquet of stout rubber tubing applied to the limb to permit rapid operation without excessive blood loss.

Open amputation below knee

Open amputation below the knee is usually done in an effort to control invasive infection that has not been successfully managed by simple drainage or by antibiotic treatment. Semielective guillotine amputation may be performed for necrosis or for major bone or joint sepsis about the ankle. Fortunately, such procedures are seldom necessary. The best level for debridement procedures below the knee is just above the malleoli. Little bleeding is encountered there, and it is not necessary to divide a great deal of soft tissue. All tissue planes and tendon sheaths should be left open for drainage. Open amputation at the level of election for below-the-knee amputation and the development of flaps in open amputation should be avoided. In patients with vascular disease, slow healing leads to more prolonged morbidity than occurs with a two-stage procedure, and it is usually advisable, after adequate drainage has been established, to perform a subsequent elective definitive amputation at a higher level.

Guillotine amputation at ankle

The patient is prepared preoperatively by conservative measures, antibiotic treatments, and the other measures previously described for elective amputations wherever they are applicable. Spinal or light general anesthesia is suitable. A tourniquet is unnecessary.

Procedure

1. Make a circular incision down to the bone at the thinnest part of the leg just above the ankle malleoli. Clamp and divide the major vessels, and ligate the few bleeding vessels in the soft tissue.
2. Divide the tibia and fibula just above the malleoli.
3. Apply petrolatum gauze over the surgical wound, and hold the bulky soft gauze dressing in place with tube gauze or tubular stockinette held to the skin with tincture of benzoin.
4. Apply a posterior splint.
5. Plan an elective second-stage amputation when infection has been controlled.

Open amputation or drainage amputations in foot

Open amputations in the foot are usally indicated for suppurative infection and gangrene in conjunction with diabetes. These infections frequently involve the bone or the metatarsal-phalangeal joint and invade the plantar space along the tendon of the flexor muscle. The operation must be designed to include removal of the infected toe along with the tendon and bone complex. Fortunately, patients suffering from diabetic neuritis frequently have pedal pulses and adequate circulation.

Preoperative preparation consists of minor debridement, incision, and probing of drainage tracts. Such preoperative investigation is usually painless and assists the surgeon greatly in appraising the problem and in planning the operation.

Open transmetatarsal amputation

The incision used for elective transmetatarsal amputation of the entire front of the foot is not adquate to drain tendon sheaths of the flexor muscles even if the flaps are left open. Open transmetatarsal amputation, however, can be done when there is extensive plantar space abscess if the plantar flap is widely undermined. This requires an extensive incision along the medial side of the foot. In severe cases, the abscess frequently extends to the tarsal bones. As a rule, only one or two tendon-joint complexes are involved, and a wedge type of amputation may be employed.

Wedge amputation of toe and metatarsal

Wedge amputation is indicated for infection and gangrene involving the proximal phalanx, a web space, or a metatarsal-phalangeal joint along with the metatarsal bone.

Anesthesia

Spinal or light general anesthesia is suitable.

Preoperative preparation

Preoperative preparation is conservative and is described on p. 479.

Procedure

1. Place the patient in the supine position.
2. Use a V-shaped incision (Fig. 19-13, *A*). The dorsal skin may overhang the end of the bone somewhat. Extend the incision as necessary along the sole of the foot (Fig. 19-13, *B*) in order to drain the deep plantar space and the associated tendon sheath of the flexor muscle. One plantar incision will also suffice if two adjacent toes with metatarsal heads are to be resected.
3. Cut between the metatarsals with the knife blade directed against the joint to be resected, thus avoiding opening into the neighboring normal joint only a few millimeters away.
4. Transect the tendon of the flexor muscle.
5. Cut the metatarsal bone, beveling the edge, so that drainage is not obstructed (Fig. 19-13, *A*). In the big toe, use the Gigli saw to divide the metatarsal. Also resect the sesamoid bones in this location.
6. Pack the open wound lightly with dry gauze or iodoform gauze. Do not suture the wound.
7. When the wound is clean and healthy, packs are removed or lessened and

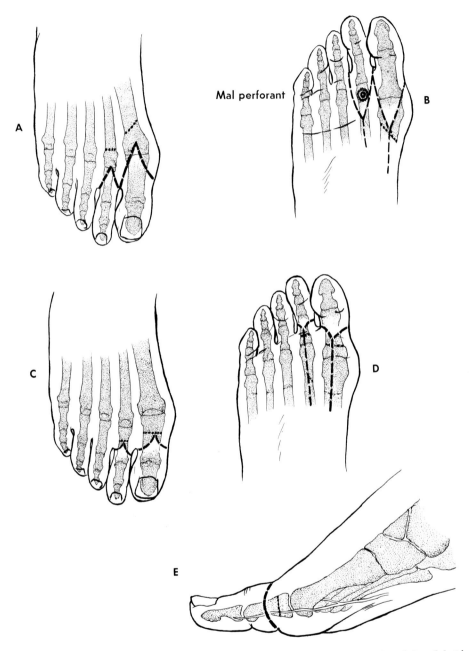

Mal perforant

Fig. 19-13. A and B, Open wedge amputation of toe and metatarsal head for debridement and drainage. A, Dorsal incision. B, Plantar incision is longer. C to E, Open transphalangeal amputation of toes. C, Dorsal incisions. D, Plantar view with incision extended proximally to drain tendon sheath. One plantar incision suffices for two adjacent toes. E, Lateral view. Digital artery extends to tip of flap.

489

the foot is bandaged so that the sides of the defects created by the surgical procedure are coapted. Healing occurs by secondary intention.

Transphalangeal toe amputation

Suppurative infection with gangrene of the toe that has not extended proximally may be controlled by open transphalangeal amputation (Fig. 19-13, *C* to *E*). Such a procedure is frequently elected for infected hammer toes, corns, and moist gangrene of the tips of the toes. The surgical technique is identical to that used for elective closed amputation except that the incision is left open. The incision may be extended proximally onto the plantar surface of the foot (Fig. 19-13, *D*) for drainage of associated tendon sheaths that may be invaded.

F.B.H.

References

Burgess, E. M., et al.: The management of lower extremity amputations: surgery, immediate post surgical prosthetic fitting and patient care, TR 10-6, Aug. 1969, Superintendent of Documents, U. S. Government Printing Office, Washington, D. C., 20402. $1.50.

Moore, W.: Amputation level determined by skin blood flow using xenon 133. Paper presented at International Cardiovascular Society, Toronto, June 22, 1973.

Appendix

BUERGER-ALLEN EXERCISES

Buerger-Allen exercises attempt to increase circulation in the pulseless foot by alternate emptying and distending of the blood vessels with aid of gravity.

Indications

Pain at rest caused by ischemia may be relieved somewhat by Buerger-Allen exercises. The edema that results from prolonged and persistent dependency may also decrease. The visible changes in the feet and the indoctrination and habits developed remind and encourage the patient to give his extremities proper care.

Position 1—draining old blood out (Fig. 1, *A*)

While lying in bed, the patient elevates his feet and legs until the skin is blanched. This may take from ten to sixty seconds. Elevation must not be continued long enough to cause pain.

Position 2—letting fresh blood in (Fig. 1, *B*)

The patient sits up with his legs hanging over the side of the bed and moves his feet slowly. Color returns, the veins fill, and when maximum rubor has returned, the patient assumes position 3. A period of two to three minutes is usually required for this. Slow rhythmic movements of the feet (Fig. 1, *C*) are also performed while the feet are dependent.

Position 3—resting (Fig. 1, *D*)

The patient lies in a supine position to complete the five-minute cycle and then begins again with position 1.

COMMENT: *In some patients, faithful use of these exercises alleviates pain, and improvement will also be noted by a more rapid filling time. In other patients, the main value may be as "occupational therapy."*

Discussion

A period of five minutes or, in some instances, ten minutes is required for the whole cycle. The times in position 1 and position 2 are determined by observation of the particular patient. The time at rest in position 3 is spent merely to round out the cycle to the convenient period of five or ten minutes. The patient is instructed to begin each cycle on the even five-minute or ten-minute reading on a watch or clock. Normally, thirty-minute sessions are performed four times daily.

The patient is given instructions and thereafter performs the exercises himself. No equipment is necessary except a chair, pillow, and watch.

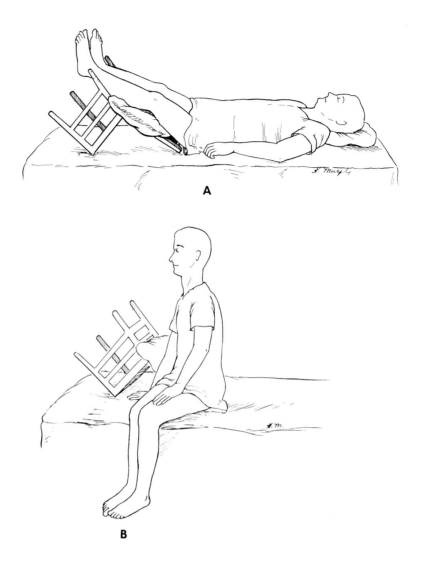

Fig. 1. Buerger-Allen exercises. **A,** Position 1—drain old blood out. **B,** Position 2—let new blood in.

DIRECTIONS FOR CARE OF FEET

Small difficulties and trivial infections and injuries can lead to serious difficulty. The following directions will help prevent injury and infections as well as blisters, corns, calluses, and other conditions that might lead to complications.

1. *Cleanliness.* The patient's feet should be washed carefully each night with soap and warm water, dried thoroughly, rubbed gently with 70% rubbing alcohol, and dried again. The skin should then be rubbed with toilet lanolin so that it is soft and moist but not sticky or greasy. The lanolin should be applied especially to any cracks, calluses, or rough or dry areas.

2. *Clothing.* Exposure to cold, particulary wet cold, must be avoided. The patient should wear clean woolen socks and, if necessary, long underwear or slacks. In the summer, clean cotton socks are sufficient. Shoes should be of soft leather and should fit well. Occasionally, special shoes may be prescribed.

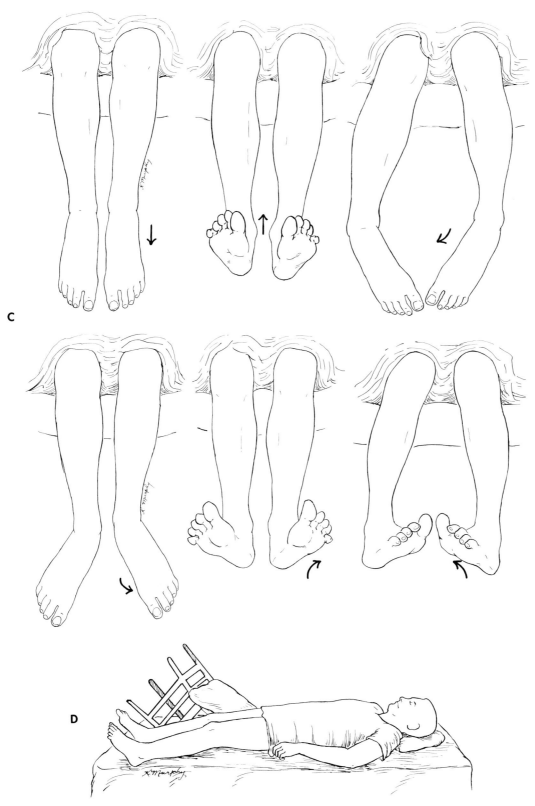

Fig. 1, cont'd. Buerger-Allen exercises. **C,** During dependency (position 2), move feet and ankles slowly as diagrammed. **D,** Position 3—rest until time to repeat cycle with position 1.

VASCULAR EXAMINATION

Name: _____ Date: _____ Age: _____

Complaint, previous surgery, diagnosis, significant past and family history:

Subjective

	RIGHT LEG	LEFT LEG	RIGHT ARM	LEFT ARM	HIP
Cyanosis					
Pain					
Coldness					
Numbness					
Redness					
Claudication					

Objective

	RIGHT LEG	LEFT LEG	RIGHT ARM	LEFT ARM
Cyanosis				
Sweating				
Redness				
Dependent rubor				
Pallor on elevation				
Ulcer				

Pulses

	RIGHT LEG	LEFT LEG	RIGHT ARM	LEFT ARM	RIGHT CAROTID	LEFT CAROTID
Dorsalis pedis						
Tibialis posterior						
Popliteal						
Femoral						
Radial						
Ulnar (Allen test)						
Carotid						

Other signs

	RIGHT LEG	LEFT LEG	RIGHT ARM	LEFT ARM
Oscillometer				
Blood pressure				
Saline wheal (sec.)				
Skin temperatures				
Swelling (cm.)				

Bruits

	RIGHT	LEFT
Femoral		
Carotids		
Abdomen		
Chest		
Aorta		

3. *Injury.* The patient should cut the toenails only after they have been softened by a footbath. A good light should always be used. When the nails are trimmed, they should be cut straight across—the corners should not be cut back. In some cases it may be necessary for the physician to trim the nails himself or to advise the patient to consult a chiropodist. The patient should not cut corns or calluses himself. He should also refrain from using strong antiseptics or chemicals on the feet, since the delicate skin can easily be injured. Sunburn of the feet, ankles, or legs must also be avoided, although gradual tanning is safe. Hot-water bottles, hot-water bags, and electric pads can be dangerous when applied to the feet. If the feet are cold in winter, the use of loose-fitting bed socks is advisable.

4. *Circulation.* To improve the circulation, moderate exercise within the limits imposed by pain, fatigue, or cramps is helpful. The use of circular garters should be avoided. If the feet have a tendency to swell, the patient should be instructed to keep them in a horizontal position on a hassock or footstool whenever he is sitting. If the feet show marked changes in color, the exercises illustrated in Fig. 1 will be beneficial.

5. *Help and supervision.* The patient should report all trivial signs of blistering, infection, ingrown toenail, or any difficulty with bunions, calluses, or athlete's foot. In some cases it may be necessary to ask a member of the family to examine the patient's feet daily and watch for warning signs.

6. *Smoking.* In some patients lifelong abstinence from smoking is essential. This should be discussed with the patient.

VASCULAR EXAMINATION

The use of a short form (see opposite page) ensures the regular completion of a basic vascular survey.

Index

Popliteal artery—cont'd
  exploration of, in occlusive disease, 175-179, 186-188
    distal portion, 177-179
    midportion, 177
    proximal portion, 175
  exposure of distal end of, 206
  injuries to, 254
Portacaval shunts; see Portal hypertension
Portal hypertension, 336-360
  anesthesia in, 343
  emergency portacaval shunt in, through midline inci-
    sion, 342, 355-359
  end-to-side portacaval shunt in, 340, 344-350
    anastomosis in, 349-350
    caudate lobe resection in, 349
    exposure of portal vein in, 345-348
    thoracoabdominal approach in, 344-345
  indications for surgery in, 342-343
  mesocaval shunt in, 342, 359
  operations for, 340-342
  percutaneous splenoportal venography in, 336-340
  postoperative care in, 344
  preoperative care in, 343
  results of shunts in, 360
  side-to-side portacaval shunt in, 340, 350-355
  splenorenal shunt in, 342
Portal vein
  exposure of, 348
  injuries to, 256
Postphlebitic syndrome, 395-396
  subfascial ligation of communicating veins in, 411-413
Profunda femoris artery; see Femoral artery, deep
Profundaplasty, 154-158; see also Femoral artery, deep
  with bypass vein grafts to tibial arteries, 193
Prostheses, 18, 30-33
  in aneurysms of abdominal aorta, 74, 82, 83
  in aneurysms of femoral artery, 163-164
    anastomotic false aneurysm in, 166-168
  in aortic arch bypass, 334
  aortofemoral, 124-126
    complications of, 129-132, 143-145
  aortoiliac, 114-118
  axillofemoral, 139-141
    complications of, 141-142
  complications with, 34-35
  femorofemoral, 138-139
  in iliac artery, 118-121
  infected, 32-33
  for lower extremity amputations, immediate postsur-
    gical fitting of, 455-457
  patch material for; see Angioplasty, patch
  reinforcement of, by external grafting, 168-169
  reinforcing sleeve of, 94-95, 115
  thromboses in, 32
  in vascular injuries, 247
Pulmonary arteriography, 428-430
  operative, 436
Pulmonary embolism
  diagnosis of, 424-430
  lung scans in, 424-427
  pulmonary angiography in, 429-430
  surgical prevention of
    choice of operation in, 430

Pulmonary embolism—cont'd
  surgical prevention of—cont'd
    DeWeese-Adams clip in, 430, 441, 445
    indications for, 430
    midline transabdominal approach in, 447-450
    Miles clip in, 430, 445
    with Mobin-Uddin caval filter, 430, 431-441
    retroperitoneal approach in, 442-446
    right subcostal intraperitoneal approach in, 450-452
    and thrombophlebitis, 415, 417
Pulse, palpation of, 28
Pulseless disease, 390
Puncture wounds of arteries, 256-257

R

Raynaud's disease, sympathectomy in, 362
Reimplantation of limbs, 271
Reinforcement procedures
  external grafting in, 168-169
  sleeve for prosthesis in, 94-95, 115
Renal artery
  aneurysm of, 82
  anterior approach to
    distal portion, 302-304
    proximal portion, 290
  arteriography of, 288
  bypass operations for stenosis of, 296-298
  endarterectomy of, bilateral, 293
  fibromuscular dysplasia of, 288, 298-304
    intraluminal dilation in, 302
Renal vein
  exposure of, 449, 452
  injuries to, 250
  splenorenal shunt in, for portal hypertension, 342
Renovascular hypertension, 287-304
  from fibromuscular dysplasia, 288, 298-304
  indications for surgery in, 288
  surgical procedures in, 288
Reoperation
  after aortofemoral bypass, 131
  after axillofemoral bypass, 141-142
Rib resection, transaxillary approach in, 392-393

S

Saphenous vein
  femorosaphenous bypass operation in, 417
  incompetence of, 396
  phlebitis of, 415-416
  phlebography of, 398
  procurement of, for graft, 261-265
  stripping of, 405-408
Scalenectomy in thoracic outlet syndrome, 391-392
Scalenus anticus syndrome, 390
Scans, lung, in pulmonary embolism, 424-427
Scissors, 21
Seldinger technique in arteriography, 42, 59-65, 383
Sengstaken-Blakemore tube, 355
Sepsis
  of plantar space, 485-486
  and thrombophlebitis, 416
Shunts
  internal
    in carotid endarterectomy, 315-316, 317

MEDICAL
OBSERVATIONS
AND
INQUIRIES.

By a Society of Phyſicians in LONDON.

VOL. II.

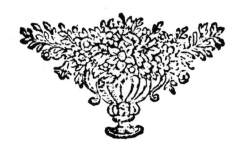

LONDON:

Printed for WILLIAM JOHNSTON,
in *Ludgate-ſtreet.*

MDCCLXII.